A practical guide to
PEDIATRIC INTENSIVE CARE

A practical guide to
PEDIATRIC INTENSIVE CARE

Editor

DANIEL L. LEVIN, M.D.

Medical Director, Pediatric Intensive Care,
Children's Medical Center;
Professor of Clinical Pediatrics,
University of Texas Health Science Center,
Dallas, Texas

Associate Editor

FRANCES C. MORRISS, M.D.

Assistant Medical Director, Pediatric Intensive Care,
Children's Medical Center, Dallas;
Staff Anesthesiologist, King's Daughters' Hospital,
Staunton, Virginia

Assistant Editor

GERALD C. MOORE, M.D.

Clinical Assistant Professor of Pediatrics,
University of Texas Health Science Center,
Dallas, Texas

Medical Illustrator

SCOTT THORN BARROWS

Second edition

with 129 illustrations

The C. V. Mosby Company

ST. LOUIS • TORONTO • PRINCETON   1984

MOSBY

A TRADITION OF PUBLISHING EXCELLENCE

Editor: Karen Berger
Assistant editor: Terry Van Schaik
Editing supervisor: Peggy Fagen
Manuscript editor: Jessica Bender
Book design: Kay M. Kramer
Cover design: Diane M. Beasley
Production: Mary Stueck, Carol O'Leary, Barbara Merritt

The C.V. Mosby Company
11830 Westline Industrial Drive, St. Louis, Missouri 63146

Library of Congress Cataloging in Publication Data
Main entry under title:

A Practical guide to pediatric intensive care.

    Bibliography: p.
    Includes index.
    1. Pediatric intensive care—Handbooks, manuals,
etc. I. Levin, Daniel L., 1943-   . II. Morriss,
Frances C., 1943-   . III. Moore, Gerald C.,
1941-   . [DNLM: 1. Critical care—In infancy and
childhood. 2. Intensive care units. WS 366 P895]
RJ370.P72 1984   618.92'0028   82-23937
ISBN 0-8016-3010-X

GW/VH/VH 9 8 7 6 5 4   01/D/069

Contributors

ALFONSO AQUINO, M.D.

Clinical Instructor of Anesthesiology, The University of Texas Health Science Center and Parkland Memorial Hospital, Dallas

DONNA BADGETT, C.R.T.T.

Supervisor, Respiratory Therapy, Children's Medical Center, Dallas

BARTON E. BERNSTEIN, M.L.A., J.D.

Attorney at Law, Hochberg and Bernstein, P.C.; Adjunct Associate Professor, Clinical Faculty, Department of Psychiatry, University of Texas Health Science Center, Dallas

MICHAEL BLAW, M.D.

Professor of Pediatrics and Neurology and Vice Chairman, Department of Neurology, University of Texas Health Science Center; Director, Division of Pediatric Neurology, Children's Medical Center, Dallas

JOHN G. BROOKS, M.D.

Associate Professor of Pediatrics, Director, Pediatric Pulmonary Medicine and Pediatric Intensive Care Unit, University of Rochester School of Medicine and Dentistry, Rochester, New York

GEORGE R. BUCHANAN, M.D.

Associate Professor of Pediatrics and Director, Pediatric Hematology-Oncology, University of Texas Health Science Center, Dallas

DONNA S. BURNS, R.N., B.S.N.

Nurse Educator (retired), Pediatric Intensive Care Unit, Children's Medical Center, Dallas

CAROLINE J. CASSELBERRY, R.R.T.

Education Coordinator of Respiratory Therapy, Children's Medical Center, Dallas

JOHN J. CHIPMAN, M.D.

Assistant Professor, Department of Pediatrics, University of Texas Health Science Center and Children's Medical Center, Dallas

JAY D. COOK, M.D.

Associate Professor of Clinical Neurology and Pediatrics, University of Texas Health Science Center; Director of Child Neurology, Texas Scottish Rite Hospital, Dallas

CYNTHIA CUNNINGHAM, M.S., R.D.

Assistant Director of Dietetics, Children's Medical Center, Dallas

WILLIAM DAMMERT, M.D.

Clinical Assistant Professor in Pediatric Surgery, University of Texas Health Science Center; Attending Surgeon, Children's Medical Center, Dallas

PATTI DUER, R.N.

Infection Control Nurse, Children's Medical Center, Dallas

GARY D. ELMORE, R.R.T.

Technical Director, Department of Pulmonary Medicine, Children's Medical Center, Dallas

DAVID E. FIXLER, M.D.

Professor of Pediatrics, University of Texas Health Science Center; Director of Pediatric Cardiology, Children's Medical Center, Dallas

MARY E. GRANDY, R.N., B.S.N.

Nurse Educator, Pediatric Intensive Care Unit, Children's Medical Center, Dallas

ALAN H. HALL, M.D.

Clinical Toxicology Fellow, Rocky Mountain Poison and Drug Center; University of Colorado School of Medicine; Denver General Hospital, Denver, Colorado

NANCY HATFIELD, C.R.T.T.

Supervisor, Pulmonary Medicine, Children's Medical Center, Dallas

KURT E. HECOX, M.D., Ph.D.

Associate Professor of Neurology and Head of Neurology, Waisman Center, University of Wisconsin Medical School, Madison

J. PATRICK HIEBER, M.D.

Clinical Associate Professor of Pediatrics, University of Texas Health Science Center, Dallas

RONALD J. HOGG, M.D.

Associate Professor of Pediatrics, University of Texas Health Science Center; Director of Renal Service, Children's Medical Center, Dallas

LARRY T. JOHNSON, C.R.T.T., E.M.T.

Assistant Technical Director of Pulmonary Medicine, Children's Medical Center, Dallas; Faculty member, Dallas Chapter of the American Heart Association

W. PENNOCK LAIRD, M.D.

Clinical Associate Professor of Pediatrics, University of Texas Health Science Center, Dallas

DANIEL L. LEVIN, M.D.

Professor of Clinical Pediatrics, University of Texas Health Science Center; Medical Director, Pediatric Intensive Care, Children's Medical Center, Dallas

KATHERINE LIPSKY, M.S.W., A.C.S.W.

Director, Department of Clinical Social Work, Children's Medical Center, Dallas

CINDY K. LYBARGER, R.N., B.S.N.

Assistant Nurse Educator, Pediatric Intensive Care Unit, Children's Medical Center, Dallas

JAMES F. MARKS, M.D.

Associate Professor of Pediatrics, University of Texas Health Science Center; Attending Physician, Children's Medical Center, Dallas

CATHERINE P. MAST, R.N.

Clinical Supervisor (retired) of Pediatric Intensive Care Unit, Children's Medical Center, Dallas

LAWRENCE J. MILLS, M.D.

Clinical Associate Professor, Department of Surgery, University of Texas Health Science Center; Vice Chairman, Thoracic Surgery, Presbyterian Hospital, Dallas

CHARLES E. MIZE, M.D., Ph.D.

Associate Professor of Pediatrics and Assistant Professor of Biochemistry, University of Texas Health Science Center; Director, Clinical Nutrition, Children's Medical Center, Dallas

GERALD C. MOORE, M.D.

Clinical Assistant Professor, Department of Pediatrics, University of Texas Health Science Center, Dallas; Co-Director, Pulmonary Services, Plano General Hospital, Plano, Texas

FRANCES C. MORRISS, M.D.

Anesthesiologist, King's Daughters Hospital, Staunton, Virginia; Assistant Medical Director, Pediatric Intensive Care Unit, Children's Medical Center, Dallas

ANNETTE MUSSELMAN, R.R.T.

Home Care Coordinator for Pulmonary Medicine, Children's Medical Center, Dallas

EDGAR A. NEWFELD, M.D.

Clinical Associate Professor of Pediatrics, University of Texas Health Science Center; Director, Cardiac Catheterization Laboratory, Children's Medical Center, Dallas

RONALD M. PERKIN, M.D.

Assistant Professor of Pediatrics, University of California, San Diego; Co-Director, Pediatric Intensive Care Unit, University Hospital, San Diego, California

PAUL R. PRESCOTT, M.D.

Assistant Professor of Clinical Pediatrics, University of Texas Health Science Center; Medical Director, Child Abuse and Neglect Program, Children's Medical Center, Dallas

TERRY RAUSCHUBER, R.N., B.S.N.

Clinical Nurse, Pediatric Intensive Care Unit, Children's Medical Center, Dallas

BARRY H. RUMACK, M.D.

Professor of Pediatrics, University of Colorado School of Medicine; Director, Rocky Mountain Poison and Drug Center, Denver

RONALD M. SATO, M.D.

Assistant Professor, Plastic and Reconstructive Surgery, Stanford University Medical Center, Stanford; Director of Burn Unit, Santa Clara Valley Medical Center, San Jose, California

DEBRA A. SAYLES, R.N., C.C.R.N.

Cardiac Nurse Educator, Pediatric Intensive Care Unit, Children's Medical Center, Dallas

JANE D. SIEGEL, M.D.

Assistant Professor of Clinical Pediatrics, University of Texas Health Science Center; Attending Physician, Children's Medical Center and Parkland Memorial Hospital, Dallas

FREDERICK H. SKLAR, M.D.

Clinical Associate Professor of Neurosurgery, University of Texas Health Science Center; Director of Pediatric Neurosurgery, Children's Medical Center, Dallas

ALAN D. STRICKLAND, M.D.

Clinical Assistant Professor of Pediatrics, University of Texas Health Science Center; Attending Physician, Children's Medical Center and Parkland Memorial Hospital, Dallas

BETSY COHEN TEITELL, R.N., M.S.

Nutrition-Clinical Nurse Specialist, Children's Medical Center, Dallas

GARY R. TURNER, M.D.

Assistant Professor of Pediatrics, University of Texas Health Science Center; Attending Physician, Pediatric Intensive Care Unit, Children's Medical Center, Dallas

RICK VINSON, C.R.T.T.

Pediatric Intensive Care Unit Coordinator, Department of Pulmonary Medicine, Children's Medical Center, Dallas

THEODORE P. VOTTELER, M.D.

Clinical Associate Professor, Department of Surgery, University of Texas Health Science Center; Director of Surgical Services, Children's Medical Center, Dallas

PATRICIA WALTERS, C.R.T.T.

Educational Coordinator, Cardiopulmonary Department, Children's Hospital, Fort Worth, Texas

KENNETH M. WIGGINS, M.D.

Formerly Professor and Director of Child and Adolescent Psychiatry, University of Texas Health Science Center; Director of Psychiatry, Children's Medical Center, Dallas

To
Our families who nurture us
Our colleagues who teach us
Our patients who make it all worthwhile
and especially to
Micah, Brendan, Erin, Laura, Ashley, and Graham

Foreword

Over the past 15 years intensive care units have become integral and essential components of medical facilities providing care to infants and children. The special focus of these units on therapies and support of children with acute problems has offered new hope to families and children with life-threatening disease. Those engaged in acute care medicine, be it for newborns or for older children, are in a very real sense acute care generalists. The expertise required of those caring for patients in intensive care units cuts across virtually every medical specialty. The modern pediatric intensivist is a chimera of cardiologist, pulmonologist, gastroenterologist, neurologist, hematologist, and surgeon. Problems encountered in our intensive care units cover the spectrum of acute pediatric insult. Drowning, poisoning, trauma, and shock from a variety of causes are common problems. Medical advances are occurring so rapidly that the intensivist must engage in an ongoing educational process. There is a constant need for thorough understanding of normal clinical physiology during growth and development.

While the intensivist leans heavily on modern technology and an intimate knowledge of clinical pathophysiology to treat the diverse problems encountered in ICUs, there are other important aspects of patient care that have to be developed by intensivists to make them effective care givers. The modern intensivist must be an effective communicator who has the ability to call upon subspecialty experts when a particular expertise is required. He or she must be able to translate conflicting recommendations into an effective treatment plan. The modern intensivist must also resist the temptation to hide behind an often awesome display of technology and be able to deal sensitively, patiently, and empathetically with families and patients frequently bewildered and confused by the very nature of acute illness. Modern intensivists must be able to work effectively with nursing personnel who are the bulwarks and the pillars of strength in modern intensive care units. The importance of emotional nurturing and support by social workers and other caretakers must be recognized as an integral component of any effective intensive care facility. The intensivist should be prepared to deal with every question faced by emotionally distraught families of children with devastating illness.

The contents and organization of this book on principles of intensive care reflect both the complexity and the scope of problems encountered in pediatric intensive care units. Dr. Levin and his colleagues have done an outstanding job of providing the physician caring for the critically ill child with an effective guide to therapy and management of acute, life-threatening diseases. This book should be useful for the general pediatrician providing interim care for the acutely ill child until transport to a regional specialty center can be carried out. It is also an invaluable resource for house staff, fellows, nurses, and therapists caring for children requiring intensive care. The promise of the many effective therapies and interventions outlined in this book offer hope to critically ill children and their families.

Joseph B. Warshaw, M.D.
Professor and Chairman
Department of Pediatrics
University of Texas Health Science Center
Dallas, Texas

Preface

to second edition

Although we faced the publication of the first edition of *A Practical Guide to Pediatric Intensive Care* with much trepidation as to how the book would be received and used, in general we have been greatly satisfied with the result. We perceived at the time that many good textbooks dealt with the various aspects of pediatric intensive care, but no one book seemed to answer many of the questions of our house staff, referring physicians, and nursing and respiratory therapy staff concerning practical, minute-to-minute and day-to-day management of patients in a pediatric intensive care unit. These questions focused primarily on physiology, monitoring, management, and equipment and techniques. We sought to fill that gap in readily available material with the first edition of this book.

We believe that those who have perceived the book as a day-to-day practical resource and have used it as such have found it to be a valuable guide. We have therefore sought to update the material, and we have added several new chapters to increase the usefulness of the book, as requested by individuals who have been using it. We hope that readers will specifically review the new chapter entitled "How to Use This Book" before referring to other chapters. We especially appreciate the assistance of Mrs. Jean Pitzer in the preparation of this book.

Daniel L. Levin

Preface

to first edition

Since developing the pediatric intensive care unit service at Children's Medical Center, Dallas, my coauthors and I have become increasingly aware of the lack of textbook material that specifically addresses the problems of critically ill children. Although many good texts deal with various aspects of pediatric intensive care, no one book seemed to answer many of the questions our house staff, referring physicians, and nursing and respiratory therapy staff asked concerning practical matters in the unit. These questions focused primarily on physiology, monitoring, management, and equipment and techniques. We have therefore attempted to supply detailed information regarding these points. We have written extensive sections on problems caused by system failures and on equipment and techniques because we believe that if the staff understands the physiologic principles of organ dysfunction and is familiar with the techniques available in pediatric intensive care, the immediate life-threatening situations can be identified and stabilized until more thorough investigations and specific therapeutic maneuvers can be instituted. In addition, we have presented those types of medical-surgical problems that are commonly seen in a pediatric intensive care unit, except for major trauma and burns, which are dealt with extensively in other texts. It is our hope that physicians, nurses, and respiratory therapists will utilize this book as a day-to-day practical resource in understanding and managing critically ill children.

We are grateful to Dr. Heinz Eichenwald for his support of this work. We also appreciate all the work of Gwen Jarrett, Mannya Sakowski, and Dawn Miller in the preparation of the manuscript.

Daniel L. Levin

Contents

PART TWO **Specific problems**

Neurologic

Appendixes

List of tables

INTRODUCTION

1 The pediatric intensive care unit concept

DANIEL L. LEVIN
CATHERINE P. MAST

The goal of the pediatric intensive care unit (PICU) is to provide optimum care for critically ill infants and children. Patients admitted to the PICU are those who are unstable or potentially unstable and need the specialized personnel and equipment available in the PICU. Personnel and facilities in the PICU should be such that continuous, repetitive, and anticipatory monitoring of patients, intervention on their behalf, and assessment of the results of intervention can be performed rapidly and accurately so that each patient entering the PICU is given the maximum opportunity to leave and thrive.

It is assumed that patients in the PICU have severe involvement of their disease process and are therefore in a potentially life-threatening situation. *Consequently, the monitoring recommended is often invasive and involves significant risk to the patient.* Therapeutic recommendations for immediate life-threatening situations are also often invasive and involve significant risk. Therefore, the recommendations presented in this book are not to be applied to mildly or less severely ill patients cared for in a routine hospital setting.

STAFF
Physicians

The medical director of the PICU is responsible for implementing the goals of the service by arranging for continuous medical and paramedical coverage, for certifying that the quality of care meets standards of excellence desired by the community, and for seeing that the facilities are used to the maximum benefit of the community.

In some programs PICU fellows should be integrated into the medical care, teaching, and research functions of the service in order to provide these fellows with the advanced training necessary for becoming certified intensivists. These individuals are usually pediatricians and/or anesthesiologists, many of whom have advanced subspecialty training in complementary areas (e.g., pulmonary, cardiology, neonatology).

Pediatric, anesthesia, and surgical house officers should be assigned to PICU duty, and during this period they should have no other clinical responsibilities. The necessary number and experience of such individuals depend on the number and types of patients seen in the unit. Every patient admitted to the PICU should have an attending physician and a resident physician from the PICU service both of whom may act in either primary or consultant roles. A physician should be in the unit or immediately available at all times.

Nurses

The nurse supervisor in the PICU should be directly responsible to the medical director and should work with the director to provide the proper environment for delivery of care to the patient. There should also be a head nurse

3

and assistant head nurses responsible for patient care and an educational nurse whose responsibilities are the orientation of new nurses entering the PICU and the ongoing education of nurses already in the unit. Clinical specialists may be desirable for education in specialized areas (e.g., cardiology). The level of responsibility of the PICU nurse is extraordinary. These nurses should be taught how to manage complex equipment and provide supportive measures used in the care of patients, and they should have an in-depth knowledge of the pathophysiology of many disease entities and the treatment required. Nursing ratios should be set by the types of patients that are seen. It is usually advisable to have a mixture of ratios so that patients requiring a high level of care will have one-to-one nursing and other patients requiring less care will have one-to-two or one-to-three nursing. Nurses should not be given permanent assignments for one type of patient (e.g., postoperative cardiac patients). Each nurse should be expected to develop the understanding and skills necessary to care for any patient admitted to the unit.

Paramedical support

Personnel specifically trained to assist in the care of critically ill infants and children should be immediately available to provide equipment and support. Respiratory therapists should be assigned to the PICU on a permanent basis so that other responsibilities will not interfere with their PICU duties. They should have a thorough understanding of the principles of respiratory care and of the equipment involved. In addition to therapists, competent laboratory, pharmacy, and radiology support must be immediately available. Finally, social service support is essential.

PHYSICAL SETTING

The number of beds available in the PICU is determined by the needs of the community. A certain number of beds should be designated for maximum intensive care, a lesser number for intermediate care, and a small number designated for isolation. The details of equipment and facilities that should be available at each bed site are presented in Chapter 81.

ADDITIONAL READING

Committee on Guidelines of the Society of Critical Care Medicine: Guidelines for organization of critical care units. In Weil, M.H., and Shubin, H., editors: Critical care medicine: current principles and practices, New York, 1976, Harper & Row, Publishers, Inc.

Grenvik, A., Leonard, J.J., Arens, J.F., and others: Critical care medicine: certification as a multidisciplinary subspecialty, Crit. Care Med. 9:117-125, 1981.

Weil, M.H., Shubin, H., and Carlson, R.W.: The new practice of critical care medicine. In Weil, M.H., and Shubin, H., editors: Critical care medicine: current principles and practices, New York, 1976, Harper & Row, Publishers, Inc.

2 How to use this book

DANIEL L. LEVIN

Although our goal in creating this book was to supply practical guidance in a format which was easily assimilated by quick reference in a PICU setting, we felt that instructions for monitoring, management, and procedural skills could not be meaningfully given or used without at least modest background material being presented as well. Therefore, although the emphasis in this text is on practical guidance, we have endeavored in each instance to present the material in a context which will allow the reader to understand the reasoning behind the advice. This is both a reading text and a quick reference, and the quick reference aspect of the book will best be utilized by the health professionals who take the time to read the text concerning definitions and physiology in advance of the time they must rapidly respond to PICU emergency situations.

Part One is an approach to pediatric intensive care on the basis of system failure. It is our belief that most patients can be successfully managed initially if the physicians and nurses understand the physiology of system failure, regardless of whether the exact diagnosis has been established. In Part Two the most commonly seen problems are presented, and the emphasis is on the short-term, urgent needs of patients. In addition to information on basic, minimal monitoring and daily care, the complete and ideal monitoring for each disease process is outlined in these chapters. Items in the monitoring sections are listed in order of importance and feasibility, so that more complex or sophisticated techniques appear after the most standard ones. The type and extent of monitoring should be individualized to each patient depending on age, severity of disease process, instability of vital signs, availability of appropriate nursing care, and physician familiarity with any specific technique. The frequency of monitoring is not intended to be applied for the duration of the patient's hospitalization but only until the patient is improved and stable. Part Three is devoted to equipment and techniques and presents the equipment we use and the way we do things. It is not intended to present all possibilities. Aspects of diagnosis, monitoring, management, and equipment that are especially pertinent to PICU nurses are presented in the text. The appendixes include reference data for normal values and a quick reference for drug dosages.

The ideas and suggestions in this book are intended for patients in the PICU who are therefore presumed to be unstable or potentially unstable. Basic, minimal monitoring needs are presented in Chapter 4 and in the interest of space are not repeated elsewhere. When devising a monitoring plan, the suggestions in Chapter 4 should always be reviewed. Specific monitoring suggestions in all other chapters are considered to be thorough and optimal for the sickest of patients during the height of their illnesses. They are not intended to be continued at the same frequency or depth during less intensive phases of the illness, either in the PICU or in the regular hospital setting. This is equally true for therapeutic suggestions. We feel strongly that salvageable patients who are extremely ill are frequently lost by a timid approach to monitoring and management during the early phases of their illness. Alternatively, it is probably true that harm to patients occurs because health care givers do not recognize when to withdraw judiciously the aggressive monitoring and management techniques when the patient is improved.

All monitoring and management suggestions as well as specific procedural techniques are presented as a way (we hope a good way) of doing things. We do not profess that this is the only way to do things. Even within our own unit we attempt to use these protocols as a basis for discussion and if a physician, nurse, or therapist is familiar with the recommended way of doing things but can present a rational, well-thought-out alternative plan, then different approaches can be attempted.

3 Admission of newborn infants and pediatric patients

DONNA S. BURNS
TERRY RAUSCHUBER

ROUTINES FOR NURSING CARE IN THE PEDIATRIC INTENSIVE CARE UNIT

Thorough initial and continuing observations are the key to successful management of critically ill, unstable infants and children. Routines that generate interpretable, complete, recorded evaluations are the practical frame of reference in which to view monitoring of the PICU patient. These routines must be thorough enough to include all major organ systems and high-risk problems for a particular population (e.g., small premature infants) but flexible enough to include patients with special problems (e.g., increased intracranial pressure, pulmonary arterial hypertension). The nurse who first admits the patient to the PICU and spends several hours observing the same patient is best suited to make and record these observations and to alert the physician to potential problems. Throughout this book, special observations and recording sheets (e.g., for cardiopulmonary resuscitation, neurologic signs, diabetic ketoacidosis [DKA]) are presented with discussion of appropriate subjects. This chapter presents protocols for admission and daily observations in newborns and older children. Special observations indicated by the patient's disease should be added to these routines.

INITIAL MEASUREMENTS AND OBSERVATIONS

Newborn infants vary greatly in body weight and other physical dimensions. A great deal of diagnostic information is available from accurate initial body measurements. In addition, many procedures performed on newborn infants require various body measurements for proper completion (e.g., placement of umbilical artery catheter), and whenever possible this information should be obtained as soon as the patient arrives in the PICU and before the urgent need for such measurements. Intake, output, and medication dosages are based on body weight or surface area, and if inaccurate, these measurements can lead to disastrous miscalculations. Changes in body weight after admission are important in gauging the success of fluid and feeding management, and therefore an accurate weight should be carefully recorded at the time of admission.

Newborn infants may have alarmingly few specific signs for many diverse abnormalities. For example, hypoglycemia may cause an infant to appear cyanotic. Alternatively, many infants with a specific disease, such as cyanotic congenital heart disease, may develop a secondary abnormality, such as hypoglycemia. Other abnormalities, such as hypotension, may be easily missed by the casual observer who does not make the effort to objectively quantitate and record all of the patient's vital signs.

Since infants can be extremely unstable if they are cold or require ventilatory support or fluid therapy, these measurements and observations must be made quickly, with particular attention to maintaining the stability of the in-

7

fant. Always make an initial, quick, overall assessment of the patient's condition and delay routine admission measurements if he appears to require immediate attention for cardiorespiratory distress.

The older child is admitted to the PICU either electively in the postoperative period or as an emergency. Although attention to basic vital functions is the essential feature for any PICU patient, in each of these circumstances the emphasis is different. Routines for children who have undergone gastrointestinal surgery, cardiothoracic surgery, or neurosurgery are detailed in other sections. Unscheduled admission of patients in emergency circumstances involves children with a large variety of disease entities, frequently involving multiple organ systems. This necessitates extensive yet rapid evaluation of the cardiorespiratory, neurologic, and renal-metabolic systems. Since these patients are unstable and may require the use of a large number of monitoring and treatment devices, emphasis must be placed on the PICU team's ability to provide the patient with the equipment rapidly, safely, and properly.

PROCEDURE
Preparation for the patient's arrival

1. Prepare the bed, radiant warmer, or incubator and the patient's bedside area (Table 3-1).
2. Assemble equipment and check to see that everything functions properly.
   a. Every patient should have emergency resuscitation equipment (oxygen, suction, bag, and mask) at the bedside.
   b. Assemble equipment specific for the anticipated problem (e.g., mechanical ventilator, infusion pump, thoracentesis tray, metabolic scales, pressure transducers).

Admission assessment

1. Recognize the severely depressed or distressed patient and initiate appropriate measures immediately (e.g., intubation,

ventilation, intravascular catheter placement, medications).
2. If the patient does not require immediate assistance, obtain his vital signs while he is still in the transport bed or incubator. Remove all clothing except diapers to facilitate complete assessment.
   a. Obtain apical pulse (1 full minute) and note regularity of heart rate. While listening to heart rate, note the presence of heart murmurs.
   b. Check peripheral pulses (right and left, arm and leg), noting strength and character. Check capillary filling.
   c. Obtain auscultatory or palpated systemic blood pressure using a cuff that is two-thirds the size of the upper arm.
   d. Obtain respiratory rate (1 full minute).
   e. Note color of skin, mucous membranes, and nail beds.
   f. Determine if upper airway is clear of secretions and note the character of the respiratory effort. Note if there is alar flaring, grunting, audible wheezing, retractions, and/or asymmetrical chest movement. Listen to see whether air can be heard entering the chest bilaterally. While listening to the chest, note if the patient has rhonchi, rales, or wheezes.
   g. Obtain axillary temperatures on babies less than 1 month of age or weighing less than 2,500 g since a rectal thermometer can perforate the rectum. Obtain a rectal temperature in older and larger infants and children.
3. Remove the patient from the incubator and weigh him on a prebalanced scale. Transfer him immediately to a prewarmed radiant warmer or incubator or to a bed.
   a. Continue to supply the patient's oxygen requirements by holding the oxygen mask over his face or, if he is intubated, by hand-ventilating him during weighing.

Table 3-1. Patient admission equipment and supply list

1. In bedside drawers
   a. Alcohol swabs
   b. Povidone-iodine (Betadine) swabs
   c. Lancets
   d. Band-Aids
   e. Cotton balls
   f. Temperature probe pasties
   g. Electrodes
   h. Tape measures
   i. Finger cots
   j. Rubber bands
   k. Safety pins
   l. Wisk adhesive remover
   m. Syringe adapters
   n. Injection site caps
   o. Hematocrit tubes
   p. Blood specimen tubes
   q. Tape
   r. Dextrostix, 1 bottle
   s. Labstix, 1 bottle
   t. Sterile lubricant packets
2. On counter
   a. Complete supply of syringes
   b. Needles
   c. Septisol foam
   d. Suction catheters
   e. Sterile saline suctioning packets
3. For infusion pumps
   a. Cassette
   b. In-line Metriset
   c. Secondary set
4. Bed, incubator, or radiant warmer
5. On bed
   a. Restraints
   b. Urine collection bag
   c. Culture swabs
   d. Gavage tray or nasogastric tube
   e. Lead wires for monitor
   f. Disposable diapers
   g. Stethoscope
   h. Blood pressure cuff and manometer
   i. Anesthesia bag and mask (check for appropriate size)
6. At bedside
   a. Monitor (ECG, respiratory, pressure modules)
   b. Suction regulator, suction canister, and tubing
   c. Oxygen blender
   d. Mechanical ventilator (when indicated)
   e. Thoracentesis tray
   f. Infusion pumps
   g. Blood pressure transducers
   h. Arterial and venous catheter equipment (see Chapters 87 and 89)
   i. Procedure cart
   j. Patient chart
   k. Clipboard
      (1) Flow sheet/nurses' notes and admission sheet
      (2) Doctor's order sheet
      (3) Graphics/medication sheet
      (4) Respiratory therapy sheet
   l. Linen
   m. Scales

b. Do not waste time during this procedure. The patient may be in a precarious situation.
4. After placing the patient in his new environment, place the electronic monitoring leads, make certain the monitors are functioning properly, and set the monitor alarms (see Chapter 82).
5. Obtain blood sample by heel stick or from arterial catheter (0.2 ml) for hematocrit (Hct), total serum protein (TSP) (from hematocrit capillary tube), and Dextrostix de-

terminations. Always chart the site, since normal Hct values vary with the location from which they are obtained.
6. Assess patency of any intravenous (IV) infusions the patient may have. If Dextrostix is low (≤ 45 mg/dl), start IV immediately with a dextrose solution to raise the serum glucose.
7. Suction nose, mouth, pharynx, and, if present, endotracheal tube. Note color, quantity, and character of secretions.
8. Obtain body measurements (Fig. 3-1).

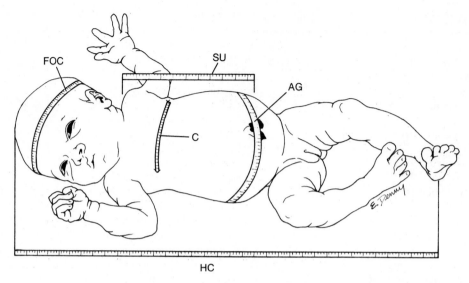

Fig. 3-1. Infant measurements: *FOC,* frontal-occipital circumference; *SU,* shoulder-umbilicus; *AG,* abdominal girth; *HC,* heel-crown; *C,* chest.

a. Heel-crown (HC). This is used in calculating proper nasotracheal tube length (HC × 0.21 + 1.0 cm).

b. Shoulder-umbilicus (SU). This is used in calculating proper length for umbilical artery catheter placement in infants (SU × 0.65).

c. Frontal-occipital head circumference (FOC). Serial measurements are needed to diagnose hydrocephalus.

d. Chest circumference (C) (at the nipple line)

e. Abdominal girth (AG) at the level of the umbilicus. Serial measurements are needed to diagnose necrotizing enterocolitis in infants and intra-abdominal pathologic conditions in older infants and children.

9. Empty stomach contents using gavage tube or nasogastric (NG) tube and syringe. Aspirate gently. Note the quantity, consistency, and color of contents.

10. Apply urine collection system to obtain specimen for urinalysis, specific gravity, and Labstix.

11. Obtain cultures (see Chapter 40).
    a. Nasopharyngeal
    b. Tracheal (in intubated patients)
    c. Rectal
    d. Skin (umbilical cord)

12. Observe the patient's behavior, noting general activity, muscle tone, response to painful and auditory stimuli, and jitteriness or seizure activity. Assess his level of consciousness.

13. Observe the skin for signs of trauma, petechiae, or poor turgor.

14. Collect in a central location any charts, roentgenograms, or laboratory specimens that have been sent with the child. Make certain they are accurately labeled.

These initial observations may be immediately life-saving and are therefore critically important. In addition, these observations generate the continued data collection necessary for proper care of critically ill pediatric patients.

4 Basic, minimal intensive care monitoring and routine daily care

DANIEL L. LEVIN
DONNA S. BURNS

After the initial observations are made, continuing anticipatory measurements are necessary to detect patient problems at the earliest possible moment. Although the collection and recording of a large number of observations may seem excessively time-consuming for patients who do well, this must be weighed against those instances in which disasters are averted because of such routine observations. All patients admitted to the PICU are critically ill or have conditions that are potentially life-threatening; routine observations are often the only manner by which potentially serious changes are detected before irreversible problems occur. (See Fig. 4-1.)

PROCEDURE (Fig. 4-1)
Renal-metabolic system

1. Weigh the patient daily. More frequent weighings may be necessary in some patients (e.g., dialysis), and in these cases a metabolic bed is useful. Calculate weight gain or loss.
2. Intake. Carefully record all blood products and intravascular and dietary fluids given to the patient. Include all flush solutions and the volumes of medications given as IV piggyback. Record these hourly and as needed and calculate the totals for every 8-hour shift and every 24 hours.
3. Output. Record urine, NG tube, chest tube, and intracranial drain losses or other drainage losses every hour. Record all other losses including stools, vomitus, blood lost from bleeding and sampling, and wound drainage. Most critically ill patients require an indwelling bladder catheter. In infants, weighed diapers can be used to estimate urine output by equating 1 g of diaper weight gain with 1 ml of urine output.
4. Measure urine specific gravity; use Labstix to check for blood, protein, and glucose; and measure pH once every 8-hour shift.
5. Measure and record patient's temperature every 2 hours. In patients less than 1 month old or less than 2,500 g avoid the risk of rectal perforation by taking axillary temperatures. More frequent temperatures may be needed in cases of abnormally high or low temperatures. Also record incubator temperature.
6. Check blood with Dextrostix every 8 hours in the more critically ill patients and once a day in the less critical, more stable patients unless you get an abnormal result; then more frequent checking is necessary until the patient's Dextrostix is stable. Blood glucose determinations may also be necessary if extreme deviation from normal occurs. Also check to determine if Dextrostix are fresh. Old materials may give misleading results.

11

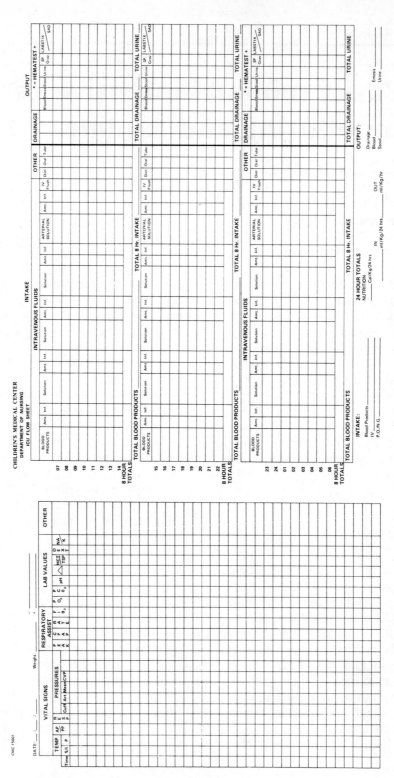

Fig. 4-1. Nursing flow sheet for daily record of vital signs, laboratory values, and intake and output.

7. Measure serum Na, K, and Cl at least once every day if patient is receiving only IV fluids.
8. Measure serum Ca initially once every day if the patient is receiving only IV fluids. In sick neonates, patients in shock, patients given frequent doses of diuretics, patients with Reye's syndrome, and patients with abnormal serum Ca values, check the level more frequently.

Cardiorespiratory system

1. Display heart rate continuously and measure apical and peripheral pulse rates (1 full minute) every 2 hours.
2. Maintain continuous electrocardiogram (ECG) monitoring.
3. Measure systemic arterial blood pressure both by indwelling arterial catheter with transducer (if catheter is present) and by blood pressure cuff, preferably by auscultation, every 2 hours. Record systolic, diastolic, and mean pressures; indicate cuff pressures obtained by palpation.
4. If catheters are present, measure central venous blood pressure (CVP) and all other blood pressures (right atrial, left atrial, pulmonary arterial, pulmonary capillary wedge) every 2 hours. Specify systolic, diastolic, and mean pressures.
5. Calibrate low-pressure (venous, intracranial) transducers every 4 hours and high-pressure transducers every 8 hours, check the levels of the transducers, and note the time of calibration on the flow sheet.
6. Display respiratory rate continuously and auscultate (1 full minute) and record every 2 hours.
7. Note quantity, character, and color of oral and tracheal secretions.
8. A daily chest roentgenogram is usually indicated during the acute phase of the disease, especially when assisted ventilation is used.
9. Obtain a chest roentgenogram after endotracheal intubation, extubation, or repositioning of the tube.

10. Analyze and record oxygen and ventilatory assistance settings every 2 hours.

Neurologic system

1. General. Note the patient's level of consciousness, muscle tone, and responsiveness to stimuli, and record every 4 to 8 hours.
2. Specific. In many patients, observation of neurologic signs will be ordered. Use a neurologic observation sheet (see Chapter 6).
3. Measure FOC every day in newborns less than 1 month old and/or less than 2,500 g.

Hematologic system

1. Obtain Hct every 8 hours. Record the sampling site, e.g., central (arterial catheter) or peripheral (heel or finger stick).
2. Check TSP every 8 hours. Use serum in hematocrit capillary tube and total serum solids meter on urine refractometer to estimate TSP every time an Hct is done.

Gastrointestinal system

1. Measure AG just above the umbilicus every 8 hours in newborns less than 1 month of age and/or less than 2,500 g.
2. Check a stool specimen for blood (Hematest or guaiac) when blood is noted in the stool, when AG increases, or when small infants fail to tolerate their feedings. If blood is noted, check each stool for blood until blood is no longer detected.
3. Check for and quantitate gastric residuals before all gavage feedings.
4. Note amount and character of NG secretions. Perform a Hematest on secretions if coffee ground material is noted.

• • •

One must know the normal values for a patient (e.g., systemic arterial blood pressure) to interpret the findings. Almost certainly the nurse or house officer will be the first person to document abnormalities. Be alert and identify problems before they result in severe morbidity or mortality.

PART ONE
Problems caused by system failures

5 Resuscitation of vital organ systems following cardiopulmonary arrest

FRANCES C. MORRISS
CATHERINE P. MAST
JAY D. COOK

DEFINITION AND PHYSIOLOGY

Cardiopulmonary arrest is the sudden and unexpected cessation of functional ventilation and circulation in a person otherwise not expected to die. Cardiopulmonary resuscitation (CPR) consists of simple techniques, the use of which can maintain life. These techniques should always be instituted in the event of sudden, unexpected death. For children in whom death is neither sudden nor unexpected, a decision about the initiation or extent of CPR can be made by the physician and family and communicated to the personnel caring for the child. Once CPR is begun, it should be continued until (1) the patient recovers, and spontaneous respiration and circulation are restored; (2) the rescuer is relieved by someone competent to continue CPR; (3) the physician conducting the resuscitation decides to discontinue CPR; or (4) the rescuer is alone, exhausted, and unable to continue CPR.

When sudden death occurs in children, respiration ceases while the heart usually continues to beat for a short period. In the absence of gas exchange, there is enough oxygen in the blood being circulated to sustain life for several minutes. The length of the critical time period is determined by the need of the brain for oxygen. CPR instituted less than 4 minutes after arrest has an excellent chance of being successful. However, after 6 minutes have elapsed, brain damage usually occurs unless the patient is hypothermic (less than 32° C).

With cessation of heart action, circulation ceases in the periphery, profound muscle relaxation and loss of consciousness occur, and metabolism changes from aerobic to anaerobic, with production of lactic acid. Thus, the consequence of the lack of energy sources (glucose, oxygen) is acidosis. The goal of CPR is prompt delivery of oxygen to the tissues, especially the heart and brain, by (1) reinstituting ventilation, (2) reestablishing effective circulation, and (3) correcting the metabolic abnormalities that are the result of an arrest.

IDENTIFICATION OF PATIENTS AT RISK

All patients in the PICU are at risk of cardiopulmonary arrest because they have life-threatening diseases or physiologic conditions that are potentially unstable. In the following discussion infant refers to a child less than 1 year of age and child to a patient 1 to 8 years of age. The highest risk situations are:
1. Patients with an unstable cardiovascular status (e.g., hemorrhage, intractable congestive heart failure, hypotension, recurrent dysrhythmias).

2. Patients with rapidly progressive pulmonary disease (e.g., asthma, croup, severe pneumonia, hyaline membrane disease).
3. Patients in the immediate postoperative period. General anesthetics or heavy sedation significantly alter a child's reflex ability to respond appropriately to a variety of stressful physical stimuli.
4. Any patients with an artificial airway, since respiratory status depends directly on airway patency.
5. Patients with a worsening neurologic status, such as the comatose patient who may not have sufficient respiratory drive to sustain adequate ventilation.

There are a number of stressful procedures that may precipitate an arrest in the high-risk patient. These include:

1. Suctioning, which can cause hypoxemia, atelectasis, and reflex bradycardia.
2. Chest physiotherapy, which may mobilize excessive secretions, thus blocking the airway, or which may fatigue a patient.
3. Withdrawal of any form of respiratory support (e.g., decreasing the fractional concentration of inspired oxygen [FI_{O_2}], extubation, cessation of ventilation or continuous positive airway pressure [CPAP]). The patient now has to perform a respiratory function that previously had been provided for him.
4. Addition of sedative medication (e.g., narcotics, barbiturates, cough suppressants), which may depress respiratory drive.
5. Procedures associated with Valsalva maneuvers or breath-holding, such as lumbar puncture (LP) or restraint for venipuncture.
6. Procedures associated with vagal stimulation and bradycardia, such as passage of NG or feeding tubes and airway manipulation. Feeding, which involves coordination of breathing and swallowing, can be hazardous in the high-risk infant.

Personnel who perform these maneuvers must be especially alert to signs of decompensation, including poor peripheral perfusion, bradycardia, apnea or change in respiratory pattern, cyanosis, and restlessness or decreased response to stimuli. The presence of any of these signs is sufficient reason to abort the procedure and institute support.

TECHNIQUES OF RESUSCITATION
(see Table 5-1)
Basic life support

1. Recognition: attempt to arouse the patient by stimulation (e.g., shaking, slapping heels).
2. Call for help.
3. Gently position the patient to allow access to airway and upper chest. To protect the spine, the head and neck must be moved as a unit.
4. Open the airway to lift the relaxed soft tissues and tongue away from the posterior pharynx.
   a. In infants place one hand beneath the shoulder blades and lift while pressing down with a hand placed on the forehead. In older children place one hand under the neck rather than under the shoulder blades.
   b. Instead of lifting the neck while tilting the head, lift the chin. Place the tips of the fingers that had been under the neck on the bony prominence of the chin and lift it forward. Do not close the mouth completely or press down on the soft tissue of the neck.
   c. Check for signs of breathing. Observe chest movement, auscultate the chest, or listen for breath sounds over mouth and nose.
   d. Suction the mouth.
5. Institute artificial ventilation if there is no breathing or ineffective breathing.
   a. Maintain head tilt.
   b. Seal the airway by pinching the nose closed (child) or covering the mouth and nose with your mouth (infant).
   c. Give four short breaths while observing the chest for movement. In infants inflate the lungs by using short puffs to avoid

Table 5-1. Algorithm for cardiorespiratory arrest

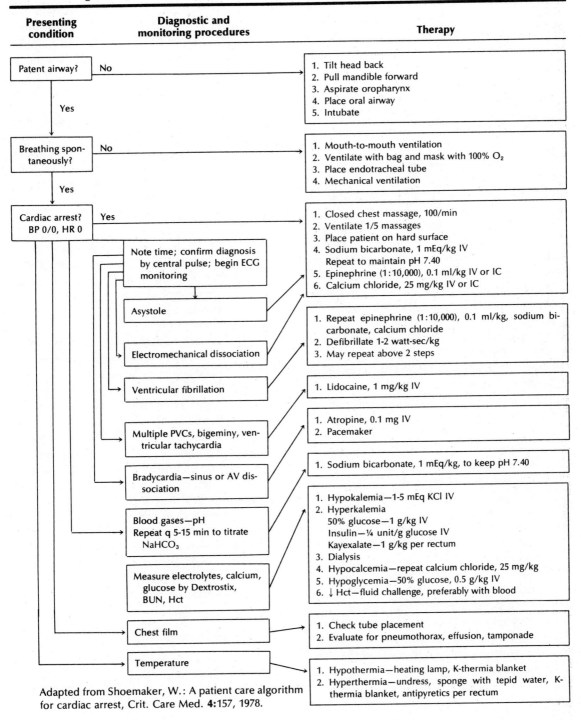

Adapted from Shoemaker, W.: A patient care algorithm for cardiac arrest, Crit. Care Med. **4**:157, 1978.

gastric distension and regurgitation of stomach contents. The volume of ventilation given should be that needed to raise the chest slightly. NOTE: Exhaled breath contains 16% oxygen and is sufficient to oxygenate the patient in cardiopulmonary arrest.

d. Switch to bag and mask technique with added oxygen as soon as possible. Be certain to maintain head tilt and a tight mask fit to prevent leaks. Insert an oral airway, if needed, to maintain airway patency.

e. Frequency of ventilation:
   (1) Infant: one breath every 3 seconds (20/min).
   (2) Child: one breath every 4 seconds (15/min).

f. See Chapter 11 for management of the obstructed airway.

6. Check for presence of adequate circulation by palpating a central pulse (specifically the carotid) or the brachial pulse in infants. Peripheral pulses may be absent with adequate central circulation.

a. The brachial pulse is located on the inside of the upper arm midway between the elbow and shoulder. Place the thumb on the outside of the arm between the elbow and shoulder and the tips of the index and middle fingers on the opposite side of the arm. Press lightly toward the bone to feel the pulse.

b. If a pulse is palpated, continue ventilatory support.

c. Assessment of circulation by palpating the precordial impulse may lead to unnecessary CPR.

7. If there is no sign of circulation, institute artificial circulation.

a. Place the patient on a firm surface.

b. Locate the ends of the sternum by palpating the xiphoid process (W- or V-shaped notch where lower ribs meet in the midline) and the sternal notch (in the midline between the clavicular heads).

c. The point of compression is the midsternum. Divide sternum in half with the hands, marking midpoint with the thumb of the upper hand. Place the first two or three fingers of the lower hand (for an infant) or the heel of the lower hand (for a child) on the point so marked. The heart now lies directly beneath the fingers, between the sternum and the spine (Fig. 5-1).

d. Depress the sternum in a perpendicular direction to force blood out of the heart into the central circulatory system.
   (1) Depth of depression:
      Infant: ½ to 1 inch
      Child: 1 to 1½ inches
      NOTE: If the force of compression is not perpendicular, ribs, lungs, stomach, spleen, or liver may be damaged.
   (2) Frequency of depression:
      Infant: 100/min
      Child: 80/min
   (3) Length of depression: apply pressure to the sternum for 50% of each cycle, since adequate filling of the heart with blood occurs during the upstroke. The compression-upstroke cycle should be rhythmical, not jerky.

8. Combine both the above techniques. Do not cease massage for respiration. Interpose a breath on the upstroke of each fifth cardiac compression.

9. Pauses in CPR may include:
   a. 5 seconds to check pulse or pupils.
   b. 15 seconds to move patient.
   c. 15 seconds to intubate patient.
   NOTE: When CPR is reinstituted, be sure to relocate the appropriate chest landmarks so that compression over the heart is reestablished.

Advanced life support

At this point in resuscitation, a delineation of responsibility is needed. The most experienced individual participating in the resuscita-

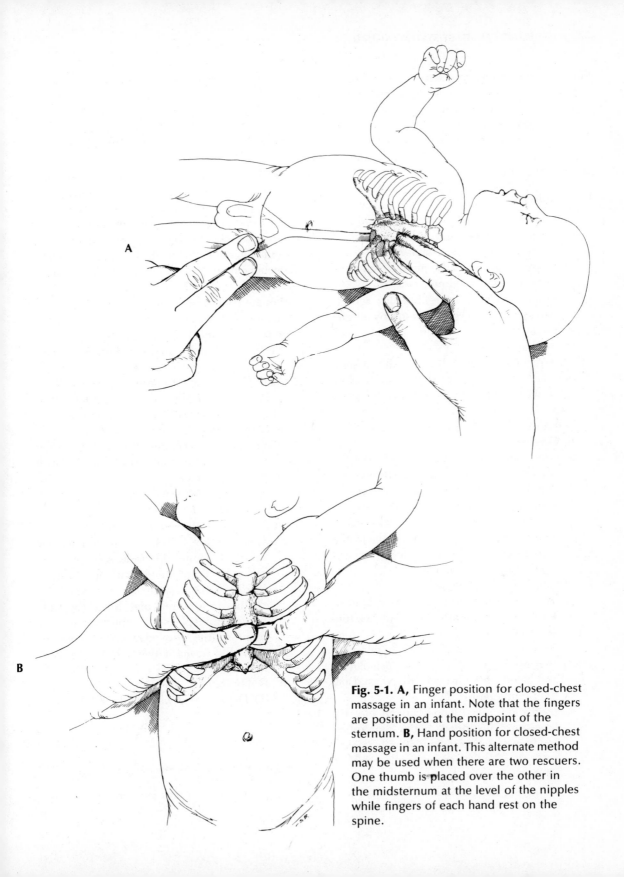

Fig. 5-1. A, Finger position for closed-chest massage in an infant. Note that the fingers are positioned at the midpoint of the sternum. **B,** Hand position for closed-chest massage in an infant. This alternate method may be used when there are two rescuers. One thumb is placed over the other in the midsternum at the level of the nipples while fingers of each hand rest on the spine.

tion should take charge and assign one person to perform each of the following functions:

1. Continue ventilation.
2. Continue closed chest massage.
3. Record further efforts.
4. Assist with drugs, monitoring, and administration of IV solutions.

Further steps

1. Monitoring:
   a. Evaluate pupils (fixed, dilated pupils indicate probable brain damage).
   b. Palpate a central pulse and measure systemic arterial blood pressure.
   c. Display ECG on a defibrillator screen.
   d. Assess adequacy of ventilation by auscultating chest and observing lips and nailbeds for cyanosis.
2. Start an IV infusion with balanced salt solution (lactated Ringer's or 0.9% sodium chloride), which supports the circulation better than a dextrose solution.
3. For correction of hypoxia and acidosis:
   a. Give oxygen.
   b. Give sodium bicarbonate, 1 mEq/kg IV, at a rate of 1 mEq/kg/min. Half this dose (0.5 mEq/kg) may be repeated every 10 minutes; after 20 minutes, check arterial blood-gas tensions and pH. Alkalosis is not tolerated as well as acidosis, and the institution of effective ventilation will rapidly correct an acidotic pH.
4. Other procedures may include:
   a. Treatment of dysrhythmias (see below).
   b. Measurement of arterial blood-gas tensions and pH.
   c. Measurement of metabolic variables: serum Na, K, Cl, Ca, glucose, osmolality, and blood urea nitrogen (BUN), and patient temperature.
   d. Intubation. This should be an elective procedure instituted under controlled conditions. Artificial ventilation by mouth or by bag and mask is usually effective while one is preparing for intubation.
   e. Emptying the stomach with an NG tube

   f. Measurement of urine output with a bladder catheter.
   g. Chest roentgenogram.

Management of life-threatening dysrhythmias

Dysrhythmias are a common cause of continued cardiovascular compromise. They are exacerbated by hypoxia and acidosis. Therefore, there must be continued oxygenation and circulation to deliver buffer (e.g., bicarbonate) and specific agents to failing heart muscle. (NOTE: Catecholamines are effective within a narrow pH range, 7.35 to 7.45; therefore, sodium bicarbonate should be administered before catecholamines). Specific therapy depends on the type of dysrhythmia:

1. Profound sinus bradycardia (Fig. 5-2): atropine, 0.01 mg/kg IV or IM.
2. Multifocal, frequent (more than 5/min) (Fig. 5-3), or coupled (Fig. 5-4) premature ventricular contractions (PVCs): lidocaine (intracardiac preparation), 1 mg/kg IV (may be repeated every 10 minutes for up to 6 doses). A continuous lidocaine infusion (30 μg/kg/min) may be necessary.
3. Ventricular tachycardia (Fig. 5-5): as in #2 or electroversion, 1 to 2 watt-sec/kg.
4. Ventricular fibrillation (Fig. 5-6):
   a. Epinephrine, 1:10,000 (dilute 1 mg in 10 ml 0.9% sodium chloride solution), 0.1 ml/kg IV. Pretreatment with epinephrine increases the chance of converting the rhythm to a normal one. Since the half-life of epinephrine is approximately 5 minutes, the dose may need to be repeated if resuscitative efforts are prolonged.
   b. Defibrillation
      (1) Dose: 1 to 2 watt-sec/kg for the first

Fig. 5-2. Sinus bradycardia.

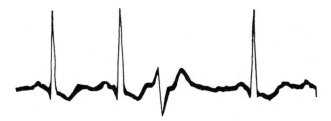

Fig. 5-3. Premature ventricular contraction.

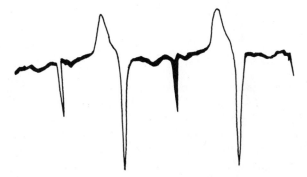

Fig. 5-4. Bigeminy (coupled premature contractions).

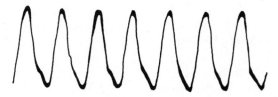

Fig. 5-5. Ventricular tachycardia.

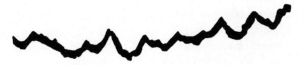

Fig. 5-6. Ventricular fibrillation.

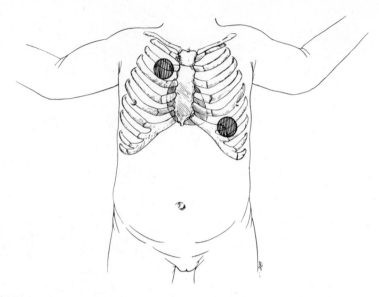

Fig. 5-7. Sites for proper placement of paddles for defibrillation: apex and base of heart.

attempt, 2 to 4 watt-sec/kg for subsequent attempts.

(2) Position: for the maximum current flow through the myocardium, place paddles at base and apex of the heart; i.e., on the upper chest to the right of the sternum just below the clavicle and to the left of the left nipple in the anterior axillary line (Fig. 5-7). Reverse paddle position if the patient has dextrocardia.

(3) Paddle size should be the largest that allows good contact with the chest over the entire area of the paddle.
Infant: 4.5 cm diameter
Child: 8 cm diameter

(4) Ensure good contact and electrical conduction by placing a saline-soaked gauze pad or specifically designed conduction jelly beneath each paddle. NOTE: If jelly is used, chest may become slippery when closed chest massage is reinstituted.

(5) Be certain to notify other personnel before discharge of the paddles so that no one is in contact with the patient or the bed.

(6) Successful defibrillation is more likely if the first shock is delivered no later than 7 to 10 minutes of recognition of the dysrhythmia and if acidosis and hypoxia have been successfully treated.

c. Closed chest massage. Reinstitute for 20 to 30 seconds before pausing to check rhythm.

d. Defibrillation. Repeat, if necessary, with higher voltage. (NOTE: Increasing the voltage excessively may produce skin or myocardial burns.)

5. Electromechanical dissociation or agonal rhythm (Fig. 5-8):

a. Calcium chloride, 25 mg/kg IV. (NOTE: Calcium chloride precipitates in the presence of sodium bicarbonate to form an insoluble substance, calcium carbonate.)

b. Epinephrine, as in #4a.

c. Atropine, 0.01 mg/kg IV.

d. Closed chest massage and ventilation.

6. Asystole: as in #5.

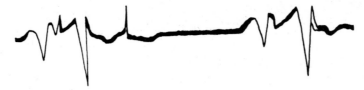

Fig. 5-8. Agonal rhythm (electrical mechanical dissociation).

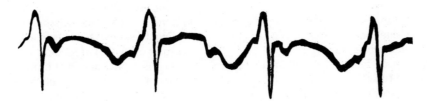

Fig. 5-9. Atrioventricular dissociation (third-degree heart block).

7. Complete atrioventricular dissociation (Fig. 5-9):
   a. Atropine, 0.01 mg/kg IV.
   b. Isoproterenol infusion, 0.1 to 1 μg/kg/min IV (see Chapter 14).
   c. Transvenous or direct electrical pacing is the treatment of choice; however, pharmacologic treatment of the dysrhythmia (steps a and b) should proceed until a pacing wire can be placed.

After restoration of palpable pulses and relatively normal cardiac rhythm, further diagnostic and supportive measures should be undertaken (cultures, CVP and arterial pressure monitoring, thoracentesis, dialysis, intracranial pressure monitoring, etc.) as indicated by the diagnosis. The patient should be transported to an intensive care area (PICU or operating room) and specialized medical and surgical consultations obtained.

ORGANIZATION OF CPR EFFORTS

The success of any resuscitation effort depends directly on the skill and training of the people involved. In any high-risk, acute care area such as the PICU it is mandatory that CPR efforts not be left to chance. A program for ensuring effective CPR should include the following:

Regular in-service training in CPR should be provided for nurses and physicians. It is highly desirable that all acute care personnel participate in the American Heart Association basic and advanced life support courses or in a similar in-hospital course. The course should include both didactic material and practical training sessions with simulated arrest situations and should be repeated at regular intervals so that CPR skills are not lost. New personnel should receive this training as soon as possible. Unscheduled simulated arrest situations may be useful in familiarizing PICU personnel with CPR procedures.

Regular checks of all resuscitation equipment should be made to ensure proper function. Defibrillators should be checked daily to determine delivered energy at both high and low levels. Performance standards should comply with the regulations of the Food and Drug Administration's Bureau of Medical Devices.

Table 5-2. Emergency resuscitation equipment

1. Cart, portable electrical suction apparatus (Gomco), and resuscitation board (30 × 50 cm)
2. Oxygen stand, portable tripod type with two E-cylinders of oxygen and a liter flow-gauge
3. Defibrillator with monitor and ECG writer
4. Ventilation equipment:
   a. One nonrebreathing partial relief (NRPR) valve with 1-liter anesthesia bag and tail clip, 8 feet of latex rubber tubing
   b. Low dead-space masks (Rendall-Baker Soucek), sizes #1 to #3
   c. One laryngoscope handle, standard size
   d. Straight laryngoscope blades, Miller, sizes #0 to #3
   e. Set of Cole endotracheal tubes (plastic), sizes #8 to #16 French
   f. Set of Portex oral blue-line tubes, sizes 2.5 to 6 mm
   g. Portex endotracheal tubes with cuff, sizes 6.0 to 7.0 mm
   h. Set of endotracheal tube connectors, sizes 3 to 7 mm
   i. Set of oral pharyngeal airways (plastic), sizes #0 to #4
   j. Nasal pharyngeal airway, Robertazzi, sizes #26 and #30 French
5. Suction equipment:
   a. Plastic suction catheter, sizes #5 and #8 French
   b. Plastic Argyle catheters, sizes #10 and #12; the red rubber tubes collapse
   c. One plastic disposable tonsil-suction tip
   d. One Sims connector
   e. One Y-type connector
6. IV equipment:
   a. One Penrose drain, tourniquet
   b. Five disposable needles, 25 gauge, ⅝ inch
   c. Five disposable needles, 21 gauge, 1 inch
   d. Five disposable needles, 20 gauge, 1 inch
   e. Five disposable needles, 18 gauge, 1½ inches
   f. Two disposable syringes, TB type
   g. Two disposable syringes, 2 ml
   h. Two disposable syringes, 10 ml
   i. Two disposable syringes, 20 ml
   j. One roll adhesive tape, 1 inch
   k. One pair bandage scissors
   l. One IV set in tray (250 ml lactated Ringer's IV solution with 1 stopcock, 1 IV tubing extension set, #21 and #23 butterfly, #16-, #18-, and #20-gauge IV catheters, and 2 povidone-iodine [Betadine] swabs)
7. Drugs:
   a. Two 50% dextrose vials, 50 ml
   b. Two sodium bicarbonate vials, 40 ml (40 mEq)
   c. One calcium gluconate vial, 10 ml
   d. One 10% calcium chloride vial, 10 ml
   e. One 0.9% sodium chloride injection solution vial, 30 ml
   f. Two atropine sulfate vials, 1 ml (0.4 mg)
   g. Two isoproterenol vials, 1 ml (0.2 mg)
   h. One diphenhydramine hydrochloride (Benadryl) vial, 1 ml (50 mg)
   i. Two diazepam (Valium) vials, 2 ml (10 mg)
   j. One hydrocortisone sodium succinate vial, 1 ml (100 mg)
   k. Two digoxin vials, 1 ml
   l. Six epinephrine vials, 1:1,000, 1 ml
   m. Two naloxone hydrochloride vials, 1 ml (0.4 mg)
   n. One lidocaine (intracardiac) vial, 20 mg/ml
8. Miscellaneous:
   a. One padded tongue blade
   b. Two small packets sterile lubricant
   c. One reusable-type needle, 20 gauge, 3-inch spinal

A

Name: _____

Hosp. no.: _____

Age: _____

Dr.: _____

Date: _____   Time started: _____   Time ended: _____   Wt.: _____

Children's Medical Center
Dallas, Texas
Nursing cardiopulmonary resuscitation report

Drugs   Time/amt
Na bicarb—ml
Ca chloride—ml
9 ml NS + 1 ml 1:1,000 Epi
Epi 1:10,000—ml
Lidocaine 1%—ml

Defibrillation
(1-2 watt-sec/kg)   Time/watt-sec

IV solutions
and drips   Time

Vital signs

Time	BP	AP	Pupils	Pa$_{O_2}$	Pa$_{CO_2}$	pH	ΔB

Additional remarks or observations:

Signature of nurse:

Participants: _____   _____   _____

Continued

Fig. 5-10. CPR flow sheet. **A,** Record of resuscitation efforts for patient chart.

DRUGS AND DOSAGES

Drug	Suggested dosage	Usual concentration
Calcium chloride	25 mg/kg IV May repeat q 10 min 0.5-1.0 g/kg/24 hr	1 g/10 ml (100 mg/ml)
Sodium bicarbonate	1-3 mEq/kg IV q 10 min × 2 then ABG	44.6 mEq/50 ml (1 mEq/ml)
Epinephrine 1:10,000	0.1 ml/kg (10 μg/kg) Drip 1 mg/100 ml D$_5$W (10 μg/ml) Small infant: 0.5 mg/100 ml D$_5$W (5 μg/ml) Start at 0.1 μg/kg/min	1:1,000 (1 mg/ml) (0.1 mg/ml or 100 μg/ml) 1:10,000 = 1 ml + 9 ml NS
Dopamine (Intropin)	100 mg/100 ml D$_5$W (1,000 μg/ml) Small infant: 50 mg/100 ml D$_5$W (500 μg/ml) Range: 2-20 μg/kg/min	200 mg/5 ml
Isuprel	1 mg/100 D$_5$W (10 μg/ml) Small infant: 0.5 mg/100 ml D$_5$W (5 μg/ml) Start with 0.1 μg/kg/min	0.2 mg/ml or 1 mg/5 ml (200 μg/ml)
Atropine	0.01-0.08 mg/kg IV	0.4 mg/ml
Lidocaine	1 mg/kg IV May repeat q 10 min × 6 Drip 50 mg/250 ml D$_5$W max. 1.5 mg/kg/hr	10 mg/ml

B

$$\text{ml/hr} = \frac{\text{kg} \times \text{μg/kg/min} \times 60 \text{ min/hr}}{\text{μg/ml}}$$

Age	ET tube size (mm)
Premi	2.5-3.0
0-6 months	3.0-3.5
6-12 months	3.5-4.0
12-18 months	4.0-4.5
2-4 years	4.5-5.5
4-6 years	5.5-6.5
>6 years	6.5-7.5

Fig. 5-10, cont'd. B, On the reverse side of the flow sheet, common drug dosages and endotracheal tube sizes are listed.

Resuscitation equipment and drugs should be arranged so that they are readily available and easily transported. An upright cart or toolbox lends itself well to this purpose. Defibrillators can be placed in strategic locations, or a portable, battery-operated unit can be stationed on the emergency cart. Equipment should be standardized throughout the hospital for ease of use. Only that equipment absolutely necessary for basic life support need be included (Table 5-2). A multiplicity of drugs and devices contributes to the confusion surrounding an arrest. The basic equipment should be sufficient to stabilize the patient until he can be transported to an area, such as the PICU, where prolonged support of various organ systems can proceed. The PICU should stock accessory equipment (such as cutdown trays, paracentesis-thoracentesis trays, mechanical ventilators, infusion pumps, dialysis equipment) and less frequently used drugs that may be needed for prolonged resuscitations. This equipment should be ready for use at all times and should be checked for proper functioning at the beginning of each shift.

Organization of CPR teams is helpful. Such a team includes specifically designated and specially trained personnel, who respond to and conduct all resuscitations. A minimum of five persons is necessary: someone skilled in ventilatory support (e.g., respiratory therapist, anesthesiologist, pulmonologist) as well as a physician who is expert in acute emergency care (cardiologist, intensivist), a senior house staff physician, an emergency room or PICU nurse, and a surgeon.

Development of a system to notify proper personnel of an arrest is essential. The general paging system can utilize a standard emergency code (stat., Doctor Blue, etc.), and direct phone lines to the emergency room or PICU or an individual beeper system may also be used.

Development of a flow sheet to facilitate accurate recording of the management of an arrest is helpful (Fig. 5-10).

Regular review of resuscitation efforts (conferences, monthly morbidity and mortality statistics) is useful in assessing the success of such efforts and in indicating weaknesses in technique and equipment.

All the above activities should be coordinated by a multidisciplinary committee that includes representatives of the following areas:
1. Nursing (preferably from the acute care area).
2. Medical staff, including cardiology, surgery, anesthesia, and the house staff.
3. Central supply or purchasing.
4. Administration.
5. Respiratory therapy.

ADDITIONAL READING

Brevick, H.: A safe multipurpose pediatric ventilation bag, Crit. Care Med. 4:32-39, 1976.

Ehrlich, R., Emmitt, S.M., and Rodriguez-Torres, R.: Pediatric cardiac resuscitation team: a six-year study, J. Pediatr. 84:152-155, 1974.

Gregory, G.: Resuscitation of the newborn, Anesthesiology 43:225-237, 1975.

Gutgesell, H.P., Tacker, W.A., Geddes, L.A., and others: Energy dose for defibrillation of children, Pediatrics 58:898-901, 1976.

Hodglien, J.E., Foster, G.L., and Nicolay, L.I.: Cardiopulmonary resuscitation: development of an organized protocol, Crit. Care Med. 5:93-100, 1977.

Kerber, R.E., and Sarnat, W.: Factors influencing the success of ventricular fibrillation in man, Circulation 60:226-230, 1980.

National Conference on Cardiopulmonary Resuscitation and Emergency Cardiac Care: Standards and Guidelines for Cardiopulmonary Resuscitation (CPR) and Emergency Cardiac Care (ECC), J.A.M.A. 244(Suppl.):453-509, 1980.

Rogers, M.C., Nugent, S.K., and Stedham, G.L.: Effects of closed chest massage on intracranial pressure, Crit. Care Med. 7:454-456, 1979.

Taylor, J.T., Tucket, W.M., Greene, H.L., and others: Importance of prolonged compression during cardiopulmonary resuscitation in man, N. Engl. J. Med. 296:1515-1518, 1977.

Todres, D., and Rogers, M.: Methods of external cardiac massage in the newborn infant, J. Pediatr. 86:781-782, 1975.

6 Altered states of consciousness

FRANCES C. MORRISS
JAY D. COOK

DEFINITION AND PHYSIOLOGY

Consciousness is a state of self-awareness that depends on the continuous interaction of intact cerebral hemispheres and activating mechanisms of the upper brainstem. The cerebral hemispheres control the content of conscious behavior, and the upper brainstem controls the degree of the patient's wakefulness. Thus, cerebral dysfunction and/or brainstem depression produce altered states of consciousness. These states may be manifested by signs of cerebral dysfunction (such as misinterpretation of external stimuli, inability to follow commands, disorientation, and memory distortion) and by signs of depressed levels of wakefulness (such as drowsiness, stupor, and coma, which is the most severe aberration of arousal). Coma is a state of complete unresponsiveness in which there is no perceivable reaction to external or internal stimuli. Two types of pathologic processes that may impair consciousness are (1) conditions that directly and widely depress or destroy functions of the cerebral hemispheres and (2) conditions that depress or destroy upper brainstem activating mechanisms.

Lesions causing the above conditions include the following:

1. Supratentorial mass lesions that interfere with cerebral function and secondarily compress the brainstem, e.g., tumor, infarct, abscess, or hematoma
2. Subtentorial mass lesions that depress or destroy brainstem function, e.g., brainstem or cerebellar tumors, infarct, hemorrhage, or contusion
3. Metabolic disorders that depress or interrupt hemispheric and/or brainstem function, e.g., ischemia, trauma, postictal states, endogenous and exogenous toxins, drugs, generalized central nervous system (CNS) infection

Supratentorial lesions are usually associated with lateralizing or focal signs. Progression of pressure-related symptoms is usually from the cerebral hemisphere to the brainstem, resulting in caudal displacement of the brainstem (herniation) with hemorrhage and structural damage. Brainstem signs appear at this point. Subtentorial lesions produce early signs relating to the brainstem, particularly cranial nerve dysfunction, and coma rapidly supervenes. Oculocephalic and oculovestibular reflexes may be absent. With metabolic abnormalities, changes in level of consciousness usually precede onset of motor signs, which, if present, tend to be symmetrical. Not all levels of the nervous system are depressed equally, and the signs of dysfunction may change from one examination period to the next. Pupillary reactivity is generally preserved. Other signs suggesting a metabolic disorder include acid-base imbalance, myoclonus, temperature abnormalities, meningismus, and unusual odors on the patient's breath. Early differentiation of the probable site of the lesion is invaluable in directing subsequent diagnostic procedures (e.g., roentgenographic vs laboratory examination) once the patient's condition has been stabilized.

MONITORING

See also Chapter 4.

Central nervous system

CNS monitoring has two objectives: to determine whether cerebral function is being preserved or is deteriorating and to assess the level of CNS involvement. A complete neurologic examination, with emphasis on the following functions, should be done at regular intervals (every 1 to 2 hours).

1. Level of consciousness: Degree of orientation to person, place, and time; tests of cognitive function such as memory or ability to obey commands.
2. Pattern of breathing.
3. Size and reactivity of pupils.
4. Oculocephalic and oculovestibular reflexes: Tests of these reflexes are based on the finding that voluntary control of eye movements, mediated by the cerebral hemispheres, is superseded by brainstem reflex control when cerebral function becomes depressed. The oculocephalic reflex is the occurrence of brisk hyperactive reflex movements of the eye that occur when the head is moved. The oculovestibular reflex, evoked by irrigating the external auditory canal with ice water, is a more sensitive test of cerebral integrity. With cerebral depression, these reflexes produce sustained conjugate lateral deviation of the eyes toward the irrigated canal or away from the direction the head was turned. Absent or sluggish reflex eye movements imply brainstem damage.
5. Skeletal muscle responses to noxious stimuli (sternal rubbing, pressure on the orbit).

Table 6-1 summarizes these patterns of reflex response and the corresponding CNS level. Specialized sheets for recording the above examination are helpful in correlating the information obtained (Fig. 6-1).

In addition, the following variables must be evaluated:

Table 6-1. Reflex responses in altered states of consciousness

Level of CNS lesion	Level of consciousness	Pupillary size and reactivity	Oculocephalic and oculovestibular reflexes	Respiratory pattern	Motor responses
Thalamus	Lethargy, stupor	Small, reactive	Increased or decreased	Cheyne-Stokes*	Normal posture, tone slightly increased
Midbrain	Coma	Midposition, fixed	Absent	Central neurogenic hyperventilation†	Decorticate,‡ tone markedly increased
Pons	Coma	Pinpoint	Absent	Eupnea§ or apneustic breathing‖	Decerebrate,¶ flaccid
Medulla	Coma	Small, reactive	Present	Ataxic breathing	No posturing, flaccid

*Cheyne-Stokes respiration: type of regular periodic breathing characterized by crescendo-decrescendo breaths interspersed with periods of apnea.
†Central neurogenic hyperventilation: hyperventilation with forced inspiration and expiration.
‡Decorticate posturing: upper extremities flexed against chest, lower extremities extended.
§Eupnea: normal breathing.
‖Apneustic breathing: rhythmical pattern of breathing in which there is cessation of respiration in inspiratory position.
¶Decerebrate posturing: arms and legs extended, with arms internally rotated, neck extended.

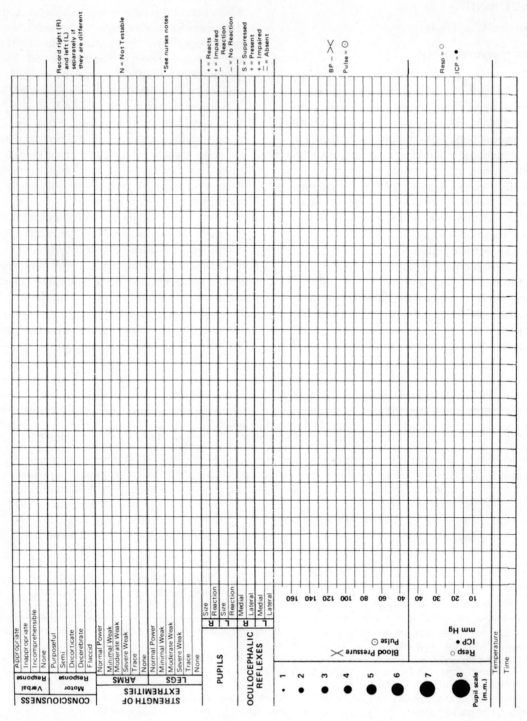

Fig. 6-1. Flow sheet for nursing record of neurologic signs.

1. Presence or absence of increased intracranial pressure (ICP) (see Chapter 10)
2. Type and frequency of seizure activity (see Chapter 9)

Respiratory system

1. Observe ability to handle secretions (this is an estimation of the patient's ability to protect his airway) as well as specific airway protective reflexes (gag, cough).
2. Measure arterial blood-gas tensions and pH initially and as needed.

Renal-metabolic system

1. Anticipate inappropriate secretion of antidiuretic hormone (ISADH) (see Chapter 51).
   a. Measure serum Na, K, and Cl and urine Na every day.
   b. Measure serum and urine osmolalities every day.
2. Perform liver and renal function tests: serum glutamic-oxaloacetic transaminase (SGOT), alkaline phosphatase, bilirubin, TSP, serum albumin/globulin ratio (A/G), prothrombin time (PT), partial thromboplastin time (PTT), serum ammonia (NH_3), BUN serum creatinine, serum acetone, and toxicology screen (when indicated by the nature of the primary pathologic process).

MANAGEMENT OF ALTERED STATES OF CONSCIOUSNESS

The management of a patient with an altered state of consciousness is aimed at preserving cerebral function (cardiorespiratory support and adequate blood glucose level) and correcting the underlying pathologic process (decreasing intracranial pressure, stopping seizures, treating infections, and correcting electrolyte and acid-base imbalances) (see Table 6-2). In addition, the functions of other vital organ systems should be closely monitored so that homeostasis is preserved until the patient can care for himself.

Table 6-2. Sequence of steps in management of altered states of consciousness

1. Preserve cerebral function
   a. Ensure adequate oxygen
   b. Ensure adequate cerebral blood flow
   c. Ensure adequate glucose
2. Correct underlying pathologic process
   a. Reduce increased intracranial pressure
   b. Control seizures
   c. Treat infections
   d. Restore acid-base and electrolyte balances

Preservation of cerebral function

Preservation of cerebral function depends on adequate delivery of energy substrate (oxygen and glucose) to the brain.

1. Keep blood oxygen tensions (Pa_{O_2}) between 100 and 150 mm Hg. It may be necessary to secure the airway with an endotracheal tube and institute mechanical ventilation. The need for an adequate airway cannot be overemphasized.
2. Keep the serum glucose level between 100 and 150 mg/dl.
3. Stabilize systemic arterial blood pressure so that it is within normal limits for age.
4. Treat seizures and increased ICP (see Chapters 9 and 10, respectively).
5. Discontinue any drugs other than anticonvulsants that are known to alter CNS function (tranquilizers, mood elevators, antidepressants).

Treatment of underlying cause

Treatment of the underlying causes of altered states of consciousness will depend on information gained from a detailed history, a thorough physical examination including a complete neurologic evaluation, and pertinent laboratory tests. The patient should be evaluated by both neurologic and neurosurgical services. If aggressive roentgenographic examination (e.g., brain scan, computerized tomography, arteriography) is necessary, plans for ongoing monitoring and close observation outside the PICU must be made. A portable ECG, resuscitation equipment including suction apparatus and oxygen, and trained personnel (PICU nurse and physician) should accompany the patient.

Prevention of damage to other organ systems

Cardiovascular system
1. Treat hypotension (see Chapter 14).
2. Treat any dysrhythmias (see Chapter 5).

Respiratory system
1. Prevent atelectasis with prophylactic chest physiotherapy; change the patient's position and suction secretions frequently. In the presence of intracranial hypertension this regimen may have to be altered (see Chapter 10).
2. Prevent inhalation of gastric contents by stopping oral intake and placing an NG tube.
3. Consider discontinuing any drugs (other than anticonvulsants) that may depress respiratory drive (narcotics, sedatives).
4. Treat associated conditions such as pulmonary edema, foreign body inhalation, or pulmonary trauma.

Renal-metabolic system
1. Maintain normal serum electrolytes by appropriate IV fluids.
2. Maintain urine output at a minimum of 0.5 to 1 ml/kg/hr.
3. Maintain temperature within normal range (35° to 37° C).

Gastrointestinal system
1. Administer antacids (Maalox, Milk of Magnesia, etc., 15 to 30 ml every 1 to 2 hours per NG tube) if gastric pH is less than 1.5.
2. Prevent constipation and fecal impaction.
3. Incontinence may be a problem.

Prevention of infection
1. Perform urinalysis every day while bladder catheter is present.
2. Inspect IV sites every day.
3. Obtain cultures of blood, urine, cerebrospinal fluid (CSF), and tracheobronchial secretions when indicated.

General supportive care
1. Prevent decubitus ulcers with a sheepskin, heel pads, and frequent position changes. Small infants may be placed on a flotation pad.
2. If patient is violent or has frequent seizures, pad bed rails and restrain him to prevent injury.
3. For eye care administer methylcellulose eye drops every hour.
4. Provide passive range-of-motion exercises.
5. If a prolonged comatose state is anticipated, nutritional requirements must be provided by appropriate tube feedings (blenderized or prepackaged diet of 1 calorie/ml given in divided amounts to provide 50 to 80 calories/kg/24 hr) or by parenteral alimentation.

ADDITIONAL READING

Plum, F., and Posner, J.: The diagnosis of stupor and coma, Philadelphia, 1980, F.A. Davis Co.

Tinsdall, R.S.A.: Evaluation and treatment of the comatose patient. In Rosenberg, R., editor: Current treatment of neurological disease, New York, 1977, Spectrum Publications, Inc.

7 Cerebral death

FRANCES C. MORRISS
JAY D. COOK

With increasing sophistication of monitoring and life-support systems, patients with irreversible brain damage can be maintained in a vegetative state for prolonged periods. Many physicians now face the distressing situation of diagnosing irreversible cerebral damage and withdrawing life-support measures. Table 7-1 summarizes four sets of criteria for the diagnosis of cerebral death. The critical criteria of brain death are clinical absence of brainstem function and laboratory demonstration (electroencephalogram [EEG]) of the absence of cerebral hemisphere function in the presence of known severe structural disease or irreversible metabolic abnormality. (Specific criteria now exist for standardizing EEG recordings for use in the diagnosis of brain death.) Whether the criteria for brain death have been met must be determined by a physician, usually a consulting neurologist, or group of physicians who are not directly responsible for the care of the patient. Another verification of absent cerebral and brainstem activity is necessary to document the irreversible nature of the process; the usual period between examinations is 12 to 24 hours, although a 6-hour interval has been suggested. The diagnosis of cerebral death cannot be entertained until all appropriate diagnostic and therapeutic procedures have been performed and stability of cardiovascular and respiratory systems has been achieved. (Therefore, a diagnosis of cerebral death is inappropriate for a patient who is being actively resuscitated.) Verification may be augmented by roentgenographic demonstration of the absence of cerebral circulation. The decision to withdraw life-support systems based on the above criteria must be in accord with family preference and whatever legal precedent may apply to the situation. Many areas have no clear-cut laws governing such a decision, and the establishment of a hospital protocol for the diagnosis of cerebral death may be helpful. Consideration of the possible donation of organs for transplantation is always indicated (see Chapter 8).

There are two important medical reasons for trying to make a diagnosis of cerebral death as early as possible:

1. It is now possible to extend the biological activity of a cerebrally dead patient at a tremendous expense, with no change in the ultimate outcome. The expense is not only to the family but also to the community. No physician wants to burden any family with a large, unnecessary bill or to use limited resources (personnel and supplies) unproductively.
2. With the advent of transplant programs and the necessity for obtaining organs before irreversible damage to usable organs has occurred, it is important to try to make a decision as early as possible.

However, there are pitfalls in making a diagnosis of brain death and it is worthwhile to review these (see Table 7-2).

Table 7-1. Summary of sets of criteria for brain death used by different investigators and clinicians

Harvard criteria	1. Unresponsive coma 2. Apnea 3. Absence of cephalic reflexes 4. Absence of spinal reflexes 5. Isoelectric EEG 6. Persistence of conditions for at least 24 hours 7. Absence of drug intoxication or hypothermia
Minnesota criteria	1. Basic prerequisite—diagnosis of irreparable cerebral lesion 2. No spontaneous movements 3. No spontaneous respiration 4. Absence of brainstem reflexes 5. Persistence of condition unchanged for 12 hours
Swedish criteria	1. Unresponsive coma 2. Apnea 3. Absent brainstem reflexes 4. Isoelectric EEG 5. Nonfilling of cerebral vessels on two aortocranial injections of contrast media 25 minutes apart
Cerebral survival criteria	1. Basic prerequisite—completion of all appropriate diagnostic and therapeutic procedures 2. Unresponsive coma 3. Apnea 4. Absent cephalic reflexes with dilated, fixed pupils 5. Isoelectric EEG 6. Persistence of the above for 30 minutes to 1 hour, and 6 hours after onset of coma and apnea 7. Confirmatory test indicating absence of cerebral circulation (optional)

From Molinari, G.F.: Review of clinical criteria of brain death. In Korein, J., editor: Brain death: interrelated medical and social issues, Ann. N.Y. Acad. Sci. **315:**62-69, 1978, with permission.

Table 7-2. Some pitfalls in the diagnosis of brain death

Findings	Possible causes
1. Pupils fixed	Anticholinergic drugs
	Neuromuscular blockers
	Preexisting disease
2. No oculovestibular reflexes	Ototoxic agents
	Vestibular suppressants
	Preexisting disease
3. No respiration	Posthyperventilation apnea
	Neuromuscular blockers
4. No motor activity	Neuromuscular blockers
	Locked-in state
	Sedative drugs
5. Isoelectric EEG	Sedative drugs
	Anoxia
	Hypothermia
	Encephalitis
	Trauma

From Plum, F., and Posner, J.B.: The diagnosis of stupor and coma, ed. 3, Philadelphia, 1980, F.A. Davis Co.

ADDITIONAL READING

Ad Hoc Committee of Harvard Medical School to Examine the Definition of Brain Death: A definition of irreversible coma, J.A.M.A. **205:**85-88, 1968.

Collaborative study: an appraisal of the criteria of cerebral death, J.A.M.A. **237:**982-986, 1977.

Jastremski, M., Powner, D., Snyder, J., and others: Problems in brain death determination, Forensic Sci. **11:**201-212, 1978.

Korein, J., editor: Brain death: inter-related medical and social issues, Ann. N.Y. Acad. Sci. **315:**1-454, 1978.

Plum, F., and Posner, J.: The diagnosis of stupor and coma, Philadelphia, 1980, F.A. Davis Co.

Silverman, D., Masland, R.L., Saunders, M.G., and others: Irreversible coma associated with electrocerebral silence, Neurology **20:**525-533, 1970.

8 Identification and preparation of organ donors

RONALD J. HOGG

The inclusion of a chapter on organ donation is intended to draw attention to the fact that just before their death, the majority of potential cadaveric organ donors are under the care of intensive care physicians. These physicians should consider the possibility of organ donation when cerebral death is apparent in their patients. It is obviously very difficult in most cases for the physician to suggest such a course of action to the grieving parents. However, the family of a deceased child may derive some consolation from the realization that the donation of their child's kidneys or other organs may save the life of another child. Certainly there are many children, and even more adults, who are being maintained on dialysis until a suitable cadaveric donor kidney is available.

The confusion regarding medical and legal definitions of cerebral death has led to the discarding of many viable organs. The diagnostic criteria of cerebral death have been considered in the previous chapter, and we will now consider the situation once cerebral death has been diagnosed. Most of the discussion will be oriented towards renal transplantation, but the possibility of donating other organs (e.g., liver, pancreas, heart) and tissues (e.g., cornea) will also be explored.

SUITABILITY OF THE POTENTIAL DONOR

Before the family is approached, some consideration should be given to whether the deceased patient is a suitable donor. It would be cruel and senseless to ask the family to consider the possibility of kidney donation if the patient has suffered tissue destruction that would necessitate rejection of the organs by the transplant service. After cerebral death has been diagnosed and before the family is approached, there should be some preliminary discussion between the primary physician and either the attending nephrologist or the transplant surgeon concerning the viability of the kidneys. The following considerations will determine the acceptability of the potential donor.

Age

It is a common misconception that kidneys of young children are unsuitable for transplantation into older individuals. It is true that attempts to transplant newborn kidneys and those from young infants have met with failure in most cases, usually as a result of thrombosis in small renal vessels. However, kidneys from older infants and young children have proven to be acceptable organs even when transplanted into older children and adults. Rapid hypertrophy of the kidney occurs following transplantation, and 6 months after transplantation the kidney will demonstrate function approximating that of an adult kidney.

DISEASE PRESENT IN THE POTENTIAL DONOR

In cases where death results from prolonged illness, there is less likelihood of the kidneys being suitable for transplantation than in patients who die from acute trauma or illness.

Therefore, the majority of viable cadaver kidneys are obtained from cases of cerebral death following either a severe head injury or an acute fulminant illness. Chronic vascular disease, hypertension, generalized infections (including hepatitis), systemic diseases involving the kidneys, and widespread neoplastic lesions eliminate the possibility of donation. The presence of a solitary brain tumor is not usually regarded as a contraindication. However, in some cases the transplantation of a kidney from a cadaver with a neoplastic lesion has led to metastases in the recipient, an occurrence that is most likely potentiated by the use of immunosuppressive agents.

The presence of acute systemic diseases that do not directly injure the kidneys does not necessarily prohibit organ donation. An example of such a disease in children is Reye's syndrome. This condition appears to be precipitated by a viral infection in many cases, but knowledge of the specific cause is lacking. Despite the abnormalities in metabolism resulting from liver dysfunction, it appears that renal function remains normal in most cases. A number of patients dying from Reye's syndrome have therefore been accepted as kidney donors with good results and no recurrence of the disease in the recipients.

Hypotensive episodes and transient periods of oliguria should not be regarded as contraindications to organ transplantation, provided that the hemodynamic and renal function status of the patient is relatively normal when cerebral death is diagnosed. Some cases remain questionable and can only be resolved by perfusion of the kidneys after removal from the cadaver. It is therefore appropriate to consult with the transplant service before rejecting a potential donor on these grounds.

MANAGEMENT OF THE POTENTIAL DONOR

Once cerebral death has been diagnosed, the management should consist of measures directed toward determining, and subsequently maintaining, the viability of the potential donor organs. No change in management that may be detrimental to the patient should be undertaken before cerebral death has been diagnosed. It is important to maintain this approach even in those patients whose disease is being treated by measures that may be detrimental to renal function. An example would be a patient who is maintained in a relatively volume-depleted state to alleviate cerebral edema. Regardless of the apparent irreversibility of the brain damage, there must be no change in management until the diagnosis of cerebral death has been established. The approach is completely different once cerebral death has been diagnosed. Under the direction of the transplant service, the volume deficit should be quickly corrected, usually with 0.9% sodium chloride solution. Additional stimulus to urine flow may be provided by mannitol or furosemide in selected cases, but the initial management should consist of measures to restore blood volume to normal. After repletion of body fluids has been achieved, the next step is to discontinue any vasoconstrictor drugs the donor may be receiving, since these may lead to renal arterial vasoconstriction.

At this stage, the management of the donor varies in different centers. A variety of tests to determine the suitability of the donor kidneys in terms of function and anatomy have been used before and after removal of the organs. The transplant service will be responsible for arranging these tests.

Crucial determinants of the viability of transplanted kidneys include the management of the donor immediately before organ removal, technical aspects of the nephrectomy, and preservation techniques used in storing the organs before transplantation. Details of these procedures are beyond the scope of this discussion, but it should be noted that many transplant centers are now equipped with mobile teams that are able to assist in the management of the donor in all these phases.

The donor is managed similarly for donation of other organs, except the cornea, which can be collected immediately after death.

ADDITIONAL READING

Chan, J.C.M.: Physiological responses of the transplanted human kidney, J. Urol. **110:**162-165, 1973.

Filoso, A.M., and Cho, S.I.: Analysis of 75 discarded cadaver kidneys, Arch. Surg. **111:**1129-1130, 1976.

Fine, R.N., Brennan, L.P., Edelbrock, H.H., and others: Use of pediatric cadaver kidneys for homotransplantation in children, J.A.M.A. **210:**477-484, 1969.

Firlit, C.F.: Reye syndrome cadaveric kidneys: their use in human transplantation, Arch. Surg. **109:**797, 1974.

Silber, S.J.: Renal transplantation between adults and children: differences in renal growth, J.A.M.A. **228:**1143-1145, 1974.

9 Status epilepticus

FRANCES C. MORRISS
JAY D. COOK

DEFINITION AND PHYSIOLOGY

Status epilepticus is one of the true medical emergencies in the care of children. The brain of a young child is more susceptible to permanent damage from prolonged motor seizure activity than that of an adult. A child is considered to be in status epilepticus if he has had three seizures without awakening or continuous motor seizure activity for more than 20 minutes. The frequency of status among children with seizures is 8%; the frequency of disability post status is 56% (transient disability, usually hemiplegia, 43%; permanent disability, 13%).

Seizures originate in small groups of abnormal neurons that spontaneously emit large numbers of repetitive discharges. Any event that causes depolarization of cellular membranes may irritate such neurons, but the exact cellular mechanism underlying seizures is unclear. Postulated causes are (1) chemical abnormalities of membranes, particularly of the sodium-potassium pump that maintains membrane polarity, (2) mechanical deformation of membranes secondary to scarring, and (3) synaptic disorders that lead to self-excitation phenomena. The repetitive discharges propagate via physiologic neural pathways so that adjacent or remote areas of the brain may be involved.

Sustained seizure activity increases adenosine triphosphate (ATP) requirements by a factor of 2.5 or more; ATP is the high-energy substrate that sustains the sodium-potassium pump, which maintains membrane integrity and polarization. Synthesis of ATP requires adequate supplies of oxygen and glucose and, by inference, an adequate delivery system (cerebral blood flow). If cerebral blood flow cannot increase to supply extraordinary metabolic needs as may be seen with continuous seizures, energy sources in the brain are quickly exhausted and neuronal death occurs. Repetitive seizures, especially those of the tonic-clonic type, commonly cause apnea, hypoxemia, and hypoglycemia. In addition, constant muscle contraction associated with status epilepticus increases oxygen consumption and produces lactic acidosis. Even with adequate oxygenation, the metabolic requirements of status epilepticus may exceed the maximum that can be supplied by an increased flow of blood to the CNS. Autopsy evidence reveals cerebral anoxic-ischemic changes in patients who died after episodes of status epilepticus; whether these changes are secondary to the systemic problems accompanying unremitting seizures or due to the seizures themselves is unknown. Experimental evidence demonstrates that even with normal cerebral oxygenation, neurons fail to respond normally once the seizure is ended. Hyperpyrexia, hypoxia, hypotension, acidosis, and hypoglycemia occurring before or as the result of prolonged seizure activity greatly increase the likelihood of neuronal damage. In addition to permanent neurologic sequelae, uncontrolled convulsions may cause anoxic injury to other organs, cardiac dysrhythmias, inhalation of stomach contents resulting in pneumonitis, lactic acidosis, and traumatic injuries such as bruising, tongue laceration, or cerebral concussion.

The most common cause of status epilepti-

41

cus in children is an inadequate serum concentration of anticonvulsant medication due to noncompliance. Sudden withdrawal of anticonvulsants or administration of phenothiazine or tricyclic tranquilizers may precipitate seizures. Other causes of status epilepticus can be categorized by patient age:

1. Neonates: congenital or acquired metabolic disorders (e.g., hypoglycemia, disorders of amino acid metabolism) perinatal cerebral hypoxic injury, congenital malformations, and CNS infection, either acquired or intrauterine, (e.g., neonatal meningitis or herpes encephalitis).
2. Children: all of the above plus neurocutaneous syndromes, toxins, and idiopathic epilepsy (most common).
3. Adolescents: metabolic disorders (including drug withdrawal and uremia), toxins, CNS tumors, head injury, idiopathic epilepsy, and drug overdoses. Hypertensive encephalopathy and cerebrovascular disease are additional causes.

MONITORING

See also Chapter 4.

Central nervous system

1. Close observation. A patient in status epilepticus should never be left unattended. Once control is achieved, continue close observation for 24 hours (status epilepticus may recur).
2. Neurologic examination every hour including level of consciousness, pupillary reflexes, pattern of respiration, oculomotor and oculovestibular responses, and motor responses to noxious stimuli.
3. Diagnostic procedures may include as indicated:
    a. EEG.
    b. Skull roentgenograms.
    c. Lumbar puncture (contraindicated in the presence of suspected increased ICP).
    d. Computerized tomography and cerebral arteriography.

Respiratory system

Arterial blood-gas tensions and pH initially and every 2 to 4 hours. Consider placing an indwelling arterial catheter.

Renal-metabolic system

1. Toxicology screen (serum and urine).
2. Serum glucose level initially and sequentially until normal.
3. Electrolytes: Na, K, Cl, HCO_3, Ca, PO_4, and Mg initially and sequentially until normal.
4. Liver function tests: SGOT, bilirubin, alkaline phosphatase, serum ammonia (NH_3), TSP, A/G, PT, PTT.
5. Anticonvulsant levels initially and until therapeutic range is achieved.
6. Abnormalities found in the initial screening should be followed sequentially.
7. Urine and serum amino acids, if appropriate.

Infection

1. Complete blood count (CBC) with platelet count.
2. Blood culture.
3. CSF culture when infection is suspected.
4. Neonates: serum and urine screening tests for congenital infection.
5. Viral cultures: CSF, stool, and nasopharyngeal secretions as indicated.

MANAGEMENT

The goals of management are to ensure CNS energy needs (oxygen, glucose, and adequate cerebral blood flow) and to halt seizure activity. Diagnostic procedures and treatment of related problems can then follow.

1. Establish an airway. Supplemental delivery of oxygen can be aided by using one of the following methods to ensure an adequate airway:

a. Tongue blade (only if oral airways are not available).

b. Oral airway.

c. Endotracheal tube. Intubation by an anesthesiologist may have to be done if the use of short-acting muscle relaxants (succinylcholine) is necessary. Intubation should be considered if there is any evidence of respiratory compromise such as cyanosis, long periods of apnea, or evidence of inhalation pneumonitis.

2. Secure an IV route for glucose and drugs, preferably with a catheter. The rate of glucose administration while the patient is convulsing should be at least 100 to 150 mg/kg/hr (Dextrostix, 175 to 250 mg/dl, or serum glucose, 150 mg/dl), preceded by a bolus of $D_{50}W$, 0.5 g/kg (1 ml/kg). When seizures are controlled, give an IV solution containing D_5W at a rate of 80% maintenance (e.g., D_5 0.25% sodium chloride solution).

3. Maintain systemic arterial blood pressure within normal limits for age (hypotension is probably more harmful than hypertension in terms of ensuring an adequate cerebral blood flow).

4. Give anticonvulsants. There are many drug regimen protocols for treating status epilepticus. There is poor documentation in the literature as to the efficacy of one regimen as compared to another with the exception that lorazepam (which is not approved for children) has been documented to be superior to diazepam (Valium) in status epilepticus in adults. In spite of the lack of agreement as to a general protocol, some general principles are commonly agreed

Table 9-1. Initial anticonvulsants to control status epilepticus

Drug	Dose	Infusion rate	Onset of action	Hazards
Diazepam (undiluted)	0.25 mg/kg, up to 0.5 mg/kg	1 mg/min	1-2 min	Respiratory depression Synergistic action with other respiratory depressants (see text) Thrombophlebitis
Phenobarbital (65 mg/ml)	10 mg/kg IV initially (respiratory depression occurs at doses greater than 18 mg/kg)	30 mg/min	10-12 min	Respiratory depression
Paraldehyde (IV, must be diluted to 1:20 with saline in *glass* syringe)	0.15 mg/kg IV (may be repeated in 20-40 min)	Total time, 4 min	1-2 min	Very low therapeutic to toxic index Contraindicated in hepatic, lung, or renal disease
Phenytoin 50 mg/ml (diluted in 0.9% sodium chloride solution; 1:10; 5 mg/ml)	10 mg/kg, up to 1000 mg	20-50 mg/min	>1 hr	Cardiac conduction block High levels may damage cerebellum

upon. These include: (1) medication to achieve initial control should be given intravenously rather than intramuscularly or orally; (2) drugs that have serious synergistic side effects (e.g., diazepam and phenobarbital) should be avoided unless one is equipped to support respiration; (3) it is not unusual to have to use two or three medications to obtain both control of the status and prevention of its recurrence (see Table 9-1). Drugs listed below are given in order of preference.

a. Diazepam (Valium) 0.25 mg/kg IV. Because of its rapid effect, diazepam is the drug of choice in status. There is a synergistic effect between diazepam and other respiratory suppressants, e.g., phenobarbital. Since most children who go into status have had a previous seizure and thus may be on phenobarbital, the use of this drug is certainly contraindicated in settings with no available respiratory support. Diazepam's duration of action for controlling seizures is much shorter than that of the other agents. This drug should not be diluted because a precipitate may form, and it should be infused slowly at a rate not greater than 1 mg/min to minimize respiratory effects. After the seizures are controlled with diazepam, it is advisable to start another drug with a longer duration of action, such as phenytoin, which can be given intravenously (see below).

b. Phenobarbital, 10 mg/kg IV initially. The onset of action of this drug is 10 to 20 minutes. Phenobarbital can cause severe respiratory depression when the total dose exceeds 18 mg/kg.

c. Paraldehyde, 0.3 ml/kg rectally or 0.15 ml/kg IV, diluted 1:20 with 0.9% sodium chloride solution (in a glass syringe only). The therapeutic to toxic index for this drug is extremely low. It should never be used in anyone with pulmonary, hepatic, or renal disease.

d. Phenytoin (Dilantin), 10 mg/kg IV. Phenytoin can also be given via an NG tube to a total dose of 10 mg/kg (maximum single dose of 1 g), which will give blood levels at the end of 8 hours equal to those from a comparable IV dose. The young cerebellum is extremely sensitive to high levels of this drug. Very high doses given rapidly may cause permanent damage. Because of the effect on the cardiac conduction system (block), the drug must be given slowly, at a rate not exceeding 20 to 50 mg/min. The maximum IV dose should not exceed 1,000 mg. Phenytoin should never be given with dextrose, since a precipitate of the drug forms immediately; therefore, it should be given as a slow injection, in a catheter, with a saline infusion.

5. If the seizures are refractory to repeated use of one or several of the drugs listed above, four options are available:

a. Use a short-acting barbiturate, thiopental sodium (Pentothal), dose 2 to 4 mg/kg IV. Since this is an anesthetic agent, its use should be supervised by an anesthesiologist.

b. Use a continuous infusion of:
   1) Lidocaine, 4 mg/kg/hr (mixed in IV fluid at a concentration of 2 mg/ml.
   2) Thiopental sodium, 1 to 2 mg/kg/hr. Respiratory support (intubation and mechanical respiration) is mandatory.

c. Assess the clinical situation for untreated metabolic derangement which may have progressed or not improved by the current mode of therapy, i.e., water intoxication from antidiuretic hormone (ADH) combined with intravenous D_5W.

d. Use general anesthesia and mechanical respiratory support.

6. Patients with refractory status epilepticus

Table 9-2. Maintenance anticonvulsants to control status epilepticus

Drug	Dose	Preparation available	Time to stabilize	Therapeutic blood level	Early significant toxic effects
Phenobarbital	3-5 mg/kg bid or tid	Elixir: 20 mg/5 ml Tablet: 15, 30, 50, 60, 90, 100 mg	1-2 wk	17-40 μg/dl	Sedation Hyperactivity
Phenytoin	4-6 mg/kg bid or tid	Suspension: 30 mg/5 ml, 125 mg/5 ml Tablets: 50 mg Capsules: 30, 100 mg	1-5 wk	10-20 μg/dl	Ataxia
Carbamazepine	10-20 mg/kg bid to qid	Chewable tablet: 100 mg Tablet: 200 mg	>2 wk	4-12 μg/dl	Ataxia Sedation Bone marrow suppression
Valproic acid	10-50 mg/kg pc.	Elixir: 250 mg/5 ml Capsule: 250 mg	1-7 days	10-100 μg/dl	Hepatic damage

may require mechanical ventilation to ensure cerebral oxygenation during aggressive therapy. If the patient develops shallow respiration or a periodic respiratory pattern, an endotracheal tube should be placed as a prophylactic measure.

7. After the seizures are controlled, start maintenance anticonvulsant therapy (see Table 9-2). A single drug is preferred, although some patients may require more than one anticonvulsant. Choices for long-term anticonvulsant therapy are in order of preference.
   a. Phenobarbital, 3 to 5 mg/kg/24 hr, either intravenously or orally. This is the drug of choice for neonates with a seizure disorder or barbiturate withdrawal.
   b. Phenytoin, 4 to 6 mg/kg/24 hr. One can achieve as high a blood level in 8 hours by oral administration of 10 mg/kg (2 mg/kg/hr) as by giving 10 mg/kg as an intravenous bolus. The oral route for achieving these high blood levels is preferable since one does not subject the nervous system to potentially toxic levels of the anticonvulsant. Phenytoin is never to be given intramuscularly.
   c. Carbamazepine, 10 to 20 mg/kg/24 hr orally. This is particularly effective in children with partial complex seizures (i.e., combination of very generalized seizures with absence spells).
   d. Valproic acid, 10 to 30 mg/kg/24 hr orally. This drug achieves therapeutic blood levels within a very short period of time; however, it has been associated with a fatal hepatitis syndrome in a small percentage of patients, particularly those children who have suffered congenital insults, e.g., congenital encephalopathy.

8. Protect patient from injury to head, extremities, and tongue during the seizure. Several people may be needed to restrain patient adequately.

9. Empty the stomach with an NG tube.

10. Treat any underlying conditions.
    a. Give antibiotics for documented infections.
    b. Correct electrolyte abnormalities.
    c. Give antipyretics and use cooling measures: remember that fever increases systemic and cerebral oxygen and glucose requirements.

   d. Correct metabolic acidosis with sodium bicarbonate.

   e. Identify and treat surgical lesions.

   f. Dialyze patients in renal failure.

11. Obtain a drug history from the family, including current anticonvulsant therapy.

12. Continue mechanical ventilation until the patient is conscious, has appropriate reflexes for protection of the airway, and ventilation is adequate (see Chapter 12).

ADDITIONAL READING

Dodson, W.E., Prensky, A.L., DeVivo, D.C., and others: Management of seizure disorders: selected aspects, part I, J. Pediatr. 89:527-540, 1976.

O'Donohoe, N.V.: Epilepsies of childhood, Boston, 1979, Butterworth (Publishers), Inc.

Solomon, G., and Plum, F.: Clinical management of seizures, Philadelphia, 1976, W.B. Saunders Co.

10 Increased intracranial pressure

FRANCES C. MORRISS

JAY D. COOK

DEFINITION AND PHYSIOLOGY

Intracranial pressure (ICP) is the pressure exerted by the contents of the cranium, a rigid structure of fixed volume encompassing brain tissue, CSF, and blood. Since the intracranial contents are almost incompressible, an increase in the volume of one of the components requires a reciprocal change in the volume of one of the others or there will be a rise in ICP. Initially, increases in the intracranial volume will be compensated for so that ICP stays within a normal range (<10 to 15 mm Hg) until a critical volume is reached. At this critical volume, compensatory mechanisms fail, and even small changes in intracranial volume will cause large changes in ICP. Compensatory mechanisms for maintaining ICP within a normal range include reduction of intracranial volume of CSF which is translocated into the distensible spinal sac and reduction of cerebral blood volume by decrease in venous capacity and redistribution of blood to arteriolar vessels. In infants and young children in whom complete fusion of the cranial sutures has not occurred, expansion of the skull (manifested as increasing cranial circumference) is a major mechanism of compensation for slowly occurring increases in ICP. The goals for controlling increases in ICP are (1) to ensure adequate cerebral perfusion and hence delivery of energy substrate, oxygen, and glucose to neural tissue and (2) to prevent shifts in brain tissue from one compartment of the intracranial space to another. Cerebral perfusion pressure (CPP) equals systemic arterial mean blood pressure minus mean ICP (e.g., CPP 80 mm Hg = BP 90 mm Hg − ICP 10 mm Hg). In the undamaged brain, perfusion pressures of 40 to 50 mm Hg are sufficient to maintain normal blood flow and adequate delivery of energy substrates.

Causes of ICP are those that increase the volume of any of the intracranial compartments or any lesions that are space occupying. This is illustrated by the following equation:

$$V_{ic} \text{ (constant)} = V_{csf} + V_{brain} + V_{blood} + V_{lesion}$$

where V_{ic} = intracranial volume, V_{csf} = volume of CSF, V_{brain} = volume of brain tissue, V_{blood} = intracranial blood volume, and V_{lesion} = volume of a space-occupying lesion.

The causes of increased ICP can be outlined as follows:

1. Impaired CSF dynamics.
   a. Communicating hydrocephalus, obstruction of CSF flow outside the ventricular system (trauma, infection, congenital anomalies, subarachnoid hemorrhage).
   b. Obstruction of CSF flow within the ventricular system (congenital anomalies, infection, tumor, intraventricular hemorrhage [IVH]).
   c. Choroid plexus abnormalities.
   d. Impaired CSF absorption (pseudotumor cerebri).
2. Increase in volume of brain tissue.
   a. Generalized edema (trauma, toxins,

metabolic disturbances including hypoxia, infection, pseudotumor cerebri).
  b. Focal edema (focal trauma, edema adjacent to a space-occupying lesion).
3. Increase in cerebral blood volume.
  a. Obstruction of venous return (superior vena cava syndrome, thrombosis of major venous sinus system).
  b. Metabolic variables increasing cerebral blood flow (hypoxia, hypercarbia).
  c. Hypertension.
  d. Hypervolemia.
  e. Failure of autoregulatory responses (trauma, tumor, cerebral ischemia, severe hypertension or hypotension).
  f. Inhalation anesthetics (e.g., halothane).
4. Mass lesions (abscess, tumor, hemorrhage).

Autoregulation of blood flow is the change in the diameter of blood vessels in an organ or in tissue so that a constant flow of blood is maintained within a wide range of systemic arterial blood pressures. Thus, adequate blood flow and delivery of energy substrate to an organ or tissue are assured despite changes in perfusion pressure. One of the possible mechanisms producing autoregulation in the brain is pH changes in tissues adjacent to cerebral vessels, causing vasodilation or vasoconstriction and corresponding changes in blood flow.

Neurogenic and myogenic control systems have been described also. In addition to local tissue metabolic changes, several systemic variables can influence cerebral vasomotor tone and the magnitude of cerebral blood flow (Table 10-1). The cerebral vessels are exquisitely sensitive to the partial pressure of carbon dioxide (Pa_{CO_2}). Hypercarbia (and acidosis) causes dilation of the cerebral vascular bed and increased cerebral blood flow. Hypocarbia (and alkalosis) produces the opposite situation (decreased cerebral blood flow). At a Pa_{CO_2} of 20 to 60 mm Hg, cerebral blood flow is almost linearly related to Pa_{CO_2}; at a Pa_{CO_2} less than 20 mm Hg, reduction of flow secondary to vasoconstriction is so great that local tissue ischemia occurs. This produces secondary vasodilation, and blood flow then increases. A second variable that affects cerebral vasomotor tone is the partial pressure of oxygen in arterial blood (Pa_{O_2}). Hypoxia (Pa_{O_2} less than 50 mm Hg) increases cerebral blood flow. At a low Pa_{CO_2} (<20 mm Hg), a lower Pa_{O_2} (35 mm Hg) can be tolerated before cerebral blood flow increases. Under normal conditions (i.e., intact autoregulatory mechanisms), systemic arterial blood pressure is not a determinant of cerebral blood flow until significant hypotension or hypertension occurs.

Table 10-1. Autoregulation of cerebral blood flow

Factors affecting cerebral blood flow	Autoregulation intact		Damaged autoregulation	
	Cerebral blood volume	Cerebral perfusion	Cerebral blood volume	Cerebral perfusion
↑Local tissue pH	↓	Adequate		
↓Local tissue pH	↑	Adequate		
↑Pa_{CO_2}	↑	Adequate	↑	Inadequate
↓Pa_{CO_2}	↓	Adequate	↓	Inadequate
↓Pa_{O_2}	↑	Adequate		Inadequate
↑P_{Sa}	Normal	Adequate	↑	Inadequate
↓P_{Sa}	Normal	Adequate	↓	Inadequate
↑ICP	↓	Adequate initially, inadequate late	Variable	Compromised

P_{Sa}, Systemic arterial blood pressure.

Changes in vessel diameter that occur with changes in blood flow account for significant changes in intracranial blood volume, which can contribute to the compensatory process. With impaired autoregulation, cerebral blood flow may vary passively with CPP. Under these circumstances, both systemic arterial blood pressure and ICP can alter cerebral blood flow. The contribution of normal mechanisms for regulating cerebral blood flow (pH, Pa_{CO_2}, and local metabolic changes) to actual volume of blood in a damaged brain is unpredictable. Thus, normal control of cerebral blood flow allows some compensatory volume changes to occur in the presence of increased ICP. With cerebral vascular damage such as may occur with CNS infection, trauma, or space-occupying lesions, changes in cerebral blood flow caused by changes in blood pressure may be detrimental. Increases in cerebral blood flow may augment increased ICP and decreases may produce local tissue hypoxia at levels of systemic arterial blood pressure that would otherwise be considered safe.

Because the absence of papilledema does not exclude the diagnosis of increased ICP, direct measurement of ICP is necessary for diagnosis and rational therapeutic planning. When ICP differences occur across rigid structures such as the foramen magnum or the tentorium, shifts and distortions of the brain referred to as herniation syndromes may occur. Signs and symptoms of herniation usually relate to brainstem and hemispheric compression, which can be fatal if untreated.

MONITORING

See also Chapter 4.

Central nervous system

1. Perform neurologic examination, including state of consciousness, pattern of respiration, cardiac status, ocular reflexes, oculocephalic-oculovestibular responses, funduscopic examination, and motor responses to noxious stimuli. These should be repeated by the same observer on a daily or twice-daily basis.

Nursing personnel should evaluate ocular reflexes and state of consciousness every hour.
2. Record frequency and type of seizure activity.
3. Measure ICP continuously by subarachnoid bolt or intraventricular catheter. These devices are placed by a neurosurgeon in the PICU using local anesthesia (see Chapter 92). The pressure transducer should be placed at the level of the midcranium. CPP can be rapidly calculated as the difference between systemic arterial mean blood pressure and ICP.
4. Additional diagnostic evaluations may include:
   a. EEG.
   b. Computerized tomography.
   c. Arteriography.
5. Measure systemic arterial mean blood pressure continuously. An intra-arterial catheter facilitates the continuous measurement of blood pressure, which is mandatory if changes in CPP are to be diagnosed and treated rapidly.

Cardiovascular system

If volume restriction is necessary, a central venous or pulmonary arterial catheter should be placed to allow measurement of filling pressures and/or cardiac output.

Respiratory system

1. Check arterial blood-gas tensions and pH every 1 to 4 hours.
2. Jugular venous Po_2 may be helpful.

MANAGEMENT

The management of increased ICP should be directed toward reduction of the volume of the intracranial compartments, preservation of cerebral metabolic function, and avoidance of situations that increase ICP.

Intracranial pressure should be kept within the normal range, or at least less than 20 mm Hg. Treat the following situations:

1. ICP 16 to 20 mm Hg lasting more than 30 minutes. After 30 minutes, changes in CSF volume cannot buffer ICP changes.
2. ICP greater than 20 mm Hg for longer than 3 minutes.
3. Any increase in ICP associated with a decrease in heart rate or with pupillary dilation.
4. Remember that increases in ICP associated with painful stimulus but sustained after that stimulus is withdrawn indicate that intracranial compliance is low.

Reduction of CSF volume

If an intraventricular catheter is present, fluid should be withdrawn when ICP exceeds 50 mm Hg. The volume withdrawn should be enough to bring pressure to 20 to 30 mm Hg. With a small or slitlike ventricular system, CSF withdrawal may be impossible and other measures of control must be employed.

Reduction of cerebral mass

Cerebral mass may be reduced by the use of:
1. Euvolemic fluid restriction. 50% to 60% of daily fluid requirements. Adjust daily fluids to maintain low-normal CVP (8-10 mm Hg), urine output of 0.5-1 ml/kg/hr, normal serum electrolytes, serum osmolality of 300-310 mOsm, and normal (for age) blood pressure and cardiac output. When necessary, blood volume should be expanded with packed red blood cells (RBCs) if Hct is less than 30% or with a colloid solution (Plasmanate, 5% albumin, or fresh frozen plasma [FFP]). Note that the free fatty acid content of FFP may be associated with increases in ICP.
2. Osmotic therapy
   a. Mannitol, 0.5 to 1 g/kg IV over 30 minutes every 4 to 6 hours or when ICP is greater than 20 mm Hg for more than 3 minutes.
   b. Glycerol, 1 g/kg IV over 30 minutes every 2 hours (concentration, 1 g/dl IV fluid).

3. Potent tubular diuretics may effectively decrease ICP by decreasing total body water, venous tone, and CSF production. Give furosemide 1 mg/kg IV.
4. Steroids, which reduce cerebral edema and restore membrane integrity in the presence of space-occupying lesions or surgically induced trauma. Give dexamethasone 1 mg/kg/24 hr IV in 4 doses. Dosage may be tapered when ICP is controlled. Steroids are not thought to be helpful in reducing edema caused by hypoxia or other metabolic insults.

Reduction of cerebral blood volume (induced hypocarbia)

1. Careful nasal intubation with a muscle relaxant and a short-acting barbiturate (thiopental sodium) and institution of mechanical ventilation may be used. In the presence of decreased cerebral compliance, the hypertension associated with intubation can be very hazardous; therefore, it is imperative that the patient be anesthetized and hypocarbic when intubation is done.
2. Maintain Pa_{CO_2} between 20 and 25 mm Hg (at Pa_{CO_2} less than 20 mm Hg, cerebral perfusion may be reduced by as much as 60% and can result in local tissue hypoxia). Change the rate on the ventilator rather than the tidal volume to obtain optimal Pa_{CO_2} (see below).
3. To facilitate ventilatory control, institute muscle paralysis with d-tubocurarine, 0.5 to 0.7 mg/kg IV initially and 0.1 to 0.25 mg/kg as needed (usually every hour or by constant infusion) when patient movement is noted. Pancuronium (0.1 mg/kg) may also be used. The d-tubocurarine releases histamine, a local vasodilator, and pancuronium causes a centrally mediated tachycardia, which may raise blood pressure; either agent may therefore increase ICP. The first signs of inadequate paralysis may be isolated tachycardia or a jerking movement of the diaphragm; these signs are often accompanied by an increase in ICP.

4. With acute increases in ICP, hyperventilate the patient manually until ICP decreases to 20 mm Hg. If hyperventilation is being used frequently to control ICP, another form of therapy should be used, since constant or nearly constant hyperventilation will decrease Pa_{CO_2} to less than 20 mm Hg and cause cerebral hypoxia (as measured by jugular venous PO_2) secondary to inadequate perfusion.

5. Use of muscle relaxants will interfere with evaluation of many of the neurologic variables that need to be followed. *d*-Tubocurarine (or pancuronium) can be discontinued 4 hours before the scheduled time of the neurologic examination. Reversal of muscle relaxants with anticholinesterases (pyridostigmine, neostigmine) is probably not desirable because of the rapidity of the process and the possibility of detrimental side effects, including bradycardia, increased secretions, and coughing.

Assurance of cerebral venous return

1. Keep patient in a 30° head-up neutral position. Placing the head in either lateral position may obstruct jugular drainage and increase ICP.

2. For pressure ventilators, the inflating pressure should be as low as possible to maintain adequate ventilation (approximately 20 cm H_2O if there is no pulmonary disease). If volume ventilator is used, select the lowest tidal volume (TV) that will inflate the lungs adequately.

3. Use minimal positive end expiratory pressure (PEEP) (2 cm H_2O), since increased intrathoracic mean pressure may impede cerebral venous return and may contribute to an increase in ICP. Remember that the complete absence of end pressure is nonphysiologic.

Preservation of cerebral metabolic function

1. Maintain oxygenation at a Pa_{O_2} of 90 to 110 mm Hg. Hyperoxia following a hypoxic cerebral insult may increase the extent of the damage.

2. Maintain systemic arterial mean blood pressure at a level 50 mm Hg greater than ICP. Periodic blood volume expansion may be necessary.

3. Give a glucose-containing solution to maintain the serum glucose level normal for age (glucose 100 to 150 mg/dl; Dextrostix 90-130 mg/dl; see Chapter 16). Hyperglycemia may be harmful in the same way that hyperoxia is.

4. Maintain serum phosphate between 4.2 and 6.7 mg/dl through the use of K phosphate.

5. Give a short-acting barbiturate (sodium thiopental), 1 mg/kg IV, before stressful procedures (see #2 in next section). Measure thiopental levels daily. High levels may occur with this regimen.

6. As elevated ICP returns to normal, the patient may become conscious. Consciousness coupled with paralysis can be stressful. The primary signs of this state are tachycardia and hypertension when parents visit or the child is approached by nursing personnel. The hypertension may be harmful (i.e., increases ICP) and should be avoided.
   a. Talk to the patient and explain procedures.
   b. Cassette tapes of parents reading favorite stories or a radio with an earplug may be soothing.
   c. Consider sedation with diazepam (Valium), 0.1 mg/kg IV every 2 to 4 hours or by constant infusion. If blood volume is fairly stable, morphine 0.1 mg/kg/hr by constant infusion may be used.

7. Vigorously treat any fever (temperature higher than 38.6° C or 100.5° F) with antipyretics and a cooling blanket (see Chapter 18). Avoid production of shivering. Although it will stop shivering, thorazine is a potent peripheral vasodilator and is often associated with profound decreases in systemic arterial blood pressure in the volume-constricted patient.

8. Vigorously treat any seizure activity either

by normalizing abnormal metabolic variables or by using appropriate anticonvulsants (see Chapter 9).

9. The techniques of constant barbiturate infusion and production of moderate hypothermia to protect the brain by decreasing cerebral metabolic processes have been used but will not be detailed here since they are not yet firmly established therapeutic procedures.

Avoidance of situations that increase ICP

1. Chest physiotherapy is poorly tolerated and contraindicated unless pulmonary problems (infiltrate, atelectasis) are present. Gentle vibration should be tried first if treatment is necessary.
2. Suctioning acutely increases ICP by increasing systemic arterial blood pressure, it should be preceded by manual hyperventilation and the use of an agent that will decrease ICP or prevent the adrenergic airway response.
   a. Thiopental sodium, 1 mg/kg IV. Cerebral uptake and redistribution occurs 1 to 5 minutes after IV dose, so control does not occur immediately.
   b. If the serum thiopental level is high or barbiturates are unsuitable, use lidocaine, 1 mg/kg IV.
3. Institute muscle paralysis with d-tubocurarine (or pancuronium) to prevent Valsalva maneuvers and coughing.
4. Avoid rapid changes in head position.

Withdrawal of support

When ICP has been maintained at 15 to 20 mm Hg for at least 24 hours, discontinue therapeutic measures sequentially. After each step, allow a 6- to 12-hour period to observe any changes in ICP before withdrawing the next form of support.

1. Sequentially decrease ventilation to allow Pa_{CO_2} to increase by 5 mm Hg every 4 to 8 hours.

2. Discontinue muscle relaxant.
3. Decrease frequency of mannitol infusions.
4. Taper steroid dose by 50% daily.
5. Discontinue mechanical ventilation.
6. Remove ICP measuring devices when most forms of therapy have been discontinued.
7. Discontinue sedation.
8. Discontinue supplemental glucose and oxygen.
9. This sequence of events should begin after specific therapy for the underlying cause of increased ICP has been completed (e.g., correction of metabolic defect, institution of antibiotic therapy, surgical intervention).
10. If the patient seems to be recovering inappropriately or more slowly than anticipated consider:
    a. Thiopental overdose (measure level).
    b. Anticonvulsant overdose (measure levels).
    c. CSF infection from indwelling ICP catheter.
    d. Undiagnosed cerebral event (hemorrhage, effusion, seizures, etc.).
    e. Premature withdrawal of ICP control.

General supportive measures

1. Respiratory system
   a. Suction every 2 to 4 hours (see Chapter 100 for technique and avoidance of situations that increase ICP).
   b. Turn patient side to back to side every 2 hours (especially important since vigorous physiotherapy is contraindicated).
   c. Consider transfusion when hemoglobin (Hb) is less than 10 g/dl, to maintain adequate oxygen-carrying capacity.
   d. Ensure endotracheal tube stability by routine retaping.
2. Chronic use of muscle relaxants may cause varying degrees of bladder dysfunction, so a bladder catheter should be used.
3. Gastrointestinal system
   a. Institute antacid regimen as prophylaxis for gastrointestinal hemorrhage (Maalox, Milk of Magnesia, etc., 15 to 30 ml per

NG tube when gastric pH is less than 2.5). Be aware that concretions, diarrhea, hypermagnesemia, and phosphate binding may occur with chronic use of antacids.

b. Prevent constipation and fecal impaction, particularly if muscle relaxants are used.
   (1) Give dioctyl sodium sulfosuccinate (Colace), 5 mg/kg/day per NG tube in 3 doses.
   (2) Give a glycerine suppository for constipation.
   (3) Give a gentle mineral oil enema if there is no stool within 24 hours of the above measures.

4. Perform passive exercise of joints every day for a comatose or paralyzed patient. Place joints in physiologic positions; when muscle relaxants are used, joint dislocation is made more likely. Consider the use of footboards and splints to prevent contractures.

5. Skin care.
   a. Change all dressings regularly.
   b. Inspect IV and ICP monitor sites every day.
   c. Inspect pressure points regularly; use sheepskin and heel pads. Cutaneous pressure damage is more likely in patients with severe volume restriction.

6. Mouth care.
   a. Remove excess mucus and intraoral material with lemon glycerine swabs twice every day.
   b. Intraoral lesions may be gently debrided with lemon glycerine swabs, and healing will occur without further treatment.
   c. If grinding of the teeth is a problem, insert a mouth guard.
   d. If the patient is febrile, moisten the lips and intraoral tissue with a wet sponge.

7. Eye care
   a. Inspect the eyes daily for conjunctivitis and corneal scarring.
   b. Instill methylcellulose eye drops every hour to prevent corneal drying.
   c. If patient is paralyzed, the eyelids may not close, and taping may be necessary in addition to eye drops.

8. Consult the medical, surgical, or social services for specific therapy for underlying or ongoing problems.

ADDITIONAL READING

Bell, W., and McCormick, W.: Increased intracranial pressure in children, Major Probl. Clin. Pediatr. 3:49-115, 1972.

Bradford, R.F., Persing, J.A., Pobareskin, L., and others: Lidocaine or thiopental for rapid control of intracranial hypertension? Anesth. Analg. (Cleve.) 59:435-437, 1980.

Bruce, D.A., Berman, W.A., and Schut, L.: Cerebrospinal fluid pressure monitoring in children: physiology, pathology and clinical usefulness, Adv. Pediatr. 24:233-290, 1970.

Marshall, L.F.: Treatment of brain swelling and brain edema in man, Adv. Neurol. 28:459-469, 1980.

Marshall, L.F., Shapiro, H.M., Rauscher, A., and others: Pentobarbital therapy for intracranial hypertension in metabolic coma, Crit. Care Med. 6:1-5, 1978.

McGraw, C.P.: Continuous intracranial pressure monitoring: review of techniques and presentation of method, Surg. Neurol. 6:149-155, 1976.

Mickell, J.J., Reigel, D.H., Cook, D.R., and others: Intracranial pressure: monitoring and normalization therapy in children, Pediatrics 59:606-615, 1977.

Miller, J.D., and Leech, P.: Effects of mannitol and steroid therapy on intracranial volume-pressure relationships in patients, J. Neurosurg. 42:274-281, 1975.

Nilsson, B., Norber, K., and Siesjo, B.K.: Biochemical events in cerebral ischaemia, Br. J. Anaesth. 47:751-760, 1975.

Raphaely, R.C., Swedlow, D.B., Downes, J.J., and others: Management of severe pediatric head trauma, Pediatr. Clin. N. Am. 27:715-727, 1980.

Risberg, J., Lundberg, N., and Inguar, D.H.: Regional cerebral blood volume during acute transient rises of the intracranial pressure (plateau waves), J. Neurosurg. 31:303-310, 1969.

Shapiro, H.M., Wyte, S.R., and Loeser, J.: Barbiturate-augmented hypothermia for reduction of persistent intracranial hypertension, J. Neurosurg. 40:90-100, 1974.

Shaywitz, B.A., Leventhal, J.M., Kramer, M.S., and others: Prolonged continuous monitoring of intracranial pressure in Reye's syndrome, Pediatrics 59:595-605, 1977.

Smith, A., and Wollman, H.: Cerebral blood flow and metabolism: effects of anesthetic drugs and techniques, Anesthesiology 36:378-400, 1972.

11 Airway obstruction

FRANCES C. MORRISS

DEFINITION AND PHYSIOLOGY

The airway conducts inspired air to the terminal respiratory units, the alveoli, where gas exchange takes place. The airway components are the nasopharynx, oropharynx, ancillary structures (eustachian tubes, orifices of the sinus system), larynx, trachea, bronchi, and bronchioles.

In addition to conducting air to and from the lungs, the airway warms and humidifies air, filters particulate matter from incoming gas, and prevents entry into the lungs of noxious substances such as fluids, foreign bodies, and irritating inhalants. This last function depends on intact neural reflexes. When vagal receptors situated around the larynx are stimulated, reflex closure of the cords and covering of the glottic orifice by the epiglottis isolate the lower airway from the oropharynx.

Obstruction of the airway occurs in two forms, acute and chronic. Acute total obstruction of the airway, particularly the larynx or the trachea, represents an urgent situation. Hypoxemia, hypercapnia, bradycardia, and cardiac arrest ensue promptly. Chronic obstruction, which tends to be partial and of varying degrees of severity, may lead to carbon dioxide retention, hypoxemia, or cor pulmonale. Varying degrees of cerebral damage and dysfunction can result from prolonged intermittent obstruction. Factors that predispose a person to develop airway obstruction include:

1. Abnormal facial and palatal anatomy.
2. Macroglossia.
3. Malocclusion.
4. Age. In a young child, airway diameter relative to the child's size is small, and the airway is more susceptible to occlusion by edema, particulate matter, or viscid secretions.
5. History of previous airway instrumentation, especially prolonged intubation or previous tracheotomy.
6. Persistent voice abnormality or progressive hoarseness.
7. History of severe allergic reactions.
8. Presence of an artificial airway.
9. Dehydration with development of tenacious secretions.
10. Swallowing abnormalities.
11. An extrinsic mass, such as subcutaneous emphysema of the neck, goiter, hypertrophied lymph tissue (e.g., tonsils, hilar nodes), or tumor.
12. Surgical manipulation of the airway (e.g., polypectomy, palatoplasty, bronchoscopy).
13. Any inflammatory process affecting the respiratory epithelium (e.g., laryngotracheobronchitis).
14. Head and neck trauma.
15. Ingestion or inhalation of toxic substances (e.g., caustic substances, smoke, steam).

Acute airway obstruction produces signs and symptoms of respiratory distress as well as those of cardiovascular compromise. Tachypnea, use of accessory muscles of respiration with suprasternal retractions, and inability to tolerate a horizontal position are usually present. With the advent of hypoxia, one may see restlessness, anxiety (air hunger), and cyanosis, which is a late finding. Breath sounds may be difficult to hear. With continued respiratory compromise, the patient becomes tachycardic and pale, and capillary filling is prolonged. Finally, bradycardia and cardiopulmonary arrest occur. Certain findings relate to the specific portion of the airway affected and may aid in identifying the site of obstruction. Nasopharyngeal obstruction causes persistent mouth breathing, nasal discharge, and snoring, and direct examination may reveal nasal septal deviation, stenosis, a foreign body, or a mass. Drooling and inability to swallow characterize lesions of the oropharynx, often identified by a decreased air shadow on a lateral neck roentgenogram. Clinical correlates of laryngeal compromise are inspiratory stridor, hoarseness, and aphonia. Subglottic stenosis is also characterized by inspiratory stridor as well as expiratory stridor if the lesion is fixed. Lower respiratory tract abnormalities may be characterized by prolonged expiration and unequal or abnormal breath sounds (e.g., rales, wheezes). Comparison of inspiratory and expiratory roentgenograms may show persistent overexpansion of one segment of the lung caused by a ball-valve type of lesion in a bronchus. Inhaled particulate matter or masses may be discovered by bronchoscopy. Maximum expiratory flow volume curves may be helpful in localizing the obstruction.

MONITORING

See also Chapter 4.

When signs of airway obstruction are present or the patient is in a high-risk group, institute the following procedures:

1. Close observation by personnel experienced in dealing with airway problems is mandatory.
2. Check heart rate and respiratory rate continuously, and auscultate the chest every hour.
3. Bring anxiety, retractions, and cyanosis to the attention of the primary physician.
4. Obtain arterial blood-gas tensions and pH initially and every 4 hours.
5. Obtain initial chest roentgenogram and repeat if indicated. Severe upper respiratory

tract obstruction may be complicated by sudden onset of fulminant pulmonary edema.
6. Check serum Ca. Laryngospasm can be associated with hypocalcemia.

MANAGEMENT
General measures

1. Have emergency resuscitation equipment available: oxygen, bag and mask, intubation equipment, and suction apparatus.
2. Remove oral, nasal, and pharyngeal secretions as needed.
3. Consider use of racemic epinephrine by aerosol for laryngotracheobronchitis, for postintubation edema, or in patients with prominent wheezing (see Chapter 29). The frequency of administration will depend on the length of time the patient remains symptom-free after a treatment. If symptoms reappear in less than 1 hour after treatment, repeat the inhaled sympathomimetic hourly if necessary.
4. Airway support of various types may be needed depending on the site of the obstruction.
   a. Nasopharyngeal airway. This is particularly helpful to bypass tonsillar hypertrophy or palatal edema secondary to surgery.
   b. Oral airway.
   c. Dental prostheses are useful to displace the tongue.
   d. Endotracheal tube. The endotracheal tube should be placed by someone experienced with intubation. If time permits before intubation, an IV should be started and the stomach emptied. A surgeon should be immediately available since it may not be possible to insert the endotracheal tube and a tracheotomy may be needed. Once an artificial airway has been placed, 24-hour nursing at the bedside is mandatory to ensure patency of the tube (see Chapter 95).
   e. Tracheotomy. This may be necessary for

long-term airway management or when the size of a previously placed endotracheal tube is grossly inadequate (see Chapter 104).

5. Consider the following ancillary measures:
   a. Since fever increases oxygen consumption and the work of breathing, administer antipyretics for a temperature greater than 38° C.
   b. Transfuse the patient with packed RBCs to increase oxygen-carrying capacity if hemoglobin is less than 10 g/dl.
   c. Discontinue cough suppressants, sedatives, and antihistamines.
   d. Hydrate the patient to liquefy pulmonary secretions. The volume necessary is generally 1.5 to 2 times greater than maintenance requirements.

Specific measures

1. Give antibiotics for infection.
2. Treat severe allergic reaction with epinephrine, diphenhydramine hydrochloride (Benadryl), and steroids.
3. Perform chest physiotherapy for clearance of tenacious secretions.
4. Surgical intervention may be necessary (e.g., incision and drainage of abscess, polypectomy, evacuation of hematoma, excision of mass lesion).
5. Correct underlying cardiovascular compromise.
6. Consider bronchoscopy.

Inhalation of a foreign body

One type of acute airway obstruction that warrants more detailed discussion is inhalation of a foreign body. Croup, epiglottitis, and postintubation sequelae are discussed in separate chapters.

Acute obstruction secondary to foreign body inhalation may occur while the patient is eating and is preceded by sudden coughing or a choking spell. An infant will often have been observed playing with small objects such as coins

prior to choking. If the obstruction is partial and the patient can exchange air, his own attempts at expelling the foreign body should be encouraged. If respiration becomes labored and distress suggesting complete obstruction intervenes (stridor, ineffective cough, wheezing, retractions, cyanosis), one of several maneuvers may be attempted.

1. Back blows and chest thrusts are most appropriate for infants; abdominal thrusts are no longer recommended.
   a. Place infant face down astraddle rescuer's arm with the head lower than the trunk. Support the head by placing a hand around victim's chest and jaw. Rescuer should rest the forearm on the thigh for further support (Fig. 11-1).
   b. Deliver 4 blows in rapid succession with the heel of the free hand between the infant's shoulder blades.
   c. Place the free hand on the infant's back so that the infant is sandwiched between rescuer's hands, one hand supporting the back and the other supporting the head and neck. Turn infant over and place him on rescuer's thigh, with the head lower than the trunk.
   d. Deliver 4 chest thrusts in rapid succession in the same manner as the external chest compressions for CPR.
2. A similar maneuver is performed on children (i.e., more than 2 years of age).
   a. Kneel on floor and drape victim face down across thighs, with the head lower than the trunk.
   b. Deliver 4 back blows in rapid succession between the shoulder blades, using somewhat greater force than is used for an infant.
   c. Support head and back and roll victim over onto floor.
   d. Deliver 4 chest thrusts.
3. Attempts to dislodge the object with blind probing of the airway are to be avoided since the foreign body may be pushed farther into

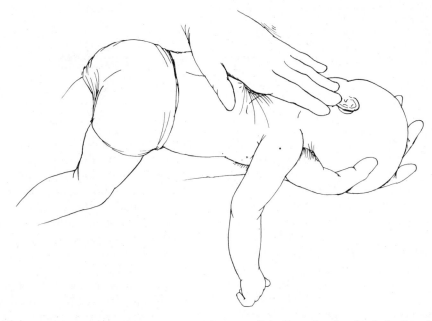

Fig. 11-1. Correct hand position for back blows to dislodge a foreign body in the airway.

the airway. The victim may expell the foreign body by coughing. If the child is unconscious, lift the tongue and lower jaw forward to open the mouth. Place the thumb in victim's mouth, over the tongue, while the other fingers are wrapped around victim's jaw. If the foreign body is seen when the mouth is opened, remove it with fingers.

4. Institute emergency breathing if patient is apneic. Repeat the preceding sequence of back blows and chest thrusts if the airway is still obstructed.

When anoxia and muscle relaxation occur, artificial ventilation may be effective because complete obstruction is converted to partial obstruction. The patient should be seen as soon as possible by an endoscopist, who can examine the airway under direct visualization and complete the removal of the foreign matter.

ADDITIONAL READING

Blanc, V.F., and Tremblay, N.A.G.: The complications of tracheal intubation: a new classification with review of the literature, Anesth. Analg. (Cleve.) **53**:202-213, 1974.

Bland, J.W., Edwards, F.K., and Brunsfield, D.: Pulmonary hypertension and congestive heart failure in children with chronic upper airway obstruction, Am. J. Cardiol. **23**:830-837, 1969.

Eavery, R.D., Casagrande, A., Blasberg, B., and others: Relief of chronic upper airway obstruction using a dental prosthesis: a nonsurgical approach, Pediatrics **59**:288-292, 1977.

Fink, B.R.: The etiology and treatment of laryngospasm, Anesthesiology **17**:569-577, 1956.

Heimlich, H.J.: A life-saving maneuver to prevent food choking, J.A.M.A. **234**:398-401, 1975.

Jordan, W.S., Graves, C.L., and Elwyn, R.A.: New therapy for postintubation laryngeal edema and tracheitis in children, J.A.M.A. **212**:585-588, 1970.

Law, D., and Kosloske, A.M.: Management of tracheobronchial foreign bodies in children: a re-evaluation of postural drainage and bronchoscopy, Pediatrics **58**:362-367, 1976.

National Conference on Cardiopulmonary Resuscitation and Emergency Cardiac Care, J.A.M.A. **244**:453-509, 1980.

Wilson, R.D., Putnam, L., and Phillips, M.T.: Anesthetic problems in surgery for varying levels of respiratory obstruction in infants and children, Anesth. Analg. (Cleve.) **53**:878-885, 1974.

12 Acute respiratory failure

GERALD C. MOORE

DEFINITION AND PHYSIOLOGY

Respiratory failure is defined as arterial blood-gas tension abnormalities that reflect severe respiratory dysfunction resulting in hypoxemia and hypercapnia, which significantly impair vital organ function. The patient with a Pa_{O_2} of less than 50 mm Hg and a Pa_{CO_2} of greater than 50 mm Hg (room air, sea level) is in respiratory failure. Clinical correlates include a decrease or absence of breath sounds, severe retractions and use of accessory muscles during inspiration, and a decreased level of consciousness.

Hypoxemia is defined as a blood oxygen level that is less than normal. This level may or may not be adequate to meet the body tissue needs. Hypoxia occurs when the tissue needs for oxygen are not met and may be seen at low or even at normal blood oxygen levels when severe anemia or congestive heart failure compromises oxygen transport. The level of circulating oxygen, as measured either by arterial blood-gas tension or by hemoglobin-oxygen saturation, varies depending on the clinical situation; however, a Pa_{O_2} of approximately 50 mm Hg is dangerously low. The components of the oxygen transport system are ventilation, diffusion, transport of oxygen in the blood, and circulation of blood to the tissues.

When 1 g of hemoglobin is fully saturated with oxygen, it will contain 1.39 ml of oxygen (e.g., 15 g/dl contains 20.9 ml of oxygen). In addition, 0.3 ml of oxygen will be dissolved in 100 ml of circulating plasma per 100 mm Hg oxygen tension (37° C). The total amount of hemoglobin is regulated by a renal sensing mechanism that seeks to maintain a balance between oxygen supply and requirement. This mechanism is mediated by erythropoietin, which increases during hypoxemia and, in turn, can cause a doubling of the daily red cell production (limited by the available iron). Assuming normal body temperature and pH, the oxygen-hemoglobin dissociation curve is unique in that oxygen association is little affected by large changes in Pa_{O_2} at the upper portion of the curve, i.e., oxygen tensions of 70 to 100 mm Hg (Fig. 12-1). In the steep portion of the curve, with oxygen tensions of approximately 10 to 40 mm Hg, the release of oxygen from the hemoglobin molecule to the tissues is facilitated with relatively small changes in Pa_{O_2}. The P_{50} value defines the Pa_{O_2} at which 50% of the hemoglobin is saturated at standard conditions of temperature and pH. Thus, a high P_{50} (e.g., 36 mm Hg; normal is 26 mm Hg) means a low hemoglobin affinity for oxygen. Increased hydrogen ion concentration, Pa_{CO_2}, temperature, and 2,3-diphosphoglycerate (2,3-DPG), which stabilizes the deoxygenated form of the hemoglobin molecule, favor oxygen release and increase the P_{50}.

When the oxygen supply is limited or oxygen consumption is increased, blood flow decreases in those tissues where low oxygen extraction occurs in favor of tissues that extract large amounts of oxygen. High-flow, low-extraction tissues constitute sources of oxygen reserve, and eliminating such tissues from the effective circulation may compensate for as much as a one-third decrease in cardiac output or a one-half increase in oxygen requirements. Coronary blood flow closely parallels changes in cardiac work, as does blood flow to exercising

58

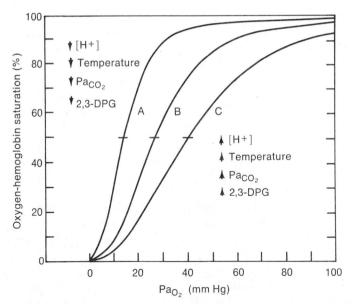

Fig. 12-1. Oxygen-hemoglobin dissociation curve. *B,* Normal. Abnormalities that result in an increased, *A,* or a decreased, *C,* affinity of the hemoglobin molecule for oxygen are shown beside the outer curves. The P_{50} value for each curve is represented by a horizontal dash at the 50% saturation level.

muscles. Blood flow to the brain remains fairly constant with increasing demands, such as those required by exercise. Tissues with high-flow, low-oxygen extraction, where a marked decrease in blood flow is seen with increased oxygen requirements, include the skin, kidneys, and gastrointestinal tract. When tissue oxygen needs are not being met, the body has several mechanisms to increase systemic oxygen transport. These include:

1. Increased pulmonary gas exchange.
2. Increased pulmonary blood flow.
3. Improved matching of ventilation and pulmonary perfusion.
4. Increased hemoglobin affinity for oxygen.
5. Increased hemoglobin concentration.
6. Greater dissociation of oxygen from hemoglobin at the tissue level.
7. Increased cardiac output and tissue perfusion.

If oxygen inflow to the lungs is blocked for 2 to 4 minutes, the preexisting oxygen supply fails to maintain an adequate tissue oxygen tension. This occurs within 10 to 15 seconds if arterial blood supply to the nonpulmonary tissues is also occluded. When oxygen transport to the tissues is insufficient, cellular metabolism becomes anaerobic and glucose degradation stops at the stage of lactic acid formation, ultimately resulting in cell death secondary to metabolic acidosis. CNS cells are particularly susceptible to hypoxia.

Carbon dioxide (CO_2), the end product of the chemical reactions of aerobic cellular metabolism, is carried by the blood in a manner similar to oxygen. After diffusing into the blood plasma, most of the carbon dioxide enters the RBCs and undergoes chemical transformation to carbonic acid ($CO_2 + H_2O \rightleftharpoons H_2CO_3 \rightleftharpoons H^+ + HCO_3^-$). This reaction is catalyzed by the enzyme carbonic anhydrase, which is present in high concentrations in RBCs. Ultimately, hydrogen (H^+) and bicarbonate (HCO_3^-) ions are formed. HCO_3^- freely diffuses from the RBCs into the plasma, setting up an electrostatic difference across the cell membrane that is neutralized by the movement of chloride ions from the plasma into the RBCs (the chloride shift). Some of the hydrogen ions liberated in the RBCs as a result of hypoxia are bound to and reduce the hemoglobin molecule. The presence of reduced hemoglobin promotes the loading of carbon dioxide, whereas the oxygenation that occurs in the pulmonary capillary promotes unloading. This is known as the Haldane effect. A rise in Pa_{CO_2} causes a shift of the oxygen-hemoglobin dissociation curve to the right, facilitating the release of oxygen to tissue. This is known as the Bohr effect.

Another mechanism through which carbon dioxide influences the patient is by stimulating the respiratory centers to increase ventilation, resulting in carbon dioxide excretion with increased oxygen consumption.

Most of the autonomic effects associated with high Pa_{CO_2} (e.g., increased pulmonary vascular resistance, bronchoconstriction, increased cardiac output, and increased ventilation) are secondary to the pH change caused by the hypercapnia.

The conditions that most commonly cause respiratory failure in pediatric patients differ with age. The most common causes of respiratory failure are:

1. Newborn infant
   a. Prematurity and clinical hyaline membrane disease
   b. Asphyxia
   c. Inhalation pneumonia
2. Less than 2 years of age
   a. Bronchopneumonia
   b. Status asthmaticus
   c. Croup
   d. Congenital heart disease
   e. Foreign body inhalation
   f. Congenital abnormalities of the airways (e.g., tracheal webs, cysts, lobar emphysema)
   g. Nasopharyngeal obstruction with large tonsils or adenoids

3. More than 2 years of age
   a. Status asthmaticus
   b. Cystic fibrosis
   c. Peripheral polyneuritis
   d. Poisoning
   e. Near-drowning
   f. Encephalitis
   g. Trauma

Abnormalities in arterial blood-gas tensions sufficient to meet the criteria of respiratory failure result in significant vital organ impairment as follows:

1. Cardiovascular system
   a. Cardiac output increases with moderate hypoxemia and hypercapnia; it decreases with severe hypoxemia.
   b. Heart rate increases with moderate hypoxemia and hypercapnia.
   c. Dysrhythmias occur with moderate hypoxemia.
   d. Pulmonary vascular resistance increases with hypoxemia and hypercapnia.
2. Respiratory system
   a. Minute ventilation increases with intact peripheral and central chemoreceptor function.
   b. Use of accessory muscles occurs in progressive airway obstruction.
3. CNS dysfunction
   a. Headache.
   b. Mental confusion.
   c. Somnolence.
   d. Irritability and anxiety.
4. Kidneys
   a. Respiratory failure results in decreased sodium and water excretion.
   b. Chronic bicarbonate resorption occurs with hypercapnia.
5. Hematopoietic system
   a. There is an increase in RBC mass.
   b. The oxygen-hemoglobin dissociation curve is shifted to the right with hypercapnia (P_{50} increases).
6. Anaerobic metabolism increases lactic acid production.

An equivalent of the adult respiratory distress syndrome (ARDS) occurs in children when a set of physiologic aberrations combine to cause impairment of gas exchange, decreases in lung compliance, and physical and radiographic evidence of diffuse pulmonary infiltrates. This condition is similar and in some cases identical to clinical hyaline membrane disease (see Chapter 34), seen in the newborn period. Indeed, the principles of therapy for clinical hyaline membrane disease have been adapted from accounts of the adult entity. A greater than 50% mortality rate underscores the need for early recognition and therapy. Common precipitating events in children include profound asphyxia, shock, sepsis, postoperative complications of cardiac surgery, and chemical injury to the lung. These triggering events lead to injury of alveolar septa, increased permeability of the pulmonary vascular endothelium, pulmonary microvascular platelet aggregation, and eventually intra-alveolar edema.

MONITORING

See also Chapter 4.

Respiratory system

1. Display respiratory rate continuously in digital and waveform patterns and record rate hourly.
2. Record evidence of increasing respiratory insufficiency hourly, i.e., dyspnea, retractions (suprasternal, intercostal), nasal flaring, fatigue, and restlessness.
3. Measure Pa_{O_2}, Pa_{CO_2}, and pH frequently via an indwelling peripheral arterial catheter. Since the carbon dioxide tensions of alveolar gas and arterial blood are virtually identical in normal subjects, the Pa_{CO_2} can be used as an estimate of the adequacy of alveolar ventilation.
4. Catheter electrodes are available that permit the continuous monitoring of intra-arterial oxygen and carbon dioxide tensions, but they are not useful in children because of the catheter's size. The technique of transcutaneous monitoring of oxygen tension

($P_{TC}O_2$) has been perfected and, if strict technique is followed, it provides an accurate and painless method of monitoring arterial (capillary) oxygen. Electrodes for monitoring carbon dioxide are also now available ($P_{TC}CO_2$). End-tidal carbon dioxide ($PetCO_2$) monitoring devices that can be used for intubated children are now commercially available.

5. Pulmonary arterial blood pressure is monitored indirectly by checking for an increased jugular venous pulse, hepatosplenomegaly, peripheral edema, right ventricular heave and/or right ventricular hypertrophy, or strain pattern on an ECG. Direct measurements are made continuously by placement of a transvenous catheter in the pulmonary artery (see Chapter 88).
6. Gas exchange can be assessed by comparing the alveolar-arterial oxygen tension difference [$P(A - a)O_2$; normal value is less than 15 mm Hg]. One method of measuring the alveolar oxygen tension is mass spectrometry.
7. Adequacy of ventilation can be estimated by measuring the ratio of physiologic dead space to tidal volume (V_D/V_T; the normal ratio is in the range of 0.2 to 0.35) by applying the Bohr equation:

$$\frac{V_D}{V_T} = \frac{Pa_{CO_2} - Pe_{CO_2}}{Pa_{CO_2}}$$

The result represents the volume of the lung that does not eliminate carbon dioxide. Measurements of expired gases (Pe_{CO_2}) are required for this calculation.

8. Continuous monitoring of respiratory gases on a breath-by-breath basis has assumed more importance in managing patients with respiratory failure (e.g., $PetCO_2$).
9. Measuring esophageal pressure with a small balloon catheter will provide an indication of intrathoracic pressure. Pulmonary compliance may then be determined and used in applying oxygen and barotherapy more effectively.

MANAGEMENT

Treat the hypoxemia. Do not wait for confirmation of the diagnosis by drawing an arterial blood-gas sample in room air when the clinical signs of respiratory failure are already present. Once the hypoxemia is treated, the underlying cause of the respiratory failure must be aggressively diagnosed and corrected (e.g., reversal of narcosis, shock, congestive heart failure, status asthmaticus). Decide whether airway intervention and mechanical ventilation are needed. This decision must include an assessment of the patient's clinical status and of the arterial blood-gas tension abnormalities. Specific indications and technique for intubation are detailed in Chapter 95.

The choice of which device to use for mechanical ventilation will not be discussed in detail (see Chapter 97). Generally, patients with poor pulmonary compliance (e.g., status asthmaticus, ARDS) are better managed by a volume rather than a pressure ventilator. Whether a volume or pressure ventilator is used, the rate and volume or pressure should be adjusted to achieve an adequate minute ventilation (the amount of air breathed per minute). Rapid ventilator rates may not allow for adequate exhalation time and may result in air trapping. The patient's respiration may be totally controlled or assisted if he is breathing spontaneously. Assistance can be provided by intermittent positive pressure ventilation (IPPV), which allows the patient to initiate a mechanical breath and receive a preset volume. It can also be provided by intermittent mandatory ventilation (IMV), which allows the patient to receive a continuous fresh gas supply, so that he breathes at his own tidal volume and intermittently receives a pre-determined number of breaths per minute at a preset volume or pressure. PEEP or CPAP is useful in any condition characterized by a decrease in functional residual capacity (e.g., pulmonary edema, hyaline membrane disease). This addition to therapy is particularly important in treating ARDS. High levels of PEEP/CPAP may be required to improve Pa_{O_2}. The inspired oxygen concentration should be adjusted to achieve a normal blood oxygen tension. Under most circumstances, a Pa_{CO_2} of 35 to 45 mm Hg is desirable.

Uniform criteria should be followed in weaning patients from mechanical ventilation (see Chapter 97, Table 97-3).

ADDITIONAL READING

Bone, R.C., editor: The adult respiratory distress syndrome, Clin. Chest Med. 3(1):1-215, 1982.

Cotton, E.K., and Parry, W.: Treatment of status asthmaticus and respiratory failure. Pediatr. Clin. North Am. **22:**163-171, 1975.

Downes, J.J., Fulgencio, T. and Raphaely, R.C.: Acute respiratory failure in infants and children, Pediatr. Clin. North Am. **19:**423-445, 1972.

Lyrene, R.K., and Troog, W.E.: Adult respiratory distress syndrome in a pediatric intensive care unit: predisposing conditions, clinical course, and outcome, Pediatrics **67:**790-795, 1981.

Petty, T.L., and Ashbaugh, D.G.: The adult respiratory distress syndrome, Chest **60:**233-239, 1971.

Rodgers, R.M., and Juers, J.A.: Physiologic considerations in the treatment of acute respiratory failure. In Pierce, A.K.: Basics of RD, vol. 3, no. 4, New York, 1975, American Thoracic Society.

Salm, S.A., Lakshminarayan, S., and Petty, T.L.: Weaning from mechanical ventilation, J.A.M.A. **235:**2208-2212, 1976.

Zwillich, A.W., Pierson, D.J., Creagh, C.E., and others: Complications of assisted ventilation, Am. J. Med. **57:** 161-170, 1974.

13 Congestive heart failure

DANIEL L. LEVIN

DEFINITION AND PHYSIOLOGY

Congestive heart failure occurs when the heart does not provide circulation adequate to meet tissue needs without compensatory mechanisms causing difficulties. Heart failure may be due to excessive preload (myocardial end diastolic fiber length or ventricular filling volume), excessive afterload (increased ventricular wall tension during systole, primarily increased vascular resistance), decreased myocardial contractility (muscle dysfunction), or dysrhythmias, or to a combination of these factors.

1. *Increased preload.* An increased volume load can be due to large left-to-right shunts (e.g., ventricular septal defect [VSD], patent ductus arteriosus [PDA]), incompetent valves (aortic, mitral, pulmonic, or tricuspid insufficiency), arteriovenous fistulae, anemia, renal failure with fluid retention, or administration of excessive parenteral fluids. The age of onset of congestive heart failure depends on many factors. Preterm infants with left-to-right (L → R) shunts, usually due to a PDA, rapidly develop congestive heart failure during the first few days of life because of inadequate myocardial reserve and a cardiac output highly dependent on heart rate alone. This is usually complicated by excessive fluid administration. Full-term babies with simple VSD or PDA usually do not develop heart failure for 6 to 8 weeks because of a gradual fall in the normally high pulmonary vascular resistance present at birth. The elevated pulmonary vascular resistance decreases L → R shunting. Patients with multiple shunts (atrial septal defect [ASD] and VSD); obligatory or high to low pressure shunts (en-docardial cushion defect with left ventricular to right atrial shunt, arteriovenous malformation); complex cardiac lesions with large L → R shunts and valvar regurgitation or right-to-left (R → L) shunts with hypoxemia (or both); severe anemia (erythroblastosis or twin to twin or fetal to maternal transfusions); or iatrogenic volume overload develop congestive heart failure rapidly after birth. Patients with volume overload due to regurgitant valves, especially those proximal to the high resistance pulmonary vascular bed (pulmonic or tricuspid insufficiency), also develop heart failure rapidly after birth.

2. *Increased afterload.* Increased left ventricular afterload may be due to systemic hypertension (e.g., due to renal disease, pheochromocytoma) or left ventricular obstruction due to aortic stenosis and/or coarctation of the aorta. The onset of signs depends on the severity of obstruction, and congestive heart failure may occur in the first few days or weeks of life. Increased afterload to the right ventricle may be due to mitral or pulmonary venous obstruction (cor triatriatum, pulmonary vein orifice stenosis, obstructed total anomalous pulmonary venous return) or pulmonary vascular obstructive disease. Pulmonary valvar stenosis increases right ventricular afterload but it is unusual for patients to have congestive heart failure.

3. *Cardiac muscle dysfunction.* Infectious myocarditis, cardiomyopathies, endocardial fibroelastosis, and myocardial ischemia due to an anomalous coronary artery or severe anemia can cause congestive heart failure. Metabolic factors such as hypocalcemia, hypomagnesemia, hypoglycemia, hypothyroidism, acidosis, sep-

sis, and asphyxia can also cause congestive heart failure and are probably common causes of heart failure in the first days of life. This is especially true for perinatal asphyxia.

4. *Dysrhythmias.* Extreme tachycardia due to paroxysmal atrial or ventricular tachycardia or extreme bradycardias, such as complete heart block with slow ventricular rate, may cause congestive heart failure. With extremely fast heart rates, the diastolic filling time is too brief to allow adequate filling of the heart, and stroke volume decreases. With extremely slow rates, even though stroke volume is increased, cardiac output may be inadequate.

The heart has a limited number of compensatory mechanisms to increase cardiac output, including cardiac dilation, hypertrophy, and increased sympathetic tone. Most of the clinical features of congestive heart failure are due to these compensatory mechanisms.

The heart is enlarged to both physical and roentgenographic examinations. Increased sympathetic nervous system activity results from stimulation of the atrial and venous stretch receptors and the aortic and carotid sinus baroreceptors secondary to reduced aortic blood and pulse pressure. Alpha receptor stimulation decreases flow to limbs, splanchnic bed, and kidneys, resulting in pale, cool extremities, weak pulses, and a decreased urine output. Beta receptor stimulation and increased circulatory catecholamines result in tachycardia and increased myocardial contractility. Stimulation of sympathetic cholinergic fibers to the skin cause increased sweating, which is generalized but is more prominent on the scalp and during exertion such as crying and feeding. Infants normally sweat just on the scalp. Reduced splanchnic and limb flow, venous congestion, and difficulty with feeding result in malaise, fatigue, and decreased appetite. Chronic congestive heart failure may result in impaired growth and cachexia. Irritability is common.

Congestive heart failure results in an increased extracellular fluid volume manifested by weight gain and eventually in peripheral edema, ascites, and pleural effusions as failure progresses. Increased extracellular fluid volume is due to decreased urinary excretion of sodium and secondary water retention because of increased secretion of antidiuretic hormone. The urinary sodium retention is due to three factors. One is a reduced glomerular filtration rate secondary to decreased renal blood flow due to either decreased renal blood pressure or increased renal vascular resistance. Renal vascular resistance is increased because of increased sympathetic tone and increased venous pressure. The second factor is an increased serum aldosterone concentration resulting from decreased removal secondary to hepatic dysfunction and from increased secretion by the adrenals. Increased adrenal secretion of aldosterone is due to decreased renal blood flow, which increases renin secretion and the renin converts plasma angiotensinogen to angiotensin I. This is converted in the lung to angiotensin II, which causes renal vasoconstriction and stimulates aldosterone secretion. The third factor causing sodium retention is a humoral factor, which may be due to vasoactive peptides or prostaglandins.

Ventricular dilation increases ventricular wall tension and radius, resulting in decreased myocardial oxygen consumption. Ventricular dilation is associated with a gallop rhythm and eventually with mitral or tricuspid regurgitation. When the atria dilate, a fourth heart sound is heard and the pressure in the veins (pulmonary and/or systemic) becomes elevated.

Pulmonary venous hypertension and pulmonary edema cause the lungs to become stiffer. This is compounded by pulmonary arterial hypertension. The work of breathing is increased and breathing becomes rapid and shallow. Greater respiratory efforts result in greater negative intrathoracic pressure, with supracostal, intercostal, and subcostal retractions. In babies with a loose pulmonary interstitium, water accumulates around the airways and causes wheezing. Edema in the bronchial mucosa also causes turbulent gas flow and wheezing. As fluid enters the alveoli, rales are heard.

Increased right atrial pressure and increased blood volume raise the systemic venous pressure, which is manifested as hepatomegaly and raised jugular venous pressure. Venous distention in the neck may be difficult to appreciate in babies. Proteinuria, ascites, and splenomegaly may occur.

MONITORING

See also Chapter 4.

The following variables should be monitored in all patients with congestive heart failure who are in an intensive care unit.

Cardiorespiratory system

1. ECG (continuously). In addition to a display of the pattern, a 12-lead ECG should be done at the beginning of the diagnostic evaluation.
2. Echocardiogram initially for diagnosis
3. Arterial blood-gas tensions and pH determinations. All children with congestive heart failure should have at least one arterial blood-gas tension and pH determination initially and this should be repeated every 4 to 8 hours when abnormalities persist.

Renal-metabolic system

1. Serum Na, K, and Cl. Measure initially and every day while the patient is receiving only parenteral fluid administration. Repeat any time there are dysrhythmias noted in association with digoxin administration. Patients given repetitive diuretic therapy should have serum Na and K determinations every 2 to 3 days.
2. Serum Ca and Mg. Measure initially, after large doses of diuretics, and at any time dysrhythmias occur. This is especially important in newborns, who develop hypocalcemia and hypomagnesemia with stress.
3. Serum glucose. Obtain Dextrostix or serum glucose determinations immediately after admission. This is particularly important in babies, who frequently become hypoglycemic with heart failure. Alternatively, hypoglycemia may be the sole cause of the congestive heart failure. Repeat every 4 to 8 hours.

MANAGEMENT

Management of congestive heart failure should be considered either general and supportive or specific and corrective. Medications should be given IV when possible, since circulation to muscle and skin may be abnormal and oral absorption erratic. The primary aims of supportive therapy are to increase tissue oxygen supply and decrease tissue oxygen consumption, to correct metabolic abnormalities, to remove excess salt and water, and to improve myocardial functioning.

General measures

1. Ensure adequate systemic oxygen transport by ensuring a normal Hct (40% to 45%) and giving supplemental oxygen.
2. Identify and correct abnormalities in serum glucose, Ca, Mg, Na, K, and Cl concentrations.
3. Restrict fluid administration to 60% to 70% of normal.
4. Treat fever with acetaminophen in older children and with cooling to decrease excessive metabolic rate associated with increased oxygen consumption.
5. Give patients nothing orally during the acute phase of congestive heart failure.
6. Digitalize the patient (Table 13-1).
7. Use the diuretic furosemide (1 mg/kg IV).
8. Treat pulmonary edema.
   a. Digitalis.
   b. Furosemide.
   c. Morphine sulfate, 0.1 mg/kg slowly IV.
   d. Intubation and CPAP at modest pressures (4 to 8 cm H_2O) may be beneficial. Excessive intrathoracic pressure may in-

Table 13-1. Digitalis administration

Patient	Dose*
Premature infant	30 μg/kg
Full-term infant <6 months	60 μg/kg
Infant 6-24 months	45 μg/kg
Older children and adults	30 μg/kg

1. Two people should individually calculate dose.
2. IM digoxin may not be picked up readily in a patient with poor circulation. Use IV.
3. Give ½ total digitalizing dose (TDD), then ¼ TDD at 8 hours and ¼ TDD at 16 hours.
4. Use ⅛ TDD as maintenance every 12 hours thereafter if therapeutic response is achieved.
5. Dose may have to be adjusted to increase or decrease digoxin in a patient.

*Oral; IV dose is ⅔ of the oral dose.

crease right ventricular afterload and decrease left atrial preload.

9. Identify and treat respiratory failure. Patients in congestive heart failure may also be in respiratory failure (see Chapter 12) and need intubation and mechanical ventilation. This may need to be done in some patients who have labored respirations or depressed states of consciousness and are at greater risk for inhalation of foreign material.
10. In some patients with normal systemic oxygen transport and increased ambient oxygen, the work of breathing may still be so great that it significantly compromises the energy stores available for cardiac work. These patients should be intubated and mechanically ventilated.

Specific measures

1. Excessive preload
   a. Correct anemia with small transfusions of packed RBCs, 5 ml/kg.
   b. Iatrogenic fluid overload can be treated with fluid restriction and furosemide, 1 mg/kg IV.
   c. L → R shunts, incompetent valves, and arteriovenous fistulae must be approached surgically.
   d. L → R shunts due to PDA in preterm infants may be corrected either surgically or pharmacologically with the prostaglandin synthetase inhibitor, indomethacin.
   e. Mechanical devices used at the time of cardiac catheterization have also been used to close both ASD and PDAs.
2. a. Increased left ventricular afterload
      (1) Systemic hypertension may be treated by antihypertensive agents (see Chapter 17) or in some cases by surgery (e.g., removal of pheochromocytoma, renal vascular reconstruction).
      (2) Coarctation of the aorta and aortic stenosis can be approached surgically.
   b. Increased right ventricular afterload
      (1) Pulmonary hypertension caused by mitral stenosis, cor triatriatum, or total anomalous pulmonary venous return may be approached surgically.
      (2) Patients with pulmonary vascular obstructive disease are frequently inoperable.
3. Cardiac muscle dysfunction
   a. Metabolic causes are usually amenable to specific treatment with glucose, calcium, magnesium, or thyroid extract.
   b. Some newborns with sepsis and congestive heart failure respond to appropriate antibiotic therapy.
   c. Most other myocardiopathies and endocardial fibroelastosis have no specific treatment.
4. Dysrhythmias
   a. Paroxysmal supraventricular tachycardias are treated with digitalis (Table 13-1), vagal stimulation, or electroversion (see Chapter 5).
   b. Ventricular dysrhythmias are usually treated with lidocaine, 1 mg/kg IV (see Chapter 5).

c. If digitalis toxicity is suspected, discontinue digoxin and make certain the serum K is normal. If multiple PVCs or PVCs close to the T wave (refractory period) occur, give phenytoin, 5 mg/kg slow IV push and then 5 mg/kg/24 hr IV in 3 divided doses.

ADDITIONAL READING

Heymann, M.A., Rudolph, A.M., and Silverman, N.J.: Closure of the ductus arteriosus in premature infants by inhibitors of prostaglandin synthesis, N. Engl. J. Med. **295:**530-533, 1976.

Hoffman, J.I.E., and Stanger, P.: Congestive heart failure. In Pascoe, D.J., and Grossman, M., editors: Quick reference to pediatric emergencies, Philadelphia, 1973, J. B. Lippincott Co.

14 Shock

DANIEL L. LEVIN
RONALD M. PERKIN

DEFINITION AND PHYSIOLOGY

Shock is an acute, complex pathophysiologic state of circulatory dysfunction, which results in a failure of the organism to deliver sufficient amounts of oxygen and other nutrients to satisfy the requirements of the tissue beds. Because of its progressive nature, shock may be divided into three phases: compensated, uncompensated, and irreversible. In compensated shock vital organ function is maintained by intrinsic compensatory mechanisms. The common denominator in this early stage is not low blood flow; flow is usually normal or increased unless it is limited by preexisting hypovolemia or myocardial dysfunction. More often blood flow is uneven or maldistributed in the microcirculation. Nonspecific measurements such as systemic arterial blood pressure, pulse rate, and cardiac output do not differentiate between the normal state and compensated shock states in spite of the important underlying physiologic derangements in compensated shock.

As shock progresses to an uncompensated state, the efficiency of the cardiovascular system is gradually undermined and microvascular perfusion becomes marginal despite compensatory adjustments. Eventually, circulatory impairment becomes self-sustained and compensatory mechanisms may actually contribute to the progression and perpetuation of the shock state. Toxic materials are elaborated that interfere with cardiac function and vasomotor adjustment. Arterioles may no longer control flow through the capillary system, allowing vasodilation in some vessels; but vasoconstriction in others may result in pooling in the capillary beds. The vascular pooling reduces the circulating blood volume, allowing platelet adhesion and coalescence of red blood cells, and in conjunction with the high level of circulating catecholamines, may produce dangerous chain reactions in the coagulation and kinin systems. Cellular function deteriorates, and disturbances in function become sequentially demonstrable in all organ systems.

Terminal or irreversible shock implies damage to key organs, such as the heart or the brain, which is of such magnitude that the entire organism will be disrupted regardless of therapeutic intervention. Death occurs even if therapy returns cardiovascular measurements to normal levels.

Hypovolemic shock

Hypovolemic shock (decreased cardiac output and decreased preload [myocardial end-diastolic fiber length or decreased filling volume]) is the most common type of shock in pediatric patients; it is due to decreased effective circulating blood volume, which may result from absolute whole blood loss (internal or external hemorrhage), relative whole blood loss (vasodilating drugs, anesthetic agents, positive pressure ventilation, sepsis), plasma loss (burns, sepsis, nephrotic syndrome, intestinal obstruction, hypoproteinemia), or fluid and electrolyte loss (vomiting, diarrhea, excessive sweating, renal).

Cardiac and peripheral compensatory adjustments may suffice to restore cardiac output, systemic arterial blood pressure, and organ perfusion to normal or near normal levels, although they do so at the expense of altered intracardiac and systemic venous blood pressures and changes in blood flow to various regional circulations.

Compensated phases of hypovolemic shock are characterized by decreases in CVP, stroke volume, and urine output with increases in heart rate, systemic vascular resistance, and myocardial contractility. Systemic arterial blood pressure is frequently normal, the result of increased systemic vascular resistance. Neurologic status is normal or only minimally impaired. The extremities are pale and cool.

With continued loss of blood volume or with delayed or inadequate blood volume replacement, the intravascular fluid losses surpass the body's compensatory abilities and decompensated phases appear. The pronounced systemic vasoconstriction and hypovolemia produce ischemic and stagnant hypoxia in the visceral and cutaneous circulations. Altered cellular metabolism and function occur in these areas, resulting in damage to vessels, kidneys, liver, pancreas, and bowel. Patients are hypotensive, acidotic, lethargic or comatose, and oliguric or anuric. Stroke volume and cardiac output are further decreased. Terminal phases of hypovolemic shock are characterized by myocardial dysfunction and widespread cell death.

Cardiogenic shock

Cardiogenic shock is the pathophysiologic state in which an abnormality of cardiac function is responsible for the failure of the cardiovascular system to meet the metabolic needs of tissues. The common denominator in it is depressed cardiac output, which in most instances is the result of decreased myocardial contractility.

A common cause of cardiogenic shock in children is impaired cardiac performance following intracardiac surgery, and this type of shock is associated with significant morbidity and mortality in the early postoperative period. Other clinically important causes of cardiogenic shock in children are dysrhythmias, drug intoxication, hypoxic/ischemic episodes, acidemia, hypothermia, metabolic derangement (hypoglycemia, myopathies), extrinsic inflow or outflow obstructions (tension pneumothorax, tension pneumopericardium, pericardial effusion with tamponade), and severe congestive heart failure secondary to congenital heart disease.

Cardiac function can also be depressed in patients in shock that is not caused primarily by a myocardial insult. Myocardial dysfunction is frequently a late manifestation of shock of any etiology. Although the cause of myocardial dysfunction in such patients is not completely understood, the following mechanisms have been proposed: (1) specific toxic substances released during the course of shock have a direct cardiac depressant effect; (2) cardiac depression is secondary to exhaustion of myocardial contractility as a consequence of nonspecific shock metabolism; and (3) reduced coronary blood flow results in focal areas of myocardial ischemia and necrosis.

Intrinsic compensatory responses can have deleterious effects in patients with cardiogenic shock as opposed to hypovolemic shock. Compensatory responses are nonspecific, not precisely regulated, and in patients with cardiogenic shock they may contribute to the progression of shock by further depressing cardiac function and accelerating tissue injury. Because of this self-perpetuating cycle, compensated phases of cardiogenic shock are rarely observed and frequently only one cardiorespiratory pattern, in varying degrees of severity, is observed. The patients are tachycardic, tachypneic, hypotensive, oliguric, and acidotic. Extremities are cool and mental status is altered. Cardiac output is depressed and elevations in CVP, pulmonary capillary wedge pressure (PCWP), and systemic vascular resistance are observed.

Septic shock (distributive shock)

Abnormalities in the distribution of blood flow may lead to profound inadequacies in tissue perfusion. This may occur as a result of vasomotor paralysis, increased venous capacitance, or physiologic shunting past capillary beds. Etiologies of distributive shock in children include anaphylaxis (see Chapter 15), sepsis, central nervous system injury, and drug intoxication (barbiturates, smooth-muscle relaxants, antihypertensive medications, and tranquilizers).

Septic shock is frequently encountered, and it is associated with high mortality rates in children as well as adults. Sepsis is a systemic disease caused by microorganisms or their prod-

ucts in the blood. When sepsis leads to circulatory insufficiency and inadequate tissue perfusion, shock is present. The most common offending organisms are gram-negative bacteria; however, septic shock may occur after infection with gram-positive bacteria, fungi, rickettsiae, and viruses. Regardless of the offending organism, there are similar cardiorespiratory responses, which appear to be host dependent. Sepsis with consequent shock often complicates other forms of shock. Moreover, lesions in the heart or intestines in septic shock may be sufficiently severe to induce fatal cardiogenic or hypovolemic shock even though the infection is controlled.

The precise mechanisms causing circulatory

Table 14-1. Stages of septic shock

Early: hyperdynamic	Late: cardiogenic
Bedside observations	
Tachycardia	Tachycardia
Tachypnea	Respiratory depression
Fever	Hypothermia
Warm extremities	Cool, pale extremities
Bounding pulses	Decreased pulses
Normal capillary refill	Prolonged capillary refill
Normal or elevated systemic systolic blood pressure	Hypotension
Wide pulse pressure	Narrow pulse pressure
Elevated cardiac index	Depressed cardiac index
Decreased systemic vascular resistance	Increased systemic vascular resistance
Adequate urine output or polyuria	Oliguria
Mild mental confusion, occasional hallucinations	Lethargy or coma
Laboratory measurements	
Hypoxemia	Hypoxemia
Respiratory alkalosis	Respiratory acidosis
Metabolic acidosis (not always present in early phase)	Metabolic acidosis
Marked pulmonary shunt	Minimal pulmonary shunt
Narrow arterio-venous oxygen saturation difference	Wide arterio-venous oxygen saturation difference
Hyperglycemia	Hypoglycemia
Mild coagulation abnormalities	Marked coagulopathy
Normal or mild elevation of blood lactate	Markedly elevated blood lactate

From Perkin, R.M., and Levin, D.L.: J. Pediatr. **101**(2):167, 1982.

dysfunction in septic shock are not clear. However, the dysfunction appears to be the result of multiple interrelated factors, including (1) derangements of intermediary metabolism; (2) direct effect of the organism or its by-products on the cardiovascular system; (3) cardiovascular effects of secondary products, including those of the activated protein cascade systems (complement, coagulation, kallikrein) and the toxic myocardial factors; (4) liberation of other vasoactive agents (serotonin, endorphins, prostaglandins, histamine); (5) failure of oxygen extraction at the cellular level; (6) host compensatory mechanisms; and (7) underlying host factors such as preexisting cardiovascular, nutritional, and immunologic status.

It is impossible to predict the effect at the microcirculatory level of these factors, which cause and perpetuate uneven blood flow and inadequate tissue oxygenation, resulting in progressive decompensation of the capillary circulation and surrounding cells. In spite of these difficulties, definite patterns have emerged allowing clinical classification and staging. Three broad stages can be recognized: hyperdynamic-compensated, hyperdynamic-uncompensated, and cardiogenic (see Table 14-1). The early stages of septic shock are characterized by vascular tone abnormalities and hyperdynamic compensatory responses. The late, or cardiogenic, stage is manifested by a hypodynamic cardiovascular picture, because cardiac insufficiency is the most prominent feature. In this stage classic signs of circulatory collapse exist, which are indistinguishable from late shock of any etiology. All aspects of cardiac performance rapidly deteriorate, even with aggressive support. Cellular dysfunction originating in the early hyperdynamic stages prevents survival despite efforts to return circulatory function to normal.

Sequelae of shock

Multiple organ failure, progressive organ failure, and sequential organ failure are terms used to describe problems that may develop after a period of circulatory dysfunction. Common sequelae include so-called shock lung (permeability edema), acute renal failure, hepatic dysfunction, pancreatic ischemia, disseminated intravascular coagulation (DIC), and gastrointestinal bleeding. When the CNS is injured, this often becomes the limiting factor that prevents survival.

Respiratory fatigue. In patients with shock the work of breathing is substantially increased due to hyperventilation elicited by acidemia and hypoxemia and alterations in pulmonary mechanics secondary to pulmonary vascular congestion. However, because of decreased or redistributed cardiac output, respiratory muscle blood flow may be limited to levels less than those required by the increased work of breathing. Respiratory muscle fatigue may then occur, leading to respiratory failure and circulatory collapse. This form of respiratory dysfunction responds well to early respiratory support (i.e., mechanical ventilation).

Respiratory distress syndrome. The lung is the most sensitive organ in shock, and respiratory failure can develop rapidly and is frequently the cause of death. The common denominator of respiratory distress in shock patients is increased extravascular lung water. Two mechanisms are responsible for increasing lung water. The first, hydrostatic edema, is produced by elevation of pulmonary microvascular pressure and results primarily from left ventricular dysfunction. This type of edema usually responds to cardiotonic regimens. The second, permeability edema, is quite different. It goes by many names, such as adult respiratory distress syndrome (ARDS) and shock lung. In this type of edema, there is damage to the alveolar epithelium and the pulmonary capillary endothelium. Due to cellular damage, pulmonary capillaries become permeable and proteinaceous fluid leaks into the interstitial space and the alveoli. Formation of intra-alveolar fluid is facilitated by degeneration of alveolar cells. The degeneration of alveolar type II cells results in a reduction of surfactant production, leading to atelectasis. Increased lung water, hypoxemia, and acidosis result in pulmonary vasoconstriction and increased pulmonary vascular resistance. Although the exact mechanism of pulmonary injury remains a mystery, numerous factors probably contribute, including leukocyte aggregates, activated complement components, DIC, kinases, lysosomes, histamine, platelet microemboli, fat and marrow emboli, endotoxins, prostaglandin release, transfusion and fluid overload, prolonged pulmonary hypoperfusion, and inhalation of gastric contents. The diagnosis of permeability pulmonary edema is made by measuring a low or normal left atrial pressure (LAP) or PCWP in combination with a high protein content in the pulmonary edema fluid. These findings establish that the edema is pulmonary, not cardiac, in origin. It is common to find patients with elements of both hydrostatic and permeability pulmonary edema.

Calcium homeostasis. Severe abnormalities of calcium homeostasis can occur in the course of any acute hemodynamic deterioration. Marked decreases in serum ionized calcium levels have been reported in conditions associated with inadequate tissue perfusion, regardless of etiology. The cause of this abnormality is unknown, although it may result from toxic or ischemic insult to the parathyroid gland.

Sustained decreases in ionized calcium have been associated with depressed myocardial function, tachycardia, electrocardiographic changes, hypotension, acidosis, cyanosis, temperature instability, alterations in mental status, and motor nerve excitability. For these reasons, therapeutic intervention is probably justified when serum ionized calcium levels fall below normal (less than 2.4 mg/dl). There is no predictable relationship between total and ionized calcium concentrations, and therefore, the total serum calcium concentration cannot be used as an index of the biochemically effective moiety, ionized calcium. Unfortunately, ionized calcium measurements are not readily available.

Inorganic phosphate. Phosphorus is essential to muscle, nervous system, and red and white blood cell function. It also is of importance in metabolism and in the body's entire apparatus of generating and storing energy. Consequences of severe hypophosphatemia (serum levels less than 1.0 mg/dl) include acute respiratory failure, altered myocardial performance, increased affinity of hemoglobin for oxygen, diminished phagocytosis, platelet dysfunction and hemorrhage, hemolytic anemia, hepatocellular damage, and neurologic abnormalities. Serum phosphate measurement is a reliable indicator of body phosphorus concentrations.

MONITORING

See also Chapter 4.

Patients in shock need aggressive, invasive monitoring and management. Some patients have a specific, immediately remediable cause of shock (e.g., paroxysmal atrial tachycardia with severe congestive heart failure, reversible by electroversion; hypovolemia due to diarrhea which rapidly responds to administration of fluid). These patients may not need the full extent of monitoring indicated. However, in most patients shock is not so immediately reversed and requires extensive monitoring.

Cardiovascular system

1. Test capillary filling frequently (See also Chapter 4).
2. Obtain arterial blood-gas tensions and pH initially and every 1 to 2 hours.
3. Continuously monitor systemic arterial blood pressure.
4. Continuously monitor CVP.
5. In patients who have undergone extensive intracardiac surgery or who have elevated systemic vascular resistance, pulmonary edema, or pulmonary hypertension or who require iontropic agents:
   a. Monitor LAP or PCWP (may use pulmonary arterial diastolic blood pressure if this has been shown to correlate with PCWP).

b. Repetitive measurements of cardiac output by thermodilution should be performed to make accurate status assessments and to verify the response to therapeutic interventions.

c. Determine systemic vascular resistance (SVR) and/or pulmonary vascular resistance (PVR).

$$\text{SVR (dynes} \cdot \text{sec} \cdot \text{cm}^{-5}) =$$
$$\frac{(\overline{\text{SAP}}\,[\text{mm Hg}] - \overline{\text{CVP}}\,[\text{mm Hg}]) \times 79.9}{\text{CO (L/min)}}$$

$$\text{PVR (dynes} \cdot \text{sec} \cdot \text{cm}^{-5}) =$$
$$\frac{(\overline{\text{PAP}}\,[\text{mm Hg}] - \overline{\text{PCWP}}\,[\text{mm Hg}]) \times 79.9}{\text{CO (L/min)}}$$

d. Determine degree of pulmonary shunt.

$$Q_s/Q_T\,(\%) = \frac{Cc_{O_2} - Ca_{O_2}}{Cc_{O_2} - C\bar{v}_{O_2}} \times 100$$

or

$$Q_s/Q_T\,(\%) =$$
$$\frac{0.0031 \times \text{A-a}_{D_{O_2}}}{\text{A-v}_{D_{O_2}} + (0.0031 \times \text{A-a}_{D_{O_2}})} \times 100$$

The equations in d are valid only where arterial blood is 100% saturated.

Other systems

1. Liver function tests: perform SGOT, bilirubin, and TSP initially and repeat if abnormal.
2. Coagulation status: Obtain results of PT, PTT, platelet count, fibrinogen, and fibrin split products when blood appears in urine, endotracheal tube, stools, or NG tube or when oozing occurs at venipuncture sites. DIC is often seen in shock states (see Chapter 20).
3. Check Ca and PO₄.

MANAGEMENT

Since shock is inadequate delivery of oxygen and nutrients to the tissues, the objective in treating shock is to improve oxygen and nutrient delivery by optimizing oxygen content (oxygen capacity or oxygen combined with hemoglobin plus oxygen dissolved in blood) and by ensuring as adequate a cardiac output as possible. Cardiac output may be optimized by manipulating (1) preload (myocardial end diastolic fiber length or filling volume), (2) myocardial contractility, (3) heart rate, or (4) afterload (ventricular wall tension during systole or resistance to ventricular ejection). Practically all these manipulations are accomplished by restoration of oxygen-carrying capacity, by increasing the circulating blood volume, by controlling heart rate, by pharmacologically augmenting contractility, and by changing vascular resistances.

Preload is best related to stroke volume by the Frank-Starling curve (Fig. 14-1), which shows the relationship of cardiac output to cardiac filling. The two curves in Fig. 14-1 depict normal versus decreased myocardial contractility. When a volume challenge is given, the preload increases (moving from A to B or from C to D) and stroke volume increases. When volume is diminished, as for example, with the use of diuretics, preload decreases (E to D) and stroke volume decreases. When inotropes are given and contractility improves (D to B), stroke volume increases. When vasodilators are given and afterload is reduced (D to F), stroke volume increases.

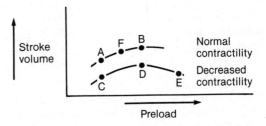

Fig. 14-1. Frank-Starling curve. $A \rightarrow B$, Increased preload (volume); $C \rightarrow D$, increased preload (volume); $E \rightarrow D$, decreased preload (venodilation, diuretics); $D \rightarrow B$, increased contractility (inotropes); $D \rightarrow F$, decreased afterload (vasodilation). (From Perkin, R.M., and Levin, D.L.: J. Pediatr. **101**(2):165, 1982.)

Contractility is an inherent quality of myocardial muscle but it may be augmented chemically with catecholamines, calcium, glucagon, and glycosides. Heart rate is reflexly controlled by the autonomic nervous system but can also be manipulated by such agents as atropine, isoproterenol, and electrical pacing. Afterload is best related to peripheral vascular resistance, which may be altered intrinsically or extrinsically by venodilation or constriction.

Recognition of the shock state is the most important step in its management. Access to the venous compartment of the vascular system must be established promptly in all patients and desired monitoring aids should be selected and instituted.

Hypovolemic shock

Fluids and minerals. Regardless of the etiology of shock, the possibility of hypovolemia must be considered and efforts taken to control ongoing losses and to restore an effective circulating blood volume (preload). Early, complete correction of hypovolemia is a major factor in the prevention of post-resuscitation complications.

Available fluids. Volume resuscitation includes the use of crystalloid and/or colloid solutions in addition to blood. Crystalloids are electrolyte-containing solutions that are distributed throughout the body because of their chemical composition and tonicity. Isotonic solutions (Lactated Ringer's, 0.9% sodium chloride) are primarily restricted to the extracellular space by the action of the cellular sodium-potassium pump. Hypotonic solutions have a percentage of water that is not associated with sodium or protein and they are therefore distributed uniformly throughout the entire body water. Hypertonic solutions (sodium concentrations in excess of 180 mEq/L) by increasing serum osmolality induce a general movement of intracellular water into the extracellular space. In general, hypotonic crystalloid solutions are never used in the early phase of fluid resuscitation of shock patients. Use of lactated solutions in patients with impaired liver function may alter acid-base balance by increasing the blood lactate concentration and causing renal loss of sodium and potassium.

Colloids used in the treatment of shock consist of plasma, prepared plasma fractions, and synthetic plasma substitutes. These solutions contain large molecules that are relatively restricted to the intravascular space, where they exert an oncotic effect upon the distribution of water. Therefore, iso-oncotic solutions, such as 5% albumin in 0.9% sodium chloride solution, fresh frozen plasma, or plasma protein fractions, produce a relatively greater plasma expansion than isotonic crystalloid solutions for the same volume of fluid infused. Hyperoncotic solutions, such as 25% albumin, tend to pull fluid into the vascular compartment from the interstitial space.

Synthetic plasma expanders, such as dextrans, gelatins, and hydroxyethyl starch (Hetastarch), are available for intravascular volume replacement. The dextrans, Dextran-40 and Dextran-70, are available either in 0.9% sodium chloride solution or 5% glucose solution. These solutions are slightly hyperoncotic with respect to plasma and therefore will expand the intravascular volume by more than the amount given. Dextrans may exert a beneficial effect upon the microcirculation in shock states by decreasing red cell aggregation and increasing oxygen transport. The major limitation of dextran is that it decreases platelet coagulability, and this results in increased bleeding time when dextran is given in volumes exceeding 10 ml/hr. Hetastarch is amylopectin in which hydroxyethyl groups are substituted. It is available as a 6% solution in 0.9% sodium chloride with a measured osmolality of 310 mOsm/L. The current recommended dose of Hetastarch is 10 to 20 ml/kg/day; however, clinical experience in children is still incomplete.

Blood loss should be replaced milliliter for milliliter with a combination of packed RBCs and fresh frozen plasma (FFP).

Fluid selection. Fluid infusion to restore

lost blood volume is the principal therapeutic goal in shock states, but considerable controversy exists over the appropriate fluids to use. Proper selection of fluid can be done only after the individual patient is assessed and the following questions answered: What type of fluid has been lost? What are the underlying physiologic problems of the specific host-disease interaction? What are the specific physiologic actions of each fluid type? Gross changes in red cell volume, colloid oncotic pressure, or serum sodium content should be taken into account when choosing initial resuscitation fluids.

An adequate oxygen-carrying capacity should be maintained by ensuring normal red cell mass. Hematocrits of 35% to 40% are most desirable, depending on the exact blood volume and cardiorespiratory status of the patient. Patients with pulmonary disease or patients who are unable to increase cardiac output should have hematocrits in the higher ranges. Hematocrits greater than 45% do not necessarily mean increased oxygen availability since increased blood viscosity may depress cardiac output and impede flow in the microcirculation (see Chapter 38).

Hypoproteinemia with a decrease in plasma colloid oncotic pressure is commonly found in severely ill patients. Hypo-oncotic states may be produced by losses of blood or plasma due to hemorrhage, traumatic injury, and surgical operation, as well as by inflammation, malnutrition, malignancy, and the infusion of large volumes of crystalloid solutions. Fluid movement between the capillary and the interstitium is governed by a balance between hydrostatic and oncotic forces as well as by the permeability characteristics of the capillary membrane. Decreased plasma oncotic pressure may result in the formation of interstitial edema in the pulmonary and systemic circulations. Maintaining colloid oncotic pressure is important for plasma volume restoration and for minimizing interstitial edema. Prevention of interstitial edema is particularly important in the lung, since accumulation of interstitial fluid leads to deterioration in gas exchange, which is a major cause of morbidity and mortality associated with critical illness. Systemic edema can also be deleterious by decreasing tissue oxygen tension, thereby increasing the infection rate and decreasing the rate of wound healing. The presence of tissue edema may also result in large fluid shifts, producing hemodynamic instability as edema fluid is reabsorbed.

In patients who are hypovolemic and hypoproteinemic or in patients with underlying cardiac, respiratory, or renal failure, plasma volume expansion is best achieved with iso-oncotic fluids. In addition, moderate amounts of noncolloid fluids may safely be used if needed for reexpansion of the intravascular space or for restoration of normal renal function. Volume replacement with only noncolloid solutions will result in a strongly positive fluid balance, which may prove unfavorable in these patients. Since hyperosmolar fluids expand the vascular space by greater than the amount infused, the threat of circulatory overload is present, especially in patients with cardiac dysfunction.

In patients with uncomplicated hypovolemia, a balanced electrolyte solution in addition to red cells, if needed, can safely be used regardless of the degree of volume deficit. When first faced with treating a patient in shock, the rapid infusion of 0.9% sodium chloride solution or Ringer's lactate should be used since these are probably the safest, cheapest, most rapidly available fluids. When using only crystalloid solutions, one must remember that it takes at least twice as much volume to accomplish the same degree of hemodynamic stability as when using a colloid solution.

Colloid solutions should not be used in patients with severe capillary leak syndromes, which occur in late or preterminal stages of shock or trauma or in the first few hours following severe burn injury. In these instances, colloid will shift into the extravascular space, where it will further deplete intravascular volume by causing an obligatory water shift into the interstitial space.

Amount of fluid. The amount of fluid necessary to restore effective circulating blood volume depends on the amount lost (deficit) and the rate of ongoing loss. The total amount of fluid given often exceeds the total volume lost because of expanded capacitance of the vascular space and dysfunction of cellular membranes. Enough fluid must be given to traverse the microcirculation, elevate the CVP, and therefore provide adequate cardiac filling pressure. An adequate filling pressure only ensures that one determinant of cardiac performance has been maximized. It does not ensure adequate perfusion of tissue beds or that the patient's heart has the functional ability to respond adequately to the volume of fluid administered.

In cases of hypovolemic shock uncompli-cated by myocardial dysfunction, the fluid resuscitation should proceed as outlined in Fig. 14-2. If improvement, as manifested by increased systemic arterial blood pressure, increased pulse pressure and peripheral perfusion, adequate urine output (0.5 to 1 ml/kg/hr), and decreased metabolic acidosis, does not occur after two infusions of isotonic crystalloid solution at 10 to 20 ml/kg of body weight and if ongoing losses are minimal, then no more fluid should be given without more invasive monitoring. Deterioration of cardiac function is a common rate-limiting factor in shock, and blood volume restoration may not restore ventricular function. In addition to placing a central venous and/or pulmonary arterial catheter, a careful search for complicating factors must be ini-

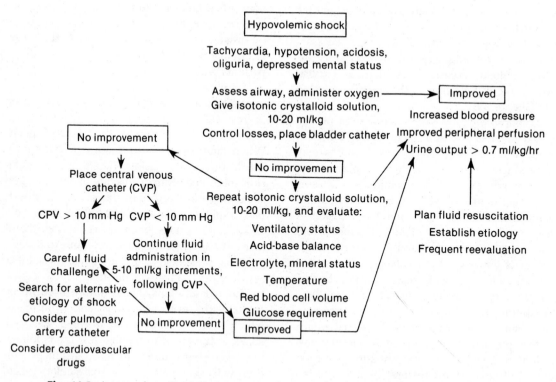

Fig. 14-2. Approach to fluid management in a child with uncomplicated hypovolemic shock. (From Perkin, R.M., and Levin, D.L.: J. Pediatr. **101**(3):321, 1982.)

tiated (hypoxemia, electrolyte or metabolic abnormalities, cardiac tamponade). Once the appropriate catheter is properly placed, a third fluid challenge may be attempted, using the guide outlined in Table 14-2. If adequate cardiovascular function is not restored by fluid administration or if elevated ventricular filling pressures preclude this approach, then the focus of the therapy should shift to pharmacologic manipulation of myocardial contractility and vascular tone (see p. 81). NOTE: CVP is not strictly an indication of the circulating blood volume nor does it demonstrate the functional efficacy of the left ventricle. The left and right sides of the heart may function disparately and fail independently. Although disparate ventricular function appears to be less common in children than in adults, it has been observed to

Table 14-2. Fluid challenge for patients in shock

1. Observe CVP or PCWP for 5 to 10 minutes.

2. If

CVP	or	PCWP	Then give following fluid
<6 mm Hg		<8 mm Hg	10 ml/kg or 200 ml over 10 min
<10 mm Hg		<12 mm Hg	5 ml/kg or 100 ml over 10 min
≥10 mm Hg		≥12 mm Hg	3 ml/kg or 50 ml over 10 min

3. Observe CVP or PCWP for 10 minutes after challenge.
4. If the CVP returns to within 2 mm Hg or the PCWP returns to within 3 mm Hg of the preinfusion value, then the fluid challenge is resumed. In each instance the pressure value immediately preceding the fluid challenge serves as the reference measurement. Fluid is administered until either the hemodynamic signs of shock are corrected or the CVP persistently exceeds 2 mm Hg or the PCWP persistently exceeds 3 mm Hg of the starting value.

occur in shock, regardless of etiology. In such patients, synchronous monitoring of PCWP and CVP is necessary in determining those who will respond to fluid administration. PCWP has been shown to reflect accurately the LAP and the mean left ventricular diastolic pressure in acute cardiac diseases and other states of critical illness. However, there are several factors that can affect the PCWP including heart rate, preload, afterload, pericardial or pleural pressure, diastolic properties of the left ventricle, and the left ventricular inotropic state.

Because of the multiplicity of factors that affect CVP and PCWP measurements, the best use of these measurements is to assess the changes in these values that occur with fluid challenge. Utilized this way, the measurement of CVP and PCWP allows detection of limitations in cardiac competence and therefore provides an important guide for volume replacement. Fluid administration should be discontinued when ventricular filling pressure rises without evidence of improvement in cardiovascular performance. (Measure increase in cardiac output if possible).

In patients with cerebral damage, efforts to provide usual fluid therapy for optimal cardiac output must be tempered by the need to keep ICP and CPP within acceptable ranges. Fluid administration, even though it improves cardiac output, may worsen cerebral edema and increase ICP. The use of inotropic agents to improve cardiac output even in the relatively hypovolemic patient may be indicated.

A controversial and frequently misunderstood period in the therapy of patients with severe shock occurs following the initial resuscitation and lasts for 36 to 72 hours. When cells are damaged, both the integrity of the cellular membrane and intracellular metabolic processes are altered. This results in sodium and water gaining access to cells and to interstitial spaces, and they are not eliminated immediately. This fluid and sodium excess further depresses cell function and may have particularly deleterious effects upon myocardial cells, causing or aggravating cardiac failure and altering ventricular compliance. Depression of cell function and consequent obligatory extravascular fluid sequestration may also lead to significant hypovolemia, which necessitates the IV infusion of large volumes of fluid even in the absence of signs of overt fluid loss. The volume of obligatory extravascular fluid expansion is directly related to the degree of cellular injury and, therefore, to the duration and severity of shock which caused the impaired cellular oxygenation. Clinically, the patients have decreased systemic arterial blood pressure, tachycardia, decreased pulse pressure, increased CVP, oliguria, weight gain, and respiratory insufficiency. The weight gain and respiratory insufficiency reflect extravascular fluid sequestration, which is obligatory and cannot be prevented by fluid restriction or diuresis. Therapeutic efforts along these lines lead to acute oliguric renal failure, which often results in death. Therapeutic efforts must be directed at simultaneously maintaining effective cardiovascular performance, adequate urine output, and intense ventilatory support. This excessive extravascular fluid is eventually mobilized after cell membranes have been repaired and an effective sodium pump has been reestablished.

Calcium. A precise definition of the optimal dose for replacement calcium is not available; however, 10 to 20 mg/kg (0.1 to 0.2 ml/kg) of 10% calcium chloride solution given by slow IV infusion through a centrally placed catheter is most usual. For patients in shock calcium chloride is preferred over calcium gluconate because the calcium is in the usable, ionized form (i.e., metabolism of the anion substrate is unnecessary). Calcium gluconate has a lower calcium ion content per volume than calcium chloride. Additional doses of calcium should be based on repeated measurements of ionized calcium (if available). Hypomagnesemia should be looked for in any hypocalcemic patient who does not respond to replacement therapy.

Common complications of IV calcium ad-

ministration are dysrhythmias (especially bradycardia) and deterioration of cardiovascular function. Calcium has membrane-stabilizing effects, which will depress depolarization of cardiac cells, and this effect is more pronounced in the presence of digitalis or hypokalemia. Exogenous administration of calcium can markedly raise calcium levels, especially if the dose is given rapidly or if the patient is hypoalbuminemic. Myocardial ischemia and necrosis can follow an abnormal elevation in intracellular calcium. Infusions of calcium must be done slowly, cautiously, and with careful hemodynamic and laboratory monitoring.

Phosphorus. Reliable recommendations for correction of phosphate deficiencies are not available. An initial dose of 5 to 10 mg/kg of potassium phosphate, if the patient is also hypokalemic, or sodium phosphate, if the serum potassium is normal, should be given IV over 6 hours. Subsequent doses should be based on clinical status and repeated measurement of serum phosphate levels to keep the phosphate level greater than 4 mg/dl. Complications of phosphate administration include hypocalcemia and hypotension.

Acid-base balance. Metabolic acidosis is a common disturbance in shock and is most frequently the result of inadequate tissue perfusion and the accumulation of acid products of anaerobic metabolism. Metabolic acidosis is usually corrected as oxygenation of tissues and renal function improve; therefore, the logical treatment is restoration of blood volume and peripheral circulation. Occasionally, the acidosis may be so severe that pH correction is necessary before tissue perfusion can be restored. Correction is indicated in serious metabolic acidosis (arterial blood pH <7.20), particularly when the acidosis arises from loss of bicarbonate from the body. The adverse effects of this degree of acidosis are impaired ventilatory response, depressed myocardial function, dysrhythmias, and altered response of autonomic receptors to exogenous drugs. Sodium bicarbonate is usually chosen as the alkali for management of systemic acidosis. Emergency therapy is given as 1 to 2 mEq/kg body weight. However, further doses should be given as a one-half correction (one-half the bicarbonate space of 0.6, or 0.3) and be based on body weight and base deficit [mEq = body weight (kg) × base deficit × 0.3].

Too rapid correction of blood pH with bicarbonate may result in paradoxical CSF and intracellular acidosis, impaired delivery of oxygen to the tissues due to alkalosis and a shift in the oxygen-hemoglobin dissociation curve to the left, and precipitous hypokalemia or hypocalcemia. Use of large amounts of bicarbonate may result in hypernatremia and hypertonicity, which may be related to intraventricular hemorrhage in the newborn period and may cause large areas of tissue necrosis due to infiltration or vasospasm. In patients with respiratory acidosis, the administration of bicarbonate may actually worsen the respiratory acidosis since it is metabolized to CO_2 and water, with a further elevation in Pa_{CO_2}.

Cardiovascular-pulmonary system

1. Correct dysrhythmias. Tachycardia is usually corrected by volume replacement. Bradycardia and irregular rhythms may be due to hypoxemia, acidemia, alkalosis, drug excesses, surgical trauma, preexisting cardiac disease, hypovolemia, fever, and pericardial fluid. Catheters within the heart (right atrium, right ventricle, pulmonary artery, left atrium) may cause dysrhythmias and may have to be repositioned or removed if another cause cannot be determined.
2. Intravascular pressures respond to volume replacement except when cardiac or renal failure has complicated the situation. Inotropic agents and fluid restriction or dialysis may be necessary.
3. Since patients in shock frequently have altered mental status, they may not maintain or protect an adequate airway, and therefore the trachea should be intubated.
4. The only known treatment for muscle fatigue is rest; therefore, critically ill patients should be intubated early and treated with positive-pressure ventilation and supplemental oxygen. If support of the respiratory system is delayed until failure is obvious, mortality is greatly increased. Once intubated, the use of paralytic and/or sedative agents may have direct beneficial effects in further reducing oxygen costs of breathing in addition to their use as adjuncts to positive-pressure ventilation (see Chapter 97).
5. Management of permeability edema, or shock lung, is difficult and usually unrewarding.
   a. Supportive measures are used since no specific therapy is known; maintain arterial blood-gas tensions, acid-base balance, and the circulation at tolerable levels while the lungs recover. Use supplemental oxygen delivered with positive pressure. Adjust mean airway pressure to provide optimal distention of alveoli to increase functional residual capacity (FRC) back to normal and reduce inspired oxygen requirements without depressing cardiac output.
   b. Remove and minimize fluid accumulation in the pulmonary interstitium. The transmicrovascular flux of small and large solutes is favorably influenced by widening the intravascular hydrostatic-colloid oncotic pressure gradient (see Fig. 102-1) either by increasing plasma oncotic pressure or decreasing microvascular hydrostatic pressure. High oncotic pressures may be achieved by diuresis, by colloid administration, or both. Mannitol and furosemide have both been used successfully to withdraw excess water from the lungs and improve oxygen delivery. If renal failure prevents diuresis, the patient should be dialyzed. Colloid administration must be done carefully, since the colloid is likely to be lost into the pulmonary interstitium; colloid solutions may increase the pulmonary hydrostatic pressures, which will increase the trans-

vascular flux of water and solute. Avoid elevations of pulmonary microvascular pressure; the lower the LAP becomes, the greater will be the ability of interstitial fluid to move back into capillaries. However, reducing the LAP may decrease cardiac output drastically.

c. Use of vasoactive and inotropic agents may improve cardiac output; however, their effect on pulmonary vascular pressures must be closely monitored.

d. Corticosteroids, heparin, nonsteroidal anti-inflammatory drugs, and protease inhibitors have also been suggested in the therapy for shock lung.

e. Extracorporeal oxygenation is utilized as a last resort in the few institutions prepared to use it expeditiously. Although the idea of placing the lungs at rest is attractive, practical limitations are discouraging.

6. Obtain a chest roentgenogram since pneumothorax, pneumopericardium, hemothorax, or tamponade may be the cause of the shock or may be a complication of treatment. Successful treatment may be impossible if these are not controlled.

Other measures

1. Maintain patient's temperature at normal levels (36.5° to 37.2° C). Moderate increases and decreases in temperature increase metabolic demands and, therefore, increase oxygen consumption.

2. Neurologic deficits improve with correction of cerebral perfusion. However, the patient may require protection of the airway from inhalation of foreign material until the level of consciousness is returned to normal.

3. Renal.
   a. Prompt and adequate restoration of plasma volume and treatment of shock and left ventricular dysfunction are required to prevent renal failure.
   b. If fluid replacement is adequate but oliguria persists, mannitol and/or furosemide can be tried in an attempt to convert oliguric renal failure into high-output renal failure.
   c. Low-dose infusion of dopamine (2 to 5 μg/kg/min) may also be helpful in improving renal blood flow and function.
   d. Failure of these measures to induce a diuresis confirms the diagnosis of established renal failure and measures must be taken to meticulously control fluid, electrolyte, and acid-base balances.
   e. Dialysis should be anticipated and performed without delay if hyperkalemia, acidosis, hypervolemia, or altered mental status occur (see Chapter 110).
   f. While oliguria in shock is more likely to lead to concern and investigation than is polyuria, the latter may be just as important and as potentially lethal. Adequate urine output is occasionally associated with inadequate circulatory blood volume and/or renal function. These patients will require appropriate fluid therapy and electrolyte, mineral, and glucose control to preserve renal function and prevent progression to an oliguric renal failure state (see Chapter 17).

4. Hepatic, pancreatic, and gastrointestinal dysfunction.
   a. Ultimate outcome in severe shock states is profoundly affected by hepatic dysfunction. Maintaining an adequate circulation will help the liver to function normally and prevent hepatocyte damage. Continuous adequate nutritional support will provide the substrate the liver needs to maintain function (see Chapter 19).
   b. There is an extraordinary incidence of major pancreatic injury (pancreatitis, focal or widespread pancreatic necrosis, and pancreatic abscess formation) in patients who have been in shock.
   c. Paralytic ileus is usually gastric in origin unless there is associated peritonitis.
      (1) Correct electrolyte disturbances,

which may contribute to paralytic ileus.

(2) The stomach should be emptied and kept evacuated with an NG tube. The tube incites gastrointestinal secretions and the continued removal of these may cause acid-base and electrolyte disturbances that need correction.

d. Stress ulceration and erosive gastritis may occur acutely in patients who are critically ill. Acute ulcerations of the stomach and duodenum commonly occur in the victims of severe trauma (including head injury), hemorrhage, shock, sepsis, major burns, operations, and intracranial disease. Factors important in the development of acute ulcerations include mucosal ischemia and tissue anoxia and altered buffering of luminal acid (see Chapter 62).

(1) Stress ulcer bleeding or perforation can almost totally be prevented by titrating for gastric acidity every hour or two and maintaining a pH of 3.5 to 4.0 or greater with antacids preferably a non–magnesium-containing agent.

(2) Whether cimetidine (the blocking agent) will play a role is still not known; however, cimetidine used alone is not adequate therapy.

Cardiogenic shock

Although volume expansion and correction of extracardiac abnormalities may enhance cardiac function temporarily, pharmacologic interventions may be necessary to improve cardiac function. This approach to treatment relies on the use of drugs having the ability to restore or augment myocardial contractility and/or improve cardiac output and bring about a restoration and maintenance of blood flow. The proper choice of drug or drugs to be used requires knowledge of the exact hemodynamic disturbance and of the pharmacology of the drugs.

The majority of these agents are administered by continuous IV infusion, which should be given into a secure, centrally placed catheter. A second catheter, which may be peripheral, should be available to switch the infusion to in case of malfunction of the primary catheter. An infusion pump should be used and the infusions should never be interrupted, since the half-life of the drugs may be only 1 to 2 minutes. This catheter should never be flushed because rapid administration of these drugs can be fatal. All drug infusions should be carefully labeled with drug name, concentration, and diluent. The secondary catheter should be used for all other drugs, blood products, and fluids.

There is no usual drug or dose in shock; instead therapy must be continually tailored to the patient's response. These drugs are extremely potent, and excessive doses may be dangerous. The infusion rate should be related in terms of $\mu g/kg/min$ (micrograms [1000 $\mu g/$ mg]) and the proper rate to administer vasoactive and inotropic drugs can be calculated by the following formula:

$$\text{ml/hr} = \frac{kg \times \mu g/kg/min \times 60\ min/hr}{\mu g/ml}$$

Myocardial contractility: inotropic agents. Depression of intrinsic myocardial function diminishes the capacity of the heart to pump blood at rates commensurate with body requirements; therapeutic measures should be directed toward improving cardiac output by augmenting myocardial contractility.

The sympathomimetic amines are the most potent positive inotropic agents available; however, their effects are not limited to inotropy (myocardial contractility). They also possess chronotropic (heart rate) effects and complex effects on the vascular beds of the various organs of the body. Therefore, their use may in some instances be complicated by undesirable vascular actions or toxic effects on the myocardium. The available sympathomimetic amines are norepinephrine, epinephrine, iso-

Table 14-3. Common cardiovascular drugs used in shock

Drugs	Mechanism	Usual dose	Comment
Norepinephrine	α and β agonist	0.05-1.0 μg/kg/min	Intense vasoconstriction may mask the myocardial stimulating effect; may dramatically compromise peripheral tissue and organ perfusion; when systolic arterial blood pressure above 90 mm Hg, usually not indicated; now rarely used
Epinephrine	α and β agonist	0.05-1.0 μg/kg/min	Positive inotropic and chronotropic effects; intensity of stimulation increases with increasing dose; may lead to renal and mesenteric ischemia; causes tachydysrhythmias and increases myocardial oxygen consumption; has potent metabolic effects ($\uparrow$FFA, $\uparrow$glucose)
Isoproterenol	β agonist	0.05-1.0 μg/kg/min	Positive inotropic and chronotropic effects; peripheral vasodilator that diverts cardiac output to noncritical tissue (skeletal muscle); dysrhythmogenic: increases myocardial oxygen consumption
Dopamine	α and β agonist; dopaminergic receptor agonist	2-20 μg/kg/min (2-10 dopa, 5-15 dopa + β, >20 α)	Stimulates cardiac beta receptors by direct and indirect mechanisms; at low doses (<10 μg/kg/min) a selective dilation of renal and mesenteric beds occurs; alpha adrenergic effects predominant at higher doses; may increase pulmonary vascular resistance; value in newborns and infants is debatable; dysrhythmogenic
Dobutamine	Selective β_1	1-10 μg/kg/min	Positive inotropic effect with minimal chronotropic effect; mild β_2 activity; possible α activity
Sodium nitroprusside	Smooth muscle relaxation	0.5-8.0 μg/kg/min	Balanced arterial and venous dilator; rapid onset, short duration (2-4 sec); may increase pulmonary ventilation : perfusion mismatch; thiocyanate toxicity with nausea, vomiting, muscle twitching, sweating; cyanide causes early persistent acidosis
Phentolamine	α antagonist	1-20 μg/kg/min	Dilation of arterial and venous beds; indirect inotropic effect; duration of action 20-40 min; may cause tachycardia; expensive.
Hydralazine	Smooth muscle relaxation	0.1-0.5 mg/kg IV q3-6hr	Duration of action 2-6 hr; pure arterial dilator; may produce tachycardia; not for continuous infusion
Nitroglycerin	Smooth muscle relaxation	N/A	Venodilator; uncommonly used in children; exact dosage requirements unknown (under investigation)

From Perkin, R.M., and Levin, D.L.: J. Pediatr. **101**(3):325, 1982.

proterenol, dopamine, and dobutamine (see Table 14-3).

Digitalis glycosides are able to augment myocardial contractility in the failing heart and thereby increase cardiac output and decrease the ventricular filling pressures. However, this inotropic effect may be opposed by direct and reflex peripheral vasoconstriction, which is most prominent in patients with normal left ventricular function and is more evident with rapid intravenous administration. Thus, digitalis may produce an increase in inotropic state that is offset by increased afterload, resulting in no change in cardiac output. Renal excretion, long serum half-life, and slowly reversible toxic effects are other major drawbacks of digitalis glycosides for patients in shock. In addition, digitalis preparations tend to be quite ineffective in the acute management of cardiac dysfunction in shock. Cardiac output is generally not increased significantly and left ventricular filling pressure decreases only slightly. Since other inotropic agents are available that can be rapidly withdrawn, patients in shock should probably not receive digitalis early in their course.

Epinephrine (Adrenalin)
Action. Alpha- and beta-adrenergic.
Effects
1. Increases:
   a. Myocardial contractility.
   b. Heart rate.
   c. Arteriolar resistance.
   d. Pulmonary vascular resistance.
   e. Myocardial oxygen consumption.
2. Decreases:
   a. Venous capacity.
   b. Airway resistance.
Dose
1. IV push (1:10,000): 0.1 ml/kg (10 μg/kg).
2. Continuous infusion, older child: 1 mg/dl D_5W (10 μg/ml). NOTE: 1 dl = 100 ml.
3. Continuous infusion, small infant: 0.5 mg/dl D_5W (5 μg/ml).
4. Start continuous infusion at 0.05 μg/kg/min and increase by 0.05 μg/kg/min until

desired effect is achieved. A positive effect is usually achieved by a dose ≤ 1.0 μg/kg/min.
Cautions and complications
1. Causes renal and mesenteric ischemia.
2. Increases myocardial oxygen consumption.
3. Inadvertent overdosage may cause cerebrovascular hemorrhage, pulmonary edema, or dysrhythmias.
4. Incompatible when mixed with alkali.
5. Do not administer simultaneously with isoproterenol since serious dysrhythmias can occur.
6. Monitor heart rate and systemic arterial blood pressure closely.

Isoproterenol hydrochloride (Isuprel)
Action. Beta-adrenergic
Effects
1. Increases:
   a. Myocardial contractility.
   b. Heart rate.
   c. Myocardial oxygen consumption.
   d. Serum glucose concentration.
2. Decreases:
   a. Arteriolar resistance.
   b. Venous capacity.
   c. Airway and pulmonary vascular resistance.
Dose
1. Continuous infusion, older child: 1 mg/dl D_5W (10 μg/ml).
2. Continuous infusion, small infant: 0.5 mg/dl D_5W (5 μg/ml).
3. Start with 0.05 μg/kg/min and increase by 0.05 μg/kg/min until desired effect is achieved or heart rate exceeds 200/min or dysrhythmias occur. The maximum dose is usually ≤ 1 μg/kg/min.
Cautions and complications
1. Produces tachycardia.
2. May produce other dysrhythmias (ventricular fibrillation).
3. Diverts cardiac output to noncritical tissue (e.g., skeletal muscle).
4. Increases myocardial oxygen consumption.
5. Do not give simultaneously with epinephrine.

Dopamine (Intropin)

Action. Dopaminergic at lower doses (2 to 10 μg/kg/min); beta-adrenergic and dopaminergic in medium doses (5-15 μg/kg/min); alpha-adrenergic in larger doses (>20 μg/kg/min).

Effects

1. Increases:
   a. Myocardial contractility.
   b. Renal, mesenteric, coronary, and intra-cerebral blood flow.
   c. Systemic vascular resistance (at higher doses).
2. Decreases: systemic and pulmonary vascular resistance at lower doses; may increase pulmonary vascular resistance at higher doses

Dose

1. Continuous infusion, older child: 100 mg/dl D$_5$W (1000 μg/ml).
2. Continuous infusion, small infant: 50 mg/dl D$_5$W (500 μg/ml).
3. Start with 2 μg/kg/min and increase dose by 2 to 3 μg/kg/min until desired effect is achieved.
4. The usual range is 2 to 20 μg/kg/min, but doses as high as 50 μg/kg/min have been used.

Cautions and complications

1. Do not add bicarbonate, since dopamine is inactivated by alkaline solutions.
2. Overdosage is manifested by excessive systemic arterial blood pressure elevation.
3. Do not administer in the face of uncorrected tachydysrhythmias or ventricular fibrillation.
4. May not work in newborn.
5. Correct hypovolemia before treatment with the drug.
6. Ectopic heart beats can occur.

Dobutamine (Dobutrex)

Action. Selective β_1-adrenergic. May have α effects.

Effects

1. Increases:
   a. Cardiac output.
   b. Stroke volume.
   c. PCWP.
2. Decreases systemic vascular resistance.

Dose

1. Continuous infusion, small infant: 50 mg/dl D$_5$W (500 μg/ml).
2. Continuous infusion, older child: 100 mg/dl D$_5$W (1000 μg/ml).
3. Start with 2.5 μg/kg/min and increase by 2.5 μg/kg/min until desired effect is reached.
4. Usual dose range: 2.5 to 10 μg/kg/min.

Cautions and complications

1. May increase PCWP and cause pulmonary edema.
2. May cause anxiety.
3. Most side effects occur at doses >7.5 μg/kg/min.
4. Better for cardiogenic than septic shock.
5. Better in children >12 months of age.

Afterload reduction: vasoactive drugs. For the following reasons, the use of vasoactive drugs is advocated in the pharmacologic management of shock: (1) improvement of ventricular function by reducing afterload and (2) redistribution of blood flow in the microcirculation.

Improvement of ventricular function. Afterload is a term utilized to express the total force opposing ejection from the ventricle. This force is composed of resistive, compliant, viscous, and inertial components. Vascular resistance is felt to represent the largest single component of the total force opposing ventricular ejection.

The dysfunctioning ventricle has a decreased ability to adapt because the contractile state is depressed and there is limited preload reserve (see Fig. 14-1). In this situation, afterload becomes the critical factor determining myocardial performance. Compensatory changes associated with ventricular dysfunction tend to increase systemic vascular resistance and therefore afterload. This increase in arterial impedance, aimed at redistribution of blood flow and maintenance of systemic arterial blood pressure, may further depress cardiac performance. Therefore, in some patients with shock and depressed cardiac function, a reduction in afterload may improve cardiac output, and this provides the rationale for using vasodilators.

A large number of vasodilators, representing

several different pharmacologic classes, have been shown to improve cardiac performance and lessen clinical symptoms by means of arterial and venous smooth muscle relaxation (see Table 14-3). Arterial relaxation should result in an increase in ejection fraction, an increase in stroke volume, and a decrease in end-systolic left ventricular volume. Alternatively, venous relaxation should shift blood into the periphery and reduce right and left ventricular diastolic volume, with attendant beneficial effects on pulmonary and systemic capillary pressure. This, in turn, ought to be reflected in decreased edema, reduced myocardial wall stress, and improved diastolic perfusion of myocardium.

Mechanisms of action as well as the site of action differ considerably among the various vasodilating drugs. Therefore, before vasodilat-

or therapy is initiated, an exact hemodynamic profile should be obtained and the mechanism resulting in elevated systemic vascular resistance should be determined. Correct hemodynamic classification will prevent adverse effects, such as the fall in cardiac output that occurs when arteriolar dilators or venodilators are used in patients with normal left ventricular filling pressures.

The use of vasodilators in shock is generally limited to situations in which cardiac dysfunction is associated with elevated ventricular filling pressures, elevated systemic vascular resistance, and normal or near normal systemic arterial blood pressure. The efficacy of vasodilators in the treatment of ventricular dysfunction provides two pharmacologic means of improving cardiac output in shock syndromes: inotropic drugs and vasodilators. Occasionally the

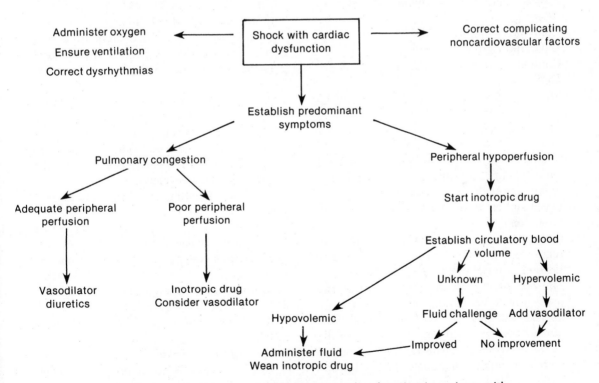

Fig. 14-3. Pharmacologic measures to improve cardiac function in patients with shock syndrome. (From Perkin, R.M., and Levin, D.L.: J. Pediatr. **101**(3):327, 1982.)

combination of vasodilator and inotropic therapy results in hemodynamic improvement not attainable with either drug alone. The proper selection of inotropic or vasodilator drug, either alone or in combination, requires knowledge of the exact hemodynamic disturbance and the mechanism of drug action (see Fig. 14-3).

Redistribution of blood flow in the microcirculation. The identification of specific etiologic mechanisms or substances that generate and sustain the lethal progression of the shock syndrome remains elusive and, therefore, treatment remains empiric. Failure of peripheral exchange-vessel or microcirculatory blood flow in the tissues remains the single common denominator in all shock syndromes.

Nitroprusside (Nipride)

Action. Smooth-muscle relaxant.

Effect

1. Decreases systemic and pulmonary vascular resistance (arterial and venous dilator).

Dose

1. Continuous infusion, older child: 10 mg/dl D_5W (100 μg/ml).
2. Continuous infusion, small infant: 5 mg/dl D_5W (50 μg/ml).
3. Start with 0.5 μg/kg/min and increase by 0.5 μg/kg/min until desired effect is achieved. The usual range is 0.5 to 8 μg/kg/min.

Cautions and complications

1. Should not be exposed to light (wrap in foil), since it is light sensitive and deteriorates.
2. Should be made fresh every 4 hours.
3. Onset and cessation of action are rapid (1 to 5 minutes).
4. Can cause a precipitous fall in systemic arterial blood pressure and close monitoring of systemic arterial pressure is mandatory.
5. The end product of metabolism is thiocyanate, which can cause nausea, vomiting, muscle twitching, and sweating. Blood thiocyanate levels should not exceed 10 mg/dl. In the presence of hepatic dysfunction or depletion of hepatic thiosulfate, the end product of metabolism is free cyanide.

6. Thiocyanate blocks the uptake and binding of iodine.
7. Monitor serum pH every 4 hours. Cyanide poisons cellular respiration and results in early persistent metabolic acidosis. (See Chapter 26 for treatment of cyanide poisoning.)

Phentolamine (Regitine)

Action. Alpha blocker.

Effects

1. Increases cardiac output.
2. Decreases systemic and pulmonary vascular resistance.

Dose

1. Continuous infusion, older child: 10 mg/dl D_5W (100 μg/ml).
2. Continuous infusion, small infant: 5 mg/dl D_5W (50 μg/ml).
3. Start with 1 μg/kg/min and increase by 1 μg/min until desired effect is achieved. The maximum dose is 20 μg/kg/min.

Cautions and complications

1. Can cause myocardial infarctions, cerebrovascular spasm, and cerebrovascular occlusions in association with marked hypotensive episodes.
2. Can cause tachycardia and dysrhythmias. Extreme tachycardia (e.g., paroxysmal atrial tachycardia, ventricular tachycardia) may cause heart failure and shock and should be treated by electroversion (see Chapter 5).

Hydralazine (Apresoline)

Action. Smooth-muscle relaxant; arteriolar dilator.

Effects

1. Increases cardiac output.
2. Decreases systemic vascular resistance.

Dose

1. Not for continuous infusion.
2. 0.1-0.5 mg/kg IV every 3 to 6 hours.

Cautions and complications. Produces tachycardia.

Nitroglycerin (Tridil)

Action. Smooth-muscle relaxant; venodilator.

Effects

1. Increases systemic venous capacitance.
2. Decreases ventricular preload.

Dose. Dose for children is under investigation.

Septic shock (distributive shock)

In septic shock one must identify and treat the infection with antibiotics and surgery when necessary. Early in the course of septic shock, the circulatory problem is usually not myocardial failure but decreased afterload secondary to increased vascular capacity and pooling of blood in the periphery. The proper treatment is to increase the blood volume as outlined in the section on hypovolemic shock (p. 74). Attempts to increase the peripheral vascular resistance with alpha stimulators such as epinephrine or norepinephrine are ineffective. Alpha stimulation decreases perfusion of the kidneys, skin, muscle, and intestines. The consequences of the decreased perfusion are a decrease in urine output and lactic acidosis.

As septic shock progresses, cardiac output decreases and systemic vascular resistance increases because of hypoxemia and acidemia. At this point, therapy should include the following measures:

1. Increase circulating blood volume with volume-expanding agents, as outlined in the section on hypovolemic shock (p. 74).
2. Use an agent that decreases peripheral vascular resistance. Isoproterenol, a beta-adrenergic agent, is most commonly used. Vascular smooth-muscle relaxants, such as nitroprusside, or an alpha blocker, such as phentolamine, may be used (see p. 86). Do not use any of these agents until volume expansion is complete.
3. Late in the course of septic shock, an inotropic agent may be beneficial. Isoproterenol both lowers systemic vascular resistance and provides an inotropic effect. If it is unsuccessful, the combination of an alpha blocker (phentolamine) or smooth-muscle relaxant (nitroprusside) and an inotropic agent, such as dopamine, may be tried.
4. Due to the possibility of subclinical adrenal insufficiency, all patients with shock that is unresponsive to other therapy should be provided at least replacement doses of adrenal corticosteroids until the status of the adrenal glands can be studied. (see *Appendix* for dosage.)

The use of large pharmacologic doses of corticosteroids in shock is not a new concept, yet its efficacy remains controversial. The mechanism of the protective action of corticosteroids is not completely understood, although several possibilities have been suggested. These are summarized in Table 14-4. The most important protective mechanisms that may enhance survival in shock are cellular. Considerable data indicate that several corticosteroid drugs sta-

Table 14-4. Suggested mechanisms of corticosteroid protection in shock

---

Circulatory
  Positive inotropic effect
  Vasodilation and improvement in regional blood flows
  Decreased production of vasoactive hormones
Metabolic
  Improved gluconeogenesis
  Antagonism of proteases
Cellular
  Increased neutrophil count
  Stabilization of cellular and intracellular membranes
  Promotion of type II pneumocyte proliferation
  Inhibition of granulocyte and platelet aggregation
  Protection against mast cell disruption
  Preservation of capillary endothelium
  Prevention of formation of toxic factors

Modified from Lefer, A.M., and Spath, J.A.: Pharmacologic basis of the treatment of circulatory shock. In Antonaccio, M., editor: Cardiovascular pharmacology, New York, 1977, Raven Press.

bilize lysosomal membranes and thereby prevent the release of endogenous proteolytic enzymes and acid hydrolases, which are responsible for tissue damage and the production of toxic factors (i.e., myocardial depressant factor).

The most recently suggested protective mechanism of corticosteroids is inhibition of complement-induced granulocytic aggregation. The plasma complement system presumably evolved as a beneficial antimicrobial mechanism; however, the complement system is activated in shock stages. Chaotic, nonmicrobial activation of complement components can be deleterious and may produce diverse tissue-damaging sequelae. Of particular importance is the complement component C5a. Generation of C5a leads to stimulation of granulocytes, and stimulated granulocytes have been shown to aggregate and cause leukoembolization and microvascular occlusion. Furthermore, complement-triggered granulocytes generate large quantities of proteolytic enzymes, arachidonic acid derivatives, and toxic oxygen radicals such as superoxide anion and hydrogen peroxide. These compounds may be responsible for endothelial and epithelial cell damage. In vitro data have suggested that high doses of corticosteroids inhibit both superoxide production and granulocyte aggregation.

Activated complement factors may also mediate platelet aggregation and embolization, platelet vasoactive amine release, and histamine and prostaglandin release. High concentration of glucocorticoids may also inhibit these deleterious consequences of complement activation.

5. If high-dose corticosteroid therapy is considered, specific steroidal agents are suggested. In general, the glucocorticoids are thought to be effective in the treatment of circulatory shock state, the mineralocorticoids are generally ineffective or aggravate the shock state. Studies suggest a higher incidence of improvement or survival or other beneficial effects when corticosteroids are given within 4 to 6 hours of presentation.

   a. Methylprednisolone, 10 to 30 mg/kg every 4 to 6 hours.
   b. Dexamethasone, 2 to 6 mg/kg every 4 to 6 hours until the patient's condition has stabilized.

6. Steroid therapy may be discontinued abruptly once the desired clinical response has been obtained as long as therapy has not lasted longer than 72 hours. Continued use of high-dose glucocorticoid therapy is not justified, since they are expensive, have numerous side effects, and their use is still controversial.

7. Principles of fluid and mineral, glucose, ventilatory, thermal, neurologic, and hepatic support are outlined in preceding sections.

ADDITIONAL READING

Altemeier, W.A.: Steroids in septic shock, Antibiot. Chemother. **31**:201-203, 1976.

Appelbaum, A., Blackstone, E.H., Douchoukos, N.T., and Kirklin, J.W.: Afterload reduction and cardiac output in infants early after cardiac surgery, Am. J. Cardiol. **39**:445-451, 1977.

Aubier, M., Trippenbach, T., and Roussos, C.: Respiratory muscle fatigue during cardiogenic shock, J. Appl. Physiol. **51**:499-508, 1981.

Barnett, J.A., and Sanford, J.P.: Bacterial shock in critical care medicine: current principles and practices. In Weil, M.H., and Shubin, H., editors: Critical care medicine: current principles and practices, New York, 1976, Harper & Row, Publishers, Inc., pp. 109-115.

Beck, J.L., editor: Handbook of critical care, Boston, 1976, Little, Brown & Co.

Behrendt, D.M., and Austen, W.G., editors: Patient care in cardiac surgery, ed. 2, Boston, 1976, Little, Brown & Co.

Bone, R.C.: Treatment of adult respiratory distress syndrome with diuretics, dialysis, and positive end-expiratory pressure, Crit. Care Med. **6**:136-139, 1978.

Bone, R.C.: Treatment of severe hypoxemia due to the adult respiratory distress syndrome, Arch. Intern. Med. **140**:85-89, 1980.

Calvin, J.E., Driedger, A.A., and Sibbald, W.J.: Does the pulmonary capillary wedge pressure predict left ventricular preload in critically ill patients? Crit. Care Med. **9**:437-443, 1981.

Carey, L.C.: Shock: differential diagnosis and immediate treatment, Hosp. Med. **11**:68-93, 1975.

Carlon, G.C., Howland, W.S., Goldiner, P.L., and others:

Adverse effects of calcium administration, Arch. Surg. 113:882-885, 1978.

Cohn, J.N., and Franciosa, J.A.: Selection of vasodilator, inotropic or combined therapy for the management of heart failure, Am. J. Med. 65:181-188, 1978.

Davidson, I., Gelin, L., and Halind, E.: Plasma volume, intravascular protein content, hemodynamic and oxygen transport changes during intestinal shock in dogs, Crit. Care Med. 8:73-80, 1980.

deLorimier, A.A.: Hypovolemic shock. In Pascoe, D.J., and Grossman, M., editors: Quick reference to pediatric emergencies, Philadelphia, 1973, J.B. Lippincott Co., pp. 5-10.

Driscoll, D.J., Gillette, P.C., and McNamara, D.G.: The use of dopamine in children, J. Pediatr. 92:309-314, 1978.

Drop, L.J., and Laver, M.B.: Low plasma ionized calcium and response to calcium therapy in critically ill man, Anesthesiology 45:300-306, 1975.

Glenn, T.: Cellular response to shock. In Skjoldborg, H., editor: Scanticon shock seminar, Amsterdam, 1978, Excerpta Medica, pp. 95-126.

Goldberg, L.I.: Dopamine—clinical uses of an endogenous catecholamine, N. Engl. J. Med. 291:707-710, 1974.

Grossman, M.: Septic shock. In Pascoe, D.J., and Grossman, M., editors: Quick reference to pediatric emergencies, Philadelphia, 1973, J.B. Lippincott Co., pp. 239-241.

Hardaway, R.M., III: Gram-negative shock, Antibiot. Chemother. 21:208-215, 1976.

Jacob, H.S., Craddoch, P.R., Hammerschmidt, D.E., and Moldow, C.F.: Complement-induced granulocyte aggregation, N. Engl. J. Med. 302:789-794, 1980.

Johnson, D.G.: Shock and its management in pediatrics, Hosp. Med. 11:22-41, 1975.

Kouchoukos, N.T., and Karp, R.B.: Management of the postoperative cardiovascular patient, Am. Heart J. 92:513-531, 1976.

Lappas, D.B., Powell, W.M.J., and Daggett, W.M.: Cardiac dysfunction in the perioperative period: pathophysiology, diagnosis, and treatment. Anesthesiology 47:117-137, 1977.

Lefer, A.M., and Spath, J.A.: Pharmacologic basis of the treatment of circulatory shock. In Antonaccio, M., editor: Cardiovascular pharmacology, New York, 1977, Raven Press, pp. 377-428.

Lowe, R.J., Moss, G.S., Jilek, J., and Levine, H.D.: Crystalloid vs colloid in the etiology of pulmonary failure after trauma, Crit. Care Med. 7:107-112, 1979.

Macklem, P.T.: Respiratory muscles: the vital pump, Chest 78:753-758, 1980.

Mason, D.T.: Afterload reduction and cardiac performance, Am. J. Med. 65:106-125, 1978.

Menquy, R.: The prophylaxis of stress ulceration, N. Engl. J. Med. 302:461-462, 1980.

Palmer, R.F., and Lasseter, K.C.: Sodium nitroprusside, N. Engl. J. Med. 292:294-297, 1975.

Perkin, R.M., and Levin, D.L.: Shock in the pediatric patient, part I, J. Pediatr. 101(2):163-169, 1982.

Perkin, R.M., and Levin, D.L.: Shock in the pediatric patient, part II, J. Pediatr. 101(3):319-332, 1982.

Shoemaker, W.C.: Cardiorespiratory patterns in various types of shock and their therapeutic implications. In Skjoldbor, M., editor: Scanticon Shock Seminar, Amsterdam, 1978, Excerpta Medica, pp. 127-144.

Shoemaker, W.C., and Hauser, C.J.: Critique of crystalloid versus colloid therapy in shock and shock lung, Crit. Care Med. 7:117-124, 1979.

Schumer, W.: Steroids in the treatment of clinical septic shock, Ann. Surg. 184:333-341, 1977.

Warshaw, A.L., and O'Hara, P.J.: Susceptibility of the pancreas to ischemic injury in shock, Ann. Surg. 188:197-201, 1978.

Weil, M.H., and Henning, R.J.: New concepts in the diagnosis and fluid treatment of circulatory shock, Anesth. Analg. (Cleve.) 58:124-132, 1979.

Weil, M.H., Henning, R.J., and Puri, V.K.: Colloid oncotic pressure: clinical significance, Crit. Care Med. 7:113-116, 1979.

Weil, M.H., and Shubin, H.: The "VIP" approach to the bedside management of shock. In Weil, M.H., and Shubin, H., editors: Critical care medicine: current principles and practices, New York, 1976, Harper & Row, Publishers, Inc., pp. 90-98.

Weil, M.H., Shubin, H., and Carlson, R.W.: Sympathomimetic and related vasoactive agents for treatment of circulatory shock. In Weil, M.H., and Shubin, H., editors: Critical care medicine: current principles and practices, New York, 1976, Harper & Row, Publishers, Inc., pp. 99-108.

Weil, M.H., Shubin, H., and Nishijima, H.: Gram-negative shock: definition, diagnosis and mechanisms, Antibiot. Chemother. 21:178-183, 1976.

Wiles, J.B., Cerra, F.B., Siegel, J.H., and Border, J.R.: The systemic septic response: does the organism matter? Crit. Care Med. 8:55-60, 1980.

Wetzel, R.C., and Rodgers, M.C.: Pediatric hemodynamic monitoring. In Shoemaker, W.C., and Thompson, W.L., editors: Critical care: the state of the art, Fullerton, Calif., 1981, The Society of Critical Care Medicine.

15 Anaphylaxis

FRANCES C. MORRISS

DEFINITION AND PHYSIOLOGY

Anaphylaxis is the term used to describe the symptom complex that occurs after the administration of an antigen to any suitably immunized subject. In this sense, it denotes all allergic reactions in humans that are manifested by systemic symptoms and signs, although most people associate it with an immediate life-threatening reaction.

The mechanism of anaphylaxis involves (1) the interaction of the antigen and an antibody, causing (2) release of pharmacologically active mediators, which elicit (3) the specific responses of various target organs. Thus, a patient must have been previously exposed to an antigen to have become sensitized to it and to have produced the antibodies necessary to initiate a reaction. The antibody involved is a heat-labile, skin-sensitizing antibody called reagin that belongs to the IgE class. This IgE antibody is located on the surface of perivascular and peribronchial mast cells and circulating basophils as well as in the serum. To induce a reaction, an antigen (often a drug) must induce an IgE response and, with subsequent administration, reach the tissue-fixed IgE antibodies.

Once the antigen reaches and combines with tissue-bound IgE, mediators are released that then act on target tissues to cause signs and symptoms. The major mediator is histamine found in mast cells, basophils, and granules located in perivascular connective tissue. Histamine produces leakage of venules, vasodilation, and a profound increase in airway resistance. Slow-reacting substance of anaphylaxis (SRS-A), a lipid material that serves as a medi-ator, is formed and released during a reaction. Its source has not been identified. It potentiates the action of histamine, causes bronchoconstriction, and enhances capillary permeability. The third mediator is eosinophil chemotactic factor of anaphylaxis (ECF-A), a preformed acidic peptide associated with mast cells. Other than the preferential attraction of eosinophils to the target organ, its actions are unknown. These three substances activate systems that release bradykinin and prostaglandins, secondary mediators in the anaphylactic reaction.

The clinical course of anaphylaxis is extremely variable. Manifestations may occur without prior occurrence of milder symptoms, and laryngeal edema or profound hypotension may be the initial manifestation. The time from antigenic exposure to onset of symptoms may vary from minutes to hours, partially depending on the route of entry. With parenteral administration, symptoms may be seen within 5 minutes and most reactions occur within 30 minutes. Duration of reaction is also variable; severity of symptoms, onset, and duration of the reaction may even vary in the same patient.

Symptoms may involve either a single organ system or several. They include:
1. Respiratory system.
   a. Rhinitis.
   b. Laryngeal edema with stridor.
   c. Bronchospasm.
   d. Pulmonary edema.
2. Cardiovascular system.
   a. Vasodilation and flushing.
   b. Hypotension with syncope.

c. Dysrhythmias: tachycardia, nonspecific ST and T-wave changes, ventricular fibrillation, asystole.
3. Skin.
   a. Urticaria with itching.
   b. Angioneurotic edema: nonpruritic asymmetrical swelling of an extremity or of the perioral or periorbital region.
4. Gastrointestinal system.
   a. Nausea and vomiting.
   b. Abdominal cramping.
   c. Diarrhea.

The patients at high risk for an anaphylactic reaction are those with:
1. History of previous allergic reaction to specific antigen.
2. History of atopy.
3. History of severe reactions in immediate family members.
4. Positive skin test (skin tests are not available for all antigens).

The most common antigens associated with anaphylactic reactions are antibiotics (penicillin), local anesthetics (procaine hydrochloride [Novocain]), analgesics (aspirin), dyes, contrast materials, hormones (insulin), vaccines, vitamins, heterologous sera, pollen extracts, insect and snake venoms, and certain foods.

MONITORING

See also Chapter 4.

Pay close attention to the patient's subjective impression. Often a patient can identify the beginning of a reaction before the onset of symptoms.
1. Cardiorespiratory system.
   a. Auscultate both lungs and over the larynx frequently to detect presence or progress of stridor.
   b. Measure systemic arterial blood pressure every 5 minutes during the reaction and hourly thereafter until patient is stable or recovered.
2. Inspect the skin for signs of rash and the face and joints for signs of swelling.

MANAGEMENT

Treatment of a systemic allergic reaction must be instituted immediately if the entire symptom complex is to be aborted. A delay to observe development of new symptoms or to start an IV may lead to a prolonged reaction or fatality. A reaction that is manifested as hypotension or laryngeal edema must be considered potentially fatal.

Specific

1. Give epinephrine, IM: 0.01 ml/kg of 1:1000 dilution up to 0.3 to 0.5 ml; IV: 0.1 ml/kg of 1:10,000 dilution (10 μg/kg). The treatment of choice is always epinephrine because its beta effect decreases release of histamine and SRS-A and causes bronchodilation; its alpha effect results in vasoconstriction of dilated capillaries.
2. Discontinue antigen administration and, if possible, isolate the site of antigen injection, bite, or sting from the systemic circulation with a tourniquet. 0.2 ml aqueous epinephrine of 1:1000 dilution may be injected into site after tourniquet is applied.
3. Increase inspired oxygen concentration.
4. The role of antihistamines is debated. Diphenhydramine hydrochloride (Benadryl), 0.5 to 1.5 mg/kg PO or IV, may be given prophylactically to a high-risk patient or to ameliorate the itching seen with skin reactions. Once histamine release has occurred, antihistamines will not reverse its effects and antihistamines have no effect on the other mediators of anaphylaxis.

Supportive

Continued observation for 24 hours is mandatory, since symptoms may reappear or wax and wane in severity.
1. Respiratory system.
   a. Continue to administer supplementary oxygen.
   b. Establish an adequate airway.
   c. For prolonged bronchospasm, consider

aminophylline or inhaled bronchodilators.

2. Cardiovascular system.
    a. Frequent heart rate, systemic arterial blood pressure, ECG monitoring, and level of consciousness.
    b. Circulatory support with fluids and pressors, preferably an alpha agonist.
    c. Treatment of dysrhythmias.
3. Skin.
    a. Diphenhydramine hydrochloride (Benadryl) may be continued until symptoms disappear. The total daily dose is 5 mg/kg, not to exceed 300 mg, either parenterally or orally.

    b. For severe reactions, consider steroids: hydrocortisone, 60 mg/m^2 IV every 4 hours or an equivalent dose of another steroid.

ADDITIONAL READING

Austen, K.F.: Systemic anaphylaxis in the human being, N. Engl. J. Med. **291**:661-664, 1974.

Committee on Drugs, American Academy of Pediatrics: Anaphylaxis, Pediatrics **51**:136-140, 1973.

Kelly, J.F., and Patterson, R.: Anaphylaxis: course, mechanisms and treatment, J.A.M.A. **227**:1431-1436, 1974.

Plaut, M., and Lichtenstein, L.: Treatment of immediate hypersensitivity reactions to drugs, Ration. Drug Ther. **8**:1-6, 1974.

16 Abnormalities in fluids, minerals, and glucose

DANIEL L. LEVIN
RONALD M. PERKIN

DEFINITION AND PHYSIOLOGY

Water is the largest single component of the body and, expressed as a proportion of total body weight, it is as much as 80% in intrauterine life and early infancy but falls progressively during the first 6 to 12 months to about 60% to 65%. After the age of 12 months total body water remains fairly constant at 65%.

The distribution of water within the body is complex. It is usual to regard body water as being divided into two major components, the intracellular fluid (ICF) and the extracellular fluid (ECF). This is a simplification since each space is divisible into several subspaces which differ in their water content. For purposes of this discussion the term intracellular water or ICF will be used to mean the total amount of water within all the cells of the body, while extracellular water or ECF will include the water in the interstitial spaces and in plasma. The ratio of ECF to ICF changes with growth such that there is a gradual increase in the ICF and a decrease in the ECF.

Maintenance fluid requirements consist of water and electrolytes, which are normally lost through the kidneys, skin, respiratory tract, and in the stool. Water turnover is an integral part of cellular metabolism and can be more accurately related to metabolic rate than to simple variables of body size. However, assuming minimal activity and the absence of abnormal thermal and other losses, a satisfactory estimate of maintenance water requirements can be made according to the scheme outlined in Table 16-1. These calculations assume renal function is not seriously impaired, so that of every 100 ml of resting water requirement approximately 55 ml will be excreted by the kidneys. In newborn infants the fluid requirements may be greater, depending upon the maturity of the baby and the ambient humidity.

The nature of the fluid to be given depends on many factors. In general, if the patient is neither depleted of nor overloaded with any particular electrolyte and renal function is normal, a maintenance solution should be used that will provide the doses of electrolytes and glucose shown in Table 16-1.

The usual maintenance requirements assume that there are no ongoing or abnormal losses of water and electrolytes via the kidney or extrarenal routes. Such losses, requiring replacement, do occur in the course of many diseases. Such patients require detailed attention to the composition and volume of the ongoing losses so that adequate replacement can be made. In critically ill patients with multi organ failure, each component of the IV solution must be calculated independently. The necessary concentrations of electrolytes and glucose are frequently provided in standardized IV solutions (see Table 16-2). Complicated fluid and electrolyte problems may require utilizing individual mixtures of the appropriate amounts of concentrated solutions (see Table 16-3). Spe-

93

Table 16-1. Maintenance fluid, mineral, and glucose requirements

Component	Weight	Dose	Example
Water*	For each kg ≤10 kg	100 ml/kg/24 hr	5-kg infant: 500 ml/24 hr
	For each kg, 11-20 kg	Add 50 ml/kg/24 hr	15-kg infant: 1250 ml/24 hr
	For each kg >20 kg	Add 20 ml/kg/24 hr	25-kg child: 1600 ml/24 hr
Electrolytes†			
Sodium (Na)		4 mEq/kg/24 hr	5-kg infant: 20 mEq/24 hr
Potassium (K)		2 mEq/kg/24 hr	5-kg infant: 10 mEq/24 hr
Chloride (Cl)		4 mEq/kg/24 hr	5-kg infant: 20 mEq/24 hr
Calcium (Ca)		50-200 mg/kg/24 hr	5-kg infant: 250-1,000 mg/24 hr
Magnesium (Mg)		0.4-0.8 mEq/kg/24 hr	5-kg infant: 2-4 mEq/24 hr
Phosphate (PO$_4$)		15-50 mg/kg/24 hr	5-kg infant: 75-250 mg/24 hr
Glucose		100-200 mg/kg/hr	5-kg infant: 500-1000 mg/hr

*Add 20% for infants placed in radiant warmers. Add 10% for infants receiving bilirubin phototherapy. Add or subtract 12% for each degree C above or below rectal temperature of 37.8° C.
†Usually infants do not require maintenance Na, K, and Cl during the first 24 hours of life. However, they frequently do require Ca during the first 24 hours of life.

cific disorders and fluid mineral and glucose balance will be discussed below.

Disorders of osmolality

Osmotic forces are important in determining the distribution of water between the intracellular and extracellular spaces. Cell membranes are more or less impermeable to most solutes but freely permeable to water so that ICF and ECF osmolality equalizes despite their different compositions. Each compartment has one major solute that, because it is restricted primarily to that compartment, acts to hold water within the compartment. Therefore, sodium salts (extracellular osmoles), potassium salts (intracellular osmoles), and the plasma proteins (intravascular osmoles) help to maintain the volumes of the extracellular, intracellular, and intravascular spaces, respectively.

The osmolality of a solution is determined by the number of solute particles per kilogram of water. Since sodium salts, glucose, and urea are the primary extracellular osmoles, the plasma osmolality and therefore intracellular-fluid osmolality can be approximated by the following formula:

Plasma osmolality =

$$2 \times [Na] + \frac{[Glucose]}{18} + \frac{BUN}{2.8}$$

where

$$[Na] = \text{Serum sodium concentration}$$
$$[Glucose] = \text{Serum glucose concentration}$$
$$BUN = \text{Blood urea nitrogen}$$

Hyperosmolality

Hypertonic states are characterized by increased concentrations of ECF solutes and net ICF volume depletion. When hypertonicity develops abruptly, osmolality equalizes primarily by water movement out of cells. The brain cells, however, protect cell volume by generating new solute intracellularly (idiogenic osmoles). The identity of these idiogenic osmoles and the speed with which they develop are functions of the cause and time course of hypertonicity, but if hypertonicity develops too rapidly, idiogenic osmoles may not form quickly enough to prevent permanent brain damage or death from intracellular volume depletion. Since it is unknown how rapidly idiogenic osmoles can be removed or

Table 16-2. Compositions of common parenteral fluid solutions

Solution	Solute	Concentration (g/100 ml)	pH	Ionic concentration (mEq/L)					Calculated osmolality (mOsm/L)
				$[Na^+]$	$[K^+]$	$[Ca^{++}]$	$[Cl^-]$	[Lactate]	
Dextrose in water									
5.0%	Glucose	5	4.7	—	—	—	—	—	250
10.0%	Glucose	10	4.6	—	—	—	—	—	505
Saline									
0.45% (hypotonic)	NaCl	0.45	5.3	77	—	—	77	—	155
0.90% (isotonic)	NaCl	0.9	5.3	154	—	—	154	—	310
Dextrose in saline									
2.5% in 0.45%	Glucose	2.5							
	NaCl	0.45	4.9	77	—	—	77	—	280
5.0% in 0.20%	Glucose	5.0							
	NaCl	0.20	4.6	34	—	—	34	—	320
5.0% in 0.45%	Glucose	5.0							
	NaCl	0.45	4.6	77	—	—	77	—	405
5.0% in 0.90%	Glucose	5.0							
	NaCl	0.90	4.6	154	—	—	154	—	310
Polyionic	Lactate	0.31							
Lactated Ringer's (RL)	NaCl	0.60	6.3	130	4	3	109	28	275
	KCl	0.03							
	$CaCl_2$	0.02							
Dextrose in polyionic									
2.5% in ½ RL	Glucose	2.5							
	Lactate	0.155							
	NaCl	0.30	5.1	65	2	1.5	54	14	265
	KCl	0.015							
	$CaCl_2$	0.01							
4.0% in modified RL	Glucose	4.0							
	Lactate	0.062							
	NaCl	0.12	5.0	26	0.8	0.5	22	5.5	280
	KCl	0.006							
	$CaCl_2$	0.004							
5.0% in RL	Glucose	5.0							
	Lactate	0.31							
	NaCl	0.60	4.7	130	4	3	109	28	525
	KCl	0.03							
	$CaCl_2$	0.02							
5% albumin	Albumin	5.0	6.9	154	1		154	—	310
(Plasmanate)	NaCl	0.9							

From Perkin, R.M., and Levin, D.L.: Pediatr. Clin. North Am. **27:**567-586, 1980.

Table 16-3. Concentrated solutions for addition to infusion fluids*

Solution	mg/ml	mEq/ml	mOsm/ml
50% glucose	500	—	2.53
3% sodium chloride	30	0.513	1.0
5% sodium chloride	50	0.855	1.7
15% sodium chloride	150	2.5	5.0
8.4% sodium bicarbonate	84	1.0	2.0
20% potassium chloride	149	2.0	4.0
10% calcium gluconate	100	0.46	0.7
10% calcium chloride	100	1.36	2.0
10% magnesium sulfate	100	0.8	0.4
50% magnesium sulfate	500	4.0	2.0

From Perkin, R.M., and Levin, D.L.: Pediatr. Clin. North Am. **27**:567-586, 1980.
*Examples: *Desired solution*   *Formula*

3.5% dextrose in 0.45% sodium chloride solution	7 ml 50% dextrose
	43 ml sterile water
	50 ml 0.9% sodium chloride solution
10% dextrose in 0.225% sodium chloride solution	70 ml 10% dextrose
	6 ml 50% dextrose
	25 ml 0.9% sodium chloride solution
15% dextrose	87.5 ml 10% dextrose
	12.5 ml 50% dextrose

inactivated, as hypertonicity is corrected, overly rapid treatment by infusion of hypotonic solutions can cause cerebral edema and seizures, which may be lethal or lead to long-term neurologic sequelae.

Hypertonicity occurs as a result of many different etiologies, indicated in Fig. 16-1.

Hypernatremia. The common denominator of hyperosmolar syndromes is depletion of intracellular water.

Hypernatremia with dehydration secondary to water loss in excess of sodium loss

1. Enteric disease. Symptoms of diarrhea, anorexia and vomiting lead to loss of water in excess of solute and to failure of water intake. Fever, hyperventilation, high solute load, and inability of the kidney to concentrate urine maximally may be contributing factors. Hypernatremia in infancy is a medical emergency, since the developing brain is highly susceptible to permanent damage or death. Clinical detection of hypernatremic dehydra-

tion can be difficult because plasma volume is maintained by the movement of water from cells; 10% to 15% of body weight can be lost before evidence of dehydration is detectable. Most patients have symptoms referrable to the CNS. If arousable, patients are irritable; however, depression of sensorium is characteristic, varying from lethargy to coma; many patients have seizures. These symptoms are related to the movement of water out of the brain cells down the osmotic gradient created by the elevation in plasma osmolality. Severity of the neurologic symptoms is related to both the degree and the rate of rise in plasma osmolality.

2. Primary water loss. Substantial water loss can occur through the lungs during marked hyperventilation and through the skin when environmental temperature is high and humidity low. Abnormal renal water loss occurs if there is a defect in the production or release of antidiuretic hormone (ISADH)

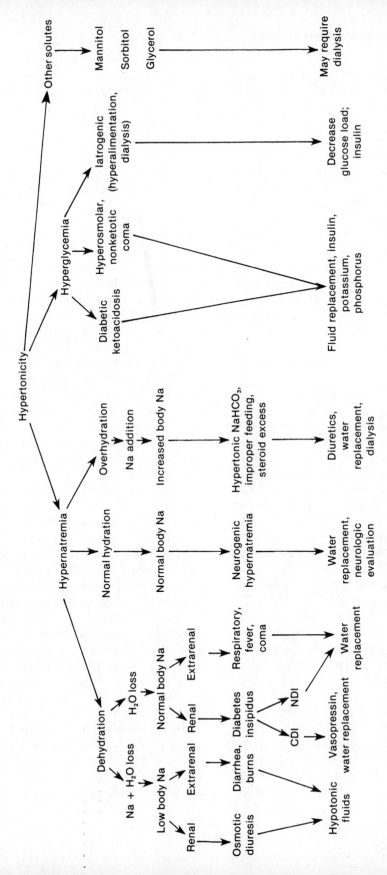

Fig. 16-1. The hypertonic state—diagnosis and approach to therapy. (From Perkin, R.M., and Levin, D.L.: Pediatr. Clin. N. Am. **27**:567-586, 1980.)

(see Chapter 51), if central diabetes insipidus (CDI) is present (see Chapter 52), or if there is a defect in the renal response to ADH, referred to as nephrogenic diabetes insipidus (NDI).

NDI is a congenital or acquired disorder in which hypothalamic function and ADH release are normal but the ability to concentrate urine is reduced because of diminished or absent renal responsiveness to ADH. Examples of acquired NDI can result from chronic renal disease, electrolyte disturbances (e.g., hypercalcemia and hypokalemia), sickle cell disease, and the use of some drugs. Hypernatremia due to NDI can be corrected with careful water replacement. Long-term therapy is usually not necessary, especially in patients in whom the defect is reversible or in whom polyuria is not a problem.

3. Osmotic diuresis. Osmotic diuresis can cause hypertonicity, whether the solute is permeable (e.g., urea) or impermeable (e.g., glucose or mannitol), because during brisk osmotic diuresis urine osmolality approaches isotonicity. Since the solute causing the diuresis constitutes a substantial fraction of the urine solute, the electrolyte concentration of the urine must be hypotonic relative to body fluids. Therefore, hypotonic losses may lead to hypertonicity in patients infused with urea or mannitol for treatment of cerebral edema and in patients with hyperglycemia and glycosuria.

Hypernatremia with normal hydration. Neurogenic hypernatremia is characterized by the absence of ECF volume depletion, a capacity to release endogenous vasopressin, and a normal renal response to vasopressin. Two types of neurogenic hypernatremia exist and they are both related to hypothalamic disorders that result in a defect in thirst (hypodipsia) and/or insensitivity of the osmoreceptors. The two types can be separated by their response to forced water intake. In one type, forced water intake is sufficient to return the plasma osmolality to normal, while in the other type, water loading is ineffective (essential hypernatremia).

Hypernatremia with overhydration. Most causes of hypernatremia with overhydration are iatrogenic or accidental. Severe hypernatremia can be produced by the acute ingestion or infusion of hypertonic sodium solutions, such as in infants given feedings with high sodium concentrations, infants given sodium bicarbonate for respiratory distress, or after the use of sodium bicarbonate during cardiopulmonary arrest. Rapid and massive increases in sodium draw water into the vascular space and may cause cerebral bleeding, pulmonary edema, and systemic hypertension.

Hyperglycemia. Hyperglycemia is a common clinical problem. Except for the unusual case in which hyperglycemia develops quickly in a hospitalized patient (e.g., during peritoneal dialysis [see Chapter 110] or total parenteral nutrition [TPN] [see Chapter 111]), most episodes of hyperglycemia take a few days to develop and result in glycosuria so that these patients will also have sodium and water loss from osmotic diuresis. There are two symptomatic, hyperglycemic syndromes: diabetic ketoacidosis (DKA) and hyperglycemic, nonketotic coma. The latter has been well documented in adults but appears to be rare in children.

Hypertonicity due to solutes other than glucose or sodium. Any ECF solute has the potential for causing hypertonicity; the most common of these substances is probably mannitol. Hypertonicity occurring because of mannitol implies either excessive doses and/or renal failure which blocks its excretion. To the extent that it is retained in the ECF, mannitol will increase the plasma osmolality and lower the serum sodium concentration in a manner similar to hyperglycemia.

Hypo-osmolality (hyponatremia). Since the serum sodium concentration is the main determinant of the plasma osmolality, hypo-osmolality usually reflects hyponatremia. Etiology, diagnosis, and therapy are outlined in Fig. 16-2.

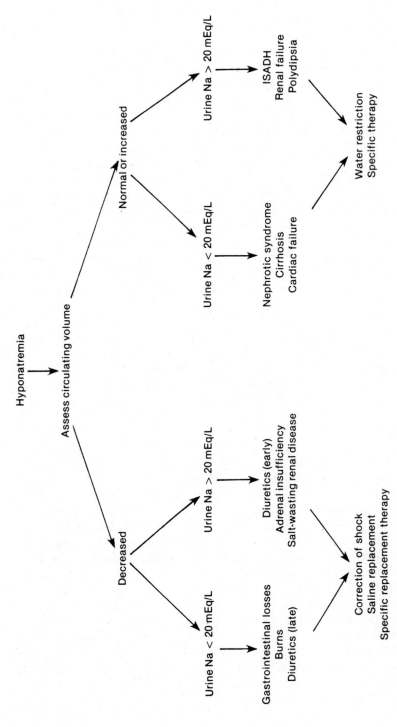

Fig. 16-2. Hyponatremia–differential diagnosis and approach to therapy. (From Perkin, R.M., and Levin, D.L.: Pediatr. Clin. N. Am. **27**:567-586, 1980.)

Since hyponatremia can occur as a result of either water retention or sodium loss or both, ECF volume may be low, normal, or high. If renal function is normal, analysis of urine sodium concentration is helpful in determining the etiology of the hyponatremia. As osmolality falls, an osmolal gradient is created across the blood-brain barrier, resulting in water movement into the brain, which is responsible for the symptoms of hypo-osmolality and hyponatremia. Symptoms depend on the etiology, magnitude, and acuteness of the condition; as the serum sodium falls to less than 125 mEq/L, nausea, vomiting, muscular twitching, lethargy, and obtundation appear; and when the serum sodium concentration is less than 115 mEq/L, the more severe symptoms of seizures and coma occur.

True hyponatremia must be differentiated from pseudohyponatremia; the latter condition exists with hyperlipidemia, hyperproteinemia, or hyperglycemia. Sodium salts are dissolved in the percentage of serum that is water (usually 90% to 93%); however, the determination of serum sodium concentration is performed on a diluted aliquot of serum. Therefore, a sodium concentration of 135 mEq/L of serum in a serum that has a water content of 90% would represent a concentration of 150 mEq/L of serum water (135/0.9). With hyperlipidemia or hyperproteinemia, the lipids or proteins may occupy a significant volume of the serum, so that the percentage of serum that is water is reduced. If the water content is reduced to 75% of hyperlipemic serum, then a sodium concentration of 150 mEq/L of serum water would correspond to a sodium concentration per liter of hyperlipemic serum of 112.5 mEq (150 × 0.75). Hyponatremia in these instances would not reflect an electrolyte abnormality or diminished effective osmolality of the water of the serum. With hyperglycemia, elevated glucose concentration increases plasma osmolality and promotes movement of water out of cells, diluting the concentration of sodium and depressing the level to the point of hyponatremia. Interpreting the hyponatremia as a decrease in plasma osmolality rather than as an increase in glucose level would be an error.

Hyponatremia with hypovolemia. Fluid losses in patients with hyponatremia and hypovolemia may have occurred by either renal or extrarenal routes. Extrarenal losses most commonly occur via the gastrointestinal tract (i.e., vomiting or diarrhea) but may be secondary to other disorders such as burns, pancreatitis, or peritonitis. The normal kidney responds to these hypovolemic states by conserving sodium and water; thus a hypertonic urine with a sodium concentration less than 10 mEq/L should be expected. A hyponatremic, hypovolemic patient whose urine sodium concentration is greater than 20 mEq/L may have adrenal insufficiency, particularly if the serum potassium concentration is elevated. The most common cause of hyponatremia with hypovolemia in the infant and young child is the salt-losing form of congenital adrenal hyperplasia. Other etiologies include congenital adrenal hypoplasia, acute infection, hemorrhage into the adrenal glands, inadequate replacement of adrenocorticosteroids, and inappropriate tapering of steroid doses.

Hyponatremia with normal volume or hypervolemia (dilutional syndromes). Hyponatremia may occur in patients with congestive heart failure, hepatic cirrhosis, and the nephrotic syndrome. These patients have an increase in total body water and thus they are hypervolemic. In patients with hyponatremia who have neither contraction of ECF volume nor expansion to the point of clinical edema, the syndrome of ISADH should be considered. Patients with ISADH have a concentrated urine in spite of hyponatremia; their urinary sodium concentration closely parallels their sodium intake and is usually greater than 20 mEq/L. Even with sodium restriction or volume depletion, these patients conserve sodium normally.

Disorders of potassium balance

Unlike sodium, which is located almost entirely in the ECF, potassium is an intracellular ion; it plays an important role in the regulation of a variety of cell functions. In addition to the absolute amount of potassium present, the ratio of the intracellular potassium concentration to the extracellular potassium concentration is extremely important because of its effect on the resting membrane potential of nerve and muscle cells (see Chapter 17). Hypokalemia increases the magnitude of the resting potential, thereby hyperpolarizing the cell membrane, making it more resistant to depolarization. Hyperkalemia, in contrast, reduces the magnitude of the membrane potential, making the cell more excitable and less able to repolarize. Even though potassium affects the resting potential, the effect of hypokalemia or hyperkalemia is still variable. Two factors responsible for this variability include (1) the speed with which the change occurred and (2) ions other than potassium including calcium, magnesium, sodium, and hydrogen that also affect membrane excitability.

Hyperkalemia. Hyperkalemia can be due to increased intake, increased movement into the extracellular space (acidosis, tissue catabolism, cell destruction), and impaired renal excretion (renal failure, adrenal insufficiency). The effects of hyperkalemia are limited to muscle weakness and abnormal cardiac conduction, the latter being the more dangerous feature. Prominent manifestations are found on the EGG (see Fig. 17-1). The earliest changes (with serum potassium levels of 6.5 mEq/L) are peaked, narrow T waves and a shortened QT interval which reflect more rapid repolarization. With increasing potassium concentration, the QRS complex widens and merges with the T wave to produce a sine-wave pattern. This is followed by ventricular fibrillation or standstill (at potassium concentrations ≥ 9 mEq/L). The cardiac toxicity of hyperkalemia is enhanced by hypocalcemia, hyponatremia, acidosis, and a rapid elevation in the serum potassium concentration.

Hypokalemia. Hypokalemia can be due to decreased intake, increased movement into the intracellular compartment (alkalosis, hypersecretion of insulin), increased urine losses (hyperaldosteronism, diuretics, renal tubular acidosis), and increased gastrointestinal losses (vomiting, diarrhea, continuous gastrointestinal suction). The symptoms of hypokalemia are related to its effects on skeletal and smooth muscle, renal function, and cardiac conduction. Typical physical findings are muscle weakness, diminished or absent bowel sounds, and abdominal distention. Polyuria and polydipsia occur due to a diminished ability to concentrate urine. Hypokalemia produces characteristic changes in the ECG: ST segment depression, decreased T wave amplitude, increased height of the U wave, and prolongation of the QU interval. These changes are primarily due to delayed ventricular repolarization). With more severe potassium depletion, increased P wave amplitude, PR interval prolongation, and QRS complex widening may occur. In addition, a variety of dysrhythmias may be present, which are increased in frequency and severity in patients taking digitalis.

Disorders of calcium balance

Calcium is the most abundant component of the skeleton and an important cofactor for neural transmission, enzyme activity, blood coagulation, and other cellular functions. Abnormalities of calcium metabolism are observed frequently in the neonatal period but are less common in older children and adolescents.

Hypercalcemia. Hypercalcemic disorders are rare in children. The differential diagnosis is limited to primary hyperparathyroidism, idiopathic hypercalcemia, immobilization hypercalcemia, and vitamin D intoxication.

The manifestations of hypercalcemia are the result of effects on multiple organ systems. Polyuria and nocturia are early signs. Other symptoms include weakness, fatigue, abdominal pain, nausea, vomiting, constipation, and lethargy; severe hypercalcemia inhibits neuro-muscular and myocardial depolarization. Cardiac contractility and irritability are increased, and concurrent hypokalemia and/or the presence of digitalis may increase the automaticity and predispose the patient to ventricular fibrillation.

Hypocalcemia. Hypocalcemia is an uncommon endocrine emergency that has multiple etiologies. It is defined as a total serum calcium concentration less than 7 mg/dl. In the PICU hypocalcemia is most frequently found in newborns, particularly those who are products of complicated pregnancies (e.g., infants of diabetic mothers) and newborns with hyperbilirubinemia, respiratory distress, cerebral injuries, or asphyxia. Other causes seen in patients in the intensive care unit are hypoparathyroidism, pancreatitis, hypomagnesemia, renal tubular acidosis, renal failure, and following parathyroid surgery, thyroidectomy, or any other surgical procedure in the neck.

Neonatal hypocalcemia is characterized by irritability, tremor, laryngospasm, twitching, and seizures. Infants may be lethargic, feed poorly, vomit, and have symptoms generally associated with sepsis. Hypotension, congestive heart failure, and renal failure may all result from hypocalcemia.

Total serum calcium levels are lower when serum protein levels are low but this may not alter ionized calcium levels.

Other common problems

Hypomagnesemia. Magnesium is necessary for a number of different enzymatic reactions involving transphosphorylation, carbohydrate metabolism, protein synthesis, and activation of adenosine triphosphate. In addition, serum magnesium concentration is an important determinant of membrane excitation; both magnesium and calcium depletion lead to increased neuronal excitability and enhanced neuromuscular transmission. Hypomagnesemia can contribute to disturbances in cardiac rhythm, especially when associated with digitalis admin-

istration. ECG changes of hypomagnesemia are a prolonged PR interval, wide QRS complexes, ST segment depression, and low T waves.

Causes of hypomagnesemia include gastrointestinal losses because of malabsorption, renal losses from diuretics, hyperaldosteronism, diabetes, and inadequate administration in patients on TPN. Hypomagnesemia is defined as a serum concentration less than 1.5 mEq/L.

Hypophosphatemia. Phosphorus is essential to muscle, nervous system, and red blood cell function; to intermediary metabolism of carbohydrate, protein, and fat; and to the body's entire apparatus of generating and storing energy. Severe hypophosphatemia (<1.0 mg/dl) can result from inadequate administration to patients on TPN, nutritional recovery after starvation, treatment of DKA, the combination of phosphate-binding antacids with dialysis, and the anabolic-diuretic state that follows severe burns. Consequences of severe hypophosphatemia include muscle weakness, acute respiratory failure, altered myocardial performance, hemolytic anemia, diminished phagocytosis, platelet dysfunction and hemorrhage, hepatocellular damage, and neurologic abnormalities including seizures, tremors, and coma. The majority of these problems are rapidly corrected by phosphate administration, and a positive correlation exists between the amount of phosphate administered and the serum inorganic phosphate levels measured.

In children the concentration of inorganic phosphate in serum varies between 4.0 and 7.0 mg/dl (1.3 to 2.3 mmol/L). In adults the concentration in serum varies between 2.7 to 4.5 mg/dl (0.9 to 1.5 mmol/L).

MONITORING (see also Chapter 4)

1. Check clinical signs every hour in severely dehydrated patients and every 4 to 8 hours in less ill patients.
   a. Skin turgor.
   b. Eyes (moisture, turgor).
   c. Anterior fontanelle fullness.
   d. Mucous membrane hydration.

e. Heart rate (continuously).
f. Capillary filling.
g. Systemic arterial blood pressure (continuously).
2. In addition to urine and serum Na, K, Cl, measure urine and serum Ca, Mg, and PO$_4$, and osmolality when appropriate. Measure BUN and serum creatinine at least every day.
3. Determine arterial blood-gas tensions and pH determinations initially in all patients and every 4 hours if abnormal.

MANAGEMENT

The components of fluid, mineral, and glucose therapy should be calculated separately using the guidelines given in Table 16-4.

Disorders of osmolality

Hyperosmolality
Hypernatremia
1. Hypernatremia with dehydration secondary to water loss in excess of sodium loss.
   a. Enteric disease
      (1) There may be a large water deficit, but rapid correction of hypernatremia with water can result in cerebral edema, seizures, and death.
      (2) Use the approach outlined in Fig. 16-3. NOTE:
         (a) The most important initial assessment is adequacy of intravascular volume. Once the intravascular volume abnormality has been corrected, one can proceed cautiously in correcting water deficits.
         (b) If the patient shows initial neurologic improvement and later deteriorates, cerebral edema should be suspected even if serum sodium concentrations and osmolality remain greater than normal. Administration of water should be stopped, and osmotherapy with hypertonic saline or mannitol should be begun and continued

until signs of cerebral edema (i.e., seizures or depressed level of consciousness) are no longer observed.
   b. Primary water loss: see Chapters 51 and 52.
   c. Osmotic diuresis: see Fig. 16-2.
2. Hypernatremia with normal hydration. In patients with essential hypernatremia, chlorpropamide has been successful in lowering the plasma sodium concentration toward normal.
3. Hypernatremia with overhydration. Since these patients are volume-expanded, the administration of water to lower the serum sodium concentration can aggravate the problem. Remove excess sodium. When renal function is normal, the sodium load may be excreted rapidly in the urine by inducing sodium and water diuresis with diuretics and replacing the urine output with water. In patients with poor renal function or in infants, peritoneal dialysis is usually required.

Hyperglycemia. Direct therapy toward each of the metabolic disturbances that may be present in the hyperglycemic patient, including hyperosmolality, ketoacidosis, potassium imbalance, and volume depletion. Since absolute or relative insulin deficiency is responsible for most of these problems, the administration of insulin and volume repletion are the mainstays of therapy (see Chapter 48).

Hypertonicity due to solutes other than glucose or sodium. If renal function is poor and sugar too slowly metabolized, dialysis may be required to remove the solute and the excessive ECF (e.g., mannitol).

Hypo-osmolality (hyponatremia)
Hyponatremia with hypovolemia
1. Expand the ECF volume with salt-containing solutions (see Chapter 14).
2. Fluid should be given to cover maintenance requirements plus deficit fluids.
3. Evaluate adequacy of replacement by physical examination and laboratory data.

Table 16-4. Correction of deficits of fluids, minerals, and glucose

Component	Deficit	Dose			Example (5-kg infant)		
Water*	5% (mild)	Maintenance plus maintenance × 0.5			500 ml + 250 ml = 750 ml		
	10% (moderate)	Maintenance plus maintenance × 1.0			500 ml + 500 ml = 1,000 ml		
	15% (severe)	Maintenance plus maintenance × 1.5			500 ml + 750 ml = 1,250 ml		
Electrolytes		Hypotonic	Isotonic	Hypertonic†	Hypotonic	Isotonic	Hypertonic
Sodium (Na)		10-12	8-10	2-4	55	45	15
Potassium (K)‡		8-10	8-10	0-4	55	45	10
Chloride (Cl)		10-12	8-10	2-6§	55	45	0-15
		(mEq/kg/24 hr)			(mEq/kg/24 hr)		
Calcium (Ca)		200 mg/kg/24 hr divided, by slow IV push every 3-4 hr (as gluconate)			≈150 mg every 4 hr		
Magnesium (Mg)		0.8 mEq/kg/24 hr in 3 divided doses, by slow IV push			≈1.3 mEq every 8 hr		
Phosphate (PO₄)		5-10 mg/kg (0.15-0.33 mmol/kg) IV over 6 hr (initial dose, then repeat measurement			≈3.75 mg over 6 hr		
Glucose		Increase by 100 mg/kg/hr repeatedly until serum glucose is 90 mg/dl (may desire higher concentrations, e.g., in Reye's syndrome)					

*Usually the first half of correction is carried out in the first 8 hours, and the second half of correction is carried out over the next 16 hours. If the patient is hypotensive or in shock, immediately give 0.9% sodium chloride or lactated Ringer's solution, 20 ml/kg. Repeat this until arterial blood pressure, capillary filling, and urinary output are restored.

†Patients with hypertonic dehydration may develop cerebral edema and seizures with rapid correction of water deficit. Correct such patients slowly over 48 to 72 hours. Never give such a patient fluid without some salt content (usually these patients are acidotic, and sodium bicarbonate can be added to D₅W to correct acidosis and provide some salt). This will help prevent the development of cerebral edema.

‡Potassium at a concentration ≤80 mEq/L at a rate ≤0.3 mEq/kg/hr.

§Balance indicates excess at the beginning of treatment.

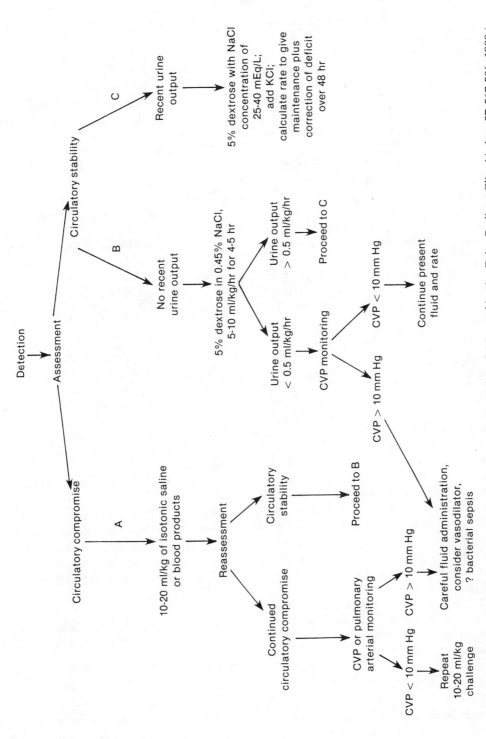

Fig. 16-3. Therapy for hypernatremic dehydration. (From Perkin, R.M., and Levin, D.L.: Pediatr. Clin. N. Am. **27:**567-586, 1980.)

4. Treat underlying disease and attempt to control ongoing losses.
5. When shock is present, give 0.9% sodium chloride solution rapidly, 10 to 20 ml/kg IV over 10 to 20 minutes.
6. Repeat this dose until systemic arterial blood pressure is restored and urine produced or until CVP is 10 to 12 mm Hg or PCWP is greater than 16 mm Hg.
7. Patients with adrenal insufficiency need glucose, potassium, and adrenocorticosteroid replacement (see Chapter 49).
8. Acute symptomatic hyponatremia is a medical emergency: use hypertonic saline (3% to 5%). NOTE: Because hypertonic saline can result in the complications of congestive heart failure or cerebral hemorrhage, use only enough hypertonic saline to correct serum sodium to a level of 120 to 125 mEq/L.
9. Calculate the amount of hypertonic saline needed using the following formula:

$$\text{mEq Na} = (0.6)(\text{body weight in kg})(120 - \text{Na})$$

where Na = serum sodium concentration in mEq/L

Hyponatremia with normal volume or hypervolemia (dilutional syndromes)
1. Direct therapy at maximal improvement of the underlying disorder.
2. Since total body sodium is already elevated, efforts to increase serum sodium through saline administration will only result in further expansion of the ECF volume and may worsen the clinical status of the patient.
3. Attempt to decrease total body water by severe fluid restriction.
4. Excess body sodium needs to be concomitantly treated by sodium restriction and judicious use of loop diuretics.
5. For treatment of ISADH see Chapter 51.

Disorders of potassium balance

Hyperkalemia (see also Chapter 17)
1. True potassium levels >7 mEq/L and/or ECG changes such as widened QRS complex, heart block, or ventricular dysrhythmias are an emergency.
2. Therapy includes (see Table 16-5):
   a. Diluting the ECF.
   b. Creating a chemical antagonism to the membrane effect of potassium by administering sodium bicarbonate and calcium gluconate.
   c. Increasing the cellular uptake of potassium by the use of glucose infusion and insulin.
   d. Removing potassium from the body by the use of potassium exchange resins or dialysis.
3. Treat the underlying disease to prevent further episodes of hyperkalemia.

Hypokalemia
1. Potassium replacement is the principal therapy. It is usually given IV, but if time and the patient's condition permits, the slower oral route may be safer.
2. Treat the underlying condition.
3. The rate of administration of potassium as well as the concentration of potassium in IV solutions must be carefully calculated. NOTE: Because cells have a limited rate at which they can restore their potassium content, rapid administration of potassium is potentially dangerous even in severely potassium depleted patients and may result in fatal dysrhythmias.
4. Monitor the ECG continuously and measure serum potassium concentration frequently.
5. Usually, infusion rates of less than 0.3 mEq K/kg/hr and concentrations of less than 80 mEq/L are adequate for replacement and are safe.
6. With alkalosis, potassium must be replaced as the chloride salt, since chloride depletion usually accompanies potassium depletion.

Disorders of calcium balance

Hypercalcemia
1. General measures
   a. Patients with hypercalcemia often have had anorexia, nausea, and vomiting for

Table 16-5. Treatment of hyperkalemia

Modality	Dose	Mechanism*	Comments
Calcium gluconate (10%)	0.5-1.0 ml/kg IV	2	Give in 2-5 minutes with ECG monitoring; the immediate improvement in ECG is a transient effect since there is no change in serum potassium concentration
Glucose	0.5-1.0 g/kg IV	1, 3, ± 4	Give as IV infusion over 15-30 minutes; follow glucose levels; insulin 0.1 u/kg SQ or IV may be required; effect begins in 1 hour, transient duration
Sodium bicarbonate	1.5-2.0 mEq/kg IV	1, 2, 3	Give over 5-10 minutes; effect begins in 30-60 minutes, transient duration
Sodium chloride	Isotonic solution (0.9%): 10 ml/kg IV or 3%: 3 ml/kg IV	1, 2, ± 3	More effective if patient is hyponatremic; transient effect
Sodium polystyrene sulfonate (Kayexalate)	0.5-1.0 g/kg per rectum (PR) or PO via NG tube	4	Give with sorbitol (70%)

From Perkin, R.M., and Levin, D.L.: Pediatr. Clin. North Am. **27:**567-586, 1980.
*1, ECF expansion
 2, antagonism to membrane effect
 3, Increased cellular uptake
 4, Removal of potassium from body
 ±, May or may not

some time prior to recognition, and severe dehydration and oliguria may be present. Rehydrate with IV fluids.

  b. Hypokalemia frequently occurs with hypercalcemia and will need treatment.

  c. If patient immobilization is the cause, mobilization and weight bearing, if possible, are effective therapy.

2. Gastrointestinal measures

  a. Reduction of the serum calcium by decreasing or eliminating dietary sources of calcium and vitamin D is simple but usually of no help in the acute situation.

  b. Administration of corticosteroids results in inhibition of calcium-absorptive mechanisms but also is of little help in the acute situation.

3. Renal excretion and dialysis

  a. Renal calcium clearance is a linear function of sodium clearance; urinary excretion of calcium can be increased by increasing urinary excretion of sodium.

  b. Use large amounts of sodium chloride solutions. If congestive heart failure or renal failure is not present, diuresis should be initiated with 0.9% sodium chloride solution and continued until the CVP reaches 10 mm Hg.

  c. Follow with infusion rates that maintain the CVP at this level.

  d. When this treatment alone is not effective, give furosemide 1 to 2 mg/kg. Furosemide is known to promote natriuresis and calciuresis even without the intermediate sodium chloride infusion.

  e. Ethylenediaminetetraacetic acid (EDTA) (50 mg/kg IV over 4 to 6 hours) increases urinary excretion of calcium by forming filterable soluble complexes that are not reabsorbed by the renal tubule.

f. Dialysis can be performed regardless of renal function and success depends solely on the calcium gradient established across the peritoneum.

4. Decrease bone resorption or increase bone formation.
   a. Corticosteroids.
   b. Mithramycin.
   c. Calcitonin.
   d. Phosphate administration.

Hypocalcemia

1. Use 10% calcium gluconate (100 mg/ml); give 2 ml/kg IV as an initial dose. (NOTE: Monitor cardiac rate for evidence of bradycardia.) Start replacement therapy (200 mg/kg/24 hr IV, divided 6 times per day. Measure serum calcium every 12 hours and increase maintenance dose as indicated (see Table 16-1) to maintain serum calcium 8 mg/dl.

Other common problems

Hypomagnesemia

1. Give 0.2 mEq/kg magnesium sulfate IM or IV every 6 hours. If IV administration is used, the dose should be diluted in a volume to be given over several hours so that hypotension is avoided.

Hypophosphatemia

1. Inorganic phosphate usually exists in serum as a mixture of two valence states, with an average valence of 1.8 at pH 7.4. Variations in serum pH are common and will alter the molar ratio and average valence of phosphate ions; therefore, the use of milliequivalents or milliequivalents per liter is confusing and may lead to large dosage errors. In contrast, the concentrations of phosphate ion in millimoles (mmol) and elemental phosphorus in milligrams (mg) are constant and independent of pH in therapeutic solutions as well as in serum, and therefore these terms are pre-

ferable. Each mmol of phosphate contains 31 mg of elemental phosphorus.

2. Maintenance requirements (i.e., hyperalimentation) for phosphorus are a dose of 0.5 to 1.5 mmol/kg/24 hr (15 to 45 mg/kg/24 hr).

3. For DKA, where hypophosphatemia is common, approximately 20 mEq/L of potassium replacement in IV solutions should be given as the phosphate salt (see Table 16-6).

4. Recommendations for correcting serum inorganic phosphate levels <1 mg/dl are not possible in a given patient, since neither the size of the body deficit nor the response to phosphorus therapy can be predicted.

5. Select an initial dose which will correct severe hypophosphatemia while minimizing side effects.

6. Hazards associated with administration of phosphate include hyperphosphatemia, leading to hypocalcemia and metastatic deposition of calcium phosphate; hypotension; hyperkalemia from excessive quantities of potassium phosphate; and dehydration and hypernatremia related to the osmotic diuretic effect of filtered phosphate.

7. Side effects are greater when phosphorus is given rapidly; therefore cautious rates of administration and low initial doses are recommended.

8. An initial dose of 5 to 10 mg/kg (0.15 to 0.33 mmol/kg) should be given intravenously over 6 hours.

9. Calcium supplements may be needed for hypocalcemia, but the addition of calcium to phosphate-containing solutions or administration through the same IV tubing causes precipitation and should be avoided.

Hypoglycemia. Give patients with hypoglycemia (<45 mg/dl) either $D_{25}W$, 2 ml/kg IV, or $D_{10}W$, 5 ml/kg IV (i.e., 0.5 g/kg). Be careful to maintain IV glucose administration with either D_5W or $D_{10}W$ thereafter to avoid reactive hypoglycemia, which can follow the administration of large amounts of glucose.

Table 16-6. Therapeutic parenteral phosphorus preparations

Preparation	Composition	pH	mOsm/kg H_2O	Phosphate (mmol/ml)	Phosphorus (mg/ml)	Sodium (mEq/ml)	Potassium (mEq/ml)
Neutral sodium phosphate	10.07 mg Na_2HPO_4 + 2.66 mg $NaH_2PO_4 \cdot H_2O$/ml	7.35	202	0.09	2.8	0.16	0
Neutral sodium; potassium phosphate	11.5 mg Na_2HPO_4 + 2.58 mg KH_2PO_4 ml	7.40	223	0.1	3.1	0.16	0.02
Sodium phosphate	142 mg Na_2HPO_4 + 276 mg $NaH_2PO_4 \cdot H_2O$/ml	5.70	5580	3.0	93	4	0
Potassium phosphate	236 mg K_2HPO_4 + 224 mg KH_2PO_4/ml	6.60	5840	3.0	93	0	4.4

From Perkin, R.M., and Levin, D.L.: Pediatr. Clin. North Am. **27**:567-586, 1980.

Glucose in a high concentration is a potent sclerosing agent and a secure large-bore IV catheter is mandatory. The umbilical vein is an inappropriate route for concentrated glucose infusion, since liver damage is a common consequence.

ADDITIONAL READING

Arieff, A.I., and Guisado, R.: Effects on the central nervous system of hypernatremic and hyponatremic states, Kidney Int. **10**:104-116, 1976.

Baumgart, S., Engle, W.D., Fox, W.W., and Polin, R.A.: Effect of heat shielding on convective and evaporative heat losses and on radiant heat transfer in the premature infant, J. Pediatr. **99**:948-956, 1981.

Berl, T., Anderson, R.J., McDonald, K.M., and others: Clinical disorders of water metabolism, Kidney Int. **10**:117-132, 1976.

Burch, G.E., and Giles, T.D.: The importance of magnesium deficiency in cardiovascular disease, Am. Heart J. **94**:649-657, 1977.

Feig, P.A., and McCurdy, D.K.: The hypertonic state, N. Engl. J. Med. **297**:1444-1454, 1977.

Finberg, L.: Hypernatremic (hypertonic) dehydration in infants, N. Engl. J. Med. **289**:196-198, 1973.

Goldsmith, R.S.: Treatment of hypercalcemia, Med. Clin. North Am. **56**:951-960, 1972.

Haddon, J.E., and Cohen, D.L.: Understanding and managing hypernatremic dehydration, Pediatr. Clin. North Am. **21**:435-441, 1974.

Hochman, H.I., Grodin, M.A., and Crone, R.K.: Dehydration, diabetic ketoacidosis and shock in the pediatric patient, Pediatr. Clin. North Am. **26**:803-824, 1979.

Holliday, M.A.: Parenteral fluid therapy in emergencies. In Pascoe, D.J., and Grossman, M., editors: Quick reference to pediatric emergencies, Philadelphia, 1973. J.B. Lippincott Co.

Kleeman, C.R., and Fichman, M.P.: The clinical physiology of water metabolism, N. Engl. J. Med. **277**:1300-1307, 1967.

Knochel, J.P.: The pathophysiology and clinical characteristics of severe hypophosphatemia, Arch. Intern. Med. **137**:203-220, 1977.

Levinsky, N.G.: Management of emergencies—hyperkalemia, N. Engl. J. Med. **274**:1076-1077, 1966.

Loeb, J.N.: The hyperosmolar state, N. Engl. J. Med. **290**:1184-1187, 1974.

Mendelssohn, S., and Rothschild, J.: Differential diagnosis of hyponatremia. In Swartz, A.B., and Lyons, H., editors: Acid-base and electrolyte balance, New York, 1977, Grune & Stratton, Inc., pp. 149-164.

Noguchi, M., Eren, N., and Tsang, R.C.: Parathyroid hormone in hypocalcemic and normocalcemic infants of diabetic mothers, J. Pediatr. **97**:112-114, 1980.

Perkin, R.M., and Levin, D.L.: Common fluid and electrolyte problems in the pediatric intensive care unit, Pediatr. Clin. North Am. **27**:567-586, 1980.

Robson, A.M.: Parenteral fluid therapy. In Vaughan, V.C.,

III, and McKay, A.J., editors: Nelson's textbook of pediatrics, Philadelphia, 1975, W.B. Saunders Co.

Root, A.W., and Harrison, H.E.: Recent advances in calcium metabolism. II. Disorders of calcium homeostasis, J. Pediatr. **88:**177-199, 1976.

Rose, B.D.: Clinical physiology of acid-base and electrolyte disorders, New York, 1977, McGraw-Hill Book Co.

Suki, W.N., Yium, J.J., Miaden, M.V., and others: Acute treatment of hypercalcemia with furosemide, N. Engl. J. Med. **283:**836-840, 1970.

Surawicz, B.: Relationship between electrocardiogram and electrolytes, Am. Heart J. **73:**814-830, 1967.

Weil, W.B., and Baile, M.D., editors: Fluid and electrolyte metabolism in infants and children: a unified approach, New York, 1977, Grune & Stratton, Inc., pp. 151-199.

Winters, R.W., editor: The body fluids in pediatrics, Boston, 1973, Little, Brown & Co.

17 Acute renal failure

RONALD J. HOGG

DEFINITION AND PHYSIOLOGY

Acute renal failure occurs when a sudden deterioration in renal function causes abnormal excretion rates of plasma constituents to the extent that disturbances in body homeostasis occur. This acute change may occur in previously normal kidneys or may be superimposed on chronically damaged kidneys. Persistence of abnormal renal function after correction of any prerenal hemodynamic abnormalities distinguishes acute renal failure from prerenal failure, a state that also results in the two cardinal features of renal failure, i.e., oliguria and azotemia.

Oliguria may be defined as a rate of urine production that is less than the volume of maximally concentrated urine necessary to maintain osmotic balance. In individuals receiving a normal diet the urine volume required to fulfill this need is approximately 300 ml/m^2/24 hr. Oliguria is therefore diagnosed when the urine flow rate is less than this volume.

Azotemia denotes an increase in the plasma concentration of nitrogenous waste products, notably urea. This condition is defined in practical terms as an elevated BUN level. Azotemia is a constant feature of acute renal failure, but other factors may also contribute to its development (e.g., high protein diet, glucocorticoids, tetracycline).

Uremia is the clinical state that develops in progressive renal failure. The condition cannot be defined precisely by laboratory values but refers to the situation in which severe abnormalities in cellular metabolism and extracellular solute concentrations lead to multiorgan dysfunction.

There are many causes of acute renal failure, but the basic defect is usually an acute reduction in the amount of plasma being filtered by the glomeruli. This may result from primary glomerular disease or may be secondary to pathologic processes that are proximal (abnormalities in prerenal or intrarenal hemodynamics) or distal (intrarenal tubular damage or postrenal obstruction) to the glomerular tuft.

Prerenal causes

The most common prerenal causes of acute renal failure are prolonged hypovolemia and/or hypoxemia associated with:
1. Burns.
2. Gastrointestinal fluid losses.
3. Hyaline membrane disease.
4. Prolonged perinatal hypoxia or hemorrhage.
5. Cardiac failure, usually associated with major cardiac surgery.
6. Septicemia.
7. Excessive use of potent diuretics, often associated with salt deprivation (a particular problem in children with chronic renal failure or nephrotic syndrome).

The extent of the renal damage produced by these abnormalities depends on the duration and severity of the underlying disorder. The age of the child is also a factor; renal vein thrombosis and medullary necrosis occur as a result of prolonged hypovolemia and/or hypoxia almost exclusively in young infants.

Another prerenal cause is major renal vessel occlusion:
1. Bilateral renal artery thrombosis; a disorder of infants that usually occurs in patients in

111

whom umbilical artery catheterization has been performed.

2. Bilateral renal vein thrombosis. As indicated above, this lesion usually occurs in hypovolemic infants. An increased incidence has also been found in infants of diabetic mothers.

Both of these major vessel disorders tend to be associated with gross hematuria, severe oliguria or anuria, and enlarged kidneys.

Intrarenal causes

Hemolytic-uremic syndrome. This is mainly a disease of infants and is characterized by hemolytic anemia, thrombocytopenia, and acute renal failure (see Chapter 47).

Rapidly progressive glomerulonephritis. This diagnosis is a descriptive term that refers to the fulminant course that may be seen in a number of glomerulopathies. In most cases, renal biopsy shows widespread crescent formation in the glomeruli, and it is common to find antiglomerular basement membrane antibodies on immunofluorescence studies. Disease entities that may produce this picture in children are lupus nephritis, membranoproliferative glomerulonephritis, Henoch-Schönlein purpura, polyarteritis nodosa, and, rarely, poststreptococcal glomerulonephritis.

Nephrotoxins. Many endogenous and exogenous substances are potentially nephrotoxic. The toxicity is dose dependent in most cases but may also represent an idiosyncratic reaction by the patient to a particular agent. The toxicity of many of these substances may be compounded in the presence of hypovolemia, because this will lead to the production of high concentrations of the substance in small volumes of urine.

Endogenous nephrotoxins

Urate nephropathy. In children, increased blood levels of uric acid are usually associated with lymphoproliferative diseases. In such cases, the turnover of leukocytes may be extremely rapid, leading to the production of large amounts of uric acid. The kidney appears to be particularly susceptible to the toxic effects of urates when urine flow rate is low. The use of allopurinol has greatly reduced the danger of urate nephropathy during leukemic remission inductions with cytotoxic agents, although occasional leukemic patients initially have high uric acid levels. Urate nephropathy has also been reported in the neonatal period.

Rhabdomyolysis and myoglobinuria. Many causes of rhabdomyolysis and myoglobinuria have been described in children. Of particular importance are hyperpyrexia associated with anesthesia and rhabdomyolysis associated with excessive exercise or septicemia. As with urate nephropathy, the contribution of hypovolemia to the nephrotoxicity of these states appears to be considerable. It is important to maintain a normal arterial blood volume in these patients.

Hemoglobinuria. There are multiple causes, and again the nephrotoxicity is augmented by hypovolemia.

Hypercalcemia. It is unusual for this electrolyte imbalance to be the primary cause of renal failure in children, but it may contribute to the acute renal failure associated with leukemia or postcardiac surgery (when large doses of IV calcium may have been given).

Exogenous nephrotoxins

Antimicrobials. Among the most common exogenous nephrotoxins are antimicrobial agents.

1. Aminoglycosides. Neomycin, gentamicin, amikacin, and kanamycin are the prototypes, but all aminoglycosides appear to be potentially nephrotoxic.

2. Cephalosporins. Cephaloridine is very nephrotoxic. The other cephalosporins are not as toxic; however, it appears that the combination of an aminoglycoside and a cephalosporin may have additive effects in terms of nephrotoxicity.

3. Penicillins. Methicillin is the most likely to cause renal damage, usually in the form of an interstitial nephritis.

4. Sulfonamides. Renal toxicity from crystal deposition can lead to acute renal failure, but this is uncommon with the newer sulfon-

amides. Care should be taken to maintain a good urine volume when using these agents.

5. Tetracyclines. Various tetracyclines and their metabolites may impair renal function in different ways, but acute renal failure is uncommon. However, the catabolic effect of these agents will result in increased azotemia in a patient with compromised renal function and may lead to uremic manifestations.

Diuretics. Aggressive use of loop diuretics may lead to oliguria and azotemia in conditions associated with increased total body water but reduced effective blood volume, as in some cases of chronic renal failure, nephrotic syndrome, and hepatic failure. Furosemide may potentiate the nephrotoxic effects of aminoglycosides when the two drugs are given together.

Other exogenous nephrotoxins. Ethylene glycol and heavy metals (e.g., mercury, lead) are nephrotoxic, as is phenytoin.

Acute pyelonephritis. This is a rare cause of acute renal failure, but it is important because it is one that is amenable to treatment when diagnosed.

Congenital renal anomalies. Acute renal failure in the perinatal period is often the result of severe structural defects in the renal parenchyma or the urinary tract. In some of these disorders there will be easily identifiable external stigmata, but this is not a constant finding. The following disorders should be considered in this category.

Multicystic kidneys. This is the most extreme form of renal dysplasia. The lesion is usually unilateral but may be associated with contralateral ureteropelvic obstruction resulting in acute renal failure.

Severe renal dysplasia. When bilateral dysplastic kidneys are present, the infant may develop severe uremic manifestations before the defective renal function is recognized.

Congenital absence of the kidneys. These patients do not survive. The deficient urine production in utero leads to the characteristic Potter facies.

Bilateral hydronephrosis and infantile polycystic kidney disease. These two disorders may also be associated with Potter facies. Both of these disorders are characterized by bilateral flank masses.

Postrenal causes

Postrenal lesions are rarely associated with acute renal failure in children. Possible causes are:

1. Ureteral obstruction
   a. Retroperitoneal fibrosis or retroperitoneal neoplasia.
   b. Calculus or tumor in patients with absence of one kidney.
2. Vesicoureteral obstruction. This may be secondary to bilateral ureteral reimplantation into the bladder.
3. Urethral obstruction by tumors, calculus, stricture, or valve.

Diagnosis

When one is confronted with a patient in whom oliguria or azotemia has developed, it is important to determine if the patient has suffered renal parenchymal damage or if there is a reversible prerenal or postrenal lesion that is responsible for the clinical presentation.

The most frequent problem is the differential diagnosis of prerenal azotemia and acute renal failure. In addition to the clinical evaluation of whether the patient is volume depleted, it is often helpful to determine the following:

	Prerenal azotemia/ oliguria	Acute renal failure
Urine sediment	Occasional hyaline casts	RBCs, coarse granular casts, RBC casts
Urine/plasma ratio of creatinine or urea	>14	<14 (often <5)
Urine osmolality	>400 mOsm	<350 mOsm
Urine Na concentration	<15 mEq/L	>20 mEq/L
Fractional Na excretion	<1%	>1% (often >3%)

The unfortunate aspect of this analysis is the fact that some overlap exists between the two groups in most of the variables. The most reliable index is the fractional sodium excretion, which is derived by the formula:

$$FEx\ Na\ (\%) = \frac{Urine\ Na\ concentration}{Serum\ Na\ concentration} \times$$

$$\frac{Serum\ creatinine\ concentration}{Urine\ creatinine\ concentration}$$

This term describes the proportion of sodium in the glomerular filtrate that is excreted in the urine and represents the renal tubular avidity and ability for sodium reabsorption. It can be determined using a random sample of urine and blood but is invalid when carried out in a patient who has recently received a diuretic or who has a chronic salt-wasting lesion on which acute renal failure has been superimposed.

In cases where doubt exists as to the presence of acute parenchymal damage and there is evidence of volume depletion, it is appropriate to institute a therapeutic trial. This trial will initially consist of volume replacement, the nature of which will depend on the composition of the fluid loss, e.g., blood for hemorrhage, saline for vomiting. Alternatively, diuretics (mannitol or furosemide) may be used, but it should be noted that a diuretic response to these agents may also be seen in cases in which early acute renal failure is present. Whether or not diuretic agents can reverse acute renal failure in its early stages is controversial. The main benefit of these drugs would appear to reside in their ability to convert an oliguric form of acute renal failure into a nonoliguric form, as discussed later.

MONITORING

See also Chapter 4.

When it has been determined that a patient with oliguria and/or azotemia has developed renal parenchymal damage, a number of variables should be monitored carefully so that complications can be treated promptly if they arise.

Renal-metabolic system

1. Accurate record of intake and output. Avoid a bladder catheter if possible.
2. Clinical assessment of hydration every 4 to 6 hours.
3. Body weight every 12 hours.
4. Serum Na, K, Cl, and HCO_3, and blood pH and Pco_2 every 4 to 8 hours.
5. BUN and serum Ca every 8 to 12 hours.
6. TSP, serum creatinine, and serum PO_4 every 24 hours.
7. Urinalysis daily when possible.
8. Urinary Na, K, and Cl every 24 hours in nonoliguric renal failure and during the diuretic recovery phase of renal failure.
9. Dextrostix or blood glucose every 8 hours, especially in patients whose fluid intake is restricted.

Cardiorespiratory system

ECG for heart rate and to detect cardiotoxicity. This is particularly important in the presence of hyperkalemia, hypocalcemia, or metabolic acidosis.

Hematologic system

1. Platelet count every 8 to 12 hours in patients with hemolytic-uremic syndrome
2. Platelet count, PT, and PTT every 12 hours in patients with DIC.

MANAGEMENT
Fluid balance

The management of a patient's fluid intake before recognition of renal failure will determine whether significant fluid overload or depletion is present at the time of diagnosis. In some cases the initial discovery of oliguria will lead to aggressive fluid administration in an attempt to push the kidneys into working again. This may eventually lead to dangerous volume overload, and the patient may develop pulmonary edema. Such a situation is particularly likely when acute renal failure is superimposed on abnormal cardiac function, as in acute renal failure occurring after cardiac surgery.

It is appropriate to attempt to induce diuresis in patients with fluid overload. This may be achieved in some cases despite the fact that renal plasma flow and glomerular filtration rate remain low. The most effective diuretic agent appears to be furosemide, a powerful diuretic whose action is achieved mainly through inhibition of chloride transport in the thick ascending limb of the loop of Henle. This agent should be used initially in a dose of 1 to 2 mg/kg, but in rare cases it is necessary to use as much as 5 to 10 mg/kg to maintain a good urine flow rate. When a response is obtained, oliguric renal failure may be converted into nonoliguric renal failure, a state in which it is much easier to manage the fluid balance.

Mannitol has also been recommended as a diuretic in acute renal failure. However, this agent, which is an effective osmotic diuretic in patients with normal or mildly impaired renal function and which can be useful in inducing diuresis in a patient with prerenal oliguria, should not be used when acute renal failure has been diagnosed. The administration of mannitol to a patient in whom renal damage has produced a significant fall in glomerular filtration rate will lead to the accumulation of mannitol in the circulation and may precipitate circulatory overload and pulmonary edema.

A more recent addition to the therapeutic agents that may be useful in prerenal oliguria is dopamine. When given in low doses as a continuous infusion (2 to 5 μg/kg/min), dopamine causes an increase in renal blood flow associated with natriuresis and diuresis without any appreciable effect on cardiac output or systemic arterial blood pressure. Somewhat higher doses (5 to 15 μg/kg/min) combine renal vasodilatory effects with cardiac stimulation, resulting in an increase in cardiac output and systemic arterial blood pressure. Dosage regimens greater than 15 to 20 μg/kg/min should be avoided because

of a paradoxical reduction in renal blood flow that results from such treatment. Whether low doses of dopamine will prove to be useful in established acute renal failure in children has yet to be determined.

Whatever the outcome of measures taken to increase the urine flow rate, it is essential to prevent further fluid overload of the patient. This may be achieved by providing the patient with a maximum fluid allowance of insensible water loss (300 ml/m^2/24 hr) plus external fluid losses, urine, stools, gastric aspirates, and blood. In most cases it is appropriate to induce a negative water balance by replacing none or only a portion of these losses. The decision regarding the fraction to be replaced will depend on the fluid-balance status of the patient. Successful management of a patient's fluid requirements depends on an accurate data base regarding fluid intake and output.

Hypertension

Hypertension is a common finding in acute renal failure, and systemic arterial blood pressure monitoring is mandatory. The frequency of measurements will depend on the status of the patient but should not be less than every 4 hours and occasionally will need to be every hour during the initial management.

The pathogenesis of hypertension varies according to the type of renal lesion. In patients with hemolytic-uremic syndrome, for example, the hypertension is associated with high plasma renin activity, whereas patients with poststreptococcal glomerulonephritis and hypertension usually have normal renin levels. The predominant cause of the hypertension is thought to be excess renin production in the former and fluid retention in the latter.

Acute elevations of systemic arterial blood pressure may result in abnormal neurologic signs and cardiovascular decompensation and should be treated vigorously. The first line of treatment is usually a potent vasodilator, but ganglion blockers and loop diuretics may also have a place in the management.

Some antihypertensive drugs to be used in parenteral therapy for acute hypertension are:

1. Hydralazine (Apresoline), 0.2 to 0.5 mg/kg/ dose IM or IV every 4 hours as necessary.
2. Diazoxide (Hyperstat), 5 mg/kg/dose IV by rapid injection. This may be repeated 30 to 60 minutes later if the response is unsatisfactory. Care should be taken when diazoxide is given after parenteral administration of hydralazine because the two drugs may potentiate each other and cause a dramatic fall in systemic arterial blood pressure.
3. Sodium nitroprusside (Nipride), 1 μg/kg/ min by continuous IV infusion.

As oral therapy for persistent hypertension, the following antihypertensive drugs may be used:

1. Hydralazine, 1 to 3 mg/kg/day, given three or four times a day.
2. Methyldopa (Aldomet), 10 to 50 mg/kg/day, given two or three times a day.
3. Minoxidil, in refractory cases, 0.1 to 0.5 mg/ kg/day, given three times a day.
4. Propranolol (Inderal), 0.5 to 2 mg/kg three times a day, in cases where excess renin activity is suspected or proved. Propranolol is not an appropriate mode of therapy for patients with acute elevations in blood pressure because it may potentiate cardiac failure.

Hyperkalemia

Electrolyte disturbances are many and varied in acute renal failure and can be adequately monitored only by frequent measurements of serum concentrations. The most serious electrolyte disturbance is hyperkalemia. When an acute accumulation of potassium occurs, the increased concentration in the extracellular fluid is not accompanied by an equal fractional increase in the intracellular fluid. This reduces the ratio of intracellular to extracellular potassium, which in turn reduces the cell rest-

ing membrane potential (normal, -88 mV) but has no effect on the threshold potential (normal, -65 mV). Since the excitability of neuromuscular tissue is defined as the proximity of the resting membrane potential to the threshold potential (normal gap, 23 mV), an acute rise in extracellular potassium may result in muscular irritability and enhanced myocardial excitability as a result of the increased proximity of the cell resting membrane potential to the threshold potential. It is the change in the resting membrane potential and the subsequent hyperexcitability of cardiac cells that presents the most dangerous potential complication of hyperkalemia.

Clinical consequences of cardiac changes produced by hyperkalemia depend on a number of factors other than the ratio of intracellular to extracellular potassium levels. The most important of these appears to be the level of serum ionized calcium. Whereas the potassium ratio dictates the resting membrane potential but has no effect on the threshold potential, the serum ionized calcium concentration is the main physiologic determinant of the threshold potential. A reduction in serum ionized calcium raises the threshold potential, thus reducing the difference between the resting membrane potential and the threshold potential and aggravating the hyperexcitability induced by hyperkalemia. Alternatively, an increase in serum ionized calcium lowers the threshold potential and reduces the excitability of the cell membrane.

This brief summary of the cardiac effects of potassium and calcium levels provides a rational basis for the treatment of hyperkalemia. When the onset of the electrolyte disturbance is acute, it is appropriate to treat it energetically, particularly if clinical and electrocardiographic evaluations demonstrate evidence of cardiotoxicity. In all patients with acute renal failure, the possibility of hyperkalemic cardiotoxicity should be evaluated and monitored by electrocardiography. Hyperkalemia may result in the following changes in the ECG: peaked T waves, widened QRS complex, prolonged PR intervals, absent P waves, and eventually complete heart block, terminating in a sine-wave pattern, ventricular fibrillation, and ventricular arrest (see Fig. 17-1). Control of the cell membrane excitability should preferably be achieved before abnormalities in cardiac rhythm occur, but if irregularities have already developed, the situation should be regarded as a medical emergency.

The cell membrane excitability may be reduced by increasing the resting membrane potential and/or reducing the threshold potential. To increase the resting membrane potential, it is necessary to increase the ratio of intracellular to extracellular potassium. This can be achieved by promoting transmembrane potassium transport into the cell or by decreasing the extracellular potassium level by measures that deplete the body of potassium. These physiologic manipulations are often attempted simultaneously.

An increase of potassium flux into cells occurs in association with (1) increased cellular uptake of glucose induced by insulin (released endogenously in response to hyperglycemia or given exogenously) or (2) increased hydrogen ion (H^+) transport out of the cell, a situation stimulated by extracellular alkalosis. The former may be achieved by IV administration of hypertonic glucose solution. Give 50% dextrose solution, 0.5 ml/kg, in combination with insulin (1 unit insulin per 4 g glucose), although endogenous insulin should be released in nondiabetic patients when hyperglycemia is induced by the administration of dextrose. Sodium bicarbonate solution will effect hydrogen-potassium exchange across the cell. This may be given as an 8.4% solution in a dose of 1 ml/kg body weight. Such treatment may be repeated once or twice if necessary.

Increased removal of potassium from the body can be achieved by the oral or rectal administration of a cation-exchange resin. Sodium

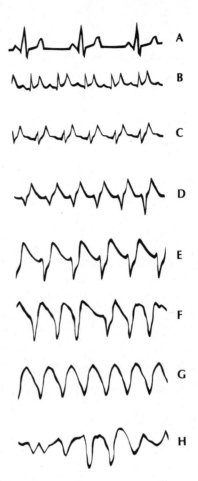

Fig. 17-1. A, Normal ECG for comparison. **B,** Rhythm strip from ECG in patient with hyperkalemia. Note peaked T waves, widened QRS complex, and prolonged PR interval. **C,** These findings progress, and, **D,** the P waves disappear. **E** and **F,** The pattern changes to a sine wave and, **G,** becomes ventricular tachycardia. **H,** Ventricular fibrillation is present.

polystyrene sulfonate (Kayexalate) is most commonly used for this purpose, in a dose of 0.5 to 1 g resin/kg body weight. A potential problem with this sodium cycle agent is that the sodium ions are exchanged for potassium to the extent that 2 to 3 mEq of sodium may be absorbed for each gram of resin administered. When sodium excess is also a problem, as it is in many patients with acute renal failure, it is important to remember this additional source of sodium ions that is being presented to the patient. When possible, give Kayexalate orally in 70% sorbitol. It is usually possible to remove 1 mEq of potassium per gram of Kayexalate.

The second method of increasing the gap between the resting membrane potential and the threshold potential, thus decreasing the hyperexcitability of cardiac cells, is to reduce the threshold potential. This may be achieved by increasing the serum calcium level. Calcium gluconate (10% solution) may be given slowly IV in a dose of 0.5 ml/kg body weight. ECG monitoring for bradycardia should be continued during this injection. If signs of cardiac toxicity persist, a second dose of calcium gluconate may be given. In each case the calcium should be given over a period of about 5 minutes.

Calcium and phosphorus imbalances

Hypocalcemia is a frequent finding in acute renal failure. The pathogenesis of this disorder appears to reside in the inability of bones to mobilize calcium even when stimulated by parathyroid hormone. This resistance to parathyroid hormone seems to occur because the active metabolite of vitamin D is necessary for the normal response of bone to parathyroid hormone; in acute renal failure the production by the kidney of the active vitamin D metabolite, $1,25 (OH)_2$ vitamin D, is impaired. Other causes of hypocalcemia may also be present, the most common being hypoalbuminemia and increased calcium deposition in damaged tissue. When significant hypoalbuminemia is present (albumin <3.0 g/dl), the protein-bound calcium will be decreased, leading to a reduction in total serum calcium level. This does not appear to have any physiologic significance provided that the ionized calcium level is normal. Increased tissue deposition of calcium is a particular prob-

lem in patients with rhabdomyolysis and myoglobinuria. In this disorder it appears that calcium is deposited in damaged muscles. Attempts to restore the calcium level to normal usually prove futile and only lead to further deposition of calcium in the damaged muscle. Hence, calcium infusion should be restricted to those patients in whom early signs of tetany are elicited.

Hyperphosphatemia is almost always present in acute renal failure and can be severe in urate nephropathy associated with leukemia and in rhabdomyolysis. The formerly held concept that hyperphosphatemia was the principal cause of hypocalcemia in acute renal failure no longer appears to be tenable. A major problem can result when hyperphosphatemia coexists with normal levels of calcium. In such cases, metastatic calcification may occur throughout the body, including vital organs. This process is occasionally fulminant and should be remembered when attempts are made to restore calcium levels to normal in the presence of high phosphate levels. Certainly the patient should be given calcium if signs of tetany (e.g., carpopedal spasm) are present; but if a patient is asymptomatic, it is prudent to treat the hyperphosphatemia before being too aggressive with calcium. The medical management of hyperphosphatemia consists of giving a phosphate-binding gel such as aluminum hydroxide (Amphojel), 15 to 30 ml every 4 hours PO or by gavage.

Nutritional aspects of management

There is now abundant evidence that the administration of essential amino acids may hasten the recovery of patients with acute renal failure. Essential amino acids induce the reutilization of urea and in addition have been shown to increase the rate of recovery of injured renal parenchyma when this tissue has been examined in vitro. The route of administration depends on the clinical status of the patient.

A number of oral preparations are commercially available and should be used if the patient has an intact gastrointestinal tract and can be given essential amino acids orally. If the oral route is not available, it is appropriate to administer essential amino acids IV. Details of the composition of commercial preparations available for oral and IV administration are given in Chapters 111 and 112. In addition to the eight amino acids that are usually provided in such mixtures, histidine and arginine should also be present in the mixtures given to uremic infants and children. Histidine has been shown to improve the nitrogen balance of uremic patients, and arginine helps to prevent hyperammonemia, a problem that may complicate parenteral nutrition. Some of the commercial amino acid mixtures include histidine and arginine in their compositions.

Nonmedical management

If medical measures are insufficient in patients with acute renal failure, it is necessary to institute peritoneal dialysis or hemodialysis. The indications for commencing dialysis are provided in Chapter 110.

Prognosis

The prognosis for children with acute renal failure resulting from primary renal disease is usually good if appropriate care is given. Patients with renal failure associated with other major organ system failures do not fare as well and the prognosis in such circumstances has improved little in recent years despite careful attention to fluid balance, normalization of electrolytes, improved nutritional support, and aggressive use of dialysis.

ADDITIONAL READING

Abel, R.M., Beck, C.H., Abbott, W.M., and others: Improved survival from acute renal failure after treatment with intravenous essential amino acids and glucose, N. Engl. J. Med. 288:695-699, 1973.

Abitol, C.L., and Holliday, M.A.: Total parenteral nutrition in anuric children, Clin. Nephrol. 5:153-158, 1976.

Driscoll, D.J., Gillette, P.C., and McNamara, D.G.: The use of dopamine in children, J. Pediatr. 92:309-314, 1978.

Ellis, D., Gartner, J.C., and Galvis, A.G.: Acute renal failure in infants and children: diagnosis, complications, and treatment, Crit. Care Med. 9:607-617, 1981.

Flinn, R.B., Merrill, J.P., and Welzant, W.R.: Treatment of the oliguric patient with a new sodium-exchange resin and sorbitol, N. Engl. J. Med. 264:111-115, 1961.

Greenhill, A.H., Norman, M.E., Cornfield, D., and others: Acute renal failure secondary to acute pyelonephritis, Clin. Nephrol. 8:400-403, 1977.

Hodson, E.M., Kjellstrand, C.M., and Mauer, S.M.: Acute renal failure in infants and children: outcome of 53 patients requiring hemodialysis treatment, J. Pediatr. 93:756-761, 1978.

Oken, D.E.: On the passive back-flow theory of acute renal failure, Am. J. Med. 58:77-82, 1975.

Porter, G.A., and Starr, A.: Management of postoperative renal failure following cardiovascular surgery, Surgery 65:390-398, 1969.

Powell, H.R., Rotenberg, E., Williams, A.L., and McCredie, D.A.: Plasma renin activity in acute poststreptococcal glomerulonephritis and the haemolytic-uraemic syndrome, Arch. Dis. Child. 49:802-807, 1974.

Seldin, D.W., Carter, N.W., and Rector, F.C.: Consequences of renal failure and their management in diseases of the kidney. In Strauss, M.B., and Welt, L.G., editors: Diseases of the kidney, ed. 2, Edinburgh, 1971, Churchill Livingstone.

Thurau, K., and Boylan, J.W.: Acute renal success, Am. J. Med. 61:308-315, 1976.

Toback, F.G.: Amino acid enhancement of renal regeneration after acute tubular necrosis, Kidney Int. 12:193-198, 1977.

Weidner, N.J., Gaum, W.E., Chou, T.C., and Kaplan, S.: Hyperkalemia—electrocardiographic abnormalities, J. Pediatr. 93:462-464, 1978.

18 Abnormalities in temperature regulation

FRANCES C. MORRISS

DEFINITION AND PHYSIOLOGY

The temperature of an object is a measure of the kinetic activity of its molecules and is proportional to the amount of heat stored in the object.

Body temperature is maintained within a narrow range (36° to 37.5° C) by the CNS where the internal thermostat is located in the preoptic nucleus of the hypothalamus. Changes in the temperature of hypothalamic tissue cause alterations in emission of impulses from these thermosensitive cells, resulting in regulation of heat loss and production.

Heat loss

Heat is lost from the body by:
1. Radiation: the direct transfer of heat from the body to the surrounding environment in the form of infrared heat rays; 60% of total heat loss is radiant. The amount of heat loss varies directly with the difference between the temperature of the body surface and the average temperature of the environment.
2. Conduction: the direct transfer of heat from the body to another surface; this accounts for 3% of total body heat loss. Conductivity in water is much greater than in air.
3. Conduction to air with convection: the direct transfer to air of body heat, which is then carried away by air currents; 12% of total body heat loss is by convection. The presence of drafts or wind increases loss by convection.
4. Evaporation: 0.58 calories of heat are lost for each gram of water that evaporates from the body surface; 22% of total heat loss is evaporative. Insensible water loss from sweat on the skin and from the lungs of an adult is 600 ml/day (200 to 400 ml/m² body surface area) or about 12 to 18 calories/hr. When the environmental temperature is greater than body temperature, the body gains heat by radiation and conduction from the environment. Under these conditions, the only means by which the body can lose heat is evaporation; therefore, any factor preventing evaporation will increase body temperature. Evaporative losses are reduced with increased humidity because sweat excreted on the body surface remains in the liquid state. Convection augments heat loss by evaporation, since air saturated with moisture from the skin moves away and is replaced with unsaturated air.

Heat production

Sources of heat in the body include:
1. Production of heat secondary to metabolic activities of tissues. Under basal conditions, 40 calories of heat/hr/m² of body surface are produced.
2. Heat from chemical reactions in contracting muscles.
3. Specific action of thyroxine on cells to increase metabolic activity.
4. Specific action of catecholamines on cells.
5. Specific action of increased temperature on cellular metabolic reactions. Because the

rate of chemical reaction increases with increasing temperature, heat production rises.

When the hypothalamus becomes overheated, heat production is decreased and heat losses are increased by:

1. Stimulation of sweating. Sweat glands, which are innervated by cholinergic fibers, are under direct control of the hypothalamic thermostat. Increased fluid on the body surface increases heat loss by evaporation.
2. Increased conduction of heat to the body surface, where it can be lost by conduction and radiation. This is accomplished by dilation of the venous plexus of the skin, producing a high flow of blood to the skin from the heat-producing internal organs. Vasodilation is controlled by the sympathetic nervous system. If blood flow from internal structures to the skin is impeded, the only way heat produced internally can be dissipated is by direct transfer of heat from one tissue to another (diffusion).

Cooling of the hypothalamus causes increased heat production via:

1. Nonshivering thermogenesis mediated by secretion of thyroxine and release of epinephrine and norepinephrine.
2. Progressive increase in muscle tone and increased oxygen consumption. At a critical muscle tone, shivering occurs, which greatly increases heat production from muscles. This is the most effective mechanism for increasing core temperature.

Cooling of the hypothalamus also causes decreased heat loss by inducing vasoconstriction and abolishing sweating.

HYPERTHERMIA

Hyperthermia is defined as core temperature greater than normal (greater than 38° C). Mild degrees of hyperthermia probably do not require treatment, but temperatures greater than 40° C warrant attention, since the body's mechanisms for temperature control may begin to fail.

Signs of extreme hyperthermia include hot, dry skin, coma, small reactive pupils, and diffuse hypertonia. Permanent neurologic sequelae are common.

Initially, the patient may be irritable, with headache, dizziness, confusion, and ataxia. With higher temperatures, seizures followed by coma occur. The EEG may show diffuse slowing.

Causes of extreme temperature include:

1. Infection, which is most often secondary to blood-borne gram-negative organisms. Lipopolysaccharides from bacteria (exogenous pyrogens) and protein breakdown products released from white blood cells (WBCs) and degenerating tissue (endogenous pyrogens) reset the hypothalamic thermostat, causing increased heat production.
2. Thermoregulatory failure from:
   a. Excessive heat production seen with hypermetabolic states such as malignant hyperpyrexia, untreated status epilepticus, thyroid storm, and narcotic withdrawal in the neonate.
   b. Impaired heat dissipation associated with heat stroke, burns, dehydration, or autonomic dysfunction secondary to spinal cord transection, congenital absence of sweat glands, or atropine toxicity.
   c. Disordered hypothalamic function associated with massive intracranial hemorrhage or CNS infection. Anticholinergics, belladonna alkaloids, phenothiazines, antihistamines, and tricyclic antidepressants can also disrupt central hypothalamic function.

The consequences of untreated high fever are:

1. Failure of heat-controlling mechanisms; at 41.6° C, heat-dissipating mechanisms are ineffective and the following events occur:
   a. Depression of hypothalamic function.
   b. Failure of sweating.
   c. Increased heat production secondary to high temperature.

d. Associated dehydration may reset hypothalamic thermostat to a higher point.

2. Parenchymal degeneration, beginning at temperatures of 41° C; CNS and muscle tissue are the most susceptible to damage.

3. A generalized hypermetabolic state, affecting all organ systems:

    a. Cardiovascular. Increased oxygen consumption may stress the cardiovascular system. There is diminished peripheral vascular resistance, with vasodilation, hypotension, and increased cardiac output, heart rate, and stroke volume. PVCs, supraventricular tachycardia, ST depression, and T-wave changes can be seen.

    b. Muscular. Generalized rhabdomyolysis may cause myoglobinuria, with subsequent renal failure and hypocalcemia secondary to calcium sequestration in necrotic muscle. Muscle cramps occur commonly.

    c. Respiratory. Hyperventilation may initially cause alkalosis and tetany. Thereafter, metabolic acidosis supervenes. The alkalosis may cause hypophosphatemia secondary to increased cellular uptake of phosphorus. In malignant hyperpyrexia, hypercarbia secondary to increased CO_2 production and hypoxia are common.

    d. Gastrointestinal. Vomiting and diarrhea may occur.

    e. Hepatic. Liver failure may be seen late in the course of extreme hyperpyrexia; enzymatic evidence of less serious damage is common in the first 2 to 3 days following the initial insult.

    f. Hematologic. Abnormalities include signs of DIC and hemolysis.

    g. Metabolic. Profound metabolic acidosis follows a respiratory acidosis. Excessive fluid losses via lungs and skin (sweat) cause disorders of volume as well as of electrolytes; insensible fluid losses increase 10% for every 1° C increase in temperature. Hyperkalemia is commonly seen with muscle tissue destruction. Glucose metabolism is disordered as well.

4. Decorticate posturing, ataxia, and seizures are common. Coma appears at 43° C. At temperatures of 43° to 45.5° C death ensues within several hours.

Monitoring

See also Chapter 4.

1. Temperature. Monitor continuously. Rectal temperature is preferred since it correlates best with core temperatures. If rectal temperatures are inappropriate, oral or axillary temperatures may be substituted. Oral temperatures are 1° C lower than rectal, and skin temperatures are 2° C lower. Measurements need to be evaluated frequently to assess the effectiveness of therapy. In the neonate continuous temperature monitoring (and control) is best accomplished via a servomechanism incorporated into most incubators. Monitoring is done with a skin probe placed over the infant's liver, an organ that accounts for about 20% of internal heat production (see Chapters 85 and 86). Record skin and incubator temperatures every hour, since in neonates temperature gradients may be as important as core temperature.

2. Musculoskeletal

    a. Serum Ca, PO_4, K, creatinine phosphokinase (CPK), and BUN initially; repeat as indicated.

    b. Urinalysis for myoglobinuria, proteinuria, and hemoglobinuria.

3. Hepatic. SGOT and serum glutamic pyruvic transaminase (SGPT) (bilirubin and alkaline phosphatase are usually normal) initially and every day for at least 3 days.

4. Hematologic. Evaluate coagulation status (see Chapter 20).

5. CNS. Serial neurologic evaluation with a repeat EEG is necessary for sustained temperatures >40° C.

6. Cardiovascular. CVP and/or pulmonary ar-

terial blood pressure (P_{pa}) and PCWP may help in determining fluid requirements.

Management

1. Undress the patient.
2. Administer antipyretics. Acetylsalicylic acid (aspirin) or acetaminophen may be given orally or rectally, 10 to 15 mg/kg/dose (1 grain/yr of age/dose), but may be ineffective for extreme hyperpyrexia (temperatures greater than 40.5° C). Do not use phenylbutazone derivatives (e.g., Pyralgin).
3. Institute surface cooling for temperatures >39.5° C and cool until core temperature reaches 37° to 38° C.
   a. Use a cooling blanket with servocontrol or manual control set between 32° and 35° C.
   b. Increase evaporative cooling by sponging the patient in tepid water (alcohol sponging may cause peripheral vasoconstriction and CNS depression secondary to inhalation of alcohol fumes; cold-water sponging induces shivering and continued heat production). Increased convective loss may occur with fanning.
   c. Pack the patient's trunk in ice, concentrating on areas of high blood flow such as the groin and axillae or submerge patient in an ice bath until rectal temperature is 38° C.
4. Inhibit shivering with chlorpromazine, 0.5 to 1.0 mg/kg IV. This may not be effective if extreme hyperpyrexia is present. This agent also increases heat loss by promoting vasodilation. NOTE: Profound hypotension may be seen with use of chlorpromazine.
5. Institute cooling of internal organs.
   a. Perform iced saline gastric lavage. (NOTE: This form of treatment may cause reflex bradycardia secondary to cold stimulation of the vagus.)
   b. Administer an iced saline enema. Use approximately 0.25 of total daily maintenance fluid requirement.

   c. Perform iced saline lavage of bladder or the peritoneal cavity.
   d. Give cool IV fluids.
   e. Cardiopulmonary bypass may be necessary in extreme situations.
6. Assure good hydration with IV fluid administation (1.5 times the maintenance requirement) to replace pulmonary and sweat losses.
   a. If the patient is hypotensive, resuscitate for shock, which may be either hypovolemic or cardiogenic in nature (see Chapter 14).
   b. Adjust fluids to correct any electrolyte or glucose abnormalities.
   c. If urinary myoglobinuria is present, initiate forced diuresis. Once good urine output is established, give mannitol, 1 g/kg IV.
   d. Correct severe metabolic acidosis (pH < 7.20) with sodium bicarbonate.
7. Assure adequate energy sources.
   a. Give supplemental oxygen.
   b. Give IV glucose. Dextrostix should measure 90 to 130 mg/dl; serum glucose, 250 mg/dl.
   c. Maintain normal systemic arterial blood pressure for age.
   d. Administer phosphorus as K_2HPO_4 to correct hypophosphatemia.
8. Treat associated conditions.
   a. Give antibiotics for infection (see Chapters 41, 42, and 43).
   b. Give anticonvulsants for seizures (see Chapter 9).
   c. Initiate beta-receptor blockade for thyroid storm (see Chapter 50).
   d. Give dantrolene sodium (1 mg/kg IV) for malignant hyperpyrexia.

HYPOTHERMIA

Hypothermia, or abnormally low body temperature, is classified as mild (32° to 37° C), moderate (26° to 32° C), deep (20° to 26° C), and profound (less than 20° C). The initial response to low temperature, beginning at a skin temperature of 33° to 34° C, consists of shivering, vasoconstriction, and signs of increased oxygen consumption (tachycardia, increased cardiac output, tachypnea). Periodic vasodilation of the extremities (Lewis phenomenon) interrupts the initial vasoconstriction and tends to protect the limbs from local cold injury. At 34.6° C heat production by cellular mechanisms is significantly depressed because of the slowing of biochemical reactions, and at 29° C all ability of the hypothalamus to regulate temperature is lost.

Causes of hypothermia include:
1. Low environmental temperature
   a. Prolonged exposure to cold.
   b. Sudden immersion in freezing water (i.e., near drowning).
   c. Artificial hypothermia, which is usually accomplished by cardiopulmonary bypass.
2. Failure of the thermoregulatory mechanism. At a temperature of 35° C core hypothermia ensues.
   a. Both hypothermia and hypothyroidism cause decreased heat production because cellular metabolic reactions are inhibited.
   b. Vasodilation associated with hypothermia causes increased heat loss from the skin. This may be drug related since one consequence of overdose may be vasomotor instability. Vasodilation is also the probable mechanism of the hypothermia accompanying sepsis.
   c. Hypothermia may be caused by central hypothalamic dysfunction, which is most often associated with brainstem trauma, mass lesions, drug-induced coma, metabolic coma, or cerebral death.

The effects of hypothermia are multiple:
1. CNS. Drowsiness (at 32° C) progresses to coma (26° C). There is no cortical activity at temperatures less than 20° C (i.e., flat EEG, areflexia, nonreactive pupils). Cerebral blood flow is reduced, conduction in peripheral nerves is slowed (with the sympathetic system being affected last), neuromuscular transmission is impeded, and responses from subcortical areas and the spinal cord are depressed. Ataxia, dysarthria, confusion, and incoordination are common early effects. Single afferent stimuli to a nerve may evoke polysynaptic reflex activity. Generalized muscle rigidity is often present, and seizure disorders are aggravated.
2. Respiratory. Respiratory rate and tidal volume diminish, causing acidosis and decreased arterial oxygenation; hypoxia then becomes the stimulus to respiration. Bronchodilation also occurs. The oxygen dissociation curve shifts to the left, so that oxygen combines easily with hemoglobin but dissociates only at low tissue oxygen levels. As hypothermia progresses, the blood carries increased amounts of dissolved oxygen and carbon dioxide, exacerbating the preexisting acidosis. For every 1° C drop in temperature below 37° C, the measured pH increases 0.015, the Pa_{CO_2} decreases 4.4%, and the Pa_{O_2} increases 7.2%. A high Pa_{O_2} does not necessarily assure good oxygenation. Death occurs at 24° to 25° C from anoxia rather than from cessation of cellular metabolic function.
3. Cardiovascular. Cold directly depresses pacemaker function, and ECG changes include increased PR interval, lengthening of the QRS complex, increased QT interval, ST segment elevation, and T-wave inversion. A J-wave (notching at the end of the QRS complex) is pathognomonic for hypothermia. The bradycardia is not responsive to atropine. Nodal dysrhythmias, PVCs, and atrioventricular block are frequent at temperatures below 28° C; at 20° C asystole or ventricular fibrillation occurs. Extreme cold also sensitizes the myocardium to abnormalities of pH or of electrolytes and to increased concentration of endogenous or exogenous catecholamines. The progressive decrease in cardiac output from cold injury to myocar-

dial muscle, rhythm disturbances particularly bradycardia, and late peripheral vasodilation result in profound hypotension at temperatures below 24° C. Direct cold injury to the microvasculature with increased capillary permeability predisposes the patient to pulmonary and peripheral edema and contributes to hypotension.

4. Renal. Hypotension leads to decreased renal blood flow and oliguria though many patients exhibit cold diuresis with hypo-osmotic polyuria. In addition, there is impaired resorption of solute in the distal tubules and consequent electrolyte loss.

5. Hepatic. Decreased basal metabolic rate and diminished hepatic blood flow depress detoxification reactions. The most significant effects are prolongation of drug half-lives and an inability to metabolize citrate. Shivering and/or exposure for more than 8 hours cause glycogen depletion.

6. Endocrine. Secretions of most endocrine glands are depressed; the calorigenic hormones (catecholamines, steroids, thyroid hormones) may become depleted. Catecholamine depletion is rapid and severe.

7. Hematologic. Blood viscosity increases as water shifts into the tissues and fluid is sequestered in peripheral vessels; peripheral perfusion becomes uneven, leading to local tissue damage and thromboembolic phenomenon. Platelets, WBCs, and eosinophils are sequestered in the liver, spleen, gut, and bone marrow. At 20° C, clinically significant bleeding occurs from thrombocytopenia; DIC has been reported.

8. Other metabolic functions. Shievering may cause hyperkalemia; potassium is released from the liver as glycogen is released to supply energy requirements. Low serum calcium and magnesium levels may also be present. Both hypercalcemia and hypokalemia may occur and each may increase myocardial irritability. When they occur together, there is a more marked effect. Metabolic acidosis is a common consequence

of a low flow state, despite decreased oxygen consumption. Hyperglycemia results from the failure of cells to metabolize glucose at temperatures less than 30° C; at 28° C the basal metabolic rate is halved. Gastrointestinal motility is decreased. Oxygen consumption decreases linearly, and there is approximately a 6% decrease in oxygen consumption per degree centigrade decrease in body temperature. However, this decrease in oxygen consumption may not be protective since intracellular oxygen requirements may not decrease concomitantly with decreased uptake. Production of carbon dioxide is also decreased in linear fashion.

9. Local tissue death (frostbite, gangrene) eventually occurs.

Monitoring

See also Chapter 4.

1. Monitor temperature continuously as suggested in section on hyperthermia (p. 122). A thermometer that registers 20° C is necessary for profound hypothermia; many standard hospital thermometers do not register temperatures less than 34° C.

2. Cardiovascular. Check circulation in the extremities hourly during rewarming. Capillary filling must be checked, and all pulses must be palpated until viability of limbs is known. Continuous ECG monitoring is mandatory. An arterial catheter, CVP, and/or pulmonary artery catheter are recommended.

3. CNS. Serial neurologic evaluations are necessary. The usual criteria for cerebral death do not apply to hypothermic patients; EEG may be isoelectric. All patients should be rewarmed and resuscitated before the diagnosis of death can be made.

4. Renal-metabolic:
   a. Obtain urinalysis. Myoglobin or hemoglobin may be present.
   b. Check serum Na, K, Cl, Ca, PO_4, Mg, and serum osmolality initially and every

24 hours. More frequent determinations are needed during active rewarming.

c. Obtain CBC, with platelet count, PT, PTT, and bleeding time initially.

5. Respiratory:

a. Arterial blood-gas tensions and pH must be corrected initially for patient's temperature. Repeat every 2 to 4 hours if abnormal.

b. Check oxygen saturation and P_{50} if available.

c. Chest roentgenogram after rewarming.

Management

Active rewarming introduces the hazard of rewarming shock, defined as circulatory collapse secondary to premature perfusion of the cold periphery, which causes chilled blood to return to the heart, resulting in another drop in core temperature. Rapid rewarming of the periphery may also cause vasodilation and decreased venous return. Myocardial function may already be compromised by hypoxia, glycogen and catecholamine depletion, increased oxygen demand secondary to rewarming, and poor perfusion. Therefore, passive rewarming should be used for mild to moderate hypothermia. A gradual return to consciousness during rewarming is expected. Vigorous CPR must accompany rewarming.

1. Rewarm at a rate of 0.5° C/hr.

a. External passive methods (for temperature >32° C):

(1) Warm blankets. Discard cold or wet clothing.

(2) Infrared heating lamp. Be certain to have lamp at the appropriate distance from the patient to avoid skin burns.

(3) Heating blanket. Set the servocontrol or manual control at 38° to 40° C.

(4) Overhead radiant heater.

(5) Immersion in warm bath at 40° C for 10 minutes. This method may interfere with CPR and monitoring and may precipitate dysrhythmias.

b. Internal methods (active core rewarming):

(1) Warm IV fluids with an immersion heater used for transfusions. Temperature of fluids should be 37° C.

(2) Peritoneal dialysis (via standard intraperitoneal catheter) with potassium-free D_5W dialysate, or D_5 Ringer's lactate warmed to 43° C in a water immersion heater set at 48° to 54° C. Six to eight exchanges of 30 minutes duration are necessary.

(3) Extracorporeal blood rewarming (40° C).

(4) Inhalation rewarming using a thermistor-controlled cascade humidifier; inhaled oxygen should be 42° to 46° C. This method is easily instituted in the field.

2. Stop warming when core temperature reaches 34° C to avoid overshoot and institute passive external methods.

3. Complications of rewarming include:

a. Ventricular fibrillation or other dysrhythmias; fibrillation can continue even after patient is warm.

b. Congestive failure secondary to fluid overload (IV fluid plus that mobilized from periphery) or cardiac depression.

c. Severe pain.

d. Cerebral edema.

e. Vomiting.

4. Care for frostbite and gangrene (occurs at environmental temperature <20° C)

a. Avoid thawing the affected extremity prior to core rewarming; reperfusion of warmed extremity with cold core blood will intensify the peripheral injury.

b. Pack extremity in ice until systemic rewarming is accomplished.

c. Immerse extremity in agitated hot water bath at 39° to 42° C water for 20 to 30 minutes or until color returns.

d. Elevate affected part to avoid edema.

e. Do not rub, debride, or apply occlusive dressings; early surgery is unadvisable.

f. Administer tetanus prophylaxis.

g. Pain is sign of viability.

5. Support the cardiovascular system (see Chapters 13 and 14).

   a. Antidysrhythmic therapy. If patient's temperature is less than 30° C, place a defibrillator at his bedside. Dysrhythmias may be refractory until the patient is warm.

   b. Vasopressors. Since depletion of epinephrine and norepinephrine occurs, adrenergic pressor support may be helpful.

   c. Treat congestive heart failure with diuretics. Both cerebral and pulmonary edema may occur.

   d. Correct electrolyte disorders (see Chapter 16).

6. Correct metabolic acidosis with sodium bicarbonate (½ correction = base deficit × 0.3 × body weight in kg given at a rate of 1 mEq/kg/min). Be certain that arterial blood-gas determination is corrected to patient's actual body temperature.

7. Consider intubation and mechanical ventilation for a comatose patient or for a patient who is to undergo active core rewarming. The inspired gases should be warmed and humidified. Use high FI_{O_2}. Carbon dioxide (5% to 10%) may be added to inspired gas to stabilize Pa_{CO_2} and pH until rewarming is accomplished, since cellular carbon dioxide production is decreased during deep hypothermia and this may result in alkalosis. Frequent arterial blood-gas tensions and pH determinations are necessary to assess ventilation. Good tracheobronchial toilet should be begun.

8. Institute specific treatment for underlying disorders other than prolonged exposure to cold. Drugs metabolized via hepatic and renal systems will have prolonged half-lives and the dosages of such drugs should be reduced.

9. Sequelae of prolonged hypothermia may include:

   a. Silent myocardial infarction.

   b. Renal failure.

   c. Hepatic failure.

   d. Dyserythropoiesis.

   e. Pancreatitis.

   f. Infection (bronchopneumonia, sepsis). Early antibiotic therapy is usual.

10. A nonenvironment source of hypothermia should be sought if the following signs are present:

   a. Absence of bradycardia.

   b. Inability to increase temperature by passive rewarming.

   c. Stupor or coma with a core temperature >32° C.

   d. Persistence of abnormal mental status after rewarming.

SPECIAL CONSIDERATIONS FOR THE NEONATE

The neonate, particularly the premature infant or infant who is small for gestational age by weight, represents special problems in thermoregulatory control. The large surface area–to–volume ratio and diminished subcutaneous fat increase transfer of heat from the interior to the body surface, where the usual methods of heat loss (conduction, convection, radiation, and evaporation) occur. Heat loss to the environment is four times that of an adult. As a consequence, the neonate is more susceptible to manipulation of the external environment than the adult.

When subjected to cold stress, usually environmental in origin, the neonate increases heat production by nonshivering thermogenesis, the effector organ being brown fat. Brown fat, which is located in sheets at the base of the neck between the scapulae, in the mediastinum, and surrounding the kidneys, constitutes 2% to 6% of body weight. Skin temperature sensors cause sympathetic stimulation and release of norepinephrine, which increases triglyceride hydrolysis in brown fat, causing production of heat. The debt incurred by this metabolic process to maintain normal body temperature is increased oxygen consumption and increased caloric expenditure. If cooling is extreme, thermoregulatory mechanisms fail and body temperature falls precipitously. Metabolic acidosis, hypoglycemia, and decreased arterial blood oxygen levels result.

When the neonate is subjected to heat stress, hyperthermia occurs rapidly, since the neonate has a lower capacity to store heat because of higher body temperature and a large surface area–to–volume ratio. The regulatory mechanisms to dissipate heat include sweating, increased skin blood flow, increased oxygen consumption, and increased calorie consumption.

The range of environmental temperatures at which body temperature can be kept constant by means of thermoregulatory mechanisms is much more limited in the neonate. At the lower end of the scale, temperature regulation can be maintained at 20° to 23° C as compared with 0° C in the adult.

Thermal neutral environment is that "set of thermal conditions at which heat production measured as oxygen consumption is minimal while core temperature is normal" (Klaus and Fanaroff, 1973, p. 59). In such an environment, fewer calories are required for heat production, and caloric intake is more effectively utilized for growth. To achieve a thermal neutral environment, an ambient temperature of 32.5° C is needed as well as absence of drafts and 50% humidity or an abdominal skin temperature of 36.5° C. At an abdominal skin temperature of 37.2° C, oxygen consumption increases 6%, and at 35.9° C it increases 10%. It is imperative in dealing with neonates that environmental thermal conditions be controlled, since a normal core temperature does not preclude heat or cold stress. It only means that the infant's thermoregulatory mechanisms are functional. The increased consumption of oxygen and calories needed to maintain a normal temperature under adverse conditions may result in chronic poor weight gain (Tables 18-1 and 18-2).

The consequences of cold injury in the neo-

Table 18-1. Incubator air temperatures, first 24 hours

Birth weight (g)	Temperatures (°C)	
	Median	Range
500	35.5	±0.5
1000	34.9	±0.5
1500	34.0	±0.5
2000	33.5	±0.5
2500	33.2	±0.8
3000	33.0	±1.0
3500	32.8	±1.2
4000	32.6	±1.4

nate are inactivity, bradycardia, respiratory distress, failure of dissociation of oxyhemoglobin (manifested as bright red color peripherally with central cyanosis), abdominal distention, peripheral edema and/or sclerema, metabolic acidosis, hypoglycemia, hyperkalemia, and oliguria. Norepinephrine secretion rises.

Rewarm the infant slowly with an ambient air temperature 1.5° C warmer than abdominal temperature (oxygen consumption is minimal when the temperature gradient between body surface and air is less than 1.5° C, even though core temperature is subnormal). Rapid rewarming increases the incidence of apneic episodes. Give oxygen, IV glucose, and IV sodium bicarbonate and withhold feedings until core temperature is 35° C. The asphyxiated infant is even more susceptible to the hazards of hypothermia; resuscitative measures with regard to prevention of cold stress should include:

1. Immediate drying to decrease evaporative losses.
2. Placement of the infant on a warm, dry blanket to eliminate conductive losses.
3. Provision of a heat-giving environment by using a radiant warmer (see Chapter 85).
4. Elimination of drafts to decrease heat loss by convection.
5. Decreasing heat loss from the lungs by warming and humidifying inhaled gases.

The consequences of hyperthermia include

Table 18-2. Ambient temperatures (°C) according to age

Age	Birth weight <1500 g			1500-2500 g		Over 36-wk gestation and >2500 g	
	Median	Range	Median	Range	Median	Range
1 day	34.3	±0.4	33.4	±0.6	33.0	±1.0
2 days	33.7	±0.5	32.7	±0.9	32.4	±1.3
3 days	33.5	±0.5	32.4	±0.9	31.9	±1.3
4 days	33.5	±0.5	32.3	±0.9	31.5	±1.3
5 days	33.5	±0.5	32.2	±0.9	31.2	±1.3
6 days	33.5	±0.5	32.1	±0.9	30.9	±1.3
7 days	33.5	±0.5	32.1	±0.9	30.8	±1.4
8 days	33.5	±0.5	32.1	±0.9	30.6	±1.4
9 days	33.5	±0.5	32.1	±0.9	30.4	±1.4
10 days	33.5	±0.5	32.1	±0.9	30.2	±1.5
11 days	33.5	±0.5	32.1	±0.9	29.9	±1.5
12 days	33.5	±0.5	32.1	±0.9	29.5	±1.6
13 days	33.5	±0.5	32.1	±0.9	29.2	±1.6
14 days	33.4	±0.6	32.1	±0.9		
15 days	33.3	±0.7	32.0	±0.9		
4 wk	32.9	±0.8	31.7	±1.1		
5 wk	32.1	±0.7	31.1	±1.1		
6 wk	31.8	±0.6	30.6	±1.1		
7 wk	31.1	±0.6	30.1	±1.1		

tachycardia, flushing, inactivity, sweating (threshold temperature equals 37.2° C), metabolic acidosis, and apnea. With prolonged hyperthermia, coma, convulsions, and brain damage are seen. Management includes undressing the infant, manipulating the ambient environment (hyperthermia may be the consequence of overheating from an incubator or other heat sources, such as a sunlight or bilirubin lights), and tepid-water sponging. Antipyretics are inappropriate for neonates. An appropriate workup for hypermetabolic states (hyperthyroidism, narcotic withdrawal, infection) should be instituted.

ADDITIONAL READING

Dinarello, C.A., and Wolfe, S.M.: Pathogenesis of fever in man, N. Engl. J. Med. 298:607-612, 1978.
Guyton, A.C.: Body temperature, temperature regulation and fever. In Guyton, A.C., editor: Textbook of medical physiology, ed. 3, Philadelphia, 1966, W.B. Saunders Co.
Hudson, L.D., and Conn, R.D.: Accidental hypothermia, associated diagnosis and prognosis in a common problem, J.A.M.A. 227:37-40, 1974.
Johnson, L.A.: Accidental hypothermia and peritoneal dialysis, J. Am. Coll. Emerg. Physicians 6:556-561, 1977.
Klaus, M., and Fanaroff, A.: The physical environment. In Klaus, M., and Fanaroff, A., editors: Care of the high risk infant, Philadelphia, 1973, W.B. Saunders Co.
Knochel, J., and Coskey, J.: The mechanism of hypophosphatemia in acute heat stroke, J.A.M.A. 238:425-426, 1977.
Silverman, W., Tertey, J., and Berger, A.: The influence of thermal environment upon survival of newly born premature infants, Pediatrics 22:876-882, 1958.
Simon, H.: Extreme pyrexia, J.A.M.A. 22:2419-2421, 1976.
Sinclair, J.C.: Heat production and thermoregulation in the small-for-date infant, Pediatr. Clin. North Am. 17:147-158, 1970.
Wadlington, W., Tucker, A., Fly, F., and others: Heat stroke in infancy, Am. J. Dis. Child. 130:1250-1251, 1976.
Zingg, W.: Cold injury. In The Surgical Staff of the Hospital for Sick Children: Care for the injured child, Baltimore, 1975, Williams & Wilkins Co.

19 Acute hepatic failure

ALAN D. STRICKLAND
CHARLES E. MIZE

DEFINITION AND PHYSIOLOGY

Acute, or fulminant, liver failure is the cessation over a few hours to a few days of the metabolic functions of the liver. This liver failure may result from viral, toxic, or intrinsic metabolic insults. Hepatitis A is perhaps the most common virus to cause fulminant hepatitis with liver failure, although hepatitis B, non-A/non-B hepatitis, Epstein-Barr virus, and less frequently other viruses (e.g., ECHO 11) can produce the same clinical picture. Toxic agents, such as carbon tetrachloride, valproate, or acetaminophen, can produce an identical clinical picture, although the hepatic morphology early in the disease may differ from that of viral hepatitis. Certain metabolic disorders such as galactosemia, fructose intolerance, and tyrosinemia can present, particularly in infancy, with acute liver failure, as can Wilson's disease in later childhood.

Under normal circumstances, the liver is supplied via the portal vein with blood from the small bowel and colon. Colonic blood is high in ammonia produced by bacterial action on urea, amino acids, shed enterocytes, and blood in the colon. The small intestine absorbs high concentrations of all of the amino acids, converts glutamate and aspartate to alanine, and delivers this to the liver. The liver deaminates the majority of the amino acids, delivering the amino nitrogen to the Krebs-Henseleit cycle for manufacture of urea. The keto acids remaining after deamination can then be used for gluconeogenesis or released into the systemic circulation. The branched-chain amino acids (valine,

leucine, and isoleucine) are not deaminated in the liver and pass unchanged into the systemic circulation. These branched-chain amino acids may enter muscle cells in response to increased insulin levels and be deaminated there. Branched-chain amino acids also compete with other neutral amino acids, such as tryptophan and phenylalanine, for entry into the brain. Blood leaving the normal liver is, therefore, high in urea, glucose, branched-chain amino acids, and alanine. In addition, the liver manufactures some molecules, such as clotting factors, uridine, and cytidine, that may be used in the brain or other organs in the body.

When an infectious or toxic agent leads to acute liver failure, all of the metabolic functions of the liver are affected to some degree. Gluconeogenesis is compromised and may cause hypoglycemia, with stupor, convulsions, and death. Urea formation is compromised, and serum ammonia levels may rise. Deamination is compromised, causing serum amino acid levels to rise. (See Table 19-1.) The greatly increased levels of phenylalanine, arginine, and tryptophan may cause increased movement of these amino acids into the brain, resulting in increases in their metabolic products, such as serotonin, epinephrine, and norepinephrine. Glutamic acid crosses into the brain and combines with ammonia to form glutamine. Cerebral oxygen consumption decreases. Although it is not known why this occurs, it is possibly due to a false neurotransmitter, which suppresses brain activity or which could cause vasoconstriction of blood vessels in the brain. Methionine degra-

Table 19-1. Serum amino acid levels in acute liver failure

Amino acid	Percentage of normal serum value
Taurine	90
Aspartic acid	100
Isoleucine	140
Valine	200
Serine	210
Glutamic acid	250
Leucine	300
Glycine	360
Tryptophan	360
Glutamine	390
Histidine	460
Threonine	490
Alanine	490
Ornithine	540
Tyrosine	580
Lysine	590
Proline	590
Cystine	620
Asparagine	700
Phenylalanine	815
Arginine	1060
Methionine	1380

dation products may produce the odor of fetor hepatis. Decreased hepatic production of clotting factors results in frequent problems (e.g., gastrointestinal hemorrhage). Significant PT prolongation and increased serum bilirubin may herald rapidly evolving hepatic necrosis associated with a sudden decrease in the size of an enlarged liver.

Sodium retention with consequent water retention and ascites formation occurs in 70% of patients with fulminant liver failure who survive for 20 days. The mechanism is probably mediated through the distal convoluted tubule, as it is in cirrhosis. Aldosterone levels increase only after sodium retention has been present for several days. Hepatorenal syndrome (oliguria, increased BUN, increased creatinine, and normal renal morphology) may follow the onset of ascites, particularly if high-dose diuretics are used. Excessive water retention usually leads to hyponatremia. Hypokalemia and hypomagnesemia are also frequent. Cardiac failure may follow the changes in blood volume. Immune function is compromised as hepatic production of immunoglobulins fails, and infections are a common final complication of acute liver failure.

Cerebral edema may follow anoxic or hypoglycemic injury to the brain, followed by respiratory alkalosis due to central hyperventi-

Table 19-2. Stages of hepatic coma

Stage	Asterixis*	Electroencephalogram	Consciousness
I	Slight	Normal	Mild confusion, slow mentation, slurred speech, altered affect or orientation
II	Easily demonstrated	Alpha waves with occasional delta spikes	Drowsiness, mentation further depressed
III	Present, but patient cooperation is poor	Alpha waves with delta spikes	Asleep or stuporous majority of time but can be aroused; mentation poor and speech incoherent
IV	Absent	Alpha waves with delta spikes	Asleep and not arousable

*Asterixis: uncontrolled flapping of flexed hands.

lation. Patients who have a fulminant illness may show delirium, deep coma, and decerebrate rigidity within 24 hours. Hepatic coma may develop and reach one of four stages of severity (see Table 19-2). The cause of the coma is not presently known, but the stage of the coma tends to correlate better with CSF glutamine than with serum ammonia. The mortality rate of persons reaching stage IV coma may be as great as 80%.

MONITORING
Hepatic system

See also Chapter 4.

1. Serum bilirubin (total/direct), SGOT, SGPT, lactic dehydrogenase (LDH), CPK, PT, PTT, alkaline phosphatase, blood ammonia, amino acids, TSP, and protein electrophoresis (for albumin, haptoglobin, ceruloplasmin, and α-1-antitrypsin) initially. Blood ammonia (preferably arterial) bilirubin, TSP, and albumin every 24 to 48 hours. Monitor SGOT, SGPT, and alkaline phosphatase every 1 to 3 days.
2. Toxicology screen for the broadest range of offending agents. These categories should include lower alcohols; acidic, neutral, and basic drugs; heavy metals; and volatile compounds. Note that in many toxicology analysis centers a special request is necessary for many agents, such as acetaminophen, chlorinated hydrocarbons, pesticides, haloperidol, hydromorphone, morphine, and alkaloid derivatives.
3. Percutaneous liver biopsy on admission if PT, PTT, and platelet count will permit needle biopsy
4. Abdominal girth and weight initially and every 12 to 24 hours. Monitor liver and spleen size. If liver size decreases and spleen size increases, this suggests portal hypertension. If liver size decreases and spleen is not palpable, this suggests resolution of the hepatitis.

Cardiorespiratory system

1. Arterial blood-gas tensions and pH initially and every 4 to 12 hours
2. Monitor respirations and agitation of the patient. Consider early intubation to prevent anoxia.
3. Consider cardiac output and vascular resistance measurements (see Chapter 14).

Neurologic system

1. See Chapters 6 and 10.
2. Monitor and record the stage of coma every 2 to 4 hours, or as needed.

Hematologic system

1. PT, PTT, Hb, Hct, and platelet count every 24 to 48 hours
2. Factor VII, fibrin split products, fibrinogen, if available, for bleeding or rapid PT prolongation
3. Blood cultures and hepatitis B surface antigen (HBsAg), hepatitis B core antibody (HBcAb), hepatitis B core antigen (HBcAg), hepatitis A antibody (IgM) (HAAb[IgM]), and cytomegalovirus (CMV) titers

Renal-metabolic system

1. Measure serum glucose and Chemstix initially. Repeat Chemstix every 1 to 2 hours and serum glucose every 12 to 24 hours.
2. Monitor serum osmolality Na, K, Cl, BUN, creatinine, Ca, and PO_4 every 12 to 24 hours.
3. Amylase initially and as needed.
4. Urine electrolytes and osmolality daily.

MANAGEMENT

Therapy for acute hepatic failure includes general as well as specific support to allow hepatic recovery and regeneration of liver tissue to occur. Therapy should be designed to prevent further liver injury, stimulate repair of damaged cells, produce new hepatocytes, and suppress untoward regenerative effects.

Hepatic coma (impending and overt)

1. Avoid the use of analgesic medications or sedatives.
2. Restrict dietary protein to less than 1 g/kg/day. With coma above Stage II, stop all protein and provide high glucose input for 4 to 7 days.
3. Decrease intestinal bacterial ammonia production or absorption.
   a. Neomycin, 100 mg/kg initially, and 50 mg/kg/day thereafter PO or via NG tube
   b. Lactulose, 5 ml every 6 hours initially. Lactulose is fermented by colonic bacteria to small organic acids. These acids aid the conversion of NH_3 to NH_4^+ (preventing NH_3 diffusion from colon to the blood) and alter the colonic environment to help suppress bacterial NH_3 formation from urea and amino acids. The osmotically active small organic acids will cause diarrhea, and the lactulose dose should be adjusted to produce one or two soft stools per day.
4. Treat gastrointestinal bleeding quickly, since blood in the intestinal tract will cause an increase in serum ammonia. Place NG tube to gravity drainage to avoid gastric mucosal trauma.
5. Avoid use of corticosteroids, since they do not effect recovery.
6. Exchange transfusions and extracorporeal liver perfusions have not been shown to offer predictable success, and significant complications can ensue. They do not presently have a place in treatment.
7. Hemodialysis does not generally offer routine advantage in toxin-induced liver failure (see Chapter 66). Its use may be considered if continued circulatory toxin can be enriched in a dialysate or for intractable hepatorenal syndrome with urea retention and/or acute tubular necrosis (see Chapter 110).
8. For cerebral edema, see Chapter 10.

Renal-metabolic system

1. Give Aquamephyton (5 mg IM) initially for prolonged PT and PTT.
2. Furnish clotting factors such as FFP if bleeding occurs after Aquamephyton administration.
3. Provide supplemental water-soluble vitamins (usually given as 2 times the required daily allowance [RDA]).
4. Ensure electrolyte balance, especially maintenance of serum potassium and phosphate (levels of 2,3-DPG must be maintained optimally). Avoid use of Ringer's lactate since lactate is normally metabolized in the liver.
5. Maintain blood glucose at 100 to 150 mg/dl with IV glucose.
6. On admission, begin sodium restriction to 1 mEq Na/kg/24 hours to help prevent sodium retention and ascites formation.
7. Moderately restrict fluids to 800 to 1200 ml/m^2/24 hours.
8. Supplement serum potassium as necessary.
9. Correct alkalosis, should it develop, to prevent movement of ammonia into cells. This is usually accomplished by changing the minute ventilation to alter Pa_{CO_2} values.
10. Avoid use of diuretics if possible.
11. Consider selective parenteral nutrition (see Chapter 111).
12. For hepatorenal syndrome, see Chapter 17.

Cardiovascular system

1. Maintain adequate hepatic and cerebral perfusion (i.e., blood pressure should be maintained within normal range for age).
2. Replace blood loss with packed RBCs. Whole-blood transfusion may increase protein intake and also compromise an already high cardiac output.
3. Consider 25% albumin infusion to maintain TSP at 5 mg/dl or greater.
4. If DIC develops secondary to bacterial infection, treat the organism isolated on the blood

culture. Prophylactic use of systemic antibiotics is not indicated since it tends to select multiply-resistant organisms.

Respiratory system

1. Provide increased FI_{O_2} to sustain Pa_{O_2} of 100 mm Hg. (NOTE: Pulmonary arteriovenous shunting may be present.)
2. Upon signs of agitation or moderate confusion, intubate the patient and control respiration with d-tubocurarine paralysis. Early institution of controlled ventilatory assistance may prevent anoxic cerebral insult.

Neurologic system

1. For hepatic coma, see above.
2. See Chapter 6.

ADDITIONAL READING

Alagille, D., and Odievre, M.: Acute liver failure in infants. In Liver and biliary tract disease in children, New York, 1979, Wiley-Flammarion, pp. 94-101.

Berk, P.D., and Popper, H.: Fulminant hepatic failure, Am. J. Gastroenterol. **69**:349-400, 1978.

Felig, P.: Amino acid metabolism in man, Ann. Rev. Biochem. **44**:933-855, 1975.

Gregory, P.B., Knauer, C.M., Kempson, R.L., and Miller, R.: Steroid therapy in severe viral hepatitis: a double-blind, randomized trial of methylprednisolone versus placebo, N. Engl. J. Med. **294**:681-687, 1976.

Levy, M.: Sodium retention and ascites formation in dogs with experimental portal cirrhosis, Am. J. Physiol. **233**:F572-F585, 1977.

Levy, M.: Sodium retention in dogs with cirrhosis and ascites: efferent mechanisms, Am. J. Physiol. **233**:F586-F592, 1977.

Nolan, J.P.: Liver disease associated with toxins and drugs. In Dietschy, J.M., editor: The science and practice of clinical medicine, New York, 1976, Grune & Stratton, Inc., pp. 316-319.

Rogers, E.L., and Rogers, M.C.: Fulminant hepatic failure and hepatic encephalopathy, Pediatr. Clin. North Am. **27**:701-713, 1980.

Vij, J.C., and Tandon, B.N.: Management of fulminant hepatitis by vigorous supportive treatment, Arch. Intern. Med. **138**:1749, 1978.

Watanabe, A., Takesue, A., Higashi, T., and Nagashima, N.: Serum amino acids in hepatic encephalopathy—effects of branched chain amino acid infusion on serum aminogram, Acta Hepatogastroenterol. **26**:346-357, 1979.

20 Disseminated intravascular coagulation

GEORGE R. BUCHANAN

DEFINITION AND PHYSIOLOGY

Disseminated intravascular coagulation (DIC), or "consumption coagulopathy," is a syndrome caused by abnormal activation of the blood clotting mechanism, leading to generalized consumption of platelets and clotting proteins with resultant deposition of platelet and fibrin plugs in the microvasculature. DIC is usually accompanied by a compensatory fibrinolytic response, i.e., the proteolytic enzyme plasmin is generated and fibrin clots are degraded. This inappropriate activation of blood coagulation is triggered by a variety of circumstances, including endothelial damage, liberation of tissue thromboplastin, circulating endotoxin, and immune complexes (Fig. 20-1). These triggering events usually accompany or are secondary to serious viral or bacterial infection, shock, or hypoxia, underlying problems that are especially common in the neonate, particularly the premature infant. One or more of these predisposing factors result in aggregation of platelets and activation of factor XII (Hageman factor), after which the coagulation cascade is activated by one of several mechanisms.

The major sequelae of DIC are:

1. Depletion of platelets and labile clotting factors, especially factor VIII, factor V, prothrombin, and fibrinogen, resulting in circulating factor levels that are inadequate to meet the requirements of hemostasis. Hemorrhage, usually generalized, follows.
2. Intravascular fibrin deposition. Thrombi or thromboemboli lodge in and may occlude blood vessels of all sizes, leading to ischemic necrosis. This thrombosis may be visible and quite obvious when it occurs in large vessels such as the femoral artery or iliac vein, or it may be clinically less apparent and result in dysfunction of one or more internal organs, such as the brain, lungs, or kidneys. In this latter instance, the fibrin and platelet thrombi are probably multiple and involve small arterioles or capillary beds.
3. Microangiopathic hemolytic anemia. This occurs secondary to mechanical fragmentation of RBCs when the red cells turbulently make contact with damaged endothelium or occluding fibrin strands.

Numerous studies have demonstrated that to a variable degree intravascular coagulation occurs in practically all infants and children with serious underlying disorders who are admitted to an intensive care unit. Fortunately, however, the excessive consumption of platelets and clotting factors is usually matched by compensatory increased production of hemostatic elements by the bone marrow and liver. When consumption occurs more rapidly than production, abnormal laboratory tests and clinical problems may occur. DIC should be suspected in all seriously ill children who develop laboratory or clinical evidence of excessive thrombosis or hemorrhage. The latter is usually manifested by oozing from cutdown and venipuncture sites, gastrointestinal bleeding, and bruising, but bleeding may occur in virtually any site.

135

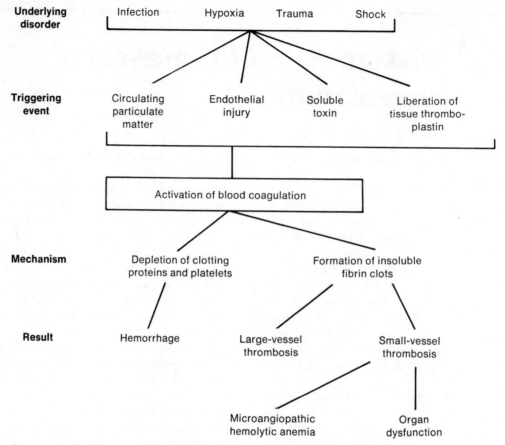

Fig. 20-1. Pathophysiology of DIC.

MONITORING

See also Chapter 4.

Monitoring of a patient with DIC primarily requires that careful attention be paid to the underlying disease and/or triggering events as well as to serial clinical and laboratory evaluation of the child's hemostatic mechanism.

Hematologic system

1. Observe for evidence of progressive bleeding.
   a. Examine the skin at frequent intervals for signs of or progression of petechiae, purpura, prolonged bleeding after venipuncture, and bleeding from cutdown or suture sites.
   b. Other sites of possible blood loss that should be carefully and frequently evaluated include the gastrointestinal tract (for occult or frank blood), the urinary tract (Labstix), and the nasopharynx.
   c. Signs of minimal bleeding elsewhere, such as hemorrhages in the retina, may be indicative of serious bleeding into a vital organ.
2. Record Hct every 6 to 12 hours, depending on the extent of hemorrhage.
3. Daily blood smears are required to assess

Table 20-1. Differential laboratory diagnosis of an acquired bleeding diathesis

Diagnosis	PT	PTT	Platelet count	Fibrinogen	Fibrin degradation products	Peripheral blood smear
DIC	↑	↑	↓	↓	↑	RBC fragments
Vitamin K deficiency	↑	↑	N*	N	N	N
Liver failure	↑	↑	N or ↓	N or ↓	N or ↑	Target cells
Mechanical consumptive thrombocytopenia	N	N	↓	N	N or ↑	RBC fragments or burr cells
Heparin effect (iatrogenic or spurious)	N or ↑	Markedly ↑	N	N	N	N
Normal values†	11-14 sec	25-35 sec	150,000-400,000/μl	150-450 mg/dl	<10 μg/ml	—

*N, normal.
†May vary, depending on laboratory used and age of patient (e.g., normal newborns have longer PTs and PTTs than older children).

the number of platelets and the extent and progression of microangiopathic hemolysis.

4. For purposes of initial screening and for following the patient with mild degrees of intravascular coagulation, only four tests (platelet count, PT, PTT, and fibrinogen) need to be performed, and they should be repeated daily as necessary. Children with grossly abnormal screening studies, particularly those who manifest hemorrhage or thrombosis, should be carefully evaluated to exclude other causes of acute coagulation disturbances, such as vitamin K deficiency, primary liver disease, or isolated mechanical thrombocytopenia.

5. Measurement of fibrin degradation products can assist in the differential diagnosis (Table 20-1), although this test is not always necessary for the diagnosis of DIC.

6. Blood samples for coagulation studies must be drawn atraumatically from a peripheral vein to obtain accurate results. Specimens drawn through plastic indwelling catheters containing even minute amounts of heparin may give spurious values.

7. Draw blood type and crossmatch specimens

as soon as the diagnosis is suspected, and keep them current as long as DIC continues.

Infection

Obtain complete cultures if infection is suspected.

MANAGEMENT
General

The signs and symptoms of DIC are often overshadowed by those of the primary disease. The high mortality in patients with DIC is usually not secondary to hemorrhage or thrombosis but is due to the underlying disorders. In most circumstances, no therapy specific for DIC is required, despite the fact that consumption may be occurring and can be documented by some of the laboratory tests just outlined. Specific therapy for DIC is warranted only when the patient is having appreciable hemorrhage or thrombosis or has grossly abnormal laboratory values, such as a platelet count less than 20,000/μl, fibrinogen less than 75 mg/dl, PT over 25 seconds, and PTT more than twice the normal values.

Replacement therapy

1. Give platelet concentrates in an approximate dose of 1 unit (10 to 50 ml) per 5 to 10 kg of body weight, and repeat every 12 to 24 hours when the clinical situation warrants. The platelet count may not dramatically increase after administration; however, clinical signs of bleeding may lessen.

2. Fresh-frozen plasma (FFP), 10 to 15 ml/kg every 12 to 24 hours, will partially replace the deficiencies of fibrinogen, prothrombin, factor V, factor VIII, and other deficient factors. Moreover, FFP contains anti-thrombin, the naturally occurring circulating anticoagulant that binds to and inactivates thrombin and other activated clotting factors; antithrombin is depleted in DIC, possibly predisposing the patient to excessive thrombosis.

3. Fresh whole blood or packed RBCs may be needed to maintain an adequate Hct (see Chapter 106).

4. For the patient, usually a neonate, who cannot tolerate the volume load of multiple infusions or platelet concentrates and FFP, exchange transfusion is an appropriate form of therapy when life-threatening hemorrhage or thrombosis occurs. After simple or exchange transfusion, the survival of the donor platelets and clotting factors is usually much shorter than normal, but clinical improvement is sometimes noted. The admonition that transfusion of clotting factors "adds fuel to the fire" and accelerates thrombosis has not been substantiated.

5. Always administer vitamin K (1 to 5 mg IV) if there is the slightest doubt about the patient's vitamin K status.

6. Prothrombin complex concentrates such as Konyne or Proplex are never indicated in the management of patients with DIC because the activated procoagulants in these compounds may accelerate the thrombotic tendency, because there is a high risk of hepatitis associated with their use, and because they lack most of the factors that are deficient in patients with DIC.

7. It is rarely necessary to administer cryoprecipitate, since FFP contains adequate amounts of both fibrinogen and factor VIII.

Heparin

About 15 years ago it was uniformly proposed that heparin was indicated for practically all patients with DIC. The basis of this recommendation was that the inappropriate activation of the coagulation mechanism could be arrested by therapeutic anticoagulation. Despite its theoretical attractiveness, heparin has been shown to possess numerous undesirable side effects, and data regarding its efficacy are limited to isolated case reports. Retrospective analysis of large numbers of patients and numerous experimental studies in animals indicate that although heparin may arrest DIC and improve laboratory values of coagulation, morbidity and mortality are unaltered. Therefore, the current consensus is that most patients can be managed without heparinization. Heparin should be administered only in those children in whom marked thrombosis has occurred and is progressing (e.g., in instances of purpura fulminans, where widespread cutaneous thrombosis is evident) and in the rare child who has massive hemorrhage that is not controlled by management of the underlying disease or by replacement transfusions.

The correct dose of heparin in these circumstances is uncertain, and therapy is therefore empirical. The most commonly recommended regimens are a continuous infusion of 10 to 20 units/kg/hr (after a loading dose of 50 units/kg) or 50 to 75 units/kg by IV push every 4 hours. Screening tests such as the PTT are useless during heparin therapy, and the patient must be monitored by other laboratory tests (such as platelet count, fibrinogen or fibrin split products) or on clinical grounds.

ADDITIONAL READING

Hathaway, W.E.: Disseminated intravascular coagulation. In Smith, C.A., editor: The critically ill child: diagnosis and management, Philadelphia, 1977, W.B. Saunders Co.

Heene, D.L.: Disseminated intravascular coagulation: evaluation of therapeutic approaches, Semin. Thrombosis Hemostasis 3:291-317, 1977.

Mant, M.J., and King, E.G.: Severe acute disseminated intravascular coagulation: a reappraisal of its pathophysiology, clinical significance and therapy based on 47 patients, Am. J. Med. 67:557-563, 1979.

Zipursky, A., deSa, D., Hsu, E., and others: Clinical laboratory diagnosis of hemostatic disorders in newborn infants, Am. J. Pediatr. Hematol. Oncol. 1:217-226, 1979.

PART TWO

Specific problems

21 Reye's syndrome

DANIEL L. LEVIN

DEFINITION AND PHYSIOLOGY

Reye's syndrome is a toxic encephalopathy that typically follows an acute febrile infectious disease in children. The infectious disease may be an upper respiratory tract infection, including Epstein-Barr virus; pneumonia; an influenzal syndrome, especially type B; acute exanthematous disease, especially varicella; gastroenteritis; pertussis; or otitis media. Reye's syndrome may also follow vaccination. Exposure to insect repellents and to aflatoxin B, possibly from eating peanut butter, have been suggested as possible causes. An increased incidence in children with influenza B or varicella who take salicylate is concerning, but the exact role of salicylate in the pathogenesis of the disease is far from certain. At present any conclusive evidence for a causal role of salicylate in the pathogenesis of Reye's syndrome is lacking. There appears to be a predominance of black infants in patients less than 6 months of age and of white males thereafter.

The prodrome may last from 1 day to 3 weeks and is followed by the onset of recurrent vomiting and hyperventilation, which are striking and may be confused with DKA. Within 1 to 2 days the child becomes irritable, restless, disoriented, and lethargic and lapses into a coma frequently complicated by seizures. The coma rapidly progresses, with the appearance of decorticate and decerebrate posturings and respiratory arrest.

Reye's syndrome is a multisystem disease affecting the liver, brain, heart, kidneys, pancreas, and skeletal muscle. Pathologic findings in the brain include cerebral edema with or without herniation; anoxic neuronal changes that are most severe in the cerebral cortex; less severe changes in the basal ganglia, periaqueductal gray matter, and brainstem; vascular congestion with lipid droplets in the capillary endothelial cells; and perineural and perivascular clear spaces in the cortex, basal ganglia, hippocampus, and brainstem. Inflammation of the meninges or brain parenchyma, microglial proliferation, demyelination, and Alzheimer's type II astrocytes are conspicuous by their absence. Electron microscopy reveals dilation of the endoplasmic reticulum and mitochondria, cytogenic edema, and lipid-containing bodies within pericytes adjacent to cerebral vessels.

The liver appears swollen and yellow or reddish yellow. Light microscopy reveals a fine vacuolization of the parenchymal cells due to intracellular lipid. Glycogen is absent, and there is no evidence of inflammation. Electron microscopy reveals mitochondrial abnormalities consisting of ameboid and spherical structural deformation, loss of dense bodies and cristae, and swelling of the mitochondrial matrix. Proliferation of the smooth endoplasmic reticulum, empty Golgi membranes, and an increase in peroxisomes are also seen.

The kidneys are pale with a slight yellowish tinge and a widening of the cortices. Light microscopy reveals fatty degeneration of the loops of Henle and proximal convoluted tubules. The glomeruli, vessels, and interstitium appear to be normal.

Examination of the heart reveals epicardial petechiae in many cases. Light microscopy reveals oil red O positive material in the ventricles and especially in the atria. Electron microscopy reveals mitochondrial swelling and fragmentation of the cristae.

Indications for treatment and evaluation of treatment regimens rely on accurate clinical assessment of the patient. To identify similar degrees of illness, several classification systems have been developed. One commonly used classification, that of Lovejoy and associates, is presented below.

NEUROLOGIC STAGING (LOVEJOY)

Stage 1. The patient has vomiting, lethargy, sleepiness, laboratory evidence of liver dysfunction, and a type 1 EEG (rhythmic slowing, dominant theta waves, rare delta waves).

Stage 2. The patient is disoriented, with delirium and combativeness, hyperventilation, and hyperactive reflexes. Appropriate responses to noxious stimuli are present. There is evidence of abnormal liver function, and a type 2 EEG is present (dysrhythmic slowing, dominant delta waves, some theta waves).

Stage 3. The patient is obtunded, with hyperventilation, decorticate rigidity, and preservation of pupillary light reaction and oculovestibular reflexes. There are abnormal liver function tests and a type 2 EEG.

Stage 4. There is a deepening coma with decerebrate rigidity; loss of oculocephalic reflexes (doll's eyes); large, fixed pupils with hippus; and dysconjugate eye movements in response to caloric stimulation of the oculovestibular reflexes. Minimal liver dysfunction can be demonstrated, and a type 3 (disorganized monorhythmic or polyrhythmic delta waves) or type 4 (isoelectric) EEG is present.

Stage 5. There may be seizures, loss of deep tendon reflexes, respiratory arrest, flaccidity, and a type 4 EEG. Hepatic function may be normal by this period.

The prognosis seems to be related to clinical neurologic stages in that the outlook is worse if patients are first seen in a more advanced stage of coma and if they progress through the stages rapidly.

Laboratory examinations reveal evidence of multisystem involvement. Younger patients are usually hypoglycemic (less than 45 mg/dl). Liver function tests are abnormal, with a prolonged PT and PTT and elevated SGOT, SGPT, CPK, and serum ammonia levels (>80 μg/dl in infants and children). The pathophysiology of hyperammonemia in Reye's syndrome is unknown, but these patients are in a profound catabolic state, resulting in a tremendous ammonia load. At the same time, ammonia disposal via urea synthesis is impaired due to decreased activity of intramitochondrial enzymes of the urea cycle, carbamylphosphate synthetase and ornithine transcarbamylase. Ammonia is taken up by the brain in patients with Reye's syndrome. Many investigators have attempted to correlate a greater severity of disease and a worse prognosis with the degree of increase in serum ammonia and a reasonable correlation exists. A serum ammonia level greater than 300 μg/dl is well correlated with a poor outcome, although there are many exceptions to this observation. Some patients survive without residua after serum ammonia levels have been documented at greater than 1,200 μg/dl. In a patient with a typical history and physical examination, an elevated serum ammonia level can be considered diagnostic of Reye's syndrome.

There is a typical serum amino acid pattern in patients with Reye's syndrome with elevations of glutamine, proline, alanine, α-amino-n-butyrate, ornithine, and lysine. There is also evidence for hypertyraminemia in these patients. Patients with partial ornithine transcarbamylase deficiency present with an illness simulating Reye's syndrome.

There is also evidence for elevations in the levels of medium-and short-chain fatty acids (propionate, butyrate, isobutyrate, isovalerate, and valerate) in patients with Reye's syndrome. The elevated free fatty acid levels are found early in the course of the syndrome, and initial levels tend to be higher in more severely ill patients. Levels tend to decrease as patients improve. These correlations do not hold in all patients.

Patients with Reye's syndrome also have hyperlactatemia that may be due to excess production by brain and muscle, impaired hepatic metabolism, hyperventilation reducing hepatic blood flow, or hypoxemia, hypoperfusion, and acidosis. Hyperlactatemia can cause hyperventilation and coma by causing systemic acidosis. Blood lactate levels are only variably elevated during the early course of the disease.

Although a generalized dysfunction of mitochondria has been suggested as the cause of Reye's syndrome, there is little evidence to support this concept. Also, this kind of dysfunction would be diffuse and cause many more abnormalities than are seen in Reye's syndrome.

Although the means by which a viral illness triggers Reye's syndrome is unknown, once the pathologic process begins, hyperammonemia results. The evidence favors a disorder of liver mitochondria in association with a massive catabolic state as the cause of the hyperammonemia. Hyperammonemia can account for the signs and symptoms seen during the early phases of the illness. Hepatic mitochondrial dysfunction causes impairment in the metabolism of fat, nitrogenous compounds, and carbohydrates, resulting in hyperfattyacidemia, hyperammonemia, hypoglycemia, and lactic acidosis. These metabolic abnormalities have been suggested as causes for the typical encephalopathy of Reye's syndrome, although the evidence best favors hyperammonemia as the cause of the cerebral edema and coma.

Rarely, other diseases (e.g., defects in urea cycle enzymes) may have a similar presentation, and therefore, a liver biopsy is necessary to confirm the diagnosis. In patients with stage 2 or greater involvement, do not delay therapy while awaiting the results of the liver biopsy. To be useful, the biopsy must be obtained within 48 hours of the onset of neurologic symptoms and antemortem.

Pancreatic involvement is reflected by an increased serum amylase level. Myocardial abnormalities are indicated by ECG evidence of dysrhythmias or myocarditis. Acute and convalescent sera for viral titers may be helpful for epidemiologic reasons.

The CSF is normal except for elevated pressure and a few lymphocytes, the CBC is not diagnostic, and the platelet count is normal. Serum sodium, potassium, and chloride may be abnormal because of vomiting and decreased intake before treatment, and serum calcium and phosphate levels are also frequently low.

MONITORING

See also Chapter 4.

The following recommendations for monitoring and management are based on experience accumulated from many authors. The cause or causes of the syndrome are unknown, and therefore specific therapy is not available. General support with specific attention to lowering elevated ICP seems indicated. However, rarely there are patients in whom ICP was continuously monitored and was never elevated and yet who have suffered brain death. There are claims for many therapeutic regimens, but no one regimen has proved obviously successful over a prolonged period. It is clear, however, that without good supportive treatment, a patient at stage 2 or more has a high risk for death or for survival with significant neurologic residua (>50% to 75%). This significant risk to the patient seems to justify aggressive supportive measures. There seems to be a greater risk for sequelae the younger the patient is and the more severe the illness (i.e., the more advanced the neurologic stage).

Stage 1

Observe patients in stage 1 closely for progression of neurologic symptoms. Since the level of therapy changes dramatically with the onset of stage 2 neurologic symptoms and since the prognosis worsens with the rapidity of advancement through the neurologic stages, patients who are even mildly ill must be carefully and repetitively evaluated. Perform serum glucose tests (or Dextrostix) every 2 to 4 hours and serum ammonia, SGOT, SGPT, CPK, and electrolyte determinations daily until normal.

Stages 2 through 5

Central nervous system

1. Check neurologic signs every hour. This should include level of consciousness, pupillary reactions, oculovestibular reflexes, deep tendon reflexes, and reflex activity.
2. Institute ICP monitoring (see Chapters 10 and 92). Since the hepatic dysfunction will resolve, the greatest risk to the patient's survival is increased ICP. Therapeutic interventions intended to lower ICP involve significant risk, and it is difficult, if not impossible, to accurately assess ICP clinically by symptoms and signs. Therefore, ICP should be measured directly in every patient who progresses rapidly to the neurologic signs of stage 2 or higher.
3. Maintain ICP monitoring until:
   a. The patient is recovering and successfully extubated, usually 3 to 4 days, *or*
   b. The patient is not recovering and there are no fluctuations in ICP, usually 4 to 6 days. In some cases this may be significantly longer.
4. Continuously display mean systemic arterial blood pressure and mean ICP. Calculate and record CPP every 2 hours and whenever ICP elevations occur (CPP = MAP − ICP) (see Fig. 21-1).
5. Obtain an EEG initially and repeat as indicated.

Respiratory system. Perform arterial blood-gas tensions and pH determinations every 2 to 4 hours.

Renal-metabolic system

1. Fluids
   a. BUN and serum creatinine initially.

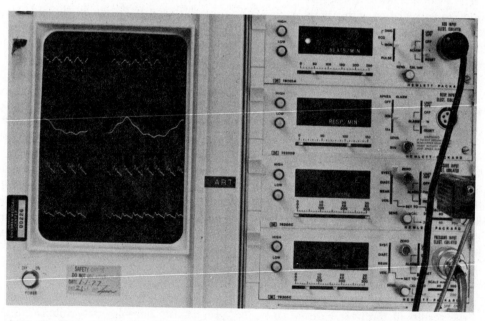

Fig. 21-1. Oscilloscopic display of ECG, respiratory waveform, systemic arterial blood pressure, and ICP *(top to bottom)* in a child with Reye's syndrome.

b. Matched urine and serum osmolalities every 4 hours for 3 to 6 days while monitoring ICP. When using osmotherapy, measure only serum osmolality.

2. Minerals
   a. Matched serum and urine Na, K, and Cl every 4 hours until ICP is no longer being measured.
   b. Serum Ca and PO_4 determinations every 4 hours until ICP is no longer being measured.

3. Hepatic-gastrointestinal monitoring
   a. PT and PTT every 12 hours for the first 2 days and daily thereafter until normal.
   b. Serum ammonia, SGOT, SGPT, and TSP daily until they return to normal. Bilirubin and alkaline phosphatase levels are not usually elevated.
   c. Serum amylase initially; repeat as needed.
   d. Dextrostix every 4 hours; serum glucose initially and every day until stable.
   e. Liver biopsy.
   f. Toxicology screen (serum and urine), including salicylate level.

   Miscellaneous

1. Infection
   a. The risk of acquired infection from invasive monitoring devices is increased in these patients. Blood cultures should be obtained frequently and all catheter tips should be cultured when removed.
   b. Perform gram stains and cultures of tracheal aspirates weekly or when tracheal secretions change in nature or when chest roentgenogram changes. The incidence of pneumonia may be as great as 90%.
   c. Obtain acute and convalescent sera for viral titers.
   d. Check all IV sites, dressings, and ICP catheter sites daily.

2. CPK initially and every day if elevated

MANAGEMENT

The goals of management are to preserve organ integrity by supplying excess energy sub-strate for cellular metabolism and to preserve organ homeostasis by treating specific dysfunctions such as elevated ICP or low systemic blood pressure.

Stage 1

Good supportive therapy is all that is required. The main objective during this stage is to identify by close observation those patients who will progress from stage 1 to more advanced stages.

Stages 2 through 5

Central nervous system. The use of gravity, mannitol, hyperventilation, volume restriction, sedation, and normothermia in the management of increased ICP is described in detail in Chapter 10. Peritoneal dialysis and exchange transfusion have been used in patients with Reye's syndrome in order to lower ICP, although proof of their efficacy is lacking. The therapy for seizures is presented in Chapter 9, and for the diagnosis of brain death see Chapter 7. Although the use of barbiturates and hypothermia to decrease cerebral metabolic needs is attractive, convincing evidence of their efficacy is lacking at this time.

Cardiovascular system

1. Maintain normal systemic arterial blood pressure according to age, since hypotension can be particularly hazardous in this condition. An acute fall in systemic blood pressure may severely compromise the cerebral circulation (see Chapter 14).
2. If urine output, CVP, and systemic arterial blood pressure all decrease, increase fluid administration to 100% maintenance.
3. Correct dysrhythmias.
4. Myocarditis is not usually severe enough to require therapy, and congestive heart failure is uncommon. Dysrhythmias can occur, however, and may be fatal.

Respiratory system

1. Maintain oxygen-carrying capacity by keeping Hct greater than 30%.
2. Hyperventilation by controlled mechanical

ventilation may be used to decrease elevated ICP (see Chapter 10).

3. If pulmonary congestion develops, perform suctioning and CPT every 4 hours after sedation (see Chapter 10). Thiopental levels may rapidly increase to high levels. If thiopental is used prior to suctioning and other procedures, blood levels should be checked and kept less than 40 to 90 μg/ml, although there is some debate as to the correct level. This is the maximum figure.

4. Turn patient every 2 hours. Remember to maintain head in neutral position. Lateral neck flexion may cause impeded jugular venous return.

Renal-metabolic system

1. Maintain temperature between 35° and 37° C. Use a cooling blanket and sponge baths for elevated temperatures. Do not use antipyretics. For treatment of hypothermia, see Chapter 18.

2. Fluids. Give the patient 75% of maintenance fluid each day as long as CVP and systemic arterial blood pressure are adequate and serum osmolality does not exceed 310 mOsm. NG losses are replaced in addition to maintenance with 0.45% sodium chloride solution. Maintain urine output at 0.5 ml/kg/ hr or greater.

3. Minerals
   a. Sodium and chloride. Give 4 mEq/kg/ 24 hr and adjust to maintain normal levels.
   b. Potassium. Because of a large glucose requirement, patients require 2 to 3 times normal maintenance (4 to 6 mEq/kg/24 hr) of potassium (given as potassium phosphate).
   c. Calcium and phosphorus. Patients usually require at least maintenance calcium, 200 mg/kg/24 hr, and phosphorus, 3 to 4 mEq/kg/24 hr (given as calcium gluconate and potassium phosphate).

4. Hepatic-gastrointestinal therapy
   a. Give FFP, 10 ml/kg, before liver biopsy.
   b. Give glucose to maintain serum glucose level at approximately 150 mg/dl. Not infrequently this requires as much as 600 to 1000 mg of glucose/kg every hour.
   c. Neomycin, 100 mg/kg, may be given orally in an attempt to prevent further increases in serum ammonia levels.
   d. Give vitamin K, 1 mg IV, as a single dose prior to liver biopsy.
   e. Other drugs metabolized in the liver may have prolonged half-lives.
   f. Avoid potentially hepatoxic drugs (e.g., nafcillin).
   g. Antacids may be needed to treat bleeding from stress ulcers.

5. ISADH and/or diabetes insipidus may complicate the picture and should be diagnosed and treated as indicated in Chapters 51 and 52.

Emotional support. Reye's syndrome is a particularly devastating and sudden illness, which usually occurs in a previously normal child. Support of the family is essential (see Chapter 75).

ADDITIONAL READING

Bartzdorf, U.: The management of cerebral edema in pediatric practice, Pediatrics **58**:78-87, 1976.

Berman, W., Pizzi, F., Schut, L., and others: The effects of exchange transfusion on intracranial pressure in patients with Reye syndrome, J. Pediatr. **87**:877-891, 1975.

Bobo, R.C., Schubert, W.K., Partin, J.C., and Partin, J.S.: Reye syndrome: treatment by exchange trasnfusion with special reference to the 1974 epidemic in Cincinnati, Ohio, J. Pediatr. **87**:881-886, 1975.

Chaves-Carballo, E., Carter, G.A., and Wiebe, D.A.: Triglyceride and cholesterol concentrations in whole serum and in serum lipoproteins in Reye syndrome, Pediatrics **64**:592-597, 1979.

Combes, B.: Reye's syndrome, medical grand rounds, Parkland Memorial Hospital, Dallas, May 8, 1975.

Corey, L., Rubin, R.J., Bregman, D., and Gregg, M.B.: Diagnostic criteria for influenza B–associated Reye's syndrome: clinical vs. pathologic criteria, Pediatrics **60**:702-708, 1977.

Corey, L., Rubin, R.J., and Hattwick, M.A.W.: Reye's syndrome: clinical progression and evaluation of therapy, Pediatrics **60**:708-714, 1977.

Cotev, S., Paul, W.L., Ruiz, B.C., and others: The effect

of PEEP on intracranial pressure, Sixth Annual Scientific and Educational Symposium of Society of Critical Care Medicine, New York, March 11-14, 1977.

DeLong, G.R., and Glick, T.H.: Encephalopathy of Reye's syndrome: a review of pathogenetic hypotheses, Pediatrics **69**:53-63, 1982.

DeVivo, D.C., Keathing, J.P., and Haymond, M.W.: Reye syndrome: results of intensive supportive care, J. Pediatr. **87**:875-880, 1975.

Faraj, B.A., Newman, S.L., Caplan, D.B., and others: Evidence for hypertyraminemia in Reye's syndrome, Pediatrics **64**:76-80, 1979.

Fleisher, G., Schwartz, J., and Lennette, E.: Primary Epstein-Barr virus infection in association with Reye syndrome, J. Pediatr. **97**:935-937, 1980.

Frewen, T.C., Swedlow, D.B., Watcha, M., and others: Outcome in severe Reye syndrome with early pentobarbital coma and hypothermia, J. Pediatr. **100**:663-665, 1982.

Gall, D.B., Cutz, E., McClung, H.J., and Greenberg, M.L.: Acute liver disease and encephalopathy mimicking Reye syndrome, J. Pediatr. **87**:869-874, 1975.

Gronert, G.A., Michenfelder, J.D., Sharbrough, F.W., and Milde, J.H.: Canine cerebral metabolic tolerance during 24 hours deep pentobarbital anesthesia, Anesthesiology **55**:110-113, 1981.

Heick, H.M.C., Shipman, R.T., Chir, B., and others: Reye-like syndrome associated with use of insect repellent in a presumed heterozygote for ornithine carbamoyl transferase deficiency, J. Pediatr. **97**:471-473, 1980.

Huttenlocher, P.R.: Reye's syndrome: relation of outcome to therapy, J. Pediatr. **80**:845-850, 1972.

Lovejoy, F.F., Smith, A.L., Bresnan, M.J., and others: Clinical staging in Reye syndrome, Am. J. Dis. Child. **128**:36-41, 1974.

Marshall, L.F., Shapiro, H.M., Rauscher, A., and Kaufman, N.M.: Pentobarbital therapy for intracranial hypertension in metabolic coma—Reye's syndrome, Crit. Care Med. **6**:1-5, 1978.

Mickell, J.J., Cook, D.R., Reigel, D.H., and others: Intracranial pressure monitoring in Reye-Johnson syndrome, Crit. Care Med. **4**:1-7, 1976.

Mickell, J.J., Reigel, D.H., Cook, D.R., and others: Intracranial pressure: monitoring and normalization therapy in children, Pediatrics **59**:606-613, 1977.

Nadler, H.: Therapeutic delirium in Reye's syndrome, Pediatrics **54**:265-266, 1974.

Nelson, D.B., Kimbrough, R., Landrigan, P.S., and others: Aflatoxin and Reye's syndrome: a case control study, Pediatrics **66**:865-868, 1980.

Reye, R.D., Morgan, G., and Baral, J.: Encephalopathy and fatty degeneration of the vicera: a disease entity in childhood, Lancet **2**:749-752, 1963.

Romshe, C.A., Hilty, M.D., McClung, H.J., and others: Amino acid pattern in Reye syndrome: comparison with clinically similar entities, J. Pediatr. **98**:788-790, 1981.

Ryan, N.J., Hogan, G.R., Hayes, A.W., and others: Aflatoxin B_1: its role in the etiology of Reye's syndrome, Pediatrics **64**:71-75, 1979.

Shannon, D.C., De Long, R., Bercu, B., and others: Studies on the pathophysiology of encephalopathy in Reye's syndrome; hyperammonemia in Reye's syndrome, Pediatrics **56**:999-1004, 1975.

Shaywitz, B.A., Leventhal, J.M., Kramer, M.S., and Venes, J.L.: Prolonged continuous monitoring of intracranial pressure in severe Reye's syndrome, Pediatrics **59**:595-605, 1977.

Shaywitz, B.A., Rothstein, P., and Venes, J.L.: Monitoring and management of increased intracranial pressure in Reye syndrome: results in 29 children, Pediatrics **66**:198-204, 1980.

Shaywitz, S.E., Cohen, P.M., Cohen, D.J., and others: Long-term consequences of Reye syndrome: a sibling-matched, controlled study of neurologic, cognitive, academic and psychiatric function, J. Pediatr. **100**:41-46, 1982.

Starko, K.M., Ray, C.G., Dominguez, L.B., and others: Reye's syndrome and salicylate use, Pediatrics **66**:859-864, 1980.

Steen, P.A., and Michenfelder, J.D.: Barbiturate protection in tolerant and nontolerant hypoxic mice: comparison with hypothermic protection, Anesthesiology **50**:404-408, 1979.

Sullivan-Bolyai, J.Z., Nelson, D.B., Morens, D.M., and Schonberger, L.B.: Reye syndrome in children less than 1 year old: some epidemiologic observations, Pediatrics **65**:627-629, 1980.

Thaler, M.M.: Pathogenesis of Reye's syndrome: a working hypothesis, Pediatrics **56**:1081-1084, 1975.

Tonsgard, J.H., Huttenlocher, P.R., and Thisted, R.A.: Lactic acidemia in Reye's syndrome, Pediatrics **69**:64-69, 1982.

van Caillie, M., Morin, C.L., Roy, C.C., and others: Reye's syndrome: relapses and neurological sequelae, Pediatrics **59**:244-249, 1977.

Vries, J.K., Becker, D.P., and Young, H.F.: A subarachnoid screw for monitoring intracranial pressure, J. Neurosurg. **39**:416-419, 1973.

Weeks, H.L.: What every ICU nurse should know about Reye's syndrome, Int. Care, July-Aug. 1976.

Wood, A.P.: Reye's concern prompts AAP to advise against salicylate use in flu-like illness, Pediatr. News, April, 1982.

Yokoi, T., Honke, K., Funabashi, T., and others: Partial ornithine transcarbamylase deficiency simulating Reye syndrome, J. Pediatr. **99**:929-931, 1981.

22 Guillain-Barré syndrome

MICHAEL BLAW

DANIEL L. LEVIN

DEFINITION AND PHYSIOLOGY

Although Guillain-Barré remains a syndrome, in the past two decades accumulated evidence strongly suggests that the pathogenesis involves an autoimmune process. This conclusion is based on clinical evidence that peripheral lymphocytes in patients with Guillain-Barré syndrome are sensitized to peripheral nervous system tissue, and it is based on the similarity between the clinical pathologic findings in Guillain-Barré and the changes produced by experimental allergic neuritis. The clinical pathologic findings reveal an acute inflammatory process of nerves and their roots, with evidence of inflammation around endoneural and epineural blood vessels. These inflammatory lesions result initially in localized areas of edematous myelin followed by segmental demyelinization. As a result of the disruption of myelin, nerve conduction is impaired, and axonal damage and degeneration may ensue. The inflammatory process is not limited to the anterior spinal root but may also involve posterior roots, dorsal ganglia, sympathetic ganglia and chain, cranial nerves, and proximal and distal peripheral nerves. Signs and symptoms will therefore be determined by the distribution and extent of the demyelinization.

Since Guillain-Barré is a syndrome, certain criteria are necessary for diagnosis. Although not all criteria are always met, the following are those most generally accepted:

1. A preceding infection, not infrequently a nonspecific upper respiratory tract infection, has occurred within 3 weeks of onset. Specific infections with chickenpox, measles, mumps, enterovirus, etc. have been documented.
2. Even though sensory complaints such as dysesthesia in hands and feet may precede paralysis, objective sensory impairment is usually minimal and transient.
3. Motor weakness with loss of deep tendon reflexes starts symmetrically in the lower extremities and progresses steadily to involve the arms and trunk. Bladder and bowel involvement is uncommon.
4. CSF analysis demonstrates an elevated protein level without significant pleocytosis.

In a study of 100 consecutive patients with Guillain-Barré syndrome, 24% had leg weakness and 74% had weakness of all four extremities at the time of admission. One patient had only arm involvement, and one patient had only face involvement. Of the cranial nerves, the facial, glossopharyngeal, and vagus nerves were involved in approximately 50% of the patients. Cranial nerve involvement above the facial nerve is much less common. Higher cortical function is preserved, although some patients will exhibit nonspecific behavioral disturbances of anxiety, irritability, depression, or lethargy. Papilledema has been observed in a small percentage of patients and is usually associated with marked increases in CSF protein.

The clinical course of the syndrome is one of increasing ascending paralysis (with or without sensory loss) over a period of several days to 3 weeks. During the initial stages of illness, autonomic nervous system disturbances include excessive or insufficient sympathetic and parasympathetic activity manifested by transient

150

periods of pallor, flushing, sweating, vasocon-striction, extremity coldness, dilated pupils, bouts of cardiac dysrhythmia, bradycardia, tachycardia, hypertension, and hypotension. Death has been attributed to these disturb-ances of autonomic function, but care must be exercised and overvigorous countertherapy avoided, since the disturbances fluctuate widely and are transient. As noted above, paralysis generally reaches a zenith by 3 weeks, with significant respiratory muscle paralysis requir-ing ventilatory assistance in up to 25% of pa-tients. Paralysis then stabilizes, and improve-ment begins in the fourth to eighth week of ill-ness. Although some patients exhibit a rapid recovery course, the average hospital stay in one clinical study was 75 days. Complete recov-ery is expected in up to 75% of patients. Signifi-cant neurologic residua are observed in 5% to 10% of patients. At this time, neither adreno-corticotropic hormone (ACTH) nor steroids have been proved to affect any aspect of the clinical course except in a small percentage of patients who run a chronic, relapsing course.

Because Guillain-Barré is a syndrome, it re-mains, for the most part, a diagnosis of exclu-sion. Of importance is the elimination of toxic neuropathies, both exogenous and endogenous. Examples include a diphtheritic polyneuritis, tic paralysis, and the polyneuropathy associated with ingestion of buckthorn (*Karwinskia hum-boltiana*). Other acute intoxications that affect the myoneural junctions (such as botulism) must be considered. Included in the differential diag-nosis are acute poliomyelitis, acute myasthenia gravis, and transverse myelitis.

MONITORING

See also Chapter 4.

Neurologic system

1. Assess proximal and distal muscle strength and cranial nerve function (speech, swallow-ing, secretions, eyelid and ocular muscle strength) every 2 to 4 hours.

2. Perform funduscopic examination every 2 to 4 hours during the acute phase.
3. Perform lumbar puncture for CSF examina-tion initially and repeat at 1 week if protein level is not elevated.
4. Autonomic nervous system.
   a. Examine skin for mottling, flushing, and diaphoresis.
   b. Check pupillary size every 2 hours.
5. Observe joints for contractures and pressure points for skin breakdown.

Respiratory system

1. Auscultate breath sounds and estimate the extent of chest wall excursion.
2. Obtain a chest roentgenogram initially and once every day early in the course, and once every week thereafter. Pay particular atten-tion to the level of the diaphragms, since these may become paralyzed and complicate respiratory care.
3. Obtain arterial blood-gas tensions and pH initially and every 2 to 4 hours during the acute phase. Obtain these measurements every 4 to 6 hours, as well as 10 minutes after every ventilatory change, when the pa-tient is started on mechanical ventilation. This may be reduced to once every day or every other day when patients are on long-term mechanical ventilation (for details of weaning from mechanical ventilation, see p. 153).
4. Assess respiratory failure:
   a. Clinical observations:
      (1) Progressive cyanosis.
      (2) Decreasing depth of respiration.
      (3) Weakening of speech.
      (4) Inability to manage secretions.
   b. Laboratory investigations:
      (1) Arterial blood-gas tension abnormali-ties as an indication of respiratory failure:
         (a) Pa_{CO_2} greater than 50 mm Hg.
         (b) Pa_{O_2} less than 50 mm Hg in an FI_{O_2} of 1.0.

(2) Forced expired volumes and flows. Mid-maximal forced expired flow (FEF_{25-75}) is an effort-independent measure of the patient's ability to expire with maximal exertion. Forced vital capacity (FVC) is the total amount of air that can be forcefully expired after a maximum inspiratory effort. Both of these variables may be measured from a single breath, and progressive deterioration compared to normal values is indicative of respiratory failure. These should be measured 3 to 4 times per day during the initial phase of the illness.

5. Assess recovery from respiratory failure.
   a. Clinical observations:
      (1) Depth of spontaneous respiration.
      (2) Strength of truncal and extremity musculature.
      (3) Maintenance of color, heart rate, and state of well-being while disconnected from mechanical ventilation.
   b. Laboratory investigations:
      (1) Maximal inspiratory force (MIF). When the patient can consistently generate more than 20 cm H_2O of inspiratory force as measured with a hand-held manometer, respiratory musculature is recovering.
      (2) Repetitive measurement of arterial blood-gas tensions and pH during withdrawal of respiratory support (see p. 153).
      (3) Improvement in mechanical lung function as described above (FEF_{25-75}, FVC).
6. Note quality and character of tracheal secretions in intubated patients. Obtain cultures and gram-stain secretions for white cells once every week and whenever the secretions change in character, the patient is febrile, or an infiltrate appears on the chest roentgenogram.

7. Obtain a blood culture if the patient is suspected of having pneumonia.

Renal-metabolic system

1. Repeat serum calcium tests twice every week in chronic patients, who may become hypercalcemic as a result of mobilization of calcium from bone. Check urine once every week for hematuria as an indication of stone formation.
2. Note character and frequency of stools. Patients tend to develop constipation or diarrhea.
3. Check frequently for bladder enlargement. Patients tend to develop urinary retention.

MANAGEMENT
Neurologic system

1. There is no treatment for the syndrome itself. Some authors recommend ACTH or steroids, although the efficacy of these has not been proved. Recent therapeutic interest has been focused on plasmapheresis.
2. Autonomic dysfunction.
   a. Do not treat tachycardia or bradycardia, hypertension or hypotension unless cardiac output (assessed by urine output, arterial blood-gas tensions, and pH) is compromised. These abnormalities tend to be transient and fluctuate; for example, hypotension may follow hypertension within a few minutes. If treatment is deemed necessary, use short-acting, quickly reversible methods of therapy, for example:
      (1) Bradycardia: use isoproterenol, 0.1 μg/kg/min as a constant IV infusion (see Chapter 14), or atropine, 0.01 mg/kg IV.
      (2) Tachycardia: attempt carotid sinus massage.
      (3) Hypotension: the problem is usually a dilated peripheral vascular bed with decreased systemic vascular resis-

tance and an increased capacity. Give fluids, 10 to 20 ml/kg IV over 30 minutes. Repeat as necessary. Avoid rapid changes in posture that may produce hypotension in this circumstance.

   (4) Hypertension: this should probably not be treated pharmacologically. If the systemic arterial blood pressure is so elevated as to be life-threatening, alpha blockade with a short-acting agent such as phentolamine hydrochloride (Regitine) may be tried (see Chapter 14).

3. Use a soft (Silastic) NG tube for constant infusion feedings in patients who have difficulty swallowing. This may occur even before or in the absence of respiratory failure.

4. Use passive range of motion and exercise programs to prevent contractures (usually parents are eager to make this contribution to care).

5. Rotate patient and massage pressure points to prevent skin breakdown and pressure (nerve) palsies.

6. Rarely, muscle pain is severe during the acute phase. Use moist heat to relieve pain.

Respiratory system

1. Intubate the patient if:
   a. Respiratory failure occurs (clinical deterioration, Pa_{CO_2} >50 mm Hg, Pa_{O_2} <50 mm Hg in FI_{O_2} of 1.0, or progressive decrease in FEF_{25-75} or FVC).
   b. The patient cannot swallow secretions and is at risk for inhalation pneumonia.

2. Use a nasotracheal tube (see Chapter 95). Do not use a cuffed tube.

3. Most patients who progress to this point will have a prolonged course requiring mechanical ventilation for 4 to 12 weeks or longer. Perform a tracheotomy after 7 to 14 days if the patient is not demonstrating significant recovery of ventilatory function.

4. Details of mechanical ventilation, CPT, and endotracheal suctioning are presented in Chapters 97, 99, and 100, respectively.

5. Weaning of these patients from mechanical ventilation is usually different from that of patients who are being ventilated for primary cardiac or pulmonary parenchymal disease. Patients with Guillain-Barré syndrome gradually recover muscle strength (including diaphragmatic), and the problem in weaning them is one of muscle fatigue. To avoid fatigue, several regimens are attempted, and combinations of these may be used in any one patient at different times.

   a. Place the patient on an IMV circuit so that he receives a preset number of breaths at a preset TV (usually 6 to 10 breaths/min and 10 to 15 ml/kg/breath). Most patients feel comfortable with this regimen since, as they develop the strength to generate spontaneous respiration, they will receive a fresh gas supply at a TV determined by their own effort in addition to the mandatory breaths. Initially, some patients who are not generating adequate negative intrathoracic pressures and therefore have small spontaneous TVs feel distressed by this regimen and prefer to return to IPPV.

   b. Slowly introduce periods of CPAP alone (2 to 4 cm H_2O). Start at 5 minutes every 2 to 4 hours. Check the arterial blood-gas tensions before and at the end of the weaning period to correlate with clinical assessment of the patient's ability to tolerate this weaning period.

   c. In conjunction with clinical assessment of peripheral muscle strength, gradually (every day or two) increase the weaning periods to 10, 15, 20 minutes and so on until the patient is spending 1 to 2 hours at a time off the mechanical ventilator.

   d. Usually at this point patients still prefer

to have mechanical ventilation on the IMV mode at approximately 6 breaths/min and 10 ml/kg/breath during sleeping hours.

e. Gradually decrease the time the patient spends on the IMV circuit during sleep by 1 to 2 hours until it is no longer required.

6. Once the patient is off mechanical ventilation consider extubation.

a. Usually the patient has a tracheotomy at this point.

b. Assess his ability to swallow secretions and food.

c. Assess his ability to cough and clear pulmonary secretions and to prevent atelectasis.

d. Assess the return of diaphragmatic function if paralysis has occurred. Diaphragmatic paralysis, especially if bilateral, will significantly impair the patient's ability to cough and clear pulmonary secretions.

e. If the patient can swallow and cough, remove the tracheotomy tube (see Chapters 103 and 104).

f. The patient may require IPPB every 4 to 6 hours while convalescing, to prevent atelectasis.

Cardiovascular system

See Neurologic system (p. 152).

Renal-metabolic system

1. Caloric intake is a major problem. Patients who are in impending respiratory failure should not be fed orally. After intubation, tube feedings can be started with a commercially prepared liquid diet (e.g., Sustical, Vivonex) or a blenderized diet. In chronic patients with significant neurologic residua, a gastrostomy may be necessary.

2. Patients tend to become constipated, and the use of stool softeners (e.g., dioctyl sodium sulfosuccinate [Colace]) or the use of laxatives or enemas may be necessary.

3. Diarrhea is frequently related to autonomic dysfunction and should not be treated except to replace fluid and electrolyte losses. It may also be related to feedings; thus, changes in diet may be required.

4. Hypercalcemia can be treated by giving or increasing IV fluids to 1.5 times maintenance.

5. Temperature instability may be a sign of autonomic nervous system dysfunction and may be treated with antipyretics or a heating/cooling blanket.

6. Fever may be a sign of infection, usually pulmonary, although urinary tract infection (UTI) and phlebitis are not uncommon.

ADDITIONAL READING

Appenzeller, O., and Marshall, J.: Vasomotor disturbance in the Landry-Guillain-Barré syndrome, Arch. Neurol. **9**:368-372, 1963.

Cook, J.D., Tindall, R.A.S., Walker, J., and others: Plasma exchange as a treatment of acute and chronic idiopathic autoimmune polyneuropathy: limited success, Neurology **30**:361-362, 1980.

Currie, S., and Knowles, M.: Lymphocytic transformation in the Guillain-Barré syndrome, Brain **94**:109-116, 1971.

Haymaker, W., and Kernohad, J.W.: Landry-Guillain-Barré syndrome, Medicine **28**:59-141, 1949.

Lichtenfeld, P.: Autonomic dysfunction in the Guillain-Barré syndrome, Am. J. Med. **50**:772-780, 1971.

Low, N.L., Schneider, J., and Carter, S.: Polyneuritis in children, Pediatrics **22**:972-990, 1958.

Moore, P., and James, O.: Guillain-Barré syndrome: incidence, management and outcome of major complications, Crit. Care Med. **9**:549-555, 1981.

Osler, L.D., and Sidell, A.D.: The Guillain-Barré syndrome, N. Engl. J. Med. **262**:964-969, 1960.

Rosenberg, R.N.: Idiopathic acute polyradiculoneuritis, Department of Internal Medicine grand rounds, University of Texas Health Science Center, Dallas, May 29, 1975.

23 Myasthenia gravis

JAY D. COOK

DEFINITION AND PHYSIOLOGY

Myasthenia (Greek: weakness) gravis (Latin: grave) is a disease characterized by pathologic fatigue (relapsing and remittent muscle weakness) resulting from a defect in the neuromuscular junction. There are three forms of the disease that affect children: neonatal, congenital, and juvenile (see Table 23-1). The neonatal form of myasthenia gravis is an autoimmune disease that is passively transmitted from a mother who has the adult form of autoimmune myasthenia gravis. The congenital form of myasthenia gravis is a nonimmunologic disease resulting from a presynaptic and/or postsynaptic structural defect. The juvenile form of myasthenia gravis is an autoimmune disease in which there are lymphocytes and antibodies directed against the postjunction receptor. All three forms meet the criteria for diagnosis of myasthenia gravis:

1. History and physical examination reveal a relapsing and remittent muscle weakness, which is better in the morning and worsens as the day progresses. The affected muscles include those of the eyes (ptosis, dysconjugate gaze, gaze paresis), face, pharynx, tongue (poor suck, dysphagia, weak speech, blank facies, oral ptosis), body (extremity weakness), and the muscles of mastication and respiration (dyspnea, shortness of breath, respiratory failure).
2. On neurophysiologic examination repetitive nerve stimulation yields a decremental response of greater than 10% at 1 to 5 Hz. At higher frequencies posttetanic facilitation is found. Single fiber study demonstrates jitter.
3. On pharmacologic examination anticholinesterase medications (edrophonium, neostig-mine, and pyridostigmine) produce a beneficial effect. Increased sensitivity to curare and lactate can be demonstrated, as well as resistance to succinylcholine.

Both the neonatal and juvenile forms of the disease may have serum antibodies that are directed against the acetylcholine receptor.

Pathogenesis

The response of the muscle to a stimulated nerve depends on the release of acetylcholine from the neuromuscular junction nerve terminal, diffusion across the synaptic cleft, and binding to the receptor membrane. The postsynaptic membrane depolarizes, resulting in further depolarization of the T tubule system of the muscle. This results in calcium release and muscle contraction. The amount of acetylcholine released and bound to the neuromuscular junction is usually far greater than necessary for postsynaptic membrane depolarization. This safety factor is felt to be 5:1. Any defect in either the amount of acetylcholine released, diffusion across the receptor cleft, or the number of receptors available for binding will result in symptoms of neuromuscular junction dysfunction, i.e., fatigability.

The various forms of childhood myasthenia gravis exhibit different pathogeneses. The congenital form is often associated with a family history, and usually there are not the marked fluctuations in muscle strength that are seen with the autoimmune disease. The congenital form is probably a result of a defect in the structure or function of either the presynaptic nerve terminal or the postjunctional muscle receptor. Recent evidence has demonstrated absence of

155

Table 23-1. Childhood myasthenia gravis

Disorder	Pathogenesis	Standard treatment	Crisis settings	Treatment of crises
Neonatal	Passive transfer of an autoimmune disease	1. Anticholinesterase drugs 2. Respiratory and pharyngeal support 3. Blood exchange	1. Within the first week of life	Same as standard treatment
Congenital	Congenital dysfunction of the neuromuscular junction	1. Ephedrine 2. Anticholinesterase drugs	1. Neonatal 2. Inhalation pneumonia 3. Infection 4. Improper medication	1. Respiratory and pharyngeal support 2. Ephedrine 3. Anticholinesterase drugs
Juvenile	Autoimmune disease directed against the neuromuscular junction	1. Anticholinesterase drugs 2. Immunosuppressive drugs 3. Thymectomy 4. Plasma exchange	1. Infection 2. Inhalation pneumonia 3. Improper medication 4. Environmental stress 5. Postoperative state 6. Menses	1. Respiratory and pharyngeal support 2. Optimize anticholinesterase dose 3. Drug holiday 4. Plasma exchange

acetylcholinesterase, small preterminal nerve endings, and abnormal postjunctional receptors in a patient with congenital myasthenia gravis.

In the autoimmune forms of the disease (neonatal and juvenile) the pathogenesis is somewhat more complex. Antibodies directed against the neuromuscular junction have been found in the sera of patients with the adult form of myasthenia gravis. Similar circulating antibodies have now also been found in both the neonatal and juvenile forms. It was originally thought that these autoimmune forms were mediated by the antibodies directly blocking the acetylcholine receptor site, thereby preventing depolarization. However, further studies found no correlation between the amount of acetylcholine receptor antibody and the disease severity. When purified antineuromuscular junction

antibody is infused directly onto the neuromuscular junction of an in vitro nerve-muscle preparation, no decremental response is seen with repetitive nerve stimulation. However, long-term passive transfer into mice did result in neurophysiologic changes similar to those seen in myasthenia gravis, i.e., decremental response. Thus, long-term exposure to the antibody was necessary to produce an abnormal physiologic response at the neuromuscular junction, suggesting that some alteration at the neuromuscular junction occurs after long-term exposure to the antibody. In experiments designed to measure the degradation and synthesis of receptors, it was found that when sera from myasthenia gravis patients were applied to muscle cells in culture, the rate of receptor degeneration was increased and the rate of receptor synthesis was decreased. Thus,

Table 23-2. Medications used to treat childhood myasthenia gravis

Agent	Preparation	Route	Dose	Onset of action	Duration of action
Anticholinesterase					
Edrophonium (Tensilon)	10 mg/ml	IV	0.02-0.2 mg/kg	1 min	10 min-4 hr
Neostigmine (Prostigmin)	1:1000, 1 mg/ml	IM or IV	0.1-3.0 mg/kg	10 min	1-3 hr
	1:2000, 0.5 mg/ml				
	1:4000, 0.25 mg/ml			1 min	
	15- mg tablet	PO	0.1-3.0 mg/kg	20-40 min	
Pyridostigmine (Mestinon)	Syrup, 60 mg/5 ml	PO	0.3-4.0 mg/kg	30-40 min	Syrup: 3-6 hr
	60-mg tablet				Tablet: 3-6 hr
	180-mg time spansule				Spansule: 6-12 hr
Acetylcholine-releasing agent					
Ephedrine	25 mg/5 ml	PO	0.4-0.8 mg/kg	15-40 min	4-6 hr
Anticholinergic agents					
Atropine	0.4 mg/ml	IV or PO	0.02 mg/kg	1 min	6-8 hr
	1-mg tablet	PO		10-20 min	6-8 hr
Glycopyrrolate (Robinul)*	0.2 mg/ml	IV or IM	0.002 mg/kg	1 min	4-8 hr
	2-mg tablet	PO	0.002 mg/kg	30 min	4-8 hr

*Not recommended for children under 12.

the total effect would result in a marked reduction in the amount of receptor, thereby producing neuromuscular junction dysfunction.

The exact role of the thymus is still not known. In the adult form of the disease, some kind of thymic pathology is found in over 70% of adult myasthenia gravis patients. Thymomas, in particular, occur in 10% of the adults with myasthenia gravis. The remission rate is greater in adult patients who have undergone thymectomy. In myasthenic patients, both cellular and humoral immune response to thymic tissue has been demonstrated. Whether this is evidence of primary or secondary response is unknown. A recent long-term follow-up study suggests that thymectomy early in the disease course results in a greater than four-fold increase in remission rate.

Rationale for treatment

Since Mary Walker demonstrated the benefit of anticholinesterase medication, these agents have been the cornerstone of therapy, until recently. In general, they are helpful to relieve symptoms of neonatal, congenital, and juvenile myasthenia gravis. These agents retard the breakdown of acetylcholine so that there is an effective increased amount of transmitter to react with the postjunctional receptor. Pyridostigmine bromide (Mestinon) or neostigmine methylsulfate (Prostigmin) are the usual drugs (see Table 23-2).

In neonatal myasthenia gravis anticholinesterase agents, respiratory and feeding support, and blood exchange transfusions are all appropriate. In congenital myasthenia gravis, only the use of anticholinesterase agents and agents promoting the release of acetylcholine (such as ephedrine) are indicated. These patients should never be subjected to immunosuppressive drugs, plasma exchange, or thymectomy. Aggressive use of thymectomy, plasma exchange, and immunosuppressive agents (prednisone or azathioprine) certainly are now considered by some as the definitive treatment for juvenile myasthenia gravis (see Table 23-1).

Clinical presentations

Emergency presentations of these three forms of myasthenia gravis result from complications of pharyngeal and/or respiratory muscle failure. It should be remembered that while all three types are treatable, they can be fatal, depending on how well respiratory and/or pharyngeal function is preserved.

Neonatal. This transient defect of neuromuscular transmission can occur in any infant whose mother has a history of autoimmune myasthenia gravis. It occurs in about 10% to 15% of such infants. The severity or duration of the infant's disorder is not correlated with the mother's clinical state at the time of birth; i.e., an asymptomatic mother's infant can be severely affected, and a severely affected mother's infant can be completely asymptomatic.

Symptoms will usually occur within the first 72 hours after birth. The child will show signs of fatigue of both bulbar and somatic muscles. These signs will usually include eye signs (ptosis and dysconjugate gaze), breathing difficulties (cyanosis, increased respiratory rate, nasal flaring, weak cry), decreased general movement (floppy infant, fluctuation in muscle tone), and feeding problems.

Congenital. This form of myasthenia gravis will usually present as an emergency, primarily as respiratory failure associated with inhalation of gastric or oral secretions and/or lower respiratory tract infection. The child will usually have a history of having been floppy from birth (no progression of weakness except daily fluctuations), with classical fatigue of both bulbar and generalized musculature. There may be a positive history of siblings, cousins, or parents being involved.

Juvenile. The autoimmune form of childhood myasthenia gravis can present as an emergency with acute pharyngeal or respiratory muscle failure resulting from three primary etiologies: (1) infection, (2) medication problems, and (3) postoperative care. In most instances, the diagnosis will already be known.

However, the child with juvenile myasthenia gravis may also present as an apparent emergency not associated with respiratory failure. Such a child presents with ptosis and diplopia. The first diagnostic consideration would be increased ICP or toxin exposure. A history of fluctuation throughout the day or involvement of other body musculature may be the only hint that the diagnosis is juvenile myasthenia gravis. Certainly the diagnostic considerations for any child with such an acute presentation must include brainstem tumor, botulism, lead intoxication, Miller-Fisher syndrome, organophosphate poisoning, or jasmine poisoning.

Infection. A child with juvenile myasthenia gravis will usually become more symptomatic when an infection is present, regardless of the site or agent (bacterial or viral). A lower respiratory tract infection poses the most serious problem because of ventilation-perfusion abnormalities secondary to the primary infection. Children who have myasthenia gravis and have never had respiratory or swallowing problems may develop severe dysphagia and/or dyspnea after developing a mild viral syndrome.

Medication problems. These can include cholinergic crises, myasthenic crises, improper use of ancillary drugs, or acute nonresponsiveness to anticholinesterase medications. Too much as well as too little anticholinesterase medication in a myasthenia gravis patient will result in weakness. Much has been made of the differentiation between these two conditions by the association of systemic symptoms. In the cholinergic crisis the patient usually exhibits diarrhea, small pupils, profuse sweating, lacrimation, increased salivation, muscle cramps, muscle fasciculations, and bradycardia. In the myasthenic crisis pupillary dilation and tachycardia secondary to the adrenalin response to stress usually occur, and muscle cramps and fasciculations are usually absent. However, the immediate treatment is identical in either situation: respiratory and/or pharyngeal support (e.g., intubation, ventilation, removal of secretions, NG feeding, alteration of food texture). Another potential danger from a pharmacologic agent is atropine poisoning, which causes altered mental status and cardiovascular dysfunction. Because of the cholinergic side-effects (sweating, salivation, diarrhea) of anticholinesterase medications, atropine may be prescribed and overused. In general, there is no role for the use of atropine-like agents on an outpatient basis; but, atropine poisoning must be kept in mind as a potential reason for a crisis.

Numerous drugs can cause acute worsening of the myasthenia gravis syndrome (see Table 23-3). The general groups of drugs are membrane stabilizers, antibiotics, and muscle relaxants.

For reasons not completely understood, patients become refractory to anticholinesterase medications. This refractoriness is often asso-

Table 23-3. Hazardous drugs in childhood myasthenia gravis

Avoid the following drugs:
Membrane stabilizers
   Procainamide
   Quinine
   Quinidine
Muscle relaxants
   Diazepam (Valium)
   Baclofen (Lioresal)
   Chlordiazepoxide (Librium)
Exercise caution when using these drugs:
Antibiotics
   Streptomycin
   Kanamycin
   Colistin
   Gentamicin
   Tetracycline
Endocrine or steroidal compounds
   Corticosteroids
   ACTH
Membrane stabilizers
   Phenytoin (Dilantin)
   Carbamazepine (Tegretol)
   Valproic acid (Depakene)

---

ciated with times of stress, infection, or menses, but there may be no significant environmental change involved. During such times the patients not only remain weak on the regular dose of medication, but do not respond to a larger dose of anticholinesterase medication.

Postoperative course. Patients who may be asymptomatic preoperatively may go into a crisis within the first 72 hours postoperatively. This may be the result of endogenous corticosteroids which (as with synthetic corticosteroids) have been shown to have an antagonistic effect at the neuromuscular junction when anticholinesterase medications are given. The response to anticholinesterase medication is erratic and careful monitoring postoperatively is mandatory.

MONITORING

In a crisis situation (acute worsening of symptoms) the myasthenia gravis patient must be monitored primarily for respiratory and pharyngeal function; the other muscle weakness is of secondary importance. The cardinal rule must be preservation of respiratory and pharyngeal function. If there is any question of dyspnea or dysphagia in the mind of the physician, the patient must be aggressively evaluated, monitored, and supported. Also, myasthenia gravis is a disease not only of weakness but of *fatigue;* therefore strength assessment must be made in reference to time: time of last medication and time of last examination.

Respiratory system

Assess for respiratory failure at least hourly.
1. Clinical observations
   a. Monosyllabic speech.
   b. Gasping.
   c. Fear.
   d. Decrease in voice volume.
   e. Poor single breath counting.
   f. Inability to handle secretions.
   g. Cyanosis.
   h. Increasing respiratory rate initially, followed by a decrease if not supported.

i. Increasing cardiac rate initially, followed by decrease if not supported.

j. Auscultation of breath sounds (decreased air movement).

2. Laboratory investigations
   a. Chest roentgenogram. Look for:
      (1) Signs of infections or inhalation of foreign material.
      (2) Level of diaphragm.
   b. Arterial blood-gas tensions and pH. Inadequate values are:
      (1) Pa_{CO_2} >50 mm Hg.
      (2) Pa_{O_2} <50 mm Hg.
      (3) pH_a < 7.30.
   c. Forced expiratory volumes
      (1) FVC (total amount of air forcefully expelled in a single breath) every 2 to 4 hours. Immediate support is indicated if FVC is less than 50% of predicted.
      (2) MIF (maximum inspiratory force) every 2 to 4 hours. Immediate support is indicated if MIF is less than −20 mm H_2O.
      (3) Continuous observation for any sign of dysfunction may be necessary in an acutely weak or stressed child.

3. Assess recovery of respiratory function.
   a. Clinical observations
      (1) Return of diaphragmatic movement.
      (2) Maintenance of color, heart rate, and state of well-being while patient is disconnected from mechanical ventilation. NOTE: There is no correlation between respiratory function and the strength of other muscle groups. There is often a disparity in clinical response between respiratory muscle function and other muscle groups' response to treatment.
   b. Laboratory investigations
      (1) MIF. Adequate when the patient can consistently generate −20 cm H_2O of inspiratory force, as measured by a hand-held manometer on an hourly basis, for a full 24 hours.
      (2) Repetitive measurement of arterial blood-gas tensions and pH during withdrawal of respiratory support (see p. 165); again, consistency on an hourly basis is most important.
      (3) Improvement in mechanical lung function, as indicated by FVC.
      (4) Careful attention should be paid to the quality and character of tracheal secretions in both nonintubated (borderline respiratory and pharyngeal functioning patients) and intubated patients.
      (5) Appropriate cultures and gram stains should be obtained routinely on a weekly basis for intubated patients and when the patient has a change in secretion character, a fever, or an infiltrate shown on a chest roentgenogram. This is important for patients on immunosuppressive agents, since the organisms of infection may be atypical.
      (6) Blood cultures should be obtained in patients suspected of having pneumonia. NOTE: Some antibiotics may compromise muscle strength (see Table 23-3).

Neurologic system

1. Assessment of oculomotor function (ptosis, dysconjugate gaze) every 2 hours
   a. Measure time to the development of ptosis or dysconjugate gaze with continuous upward gaze.
   b. Red lens test (estimation of degree of dysconjugate gaze with use of red lens in front of examined eye; two lights, one red and one white, are seen when light is shined in eye if dysconjugate gaze is present).

2. Assess motor function or other cranial nerve function and proximal and distal somatic muscle groups. Fasciculations indicate overmedication. Formal strength is helpful, but functional tests are best.

a. Time able to hold arms up (normal: longer than 1 minute).
b. Time able to hold legs off bed (normal: longer than 1 minute).
c. Number of times the wrist or ankle can be moved the full range of motion in 1 minute (normal: more than 45).
d. Ability to cough effectively.
3. Assessment of responsiveness to anticholinesterase medications:
   a. Edrophonium HCl (Tensilon) test. Edrophonium hydrochloride (Tensilon) is a short-acting anticholinesterase. It will produce a transient improvement (10 minutes to 4 hours) in myasthenic muscle groups. If time is taken prior to the introduction of needles to explain to both the parents and child what is going to be done, the test may be relatively simple. If this is not done, the test may be a disaster. It is important that the patient cooperate because of the brief time available to make pertinent observations. It is also important to decide what signs of weakness are going to be examined for improvement (respiratory function must always be one of these). In neonates and very young children, observation of feeding ability or resistance to passive motion may be substituted for more quantitative measurements of strength. There should always be resuscitation equipment and a nurse on hand to help with any difficulties (primarily respiratory, pharyngeal, or cardiac) the patient may experience during the test.
   Procedure:
   (1) Resuscitation cart and nurse are present.
   (2) Measure pretest variables (FVC or single breath counting is always included).
   (3) A butterfly needle is introduced into a vein, secured with tape, and flushed with 0.9% sodium chloride solution.
   (4) Atropine (0.01 mg/kg) is given IV.

This is infused slowly to prevent severe autonomic responses to the edrophonium hydrochloride, i.e., bradycardia, hypotension, and abdominal cramps with nausea and vomiting. The atropine should not be given more frequently than every 6 to 8 hours if repeated Tensilon tests are being done (see below).
   (5) Variables being followed may again be evaluated to test for placebo effect.
   (6) A small test dose of edrophonium hydrochloride (0.04 mg/kg is infused slowly (10 to 15 seconds) and followed with 2 to 3 ml of 0.9% sodium chloride solution.
   (7) The variables are tested after 1 minute.
   (8) If there is no dramatic improvement or worsening, then a larger amount of edrophonium hydrochloride (0.16 mg/kg) is infused.
   (9) The variables are again tested after 1 minute (see Table 23-4).
In addition to helping make the diagnosis of myasthenia gravis, the Tensilon test is useful in following the therapeutic response of myasthenic patients to other anticholinesterase medications. However, it should never be used in an emergency situation to determine whether a patient is overmedicated (cholinergic) or undermedicated (myasthenic). Respiratory functions should be stabilized and then a Tensilon test can be done to determine the state of responsiveness to the anticholinesterase agents (see Table 23-5).
   b. Assessment of the proper dose of pyridostigmine (Mestinon) to achieve maximum benefit. The optimal dose is that dose which allows the patient the greatest strength with no, or few, side effects. Different muscle groups will respond to medication differently; certain muscles may in fact be unresponsive, or choliner-

Table 23-4. Edrophonium HCl (Tensilon) test: an example of a positive test

Variables to be observed	Pretest	Post-atropine	Edrophonium HCl dose	
			0.04 mg/kg	0.16 mg/kg
Single breath counting	11	13	15	26
Arms held straight (time)	23 sec	25 sec	27 sec	43 sec
Development of ptosis with upward gaze	10 sec	9 sec	15 sec	>60 sec

Table 23-5. Use of edrophonium HCl (Tensilon) test to establish proper dose of pyridostigmine bromide (Mestinon)

Condition	Variables tested	Hours after pyridostigmine administration											
		0			1			2			4		
		PRE*	LE†	HE‡	PRE	LE	HE	PRE	LE	HE	PRE	LE	HE
Undermedi-cated	Single breath count	16	20	29	20	23	30	18	23	29	16	21	29
	Arm strength (sec)	23	25	27	29	30	50	29	30	45	23	26	29
	Upward gaze or ptosis (sec)	10	9	25	12	12	30	12	15	40	10	11	30
Optimal	Single breath count	24	25	33	33	34	35	30	31	33	26	25	34
	Arm strength (sec)	50	55	>60	>60	>60	>60	>60	>60	>60	>55	>60	>60
	Upward gaze or ptosis (sec)	40	50	55	55	>60	>60	>60	>60	>60	>60	>60	>60
Overmedi-cated	Single breath count	27	26	21	21	21	12	23	21	18	24	25	20
	Arm strength (sec)	>60	55	50	30	30	20	30	28	28	55	54	56
	Upward gaze or ptosis (sec)	>60	>60	>60	>60	50	45	55	50	50	55	55	>60

*PRE, Prior to edrophonium HCl administration.
†LE, After 0.04 mg/kg edrophonium HCl.
‡HE, After 0.16 mg/kg of edrophonium HCl.

gic, when other muscles are still myasthenic in their response. Obviously, respiratory and pharyngeal function must be given priority in adjusting the dose. The use of the Tensilon test at 0, 1, 2, and 4 hours after medication will allow one to decide how near to the optimum dose the patient is, the goal being to have the dose such that at 0 and 4 hours there will be a moderate response but that at 1 to 2 hours the response will be minimal (see Table 23-4). As mentioned above, the dose of pyridostigmine will often have to be altered because of viral syndromes, menstrual periods, variations in activities, variations of the disease, and changes in the form of medication (syrup versus pill versus IV). The length of action of the medication varies from patient to patient. The range for pyridostigmine bromide (Mestinon) is 3 to 8 hours. A time spansule (effective for 8 to 12 hours) is available, but it is a 180-mg size and can be broken easily only into halves. CAUTION: Usually edrophonium hydrochloride is pharmacologically active for 10 minutes; however, in some patients it has been shown to be active up to 8 hours. Therefore, it is possible to create a cholinergic crisis in a patient by doing repeated Tensilon tests.

4. Check for contractures and pressure sores daily in patients confined to bed.

Autonomic system

1. Observe patient for signs of anticholinesterase excess (i.e., cholinergic stimulation): profuse sweating, lacrimation, salivation, bradycardia, small pupils, diarrhea.
2. Check for signs of atropine-like agent excess: dry skin, dilated pupils, altered mental status, tachycardia, and hypertension.

Pharyngeal system

Assessment for dysphagia should be done hourly to prevent inhalation pneumonia.

1. Clinical observations
   a. Inability to handle secretions.
   b. Difficulty drinking water.
   c. Oral ptosis (inability to close the mouth and purse the lips).
   d. Dysphonia or aphonia.
2. Laboratory investigations
   a. Chest roentgenogram.
   b. Swallowing cineradiography.
   c. Time required to swallow 1 to 4 ounces of water (normal is less than 5 seconds).
3. Assessing recovery
   a. As with the respiratory system, one cannot assume any correlation between the pharyngeal muscles and the clinical course of other strength variables.

Renal-metabolic system

1. Assess recent caloric intake to ensure adequate nutrition.
2. As with any child immobilized for a long period of time, serum Ca should be monitored for hypercalcemia.
3. Character and frequency of stools should be noted in patients who are bedridden, and measures should be taken to prevent constipation or impaction.

MANAGEMENT

An often overlooked, important part of therapy is communication of the physician's confidence in the reversibility of the present clinical situation. In treating patients with myasthenia gravis, this is an important aspect of therapy since anxiety changes the patient's physiologic response to the various pharmacologic agents. As a way to communicate this confidence to the parents and the patient, the following strategy is recommended:

1. Assess the situation and stabilize the patient.
2. Develop both a short-term and a long-term plan of therapy.
3. Explain the situation to the parents and patient. Never withhold from the parents or patient the fact that this can be a fatal disease. At the same time, stress that myasthenia is completely treatable. Explain specifically the short-term therapy goals and the expected time of achievement. Then explain the long-term therapy plans.
4. As with any clinical situation, therapy plans may have to be revised, but explain thoroughly the rationale for such changes.

When the diagnosis is made, the majority of family counseling time is spent explaining the disease. However, when the diagnosis has been known for about 3 months, the patient and/or parents become quite sophisticated as to the various options for therapy. Then a great deal of time is spent explaining why the crisis has occurred and what measures are being taken to optimize therapy.

Neurologic symptoms

Neonatal myasthenia gravis. In the neonate, myasthenia gravis is a monophasic disease that usually reaches its zenith in 24 to 72 hours and then slowly improves over the next few weeks or months. The severity of symptoms dictates the extent of therapy.

If the child is only mildly affected, anticholinesterase medications are probably the best choice. Neostigmine methylsulfate (Prostigmin) may be used, since it can be given both orally and parenterally; however, it has more cholinergic side effects. The usual starting dose is 0.02 mg/kg parenterally or 0.1 mg/kg orally. Pyridostigmine bromide (Mestinon) is probably the drug of choice since it has fewer side effects, but it is available only for oral administration. Ease of administering small doses is enhanced by the fact that it is compounded as a syrup (12 mg/ml). The usual starting dose is 0.3 mg/kg every 3 to 8 hours, given a half-hour before feedings. Adjust the dose to optimize strength and minimize side effects. Medication can usually be tapered and then discontinued by age 4 to 10 weeks.

Alternatively, if the child is in respiratory or pharyngeal failure, preservation of respiratory and pharyngeal function by mechanical ventilation in addition to NG feeding is obviously appropriate. Blood exchange transfusions (two blood volumes) have been found to be quite effective. The passively transmitted antineuromuscular junction antibodies are thought to be removed. With blood volume exchange, mechanical ventilation and NG feeding can be discontinued much earlier and the difficult problem of determining the proper dose of anticholinesterase is avoided.

At least one child whose mother was on anticholinesterase medication during her pregnancy has been reported to have had severe cholinergic symptoms that persisted for the first 10 weeks of life. Because of the profuse salivation and lacrimation, atropine (0.01 mg/kg every 6 hours) was necessary to control these symptoms.

Congenital myasthenia gravis. Rarely does the congenital myasthenia gravis patient present with severe problems at birth; occasional feeding problems may be seen. Anticholinesterase medications or ephedrine (0.25 to 1 mg/kg every 8 hours) or NG feeding will be helpful. Blood exchange transfusions or immunosuppression are of no benefit. In the older child who presents in respiratory failure associated with pneumonia, mechanical support is indicated until control of the intercurrent infection is achieved by appropriate antibiotic therapy. The anticholinesterase and ephedrine dosages should be optimal.

Juvenile myasthenia gravis. Several different approaches are available to reverse the severe muscle weakness seen in these patients. All are supplementary to the appropriate pharyngeal and/or respiratory support given at the initial presentation of an emergency crisis.

1. Use the optimal dose of anticholinesterase. Determine whether the patient is overmedicated or undermedicated. If overmedicated, decrease the dose. If undermedicated, slowly increase the dose of anticholinesterase on a daily basis, monitoring muscle strength at the same time. Use frequent Tensilon tests, as described earlier, to judge the appropriate dose.

2. Drug holiday. For patients who are no longer responsive to anticholinesterase medication, withholding all anticholinesterase medications for 1 to 2 weeks may allow them to redevelop a responsiveness to these medications. Respiratory and pharyngeal function may need to be supported during that time.

3. Plasma exchange. Several one- or two-volume plasma exchanges may produce beneficial effects within 24 to 72 hours. The benefit is temporary, but exchanges can stabilize a patient who is otherwise respirator-dependent. If the patient is unresponsive to

anticholinesterase medications, an immunosuppressive agent (see below) must be added in addition to maintenance plasma exchange.

4. Immunosuppressive agents. Either prednisone (2 mg/kg every other day PO) or azathioprine (3 mg/kg every day PO) can be added. With prednisone there is usually a 2 to 4 week interval between the institution and benefit of drug therapy, and a 1 to 6 month interval exists for azathioprine. (Prednisone is my drug of choice.) The association or occurrence of lymphomas and azathioprine suggest that it should not be used until all other therapies have been tried.

5. Thymectomy. There have been no studies showing that thymectomy alone provides rapid benefit; however, anecdotal reports are frequently used to support a role for a thymectomy in an acutely ill myasthenic patient. One study has shown that plasma exchange used in conjunction with thymectomy can result in a complete remission in children. The high morbidity and mortality that occurs in myasthenic patients undergoing surgery is not the result of the surgery, but of problems with postoperative care.

   a. Preoperative care.
      (1) Working with the anesthesiologist, plan appropriate medication doses, giving particular attention to anticholinesterases, muscle relaxants, and immunosuppressive agents.
      (2) Monitor patient closely before surgery to optimize drug regimen.
      (3) Patients receiving prednisone should receive steroids preoperatively for possible adrenocortical suppression. (Dose should be equivalent to 60 mg/m² of hydrocortisone; it should be given 12 hours and 1 hour preoperatively and continued through the immediate postoperative period.)
      (4) Anticholinesterase medications may be given parenterally.
      (5) Preoperative baseline respiratory function testing (FVC, MIF) is necessary.

   b. Postoperative care.
      (1) Keep patient intubated for at least 24 to 48 hours, especially if there was evidence of respiratory insufficiency prior to surgery, i.e., reduced FVC.
      (2) Give no anticholinesterase medication in the first 24 to 48 hours. Then when it is reinstituted, follow objective variables closely for signs of overmedication.
      (3) Complications not unusual in postthymectomy patients include myasthenic or cholinergic crisis, pneumonia, collapsed lung, adverse reactions to medications.

Respiratory system

1. Intubate patient if:
   a. Respiratory failure occurs (clinical deterioration as shown by a Pa_{CO_2} >50 mm Hg or a Pa_{O_2} <50 mm Hg in FI_{O_2} of 1.0 or by a progressive decrease in FVC).
   b. The patient cannot swallow secretions. Such a patient is at risk for inhalation pneumonia.

2. Use a nasotracheal tube (see Chapter 95); do not use a cuff tube or do not inflate the cuff.

3. Most patients in respiratory failure will only require mechanical ventilation for several days, but some may require respiratory assistance for up to several months. Perform a tracheotomy after 7 to 14 days if the patient is not demonstrating significant recovery of ventilatory function.

4. Details of mechanical ventilation, CPT, and endotracheal suctioning are presented in Chapters 97, 99, and 100, respectively.

5. Weaning myasthenia gravis patients from the mechanical ventilator is totally different from weaning other patients, because of the rapid variations in pulmonary function that can occur and because of the lack of correlation between pulmonary function and other variables of strength. The patient's primary dis-

ease must be treated first and stabilized, as described in the section on the management of neurologic symptoms. A slow tapering has been found most effective for weaning these patients from mechanical ventilation, since it helps to avoid fatigue (see Chapter 22).

Cardiovascular system

Monitor for side effects of anticholinesterase medications.

Renal-metabolic system

1. Caloric intake must be maintained. Patients who are in impending respiratory failure should not be fed orally. After intubation, NG feedings can be started with either a commercially prepared liquid diet (Sustacal or Vivonex) or, preferably, a blenderized diet. Gastrostomy rarely is necessary.
2. Immobilized patients tend to become constipated, and the use of stool softeners, laxatives, or enemas may be necessary.

ADDITIONAL READING

Drachman, D.B.: Myasthenia gravis, N. Engl. J. Med. **298**:138-186, 1978.

Dunn, J.M.: Neonatal myasthenia, Am. J. Obstet. Gynecol. **125**:265-266, 1976.

Elias, S.B., and Appel, S.H.: Current concepts of pathogenesis and treatment of myasthenia gravis, Med. Clin. N. Am. **63**:745-757, 1979.

Engel, A.G., Lambert, E.H., and Gomez, M.R.: A new myasthenic syndrome with end-plate acetylcholinesterase deficiency, small nerve terminals, and reduced acetylcholinesterase, Ann. Neurol. **1**:315-330, 1977.

Pasternak, J.F., Hageman, J., Adams, M.A., and others: Exchange transfusion in neonatal myasthenia, J. Pediatr. **99**:644-646, 1981.

Rodriquez, N., Gomez, M.R., Howard, F.M., and Taylor, W.F.: Myasthenia gravis in children: long term follow-up, Ann. Neurol. **13**:504-510, 1983.

Sarnat, H., McGarry, J.D., and Lewis, J.F.: Effective treatment of infantile myasthenia gravis by combined prednisone and thymectomy, Neurology **27**:550-553, 1977.

Swaiman, K.F., and Wright, F.S.: Pediatric Neuromuscular Diseases, St. Louis, 1979, The C.V. Mosby Co., ch. 5, Diseases of the neuromuscular junction.

Zaimis, E., and MacLagen, J.: General physiology and pharmacology of neuromuscular transmission, John Walton, Disorders of muscle, Edinburgh, 1981, Churchill Livingstone, pp. 76-101.

24 Neurologic complications of hypoxia

KURT E. HECOX

DEFINITION AND PHYSIOLOGY

Of the many neurologic syndromes encountered within a PICU, hypoxic-ischemic encephalopathy is the most common. This syndrome represents a collection of clinical entities with variable expression depending on age and pathologic process. The optimal management of this entity demands knowledge of the effect of asphyxia on multiple organ systems in addition to a detailed knowledge of the brain's response.

Nearly 25% of oxygen consumption in humans is accounted for by cerebral metabolism. Approximately 90% of cerebral energy is provided by aerobic metabolism; thus, a failure of cerebral metabolism is generally due to oxygen deficit or lack of substrate or both. Previously, the irreversible damage suffered during hypoxemia was attributed to exhaustion of the limited cerebral substrate stores suitable for anaerobic metabolism. Recently, however, laboratory and clinical investigations into the underlying pathophysiology have brought this concept into question. It is now thought that much of the damage incurred from hypoxia occurs after the insulting event. This has resulted in an increased emphasis on the management of the complications of hypoxic injury, including temperature control, electrolyte management, control of increased ICP, improved airway management, and closer control of seizures. Thus, there is an increased appreciation of the multifactorial determinants of outcome, with greater emphasis on the recognition and management of general medical problems known to be involved in such disorders.

The list of causes of hypoxic encephalopathy is long, as shown in Table 24-1. The underlying pathophysiology depends on the cause, but there are a number of common principles.

If the brain is acutely deprived of oxygen, a five-fold to ten-fold increase in glycolysis rapidly ensues (this is an age-dependent number), and there is a consequent increased production of lactate associated with vasodilation, resulting in the increased delivery of substrate. Significant ischemia may interfere with this response, resulting in the poor return of blood flow (no reflow) despite the restoration of normal perfusion pressure. The relative importance of endothelial damage versus cerebral swelling in determining the posthypoxic return of blood flow is unknown. Prolonged hypoxia appears to interfere with cerebral autoregulation, which may also significantly diminish re-perfusion. In addition, localized acidosis in the region of increased glycolysis may progress to the point of inhibiting glycolysis at the level of phosphofructokinase. An unexplained feature of these events is that neural activity diminishes before significant cellular damage occurs, as if the brain were protecting itself against metabolic deprivation by decreasing metabolic demands. There is little correlation between ATP levels and the timing of the decrease in brain electrical and metabolic activity. An important corollary of these facts is that adequate oxygen and glucose should be present for optimal survival. Several

167

Table 24-1. Some causes of cerebral anoxia

Anoxic anoxia	2. Intraluminal obstruction
Decreased availability from the atmosphere	a. Inhaled vomitus or blood
1. Altitude	b. Inadequately masticated meat
2. Diving and tunneling accidents	c. Near-drowning
3. Smoke inhalation	Interference with alveolar exchange
4. Displacement in small spaces by other gas	1. Pneumonia
Decreased respiratory movements	2. Pulmonary edema
1. Neonatal apnea	3. Emphysema
2. Neuromuscular dysfunction	Cyanotic congenital heart disease
a. Myasthenia gravis	
b. Poliomyelitis	**Anemic anoxia**
c. Motor neuron disease	Hemorrhage
d. Pharmacology	Chronic anemia (involves additional factors)
(1) Curarization	Carbon monoxide (CO) intoxication (involves
(2) Cholinergic crisis	additional factors)
(a) Anticholinesterase therapy	Cyanide (CN) intoxication
(b) Pilocarpine intoxication	
(c) Organic phosphorus insecticide	**Stagnant anoxia**
poisoning	Shock
(3) Asthma	Congestive heart failure
(4) Accidental mechanical pressure	Cardiac arrest
to chest	Stenosis, occlusion, or "kinking" of carotid or
Respiratory tract obstruction	other arteries extracranially
1. Extrinsic pressure	Occlusion of intracranial arteries
a. Granuloma	"Steal" syndrome (subclavian or external carotid
b. Lymph node enlargement	occlusion)
c. Neoplasm	Cardiovascular surgical procedures
d. Hanging	

From Cohen, M.: Clinical aspects of cerebral anoxia. In Vinken, P.J., and Bruyn, G.W., editors: Handbook of clinical neurology. Vol. 27: Metabolic and deficiency diseases of the nervous system, New York, 1976, Elsevier/North-Holland Biomedical Press.

recent studies have suggested, however, that hyperglycemia and hyperoxia may be deleterious to neurologic outcome. Thus the clinician should have as the goal the restoration of age-specific *normal* oxygen and glucose levels.

Intracranial pressure (ICP) also plays a role in determining substrate and oxygen delivery. Cerebral perfusion pressure (CPP) depends on the difference between systemic arterial blood pressure and ICP. Therefore, either systemic hypotension or intracranial hypertension may interfere with oxygen or substrate delivery by decreasing cerebral perfusion. This is an area of considerable controversy in terms of the indications for monitoring and/or treatment of increased ICP. The sequence of events associated with increased ICP is a transient reduction in perfusion pressure, resulting in vasodilation, with a lowered systemic arterial resistance, followed by the Cushing effect (bradycardia, systemic hypertension, and respiratory irregularities) if ICP continues to rise. If this cycle is not interrupted, capillary flow will eventually decrease, with increased capillary leakage and stasis, resulting in increased venous resistance, leading to increased cerebral edema and vasoparalysis. Therapy is difficult and prognosis grim at this point. Preliminary evidence suggests that the control mechanisms of cerebral blood flow may not be present in the neonate, so that interventions such as hyperventilation to depress Pa_{CO_2} and decrease cerebral blood volume may not be effective in this age group.

Seizures commonly complicate the neurologic picture and must be treated vigorously. Seizures may contribute to local acidosis, loss of autoregulation, and increased metabolic demands. In addition, they may cause hypoventilation (hypercarbia) with associated increased cerebral blood flow, thus worsening coexisting cerebral edema. Seizures following hypoxia may be very difficult to control initially, and effective therapy often requires assisted ventilation and large doses of anticonvulsants for 24 to 72 hours.

The distribution of neuropathology, and thus the nature of the clinical deficits following hypoxemia depend on age. In the premature infant, the most common distribution is in the periventricular region, resulting in a predominance of lower-extremity abnormalities (spastic diplegia). In a term infant, a child, or an adult, the underlying pathologic condition most commonly results in a symmetric parasagittal distribution. These distributions are explained on the basis of the developing vascular anatomy, and both represent end-arterial zones (watershed regions), where a loss of perfusion leads to the greatest degree of damage.

Two other patterns of neuropathology are not well explained on the basis of the vascular anatomy. The first is the rostrocaudal sequence of sensitivity and the second is the brainstem-thalamic distribution. The clinical picture in the former includes early mental status changes, apathy, poor feeding, seizures, and fine-motor difficulties, while the latter is characterized by brainstem signs such as skew deviation, vertical nystagmus, and ocular bobbing. These distributions are postulated to be based on regional differences in metabolic rates, which are particularly sensitive to regional loss of perfusion.

In the newborn the time course of hypoxic encephalopathy includes an initial 12 hours in which the sensorium is markedly impaired and there are intact brainstem reflexes, with hypotonia and a few seizures. This is followed by a lightening of the stupor and the appearance of weakness, with a worsening of the seizures (which may be resistant to therapy). From 24 to 72 hours the patient's level of consciousness may deteriorate, and brainstem dysfunction may become more apparent. In older infants and children the time sequence is extended. After initial deep coma, the patient may show improvement over days 1 and 2, but usually by days 2 and 3 deterioration (if it is to occur) will begin. This phase of the progression is characterized by a worsening of the level of consciousness, sometimes associated with brainstem abnormalities. It is during this period that signs of increased ICP and many general metabolic problems (including ISADH) may appear.

A rare syndrome of delayed postanoxic encephalopathy has also been described. A patient may appear to be recovering well until several months after anoxic insult, at which time the mental status changes and seizures may become preeminent. The pathogenesis and determinants of recovery in this entity are unknown. The relationship of this entity to the delayed appearance of basal ganglia disorders, as in status marmoratus or athetoid cerebral palsy, is not known.

It is always difficult to prognosticate in neurologic disease. Infants or children who exhibit fixed and dilated pupils with absence of doll's-eye maneuvers for more than 48 hours or who are deeply comatose for more than 7 days have little hope of recovery, although they may persist in a vegetative state. In the perinatal period, absence of doll's-eye maneuvers or signs of brainstem dysfunction (skew deviation, vertical nystagmus, ocular bobbing) suggest a high likelihood of irreversible damage. In neonates the occurrence of seizures worsens the prognosis, but the EEG is poorly correlated with outcome. Prognosis in the delayed postanoxic syndrome is poor. Recent work has demonstrated the utility of certain evoked-potential measures in predicting ultimate neurologic outcome.

It is useful to explain to parents at the outset many of the possible delayed complications of hypoxic injury. This facilitates later communication and prepares the parents for dealing with any subsequent periods of deterioration. This is particularly true with respect to the many complications that arise on days 2 through 4, when cerebral edema may be at its maximum.

MONITORING

See also Chapter 4.

Neurologic system

1. Perform neurologic examinations and especially note spontaneous movements, posturing, tone, pupillomotor responses, and level of consciousness initially and every 2 to 4 hours.
2. Obtain serial EEGs as needed but at least on days 1 and 4 (after insult).
3. Immediately report any activity suggestive of seizures.

Cardiorespiratory system

1. Measure arterial blood-gas tensions and pH, preferably via indwelling arterial catheter every 2 to 4 hours.
2. Observe for signs of myocardial hypoxic damage with chest roentgenogram and serial ECGs.

Renal-metabolic system

1. Perform tests of matched serum and urine Na, K, Cl, and osmolalities at least daily, since the appearance of many abnormalities may be delayed (e.g., ISADH).
2. Observe for signs of hypoxic renal damage by obtaining urinalysis, BUN, and serum creatinine levels.

3. Fluid intake and output should be carefully monitored.

MANAGEMENT
Neurologic system

1. See Chapter 10.
2. Avoid hyperosmolar fluids in the perinatal period, but use them in older infants for signs of marked intracranial hypertension (mannitol, 0.5 to 1.0 g/kg IV push). Although there is little evidence that long-term administration of mannitol is effective for persistent lowering of ICP, in a severely ill patient with continuing signs of intracranial hypertension the administration of mannitol, 0.5 g/kg IV every 4 hours, is sometimes helpful. With the latter regimen, plasma volume, serum osmolality, and electrolytes must be closely monitored.
3. Control seizures. The initial drug of choice is phenobarbital (loading dose of 15 to 20 mg/kg IV, with a maintenance dose of 4 mg/kg). Paraldehyde (0.3 ml/kg per rectum, repeated up to three times) and phenytoin (loading dose of 20 mg/kg IV, with a maintenance dose of 5 mg/kg/day) are the two most useful adjuncts to phenobarbital. Use of paralytic agents should be considered only with significant compromise of ventilatory effort or with uncontrolled lactic acidosis.
4. Maintain normothermia.
5. Maintain the head at 30 degrees from the horizontal.
6. There are no controlled studies supporting the use of steroids.

Cardiorespiratory system

1. Maintain adequate systemic arterial blood pressure (normotension), and if there are signs of increased ICP with possible herniation, consider monitoring ICP (subarachnoid or intraventricular monitors).
2. Controlled hyperventilation may be useful in treating increased ICP (see Chapter 10) after the neonatal period.

3. Maintain Pa_{O_2} at about 100 mm Hg except in premature infants, in whom the O_2 level must be adjusted downward. Pa_{CO_2} levels should be maintained at normal levels for age unless there is evidence of raised ICP.

Renal-metabolic system

1. Keep fluids at two-thirds maintenance unless systemic arterial blood pressure becomes compromised during the first 3 to 4 days after the insult. Urine output should not be allowed to drop below 1 ml/kg/hr, and urine specific gravity should be from 1.012 to 1.018.
2. Avoid hyperthermia, since there are increased fluid requirements and seizure control is more difficult.
3. Provide glucose to maintain age-specific normal values for glucose.
4. Correct chronic metabolic acidosis slowly with bicarbonate only if pH is less than 7.30 and ventilatory control is unsuccessful.

ADDITIONAL READING

Anoxic-ischemic brain damage, symposium, Arch. Neurol. **29:**359-420, 1973.

Blackwood, W., and Corsellis, J.: Greenfield's neuropathology, Chicago, 1976, Year Book Medical Publishers, Inc.

Cohen, M.: Clinical aspects of cerebral anoxia. In Vinken, P.J., and Bruyn, G.W., editors: Handbook of clinical neurology. Vol 27: Metabolic and deficiency diseases of the nervous system, New York, 1976, Elsevier/North-Holland Biomedical Press.

Hecox, K.E., and Cone, B.: Prognostic importance of brainstem auditory evoked responses after asphyxia, Neurology **31:**1429-33, 1981.

Leech, R., and Alvord, E.: Anoxic-ischemic encephalopathy in the human neonatal period, Arch. Neurol. **34:**109-113, 1977.

Lewis, A.: Mechanisms of neurologic disease, Boston, 1976, Little, Brown & Co.

Volpe, J.: Perinatal hypoxic-ischemic brain injury, Pediatr. Clin. North Am. **23:**383-397, 1976.

25 Lightning injuries

GARY R. TURNER

DEFINITION AND PHYSIOLOGY

Although lightning discharges involve enormous amounts of electrical current (median values are approximately 25,000 amperes), lightning injuries are not invariably fatal. Two thirds of the people struck by lightning survive; the number of survivors would undoubtedly increase if immediate cardiopulmonary resuscitation were undertaken at the scene of lightning accidents (see Chapter 5).

There are three different types of lightning injuries. A person may be struck directly or may be the victim of a side flash. In a direct strike on an upright human the lightning current enters the upper part of the body and exits through the feet. A side flash occurs when lightning strikes an object with a relatively high electrical resistance, e.g., a tree. Flashover then occurs along a pathway of lower electrical resistance, e.g., a person. Either direct or side flash injuries can be fatal. The third type of lightning injury occurs when lightning strikes the ground adjacent to an area where a person is standing. A potential difference is generated between the legs, and current flows through the legs and the lower trunk (but not through the heart or brain). Death is rare in this step voltage type of injury, but temporary paralysis of the lower body can occur.

Lightning can produce injury in several ways. It can cause electrical burns, interfere with neuromuscular transmission, or produce blast injury from expanding, heated air. Victims can be injured during a fall after being knocked unconscious by a lightning discharge. The different mechanisms of lightning injury can result in numerous possible clinical and laboratory manifestations in an individual; the most characteristic effects on the specific organ systems are given below.

Respiratory system

Respiratory arrest ensues when the pathway of the lightning current includes the respiratory center in the medulla. Breathing may resume spontaneously, but often effective artificial ventilation must be initiated to sustain life. Lung contusions are thought to be secondary to the blast effect, and ARDS can occur in the postinjury period (see Chapters 12 and 14).

Cardiovascular system

The heart is frequently affected directly by the lightning discharge. An initial forceful systolic contraction is followed by a period of asystole, during which the ventricles slowly relax. Sinus rhythm resumes spontaneously, but asystole or ventricular fibrillation may occur if effective ventilation has not been established. Atrial or ventricular fibrillation may also occur directly as a result of the lightning discharge.

Myocardial injury and infarction may complicate lightning strikes. Pathologic changes include diffuse myocardial necrosis, spiral malformation of myocardial fibers, and epicardial hemorrhages. Damage may occur directly from electrical injury and the blast effect or secondary to hypoxemia. Infrequently, acute congestive heart failure can occur as a consequence of damaged myocardium.

Electrocardiographic abnormalities are common after lightning injury and may be due to electrical injury to the myocardium, to hypoxia, or to CNS injury. Abnormalities reported include T wave inversion in the chest leads and prolongation of the QT interval. The ECG abnormalities usually disappear within a week after injury, but they may persist for up to a year.

Transient hypertension and tachycardia can occur after lightning injury; they may be caused by increased endogenous catecholamine release. Vasomotor spasm in the extremities can occur, with a concomitant decrease in palpable pulses, skin mottling and coolness, and decreased sensation. This usually resolves within several hours after the injury but can cause temporary sensory derangement, e.g., paresthesias from nerve ischemia.

Neurologic system

CNS signs and symptoms may be caused by the primary electrical or blast injury, or they may be secondary to hypoxia. Early signs of CNS injury after lightning trauma include coma, convulsions, retrograde amnesia, aphasia, paresthesias, and paralysis. Paresthesias and paralysis often resolve spontaneously within hours of the injury. Subarachnoid and cerebral hemorrhage in lightning victims are probably due to the blast effect. Cerebral edema may occur, especially if there is prolonged hypoxia immediately after the injury. Late CNS manifestations of lightning injury include extrapyramidal signs, psychiatric problems, aphasia, and hemiplegia.

Auditory. The most common ear injury of lightning victims is tympanic membrane rupture, which is thought to be due to the blast of thunder close to the ear. Mastoid effusion, transient facial nerve edema, prolonged sensorineural hearing loss, and dizziness of vestibular origin may also occur.

Visual. Cataracts are the most common eye injury of lightning victims; they develop from 1 month to 2 years after the person is struck. Corneal burns, retinal detachment, and optic atrophy also occur occasionally in patients who were struck by lightning.

Renal-metabolic system

Hemoglobinuria and myoglobinuria may be observed. Myoglobinuria may have several different etiologies, including heat damage to the tissues, systemic hypoxemia, or cardiac resuscitation efforts.

Gastrointestinal system

Ileus is a frequent finding and may be caused by bowel contusion. Upper gastrointestinal bleeding may be caused by stress ulcers, as in other critically ill patients.

Integument

Burns may range in severity from mild erythema to full thickness, but they usually are not severe (see Chapter 56). They may be the result of the lightning itself or may occur secondary to burning clothing or melting metal clothing parts, e.g., buckles and zippers. Small punctate burns at the entrance and exit sites of the lightning current are common.

Lightning victims can have a pathognomonic skin sign consisting of an arborescent, macular mark that does not blanch. These Lichtenberg figures are not burns; they fade within hours without residual scars. Theories regarding their etiology include electron redistribution in a strong electric field and transmission of static electricity along the skin vasculature.

Musculoskeletal system

Lightning can cause violent muscle contractions, which can throw a victim to the ground, causing fractures of the skull or extremities. Compartmental syndromes in the arms and legs can be caused by local tissue swelling.

MONITORING

See also Chapter 4.

Respiratory system

1. Assess adequacy of ventilation by physical examination and by arterial blood-gas tensions and pH.

2. Patients requiring mechanical ventilation should have an indwelling peripheral arterial catheter, and arterial blood-gas tensions and pH samples should be taken every 4 hours.

Cardiovascular system

1. Assess peripheral pulses on admission and at least every hour when swelling of the extremities is noted.
2. Systemic arterial blood pressure should be taken at least every hour if the patient is unstable or hypertensive.
3. Obtain an ECG on all patients struck by lightning; daily ECGs should be done when abnormalities are noted.
4. Serial CPK, SGOT, and LDH isoenzymes should be studied when ECG abnormalities are noted.

Neurologic system

1. Evaluate mental status, cranial nerves, reflexes, posturing, spontaneous movement, and sensation on admission, and repeat at least every hour if abnormal (see Chapter 6).
2. Reevaluate pupillary responses and mental status every 2 hours in all patients.
3. Obtain skull roentgenograms when there is a history or physical signs of head trauma.
4. Consider an ICP monitor in patients with signs of increased ICP or in comatose patients who have suffered a prolonged period of hypoxemia.

Renal-metabolic system

1. Obtain urinalysis, BUN, and serum creatinine on admission.
2. Examine urine for myoglobin and, if positive, measure serum myoglobin.
3. Insert bladder catheter if osmotic diuretics are being used or if patient is unstable.

Gastrointestinal system

1. If bowel sounds are absent, insert a NG tube; attach NG tube to a low-pressure suction device.
2. Quantitate the amount of gastric secretions.

Musculoskeletal system

1. Obtain roentgenograms of extremities that show signs of trauma; check for the presence of fractures.

MANAGEMENT
Respiratory system

1. Intubation and subsequent mechanical ventilation should be initiated immediately in patients who are apneic.
2. Other indications for assisted ventilation include progressive hypoxemia despite high concentrations of inspired oxygen, hypercarbia (see Chapter 12), and signs of increased ICP.
3. Adjust ventilator settings to maintain the Pa_{O_2} and Pa_{CO_2} with the normal range for age, unless increased ICP is suspected (see Chapter 10).

Cardiovascular system

1. Dysrhythmias should be treated with the appropriate agent (see Chapter 5).
2. Treat congestive heart failure with furosemide and/or inotropic agents (see Chapter 13).
3. Consider beta-adrenergic blocking agents for hypertension and tachycardia, which often accompany lightning injury. These agents should not be used in patients with cardiac failure or in patients with increased ICP, who may require high systemic arterial pressure to maintain cerebral perfusion.
4. Severe peripheral vasoconstriction usually resolves without specific treatment; fasciotomy may occasionally be necessary when poor peripheral perfusion does not improve over a period of several hours and soft-tissue swelling is the cause.

Neurologic system

1. Administer anticonvulsants to control seizures (see Chapter 9).
2. Treat cerebral edema with head elevation, hyperventilation, and diuresis (see Chapter 10).

Auditory system

1. Clean auditory canal of blood and debris.
2. Test hearing once the patient has recovered from the acute injuries.

Renal-metabolic system

1. Fluid management varies with the individual patient's clinical manifestations.
2. Patients with evidence of cardiac failure or cerebral edema should receive less than maintenance fluids.
3. Patients with extensive burns, excessive gastrointestinal losses, or myoglobinuria will need increased volumes of fluid.
4. Treat myoglobinuria with mannitol to prevent myoglobin casts from forming in the renal tubules.

Gastrointestinal system

1. Treat ileus with low-pressure suctioning of gastric secretions through an NG tube.
2. Institute antacid therapy in the critically ill patient to prevent stress ulcers (see Chapter 62).

Integument

1. Treat burns according to their severity (see Chapter 56).
2. Administer tetanus toxoid when appropriate.

Musculoskeletal system

1. Treat fractures appropriately.

ADDITIONAL READING

Apfelberg, D.B., Masters, F.W., and Robinson, D.W.: Pathophysiology and treatment of lightning injuries, J. Trauma **14**:453-560, 1974.

Bartholome, C.W., Jacoby, W.D., and Ramchand, S.C.: Cutaneous manifestations of lightning injury, Arch. Dermatol. **111**:1466-1468, 1975.

Bergstrom, L.V., Neblett, L.M., Sando, I., and others: The lightning damaged ear, Arch. Otolaryngol. **100**:117-121, 1974.

Burda, C.D.: Electrocardiographic changes in lightning stroke, Am. Heart J. **72**:521-524, 1966.

Chia, B.L.: Electrocardiographic abnormalities and congestive cardiac failure due to lightning stroke, Cardiology **68**:49-53, 1981.

Death by lightning (editorial), Lancet **1**:230, 1977.

Golde, R.H., and Lee, W.R.: Death by lightning, Proc. Inst. Elec. Engineers **123**:1163-1180, 1976.

Hanson, G.C., and McIlwraith, G.R.: Lightning injury: two case histories and a review of management, Br. Med. J. **4**:271-274, 1973.

Jackson, S.H.D., and Parry, D.J.: Lightning and the heart, Br. Heart J. **43**:454-457, 1980.

Kleiner, J.P., and Wilkin, J.H.: Cardiac effects of lightning stroke, J.A.M.A. **240**:2757-2759, 1978.

Kravitz, H., Wasserman, M.J., Valaitis, J., and others: Lightning injury: management of a case with a ten day survival, Am. J. Dis. Child. **131**:413-415, 1977.

Myers, G.J., Colgan, M.T., and Van Dyke, D.H.: Lightning-strike disaster among children, J.A.M.A. **238**:1045-1046, 1977.

Noel, L.P., Clarke, W.N., and Addison, D.: Ocular complications of lightning, J. Pediatr. Ophthalmol. Strabismus **17**:245-246, 1981.

Ravitch, M.M., Lane, R., Safar, P., and others: Lightning stroke: report of a case with recovery after cardiac massage and prolonged artificial respiration, N. Engl. J. Med. **264**:36-38, 1961.

Sharma, M., and Smith, A.: Paraplegia as a result of lightning injury, Br. Med. J. **2**:1464-1465, 1978.

Strasser, E.J., Davis, R.M., and Menchey, M.J.: Lightning injuries, J. Trauma **17**:315-319, 1977.

Taussig, H.B.: "Death" from lightning—and the possibility of living again, Ann. Intern. Med. **68**:1345-1353, 1968.

Yost, J.W.: Myoglobinuria following lightning stroke, J.A.M.A. **228**:1147-1148, 1974.

26 Smoke inhalation and carbon monoxide poisoning

ALFONSO AQUINO

DEFINITION AND PHYSIOLOGY
Postburn respiratory injury

Smoke inhalation is a syndrome of acute tracheobronchitis and/or alveolitis caused by direct injury to the respiratory system following inhalation of toxic fumes or products of incomplete combustion or by direct thermal injury. Thermal injury may be produced by direct flame exposure, hot gas, or steam. Flame exposure and hot gas affect only the upper airway because efficient cooling of the upper air passages prevents damage beyond the vocal cords. Steam, however, causes lower airway injury due to its greater heat capacity. Smoke is defined as the gaseous product of burning organic materials, rendered visible by the presence of small particles of carbon. It is the particulate nature of smoke that causes the injury to be confined to the tracheobronchial tree. However, toxic fumes are often mixed with smoke and, by virtue of their not being particulate, they penetrate to the alveolar level and cause more severe damage.

The deleterious effects of toxic fumes released by combustion and mixed with smoke depend on their water or lipid solubility. Water-soluble gases, such as chlorine, sulfur dioxide, and ammonia, can cause severe irritation of mucous membranes and bronchospasm. Oxides of nitrogen, aldehydes, and phosgene exert their toxicity because they dissolve in the cellular membrane lipid fraction and cause severe epithelial damage, sloughing of the mucosa, and alveolar-capillary disruption. The clinical effects of these toxic components of smoke vary according to where they are deposited in the respiratory tract. Symptoms can include conjunctivitis, cough, wheezing, laryngeal edema, mucosal sloughing, and pulmonary edema. Stridor, hoarseness, retractions, and/or difficulty with phonation indicate the need for prompt evaluation of upper airway patency, since thermal injury to the hypopharynx or glottis may be followed by obstruction and rapid asphyxia secondary to edema. Evaluation of the upper airway depends on subjective rather than objective assessment. The diagnosis of a pulmonary burn is presumed by the presence of the following criteria:

1. Flame burns of the face and neck.
2. Scarred nasal vibrissae and/or burned oral or nasal mucosa.
3. External skin burns inflicted in a closed area.
4. Carbonaceous material present in sputum.

Injury to the respiratory tract can occur in all grades of severity but the majority of patients go through three apparent stages (or phases) of inhalation injury: the early bronchial spastic component (1 to 12 hours postburn), pulmonary edema (6 to 72 hours), and bronchopneumonia (>60 hours).

Carbon monoxide poisoning

Carbon monoxide intoxication is frequently an immediate cause of death during a fire. The burning of wood and furniture in inadequately ventilated areas results in a toxic concentration of this colorless gas, which has an affinity for hemoglobin 210 times that of oxygen. Because of this marked affinity for hemoglobin, a carbon monoxide concentration of 0.1% in room air (21% oxygen) produces equal blood concentrations of oxyhemoglobin (HbO_2) and carboxyhemoglobin (CoHb) and results in a 50% reduction in oxygen-carrying capacity. Carbon monoxide produces tissue hypoxia by shifting the oxyhemoglobin dissociation curve to the left. This shift results in an increased affinity of hemoglobin for oxygen and in decreased oxygen release to tissues for a given partial pressure of oxygen (see Fig. 12-1). The signs and symptoms of carbon monoxide intoxication are related to blood CoHb level. CNS symptoms predominate because of the extreme sensitivity of the CNS to oxygen deprivation. Headache, slight breathlessness, and diminution in visual acuity and higher cerebral functions are present at 20% to 30% CoHb. At levels of 30% to 40%, nausea, irritability, dimness of vision, chest pain, impaired judgment, tachycardia, and rapid fatigue occur. Levels of 40% to 60% produce confusion, hallucinations, ataxia, collapse, seizures, and coma. A cherry pink color of the skin, nailbeds, and mucous membranes indicates severe poisoning. CoHb levels greater than 60% usually result in death. Late onset of cerebral edema is fairly common.

MONITORING

See also Chapter 4.

Postburn respiratory injury

The early diagnosis and determination of the extent of pulmonary injury are difficult but important.

1. Roentgenographic examination of the chest in these patients is almost invariably normal in the first 24 to 48 hours. The onset of pulmonary edema may be immediate or may occur as late as 1 week after the inhalation injury. The presence of pulmonary edema clinically and by chest roentgenogram within the first few hours following injury almost always implies severe pulmonary damage and carries a poorer prognosis. Pulmonary infiltrates and respiratory failure that occur after 2 weeks comprise a distinct clinical entity, and they are almost always secondary to sepsis.

2. Endoscopy has been of assistance in making the diagnosis of upper airway injury and impending airway obstruction from laryngeal edema. Bronchoscopy may not be possible initially but may be necessary to remove mucosal sloughs later in the course.

3. A chest roentgenogram should be obtained at least every day, since pulmonary edema and bronchopneumonia appear in the latter stages.

4. An initial CoHb level and serial arterial blood-gas tensions and pH are the most useful of the laboratory data that are easily available in the PICU.

5. The initial $P(A-a)O_2$ gradient and subsequent changes in the gradient are valuable in predicting and estimating pulmonary dysfunction.

Carbon monoxide poisoning

1. CoHb concentration of blood initially and serially until the level is less than 10%.

2. Arterial blood-gas tensions may show normal Pa_{O_2} even though the patient is hypoxic; thus they do not correlate with the severity of the process.

3. Frequent neurologic evaluations should be performed.

4. CVP or PCWP monitoring may be helpful.

MANAGEMENT
Postburn respiratory injury

Management of respiratory injury resulting from smoke inhalation is largely empirical and not based on extensive experience in controlled clinical trials, so therapy is guided toward the actual stage through which the patient is progressing (bronchospasm, edema, pneumonia). Aggressive supportive care of patients with acute respiratory failure is critical.

1. Adequate airway patency. Endotracheal intubation should be done early after injury. The exact indications for early intubation in this entity are more difficult to define than in acute respiratory failure (i.e., Pa_{O_2} <50 mm Hg in FI_{O_2} 0.5 or Pa_{CO_2} >50 mm Hg). Specific indications that can be defined are facial burns associated with notable CNS depression, visible edema in the posterior pharynx, full-thickness facial burns including the nose and lips, facial burns associated with circumferential full-thickness burns of the neck, or the presence of stridor, dyspnea, retractions, wheezing, or other signs of airway obstruction. If the patient develops respiratory distress during transportation to the hospital, intubation may be technically impossible by the time he arrives. This requires a surgeon on standby for emergency tracheostomy.

2. Assisted ventilation. PEEP is essential to ensure adequate oxygenation with sufficiently low FI_{O_2} to avoid pulmonary oxygen toxicity. Mechanical ventilation will be necessary to maintain normal carbon dioxide levels. Because an alveolar-capillary leak exists, judicious administration of fluids is necessary. Although formulas and clinical criteria exist to determine IV fluid requirements in burn patients (see Chapter 56), monitoring of cardiac output, PCWP, and mixed venous oxygen content must supplement these calculations in order to minimize iatrogenic pulmonary fluid overload and guide adjustments in PEEP without causing deterioration of cardiovascular hemodynamics.

3. Pulmonary toilet. Since abundant carbonaceous secretions and continuous sloughing of the mucosa for the first few days threaten the patency of the already swollen airway, it may be necessary to intubate these infants and children to ensure adequate pulmonary toilet. Always maintain adequate humidification of inspired gases and frequent suctioning to remove such material.

4. Infection. Bronchopneumonia develops in almost all children who survive the third postburn day. Initial antibiotic coverage is directed to gram-positive cocci and gram-negative rods. (*Staphylococcus aureus, Pseudomonas*, and *Klebsiella* are the most common.)
   a. Specific antibiotics should be instituted according to culture and sensitivity tests.
   b. Maintain a clear airway.
   c. Encourage an effective cough.
   d. Use frequent nasotracheal suctioning.
   e. Use CPT.

5. Bronchodilators. If wheezing is a prominent feature during the course of the disease, after effective removal of secretions, bronchodilators such as aminophylline and aerosolized racemic epinephrine can be of value (see Chapter 28).

6. Steroids. The use of corticosteroids is contraindicated in the treatment of smoke inhalation.

Carbon monoxide poisoning

1. Remove patient from the source of carbon monoxide.

2. Administer 100% oxygen via bag and mask or endotracheal tube to increase elimination of carbon monoxide via the lungs and increase dissociation of carbon monoxide from hemoglobin. 100% oxygen should be administered until CoHb concentration is less to 10% (approximately 45 to 60 minutes for an initial concentration of 50% CoHb).

3. Hyperbaric oxygen administration has been used.

4. See Chapter 10 for management of cerebral edema.

ADDITIONAL READING

Armstrong, R.F., MacKensie, A.M., McGregor, A.P., and Woods, S.D.: The respiratory injury in burns, Anaesthesia **32:**313-319, 1977.

Bartlett, R.H., Niccole, M., Travis, M.J., and others: Acute management of the upper airway in facial burns and smoke inhalation, Arch. Surg. **111**:744-749, 1976.

Boutros, A.R., Hoyt, J.L., Boyd, W.C., and Hartford, C.E.: Algorithm for management of pulmonary complications in burn patients, Crit. Care Med. **5**:89-92, 1977.

Channock, E.L., and Meehan, J.J.: Postburn respiratory injuries in children, Pediatr. Clin. North Am. **27**:661-676, 1980.

Chi-Shing, Chu: New concepts of pulmonary burn injury, J. Trauma **21**:958-961, 1981.

Davies, M.R., Cywes, S., Van Der Riet, R.L.S., and others: A review of deaths in a paediatric burn unit, S. Afr. Med. J. **50**:1479-1483, 1976.

Head, J.M.: Inhalation injury in burns, Am. J. Surg. **139**:508-512, 1980.

Luce, E.A., Su, C.T., and Hoopes, J.E.: Alveolar-arteriolar oxygen gradient in the burn patient, J. Trauma **16**:212-217, 1976.

Mellins, R.B., and Park, S.: Respiratory complications of smoke inhalation in victims of fires, J. Pediatr. **87**:1-7, 1975.

O'Neill, J.A.: Evaluation and treatment of the burned child, Pediatr. Clin. North Am. **22**:407-414, 1975.

Schall, G.L., MacDonald, H.D., Cann, L.B., and Capozzi, A.: Xenon ventilation-perfusion lung scans, J.A.M.A. **240**:2441-2445, 1978.

Stephenson, S.F., Esrig, B.C., Polk, H.C., and Fulton, R.L.: The pathophysiology of smoke inhalation injury, Ann. Surg. **182**:652-660, 1975.

Stone, H.H.: Pulmonary burns in children, J. Pediatr. Surg. **14**:48-52, 1979.

Trunkey, D., and Parks, S.: Burns in children, Curr. Probl. Pediatr. **6**:35-41, 1976.

Vivori, E., and Cudmore, R.E.: Management of airway complications of burns in children, Br. Med. J. **2**:1462-1464, 1977.

Wroblewski, D.A., and Bower, G.C.: The significance of facial burns in acute smoke inhalation, Crit. Care Med. **7**:335-338, 1979.

27 Near-drowning

GERALD C. MOORE

DEFINITION AND PHYSIOLOGY

Near-drowning is defined as survival after submersion in a fluid medium. The condition is usually associated with asphyxia and/or inhalation. Early speculation regarding the pathogenesis of drowning was concerned with whether there were additional effects associated with inhalation of the fluid medium into the lungs. The fact that water was inhaled was not firmly established until about 100 years ago. It had been previously thought that spasm of the glottis prevented entry of water into the lungs and that cessation of the heart beat was due solely to asphyxia.

According to the present understanding of drowning, the sequence of events is as follows: After a period of time when breathholding is no longer possible, large amounts of the submersion fluid are swallowed. Excessive distention of the stomach and progressive asphyxia result in regurgitation and inhalation during active gasping. If asphyxia is not severe enough to result in unconsciousness, laryngospasm occurs automatically to prevent further inhalation of fluids. With unconsciousness, airway reflexes are abolished and fluid is passively introduced into the airway. Cardiorespiratory arrest follows shortly thereafter.

The physiologic manifestations of near-drowning are generally divided into freshwater and saltwater categories. Theoretically, in a freshwater near-drowning episode one would expect large volumes of hypotonic fluid to enter the alveoli and, because of the oncotic and hydrostatic pressure differences, to pass into the circulation. This would result in hemodilution, with lowered values for hemoglobin and circulating serum electrolytes, except that an increase in serum potassium would be expected from hemolysis. Blood volume may be expected to increase and is reflected by an increase in CVP, assuming there are no cardiac abnormalities. Observed phenomena are usually quite different from those described above. The changes in hemoglobin, hematocrit, and electrolytes are usually not great enough to require correction. There is usually a transient increase in blood volume, which is corrected by increased urine output if renal function is adequate. The patient is usually hypokalemic.

In saltwater near-drowning, hypertonic fluid (most salt water has an osmolality 3 to 4 times that of blood) enters the alveoli, draws fluid from the vascular space, and causes hemoconcentration with an increase in hemoglobin and serum electrolytes and a concomitant decrease in blood volume. Although significant hematocrit or electrolyte changes usually do not occur, the changes in blood volume are frequently significant and are directly proportional to the amount of fluid swallowed and inhaled. Hypovolemia may persist for several days and may require vigorous expansion therapy.

Abnormalities common to both types of near-drowning include combined respiratory and metabolic acidosis, hypothermia, and varying degrees of neurologic deficit, depending on the severity of the asphyxia.

The lung is the primary target organ, and pulmonary insufficiency, hypoxemia, hypercapnia, and CNS damage may be seen as a result of the insult to the lungs. A hypotonic medium

180

may cause a washing out of surfactant sufficient to increase the surface tension properties of the gas-fluid interface of the alveolar membrane. Respiratory distress syndrome develops, with alveolar collapse and atelectasis, ventilation-perfusion imbalance, and a decrease in lung compliance. The loss of surfactant is also associated with pulmonary edema, previously thought to be caused by heart failure. In saltwater near-drowning, the surface tension properties of the lungs are usually not significantly altered; however, with severe degrees of asphyxia and fluid shifts, respiratory distress syndrome may still occur. The primary mechanism for the hypoxemia seen in saltwater near-drowning is probably intrapulmonary shunting as a result of fluid-filled alveoli, i.e., pulmonary edema. Chest roentgenographic changes are usually consistent with pulmonary edema and/or respiratory distress syndrome, which, with appropriate therapy, generally clears by 3 to 5 days. Persistence of an abnormal roentgenogram or progression of infiltrates suggests superimposed infection. Barring severe neurologic sequelae, the condition is self-limited, and the patient should show definite improvement after 48 hours of appropriate therapy.

MONITORING

See also Chapter 4.

Cardiorespiratory system

1. Perform an ECG initially and repeat as necessary. Hypoxemia may injure the myocardium and result in dysrhythmias, which should be anticipated and documented on a strip recorder or by a rhythm strip.
2. Monitor arterial blood-gas tensions and pH at least hourly during the initial phase from samples taken from an indwelling arterial catheter. Expected abnormalities include a combined respiratory and metabolic acidosis, with varying degrees of hypoventilation manifested by hypoxemia and hypercapnia.

Neurologic system

1. If significant neurologic damage is thought to be present, the patient should be examined immediately by a neurologist. It may be necessary, depending on the severity of the insult, to use assisted ventilation and muscle relaxants to achieve adequate ventilation. In such a situation, adequate neurologic evaluation is practically impossible; thus an attempt should be made to perform the evaluation before the institution of such therapy. Near-drowning in subzero temperature water may cause changes in the neurologic examination; therapy should be instituted despite negative findings when the patient's temperature is very low (<34° C).
2. Record neurologic assessment every 2 hours if necessary. This should include the presence of appropriate ocular reflexes, state of consciousness, motor responses to noxious stimuli, and appropriate responsiveness to spoken commands.
3. Make a careful assessment of increases in ICP (see Chapter 10).

MANAGEMENT

The management of a child with near-drowning should be directed toward the correction of abnormalities in pulmonary function and body fluids. Since most of the patients arrive in the PICU with varying degrees of hypothermia, a heating blanket should be available (see Chapter 18). Another frequently overlooked aspect of management is the emptying of all stomach contents as soon as possible after the near-drowning episode or immediately after admission to the PICU.

Cardiovascular system

Frequently evaluate the stability of the cardiovascular system and maintenance of adequate cardiac output. Carefully watch for and treat dysrhythmias if they affect cardiac performance and tissue perfusion. Bradycardia may be a manifestation of profound hypoxemia. An adequate circulating blood volume must be maintained to ensure proper peripheral perfusion. This may be done either by volume expansion or by administration of vasoactive agents. The former is the preferred method, particularly in the saltwater victim. If a vasoactive agent is necessary, epinephrine is the drug of choice, because it possesses both alpha- and beta-adrenergic activity (see Chapter 14), which will increase cardiac output while maintaining systemic arterial blood pressure.

Respiratory system

Provide supplemental oxygen for all patients admitted to the PICU with the diagnosis of near-drowning. The burden of proof regarding adequacy of oxygenation is on the medical staff, and until such proof is obtained, oxygen must be administered. Elevations in Pa_{CO_2} are a late manifestation and are seen only with significant degrees of alveolar hypoventilation. Hypoxemia is generally seen earlier than hypercapnia. The importance of understanding this sequence is that the majority of patients will be hypoxemic but may have a normal or low Pa_{CO_2}. In one large study, all patients who required a supplemental oxygen concentration of greater than 40% to maintain a normal Pa_{O_2} subsequently required assisted ventilation. Indications for intubation and ventilation of a patient with near-drowning include hypoxemia (Pa_{O_2} of less than 90 mm Hg in an FI_{O_2} of 0.5), progressive elevation of Pa_{CO_2} to greater than 45 mm Hg, and progressive neurologic deficit including status epilepticus or coma with absence of gag and cough reflexes.

If the patient maintains adequate spontaneous ventilation, he may require only CPAP to maintain adequate oxygenation. If this is not the case, then IPPV with PEEP will be necessary. It is frequently necessary to use a muscle relaxant such as pancuronium or tubocurarine to control ventilation in a patient with an abnormal ventilatory drive secondary to CNS asphyxia. PEEP has been shown to be particularly useful in any condition associated with a low FRC, such as respiratory distress syndrome and pulmonary edema; however, its use has been associated with increases in ICP. This effect is thought to be more significant in patients with an already abnormally increased ICP.

In the treatment of freshwater victims, it is important to withdraw ventilation slowly, because although adequate ventilation may be achieved early, the patient may not have had time to resynthesize his own surfactant. These patients are usually ventilated for 48 to 72 hours. In addition, it may be necessary to maintain a low Pa_{CO_2} for the theoretical advantage of decreasing cerebral perfusion and to minimize the effects of increased ICP.

The measurement of expired gas tensions is particularly helpful when weaning patients from mechanical ventilation. By comparing the alveolar gas tensions with arterial blood samples, measurements of intrapulmonary shunting may be made (see Chapter 12).

Renal-metabolic system

Treat abnormalities in circulating volume aggressively. It is frequently necessary to administer large amounts of colloid to patients suffering from saltwater near-drowning. This may require as much as 40 to 50 ml of plasma or whole blood per kg. In contrast, brisk diuresis may be desired in treating patients with freshwater near-drowning. Administer proper electrolyte solutions in accordance with standard recommendations (see Chapter 16). ISADH is a frequent concomitant of near-drowning and presents a particularly difficult complication because of the nature of the other abnormalities observed. It should be possible, however, to administer colloid while restricting overall fluid intake if ISADH occurs.

Other

Treat convulsions aggressively (see Chapter 9). Also treat increases in ICP vigorously (see Chapter 10).

Various investigators have suggested that corticosteroids and antibiotic therapy be used routinely in the treatment of patients with near-drowning; however, there is no conclusive evidence that these potentially dangerous modes of therapy are useful. In the event that a patient is found in a contaminated pool, broad-spectrum antibiotic therapy may be indicated. This is particularly true with the possibility of *Pseudomonas* infection when near-drowning occurs in a hot tub.

With deterioration in the overall ventilatory condition, superimposed infection should be considered, appropriate cultures taken, and broad-spectrum antibiotic coverage begun (see Chapter 41).

Finally, psychologic support of the family should be provided immediately after admission, because there is frequently a tremendous amount of guilt associated with this condition and death or permanent residua are not uncommon.

ADDITIONAL READING

Cahill, J.M.: Drowning: the problem of nonfatal submersion and the unconscious patient, Surg. Clin. North Am. 48:423-430, 1968.

Calderwood, H.W., Modell, J.H., and Ruiz, B.C.: The ineffectiveness of steroid therapy for treatment of freshwater near drowning, Anesthesiology 43:642-650, 1975.

Fandel, I., and Bancalari, E.: Near-drowning in children, clinical aspects, Pediatrics 58:573-579, 1976.

Fuller, R.H.: The clinical pathology of human near-drowning, Proc. R. Soc. Med. 56:33-38, 1963.

Giammona, S.J., and Modell, J.H.: Drowning by total immersion: effects on pulmonary surfactant of distilled water, isotonic saline, and seawater, Am. J. Dis. Child. 114:612-617, 1967.

Modell, J.H.: The pathophysiology and treatment of drowning and near-drowning, Springfield, Ill., 1971, Charles C Thomas, Publisher.

Modell, J.H., Calderwood, H.W., and Ruiz, B.C.: Effects of ventilatory patterns on arterial oxygenation after near-drowning in sea water, Anesthesiology 40:376-384, 1974.

Modell, J.H., Graves, S.A., and Ketover, A.: Clinical course of 91 consecutive near-drowning victims, Chest 70:231-238, 1976.

Siebre, H., and Breivik, H.: Survival after 40 minutes' submersion without cerebral sequelae, Lancet 1:1275-1277, 1975.

28 Acute severe asthma

GERALD C. MOORE

DEFINITION AND PHYSIOLOGY

Status asthmaticus and acute severe asthma are terms that describe the same phenomenon: a prolonged severe episode of asthma, intractable in that an increase in routine outpatient medication fails to alleviate the symptoms of progressive airway obstruction. This discussion will exclude those asthmatics who die suddenly, since this is an unusual occurrence in an intensive care unit. Such episodes usually occur at home, on the playground at school, or on the way to the hospital.

The major changes that occur during an attack of severe asthma are due to extensive airway narrowing caused by bronchial constriction that is irregularly distributed, mucous plugging, and/or airway edema. The sudden decrease in airway caliber would cause complete closure of the airways between the alveoli and the lobar bronchi unless opposed by an increased distending pressure. Under static conditions, the only way the distending pressure of the intrathoracic airways can be increased is by an increase in the static transpulmonary pressure; and for a lung of given elastic properties, the static transpulmonary pressure can be increased only by an increase in lung volume. The major physiologic difference between the asthmatic and normal lung is that the asthmatic lung has closure of airways at greater than normal transpulmonary pressures. The more severe the attack, the greater the transpulmonary pressure at which the airways close; and the greater the closing pressure, the larger the lung volume must be to keep the airways open so that ventilation and gas exchange can occur. This

change results in the decrease in vital capacity (VC) seen in the acute asthmatic attack and is almost certainly due to a marked increase in residual volume (RV). During severe attacks, tidal volume (TV) composes a considerable portion of the VC, and patients breathe at a functional residual capacity (FRC) very near total lung capacity (TLC) (Fig. 28-1).

The mechanics of forced expired flow are markedly disturbed at large lung volumes. There is a tendency toward premature closure of the airways on expiration, whereas the airways may be enlarged during inspiration. Flow with maximum effort at a given lung volume is largely determined by the characteristics of the flow-limiting segment or the locus where the distending pressure of the airways has fallen to the critical level that results in airway closure. This is the point at which airway pressure is less than transpulmonary pressure and is located more distally as the condition progresses. An analysis of the pulmonary pressure, flow, and volume relationships in asthmatics shows that an increase in the critical distending pressure of the flow-limiting segment is probably due to an increase in smooth-muscle tone of the airways at that point. Thus, the major effect of the increase in smooth-muscle tone appears to be an increased closing tendency of the airways that requires breathing at larger lung volumes; but even at large lung volumes, the tendency toward closure results in flow limitation during a forced expiration. This large lung volume that is required to maintain patent airways during inspiration is probably the predominant cause of dyspnea seen during severe

184

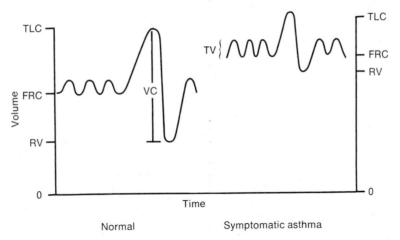

Fig. 28-1. Timed-volume spirometry. Normal curve compared with a curve from a patient with symptomatic asthma.

asthma. It was previously believed that an increase in airway resistance was the overwhelming contributor to this symptom. Dyspnea is easily reproduced when a normal individual tries to breathe at near total lung capacity, whereas little or no dyspnea occurs in patients breathing through a long, narrow tube of high resistance if a normal minute volume is preserved.

Tremendous swings in intrapleural pressure occur during inspiration and expiration. At end-expiration in a normal resting subject, the thorax tends to recoil outward, producing a slightly negative or subatmospheric intrapleural pressure. At large lung volumes, however, the thorax tends to recoil inward at end-expiration, producing a slightly positive intrapleural pressure. During an acute asthmatic attack, these modulations of intrapleural pressure are due more to marked changes in negativity during inspiration than to the degree of positivity during expiration. Furthermore, these changes are almost entirely due to the large lung volume. Compliant pulmonary vessels exposed to the marked increases in intrathoracic pressure respond to pressure changes in the intrapleural space, and there is a concomitant rise in pul-

monary arterial blood pressure with rising intrapleural pressure. This mechanism to restore pulmonary blood flow to a normal level is probably inadequate, because much of the ventilation/perfusion imbalance observed during asthmatic attacks may be due to the shunting of blood away from overly distended areas, which are being ventilated and not perfused.

Pulmonary functional abnormalities observed in an acute asthmatic attack include increases in TLC with marked increases in RV at the expense of a decrease in VC (Fig. 28-2). Dynamic lung volumes (forced expired volume in 1 second [$FEV_{1.0}$], peak expiratory flow rate [PEFR], and mid-maximal forced expired flow FEF_{25-75}) are decreased. It is important to identify which of these tests of lung function are dependent on patient motivation and cooperation. PEFR is the most effort-dependent test of forced expiration. More reproducible are $FEV_{1.0}$ and FEF_{25-75}. Resistance to air flow (R_{aw}) is markedly increased during an asthmatic attack, and lung compliance (C_L) is decreased. Because of the irregularly distributed occlusion of small and medium airways, impaired gas exchange occurs, and this results in ventilation/perfusion imbalances, hypoxemia, and early

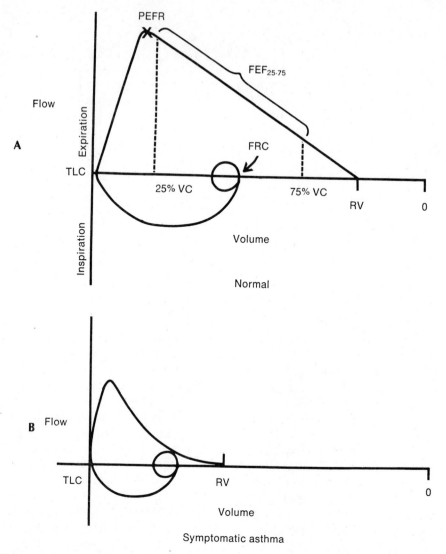

Fig. 28-2. Maximal expired flow-volume curve. Normal curve, **A,** compared with that from a patient with symptomatic asthma, **B.** Note the marked increase in RV and the effect of dynamic compression on the descending limb of the expiration curve as shown by the concave shape of this portion of the curve.

hypocapnia. A normal laboratory value for Pa_{CO_2} (35-42 mm Hg) in a patient with severe asthma should be considered elevated since the increase in ventilation usually seen during symptomatic asthma results in lower than normal Pa_{CO_2} values unless respiratory failure occurs. As ventilation becomes inefficient, use of accessory muscles increases, the work of breathing increases, and acidemia occurs. Metabolic or respiratory acidemia results in further bronchial constriction and pulmonary vascular spasm, perpetuating the cycle of airway obstruction and ventilation/perfusion imbalance. Unless this cycle can be broken, respiratory failure will occur. To underline the importance of monitoring arterial blood-gas tensions and pH during severe asthma, increases in Pa_{CO_2} are generally not observed until the $FEV_{1.0}$ falls to less than 20% of the patient's predicted normal value.

Oxygen therapy is not thought to increase Pa_{CO_2}. Since 50% of asymptomatic children with asthma have been shown to be chronically hypoxemic, it is safe to assume that any patient who is symptomatic will benefit from supplemental oxygen. Hypoxemia not only occurs acutely but frequently persists for several days after clinical remission. Because of the narrow spectrum of pH within which certain medications are effective, patients who are acidemic for whatever reason frequently fail to respond to sympathomimetics. Pulsus paradoxus will occur in patients who have an $FEV_{1.0}$ of less than 20% of their best values and in two thirds of those with an $FEV_{1.0}$ of less than 40% of their best test.

MONITORING

See also Chapter 4.

Respiratory system

1. The patient should be continually observed for retractions (suprasternal, intercostal), nasal flaring, and/or fatigue. These should be recorded every 2 hours. The quality of air movement, increase in expiratory phase of breathing, and period of respiratory cycle during which wheezing occurs should be recorded every 2 hours. An asthma score such as that shown in Table 28-1 may be useful in standardizing these observations.
2. Measure arterial blood-gas tensions and pH initially and frequently via an indwelling peripheral arterial catheter. It may be necessary to measure these variables as frequently as every 15 minutes, particularly during the administration of sympathomimetics.
3. Perform pulmonary function tests.
   a. Record static and dynamic lung volumes ($FEV_{1.0}$, PEFR, FEF_{25-75}, VC) every 2 hours and before and after each administration of rapidly acting bronchodilators.

Table 28-1. Clinical asthma score

Score	Description
1	Expiratory wheezing with tidal volume breathing
2	Inspiratory and expiratory wheezing with tidal volume breathing
3	Wheezing with tidal volume breathing plus prolonged expiratory phase
4	3 plus subcostal and lower intercostal retractions
5	4 plus intercostal and supraclavicular retractions and nasal flaring
6	5 plus diminished breath sounds

Air exchange may be indicated as a letter-suffix to the numeric score as follows:
p = poor; markedly reduced sounds
f = fair; moderate diminution
g = good inspiratory sounds

   b. If the patient should require mechanical ventilation, compare arterial blood-gas tensions with expired gas measurements (PE_{O_2}, PE_{CO_2}) to determine dead space-to-tidal volume ratio (V_D/V_T) and alveolar-arterial oxygen tension difference ($P[A - a]O_2$) (see Chapter 12).

Central nervous system

1. Anxiety may be a sign of progressive airway obstruction and hypoxemia.
2. Record the level of consciousness whenever it changes, otherwise routinely every 2 hours. Profound hypoxemia and/or hypercapnia are associated with lethargy and stupor.

MANAGEMENT
Correction of hypoxemia

1. Humidified oxygen supplementation is essential (see Chapter 98).
2. Since there is no practical way to determine accurately the concentration of oxygen being delivered to the lungs unless a cuffed endotracheal tube is inserted, control of inspired oxygen is achieved by monitoring Pa_{O_2}.

3. Administer supplemental oxygen sufficient to achieve a Pa_{O_2} of about 150 mm Hg at sea level.

Correction of acidemia

1. Adequate oxygenation may be sufficient to reverse anaerobic metabolism.
2. If treatment is considered necessary, sodium bicarbonate may be infused according to the following formula for correction of the base deficit:

mEq of bicarbonate to be infused =
$\qquad$ 0.3 × body weight in kg × base deficit

This is a one-half correction. Infusion rate should not exceed 1 mEq/kg/min. The primary indication for pharmacologic treatment of metabolic acidosis is to increase the pH to greater than 7.35, where antiasthmatic medicines are most active. It is possible to record an increase in Pa_{CO_2} following a rapid infusion of sodium bicarbonate.

Correction of fluid volume deficit

1. Administer balanced salt-containing solutions at 1½ to 2 times the usual maintenance amount. Most children who have been ill for a matter of hours will be volume depleted because of decreased intake and increased insensible fluid losses associated with tachypnea. Use either a 0.25% sodium chloride solution with 5% dextrose and added potassium or a 0.45% sodium solution with half of the anion chloride and half bicarbonate plus dextrose and potassium.
2. If parenteral fluids are required for several days and no adjustment is made in the initial infusion rate, fluid overload may occur, resulting in interstitial pulmonary edema. This edema is another form of airway obstruction, and pulmonary function tests may continue to show decreases in forced expired volumes and flows while the asthma is remitting. Therefore, if the patient is not improving as expected, a chest roentgenogram may identify the cause. If edema is present, furose-

mide, 1 to 2 mg/kg, may be given IV and repeated as necessary. A prompt improvement in pulmonary function should occur.

Correction of pulmonary abnormalities

Pharmacologic agents. *Aminophylline*, the ethylenediamine derivative of theophylline, is a methyl xanthine. The xanthines cause a number of pharmacologic actions in the body, including CNS stimulation, variable action on the heart (increased cardiac output, bradycardia, tachycardia), peripheral vasodilation, cerebral vasoconstriction, diuresis, and bronchodilation. The mechanism of this last action is based on theophylline's ability to inhibit the intracellular enzyme phosphodiesterase, thus preventing the breakdown of cyclic-3'5'-adenosine monophosphate (AMP), which in turn prevents the cellular release of mediators of bronchoconstriction, including histamine. Aminophylline is given at 5.8 mg/kg/dose IV over 30 minutes every 6 hours. This dose is equivalent to 5.0 mg of theophylline per kilogram. If the patient's dose of theophylline has been regulated by measuring serum levels during continuous outpatient use, that same dose may be given IV during the acute illness. Continuous IV infusion of aminophylline at a rate of 1.1 to 1.5 mg/kg/hr, after a bolus of 5.8 mg/kg is given, is an acceptable and in some cases desirable alternative to intermittent therapy. Improvement in lung function is linearly related to plasma levels in the range of 10 to 20 μg/ml. Toxicity is similarly related to plasma levels greater than 20 μg/ml, and symptoms include gastric discomfort, emesis, cardiac dysrhythmias, and convulsions, which usually are not seen until serum levels reach 50 μg/ml. Serum levels should be monitored frequently during administration of a constant infusion.

Concurrently give an *adrenergic bronchodilator* by aerosol (see Chapter 101). Isoproterenol (Isuprel), isoetharine (Bronkosol), epinephrine (Adrenalin), and metaproterenol (Alupent, Metaprel) may be used.

Cortisol may exert its bronchodilatory action

in a manner similar to adrenergic agents: by stimulating the catalytic action of adenyl cyclase. Methylprednisolone sodium succinate (Solu-Medrol), 1 to 2 mg/kg/dose IV, should be given every 4 to 6 hours throughout the acute illness and stopped abruptly within 3 to 5 days, if clinical improvement has occurred, and if there is no evidence of adrenal suppression or a history that shows that the patient has been receiving long-term steroid therapy. Discontinuing steroids too rapidly has been associated with sudden recurrence of airway obstruction. An acceptable alternative to methylprednisolone sodium succinate is hydrocortisone succinate (Solu-Cortef). This agent is given IV, 5 to 10 mg/kg/dose every 4 to 6 hours. Since hydrocortisone exerts more mineralocorticoid activity than does methylprednisolone, monitoring circulating blood volume and systemic arterial blood pressure is essential because of hydrocortisone's salt-retaining property. Acute gastric ulceration has been associated with the use of high-dose parenterally administered corticosteroids. This may be a direct effect of the steroids or a reflection of the clinical situation in which they are given.

If the patient exhibits progressive hypoxemia, hypercapnia (i.e., Pa_{CO_2} of 50 mm Hg), and clinical deterioration, give *isoproterenol* by constant infusion (see Chapter 14). Preexisting heart disease may preclude the use of this catecholamine by infusion. An intra-arterial catheter must be used for rapid sampling. Begin at an infusion rate of 0.1 μg/kg/min, and increase it by 0.1-μg/kg/min increments at 15- to 20-minute intervals based on clinical response and arterial blood-gas tension measurements. It is important to have an arterial blood-gas machine immediately available, because results are necessary within 2 to 3 minutes. A favorable clinical response includes increases in breath sounds, a trend toward a decrease in Pa_{CO_2} and an increase in Pa_{O_2}, less agitation, and less dyspnea. There is a significant association between heart rates of 180 to 200 beats/min and a favorable clinical response. The average total time of the isoproterenol constant infusion is approximately 40 hours. When a favorable clinical response is achieved, the period during which the patient has been receiving the infusion is subtracted from 40 hours, and the medication may be uniformly decreased over the remaining period. The occurrence of frequent PVCs or other hemodynamically significant dysrhythmias requires that the medication be discontinued.

Assisted ventilation. If the patient fails to respond to the above measures and demonstrates progressive respiratory failure, assisted ventilation will be necessary (see Chapters 12, 96, and 97). A volume-controlled ventilator is recommended because of the extremely high airway pressures often required to ventilate these patients. The patient is intubated nasally with a cuffed endotracheal tube (see Chapter 95). Peak inspiratory pressures up to 100 cm H_2O may be necessary to achieve satisfactory minute ventilation. The TV is usually set at 15 to 20 ml/kg initially and adjusted according to the arterial blood-gas tension analyses. Low levels of PEEP may be necessary. Promptly discontinue PEEP if cardiac or respiratory deterioration (i.e., hypotension, poor peripheral perfusion, and progressive hypoxemia or hypercapnia) occurs, since most patients with severe asthma are volume depleted and overly distended alveoli may aggravate intrapulmonary shunting. Satisfactory minute ventilation, which is the product of ventilatory rate and TV, may be achieved by adjusting either of these two variables, as long as standard principles of ventilation are followed. For example, adequate expiration time must be allowed to permit proper emptying of the lungs. Similarly, fast rates at low TVs can lead to atelectasis. All of the medications listed above should be continued or reduced and discontinued in an orderly fashion while the patient is receiving mechanical ventilation. In addition, it may be necessary to use a sedative such as diazepam and possibly a muscle relaxant such as pancuronium to facilitate mechanical ventilatory control. (Do not use tubocurarine, which releases histamine.) Because high inspiratory pressures are frequently required, pneumothorax may occur. The patient may be weaned from assisted ventilation while the isoproterenol infusion is being discontinued. Commonly, over the first 24 to 36 hours of assisted ventilation, inspiratory pressures required to achieve adequate ventilation will return to near normal range (30 to 40 cm H_2O). Finally, with return of Pa_{O_2} and Pa_{CO_2} to normal levels, the patient may be weaned systematically from the ventilator (see Chapter 97).

ADDITIONAL READING

Austen, K.F., and Lichtenstein, L.M., editors: Asthma: physiology, immunopharmacology and treatment, New York, 1973, Academic Press, Inc. pp. 15-24.

Burankul, B., Washington, J., Hillman, B., and others: Causes of death during acute asthma in children, Am. J. Dis. Child. 128:343-350, 1974.

Cade, J.F., Woolcock, A.J., Rebuck, A.S., and Pain, M.C.F.: Lung mechanics during provocation of asthma, Clin. Sci. 40:381-391, 1971.

Collins, J.V., Clark, T.J.H., Brown, D., and Townsend, J.: The use of corticosteroids in the treatment of acute asthma, Q. J. Med. new series 44(174):259-273, 1975.

Cotton, E.K., and Parry, W.: Treatment of status asthmaticus and respiratory failure, Pediatr. Clin. North Am. 22: 163-171, 1975.

Despas, P., and Macklem, P.T.: Site of airway obstruction in asthma and chronic bronchitis, Physiologist 14:131, 1971.

Downes, J.J., Wood, D.W., Striker, T.W., and Pittman, J.C.: Arterial blood gas and acid-base disorders in infants and children with status asthmaticus, Pediatrics 42:238-249, 1968.

Ellis, E., and Eddy, E.D.: Anhydrous theophylline equivalence of commercial theophylline formulations, letter, J. Allergy Clin. Immunol. 53:116, 1974.

Hill, D.J., Landau, L.I., McNicol, K.N., and Phelan, P.D.: Asthma: the physiological and clinical spectrum in childhood, Arch. Dis. Child. 47:874-881, 1972.

Knowles, G.K., and Clark, R.J.H.: Pulsus paradoxus as a valuable sign indicating severity of asthma, Lancet 2: 1356-1359, 1973.

Levy, G., and Koysooko, R.: Pharmacokinetic analysis of the effect of theophylline on pulmonary function in asthmatic children, J. Pediatr. 86:789-793, 1975.

McAllen, M.: Long term side effects of corticosteroids, Respiration 27:250-259, 1970.

McFadden, E.R., Jr., Kiser, R. and DeGroot, W.J.: Acute bronchial asthma: relations between clinical and physiologic manifestations, N. Engl. J. Med. 288:221-225, 1973.

Mitenko, P.A., and Ogilvie, R.I.: Rational intravenous doses of theophylline, N. Engl. J. Med. 289:600-603, 1973.

Olive, J.T., and Hyatt, R.E.: Maximal expiratory flow and total respiratory resistance during induced bronchoconstriction in asthmatic subjects, Am. Rev. Respir. Dis. 106:366-376, 1972.

Rebuck, A.S., and Read, J.: Assessment and management of severe asthma, Am. J. Med. 51:788-798, 1971.

Rees, H.A., Millar, J.S., and Donald, K.W.: A study of the clinical course and arterial blood gas tensions of patients in status asthmaticus, Q. J. Med. new series 37(148): 541-561, 1968.

Simpson, H., Forfar, J.O., and Grubb, D.J.: Arterial blood gas tensions and pH in acute asthma in childhood, Br. Med. J. 3:460-464, 1968.

Tai, E., and Read, J.: Blood-gas tensions in bronchial asthma, Lancet 1:644-646, 1967.

Weng, T.R., Langer, H.M., Featherby, E.A., and Levison, H.: Arterial blood gas tensions and acid-base balance in symptomatic and asymptomatic asthma in childhood, Am. Rev. Respir. Dis. 101:274-282, 1970.

Weng, T.R., and Levison, H.: Pulmonary function in children with asthma at acute attack and symptom-free status, Am. Rev. Respir. Dis. 99:719-728, 1969.

Wood, D.W., Downes, J.J., Scheinkopf, H., and Lecks, H.I.: Intravenous isoproterenol in the management of respiratory failure in childhood status asthmaticus, J. Allergy Clin. Immunol. 50:75-81, 1972.

Woolcock, A.J., and Read, J.: Improvement in asthma not reflected in FEV_1, Lancet 2:1323-1325, 1965.

Woolcock, A.J., and Read, J.: Lung volumes in exacerbations of asthma, Am. J. Med. 41:259-273, 1966.

29 Postintubation sequelae

FRANCES C. MORRISS

DEFINITION AND PHYSIOLOGY

There are numerous immediate complications of intubation, ranging from traumatic damage to the mouth and teeth to reflex-mediated changes in vital signs. Most of these problems can be remedied easily at the time they occur. There are, however, a number of problems that can arise as a consequence of intubation but become clinically apparent only after the tube is removed. Recent study of PICU patients showed that major complications (stridor, granuloma formation, pneumothorax, or infections) were present in 12 out of 100 patients with airway intervention. They occurred in 10% of patients with orotracheal tubes, 11% of patients with nasotracheal tubes, and 26% of patients with tracheostomy. Conditions predisposing the patient to a high rate of complications were primary diagnosis of laryngotracheobronchitis, occurrence of seizures, hypoperfusion, and presence of acquired respiratory tract infection (*Haemophilus influenzae, Pseudomonas, Klebsiella,* and *Candida albicans*). Several of the more serious of these sequelae will be discussed here.

The most common and benign sequela of intubation is sore throat, which occurs in 6% to 40% of patients, more commonly in females than in males. The postoperative incidence in nonintubated patients is 10%. Sore throat usually disappears within 48 to 72 hours without therapy, although a humidified atmosphere seems to be subjectively beneficial to these patients.

Another common problem is traumatic laryngitis, evidenced by hoarseness alone, occurring in 30% to 50% of patients. Laryngoscopic examination reveals discrete epiglottic or arytenoidal edema or edema of the posterior third of the vocal cords, although movement of the cords remains intact. This condition also disappears within 3 days without therapy, although humidity may be helpful.

Infection, specifically sinusitis secondary to obstruction of sinus orifices, can follow intubation, and the likelihood of this increases with the increasing length of intubation.

One of the most frequent problems in children is glottic edema, which can include the supraglottic, retroarytenoid, or subglottic areas and can progress to obstruction. This lesion is associated with more serious lesions, such as ulcers, granulomas, and stenosis. The loose areolar tissue on the anterior surface of the epiglottis and on the aryepiglottic folds predisposes these areas to edema. Edema posterior to the arytenoid cartilages can limit abduction of the vocal cords on inspiration. The most common cause of reintubation in infants is subglottic edema that occurs because the cricoid cartilage is circumferential and swollen mucosa cannot expand externally, so that internal airway narrowing, secondary to edema, follows. In addition, the mucosa of the subglottic region is fragile, with a loose submucosal connective tissue that is very prone to edema.

One millimeter of uniform edema at the cricoid ring can reduce the internal airway diameter by 30% to 65%, depending on the child's age (Table 29-1). Laryngeal edema is manifested

Table 29-1. Effects of 1 mm uniform edema at the cricoid ring

Age	Internal circumference cricoid ring (mm)	Percent decrease in area
<4 months	16	64%
4-6 months	19	55%
7 months	22	49%
3-5 years	25	44%
8 years	29	39%
10 years	31	36%
>14 years	38	30%

From Waterman, P.M., and Smith, R.B.: Tracheal intubation and pediatric outpatient anesthesia, Eye Ear Nose Throat Mon. **52:**175, 1973.

by hoarseness, inspiratory stridor, and croupy cough, usually within the first 8 hours after extubation although it can be seen as long as 24 hours after extubation. If edema is severe, obstruction with distress, air hunger, and ultimately airway occlusion can occur. The incidence has been reported between 0.19% and 4% in children undergoing intubation for elective surgical procedures; with intubation in the presence of a known inflammatory process, the incidence may range from 5% to 20%.

All intubations are associated with mucosal lesions, regardless of the skill of the intubator. Within 2 to 4 hours there is laryngeal irritation with congestion, followed by mucosal erosion in 6 hours. Eventually epithelial degeneration causes an ulcer covered with a pseudomembrane of fibrin and necrotic debris. By 48 hours there is bacterial invasion of the vocal processes and cricoid lamina, and by 96 hours microscopic ulcerations appear. Methylene blue staining techniques have shown that the areas of maximal damage occur on the arytenoid vocal processes, the cricoid plates, and the anterior tracheal wall. All these areas are subject to pressure necrosis secondary to entrapment of the mucosa between two rigid structures, the endotracheal tube and an underlying nonexpansible cartilage. In addition, the loose areolar tissue in these areas is subject to shearing forces from movement of the tube or of the head and neck. Postextubation reepithelialization, from a regenerating basal layer of the epithelium or from migration of cells from intact epithelium, begins within 48 hours after extubation and is complete by 100 hours. Patients with impaired perfusion have been shown to have earlier appearance of leukocytes and histiocytes and greater cytomorphologic changes in epithelial cells during cannulation. The significance of the laryngeal ulcerative lesion is that it is the common predisposing injury for the more serious lesions of granuloma, synechia, webs, and stenosis.

The incidence of laryngeal granuloma is 1 out of 800 to 1 out of 1,000 intubations; however, the incidence may be as high as 1% to 2% with prolonged intubations. Laryngeal granulomas are more common in females and adults. The location of the granuloma corresponds to that of ulcer formation, namely the vocal processes of the arytenoids, the anterior cricoid cartilage, and the anterior tracheal wall. They are usually manifested by hoarseness, dysphagia, sore throat, and signs of progressive respiratory obstruction several weeks to months after intubation. Granuloma formation should always be suspected when several efforts to remove long-term (>30 days) endotracheal tubes have failed.

Necrosis of the free edges of the cords can cause membrane formation between the posterior thirds of the cords or between the vocal processes of the arytenoids, leaving a slitlike laryngeal aperture. Such a lesion causes aphonia and obstruction but is readily amenable to surgical correction. Membranes can also form just below the vocal cords, and removal in this case can be difficult, since the epithelium is continuous with that of the laryngeal mucosa and makes recurrence common.

The most severe sequela of intubation is laryngeal stenosis secondary to fibrosis. There may be narrowing of the subglottic lumen or ankylosis of the cricoarytenoid joint, with immobilization of the vocal cords. An increasingly common phenomenon is the recognition of a silent subglottic stenosis in graduates of neonatal intensive care units several weeks to months after extubation and discharge. These children present with a mild respiratory disease complicated by a crouplike picture and on further investigation they are shown to have a circumferential subglottic scar. The incidence of this complication has been estimated at 8%. Either situation, laryngeal or subglottic stenosis, may produce severe respiratory obstruction, often requiring permanent tracheostomy. Children are more susceptible to this lesion than adults. Tracheal stenosis is relatively uncommon and usually occurs at the site where the cuff of the tube was inflated. The cause of the lesion is pressure necrosis caused by inadequate mucosal blood flow.

Etiologic factors contributing to sequelae of intubation may be divided into three types: predisposing factors, adjuvant factors, and decisive factors.

Predisposing factors consist of those conditions that render the patient more likely to develop problems with intubation.

1. Age. Although children seem to withstand prolonged intubation better than adults, they are more prone to develop symptomatic subglottic edema because of the smaller absolute size of the airway, increased likelihood of traumatic intubation secondary to anatom-

ic peculiarities of the infant airway, and in general a more delicate epithelial surface. The incidence of subglottic edema is highest in children less than 3 years of age.

2. Sex. Granulomas and sore throat are much more common in women, probably because of a slightly smaller larynx than that of the same-sized man and the consequent use of inappropriately large tubes. In addition, the laryngeal mucosa of the female is thinner than that of the male and hence more prone to trauma.

3. Fragility of mucosa. As mentioned earlier, females have a thinner epithelial surface on the larynx than males. Exfoliative cytology before and after intubation in healthy children undergoing short procedures (20 to 200 minutes) has shown that the ciliated columnar epithelium of the larynx is prone to sloughing. Pap smears made from a cotton applicator gently applied to the posteromedial aspect of one vocal cord after intubation showed sheets of desquamated cells without evidence of inflammatory reaction. This desquamative response to a foreign body was unchanged with the use of a lubricant or topical anesthesia and occurred in 100% of cases investigated.

4. Abnormal anatomic characteristics, such as cysts, tumors, and bands that predispose the patient to airway problems and also those characteristics such as short neck, micrognathia, and dental curtain that predispose the patient to traumatic intubation.

Adjuvant factors are those that if present enhance the possibility of sequelae. These include:

1. Debilitating states, such as cancer, steroid therapy, chronic anemia, and malnutrition, all of which may delay healing.

2. Circumstances favoring edema formation, such as a predisposition to allergy, cardiac failure, or hyperhydration.

3. Upper respiratory tract infection, particularly croup, in which the foreign body (the

endotracheal tube) is introduced into an already inflamed airway. The tube also violates the natural protective barrier created by the vocal cords and allows infected secretions from the upper airway easy access to the tracheobronchial tree. Loss of ciliary activity secondary to drying or the presence of the tube leads to stasis of secretions and enhances the inflammatory reaction already present.

4. State of hydration, particularly dehydration, which diminishes the volume of respiratory secretions. Exfoliative cytology has demonstrated that the degree of damage to mucous membranes is directly related to the duration of exposure of mucosa to dry gases.

5. Surgical site. Procedures involving the head and neck impart more trauma to the region in general and predispose the patient to sequelae of intubation.

6. Hypotension, with underperfusion of tracheal mucosa.

   Decisive factors are those that if present can cause sequelae.

1. Duration of intubation. The duration of intubation influences the postintubation outcome; the longer the tube is present, the more likely it is that problems will occur and the more likely that they will be severe. Many authorities recommend routine tracheotomy after 3 weeks of intubation.

2. Movement of the tube. Traction and rubbing of the tube on the larynx and trachea are always associated with the ulcerative necrotic lesions described earlier. The presence of such lesions is directly related to the tube diameter and tube shape. Most tubes do *not* conform to the natural anatomy of the airway and thus exert pressure posteriorly on the arytenoids and dorsally on the tracheal wall. Inappropriately large tubes increase such pressure. Because of the small absolute size of the airway and the small diameter at the cricoid, children are more likely to be intubated with inappropriately sized tubes.

Movement of the cords, bucking and coughing, and artificial ventilation (which imparts a pistonlike action to the tube) all increase the amount of trauma (a shearing type of stress) to the tracheal mucosa. In addition, flexion of the head increases the amount of pressure exerted by the tube to the posterior portion of the larynx.

3. Pressure from an inflated cuff. Direct, excessive pressure to the tracheal wall secondary to an occlusive high-pressure cuff correlates well with the incidence of tracheal stenosis and causes diminished capillary flow and pressure necrosis. The longer the period of occlusion, the more likely it is that an inflammatory response leading to stenosis will occur.

4. Tube material characteristics. Plastics can cause extensive tissue damage, principally from tissue reactions elicited by additives that facilitate polymerization, harden the plastic, protect against deterioration, and impart color. These materials may be leached from the tube by tracheal secretions or split off by mucosal enzymes. For this reason, all tubes should show an "IT" or "Z-79" mark on them to indicate that tissue testing approved by the Anesthesia Equipment Committee of the U.S. Standards Institute has been done. Test material from tubes is implanted in rabbit muscle or cell culture and checked for tissue toxicity after appropriate incubation. Materials so tested and marked are relatively nontoxic. Improper sterilization techniques, such as reuse of gamma-irritated tubes or improper aeration of ethylene oxide-sterilized tubes, can lead to enhanced tissue irritation secondary to release of toxic byproducts.

MONITORING

See also Chapter 4.

The most important feature of postextubation management is close observation for 24 hours or until symptoms have resolved. The patient must be cared for in an area where intubation equipment and physicians skilled in intubation are immediately available (intensive care unit, recovery room).

Respiratory system

1. Repeated evaluation for stridor, retractions, hoarseness or aphonia, anxiety, and cyanosis.
2. Hourly auscultation for breath sounds.
3. Arterial blood gas tensions and pH as indicated.

MANAGEMENT

See also Chapter 103.

Postextubation distress with croupy cough and stridor

1. Withhold oral feedings and hydrate the patient intravenously until resolution of severe symptoms occurs.
2. Withhold deep suctioning.
3. Place the patient in humidified cool mist to which oxygen may be added according to the degree of distress or for documented hypoxemia.
4. Administer racemic epinephrine by aerosol or IPPV for vasoconstriction and bronchodilation:
   a. <20 kg: 0.25 ml in 3 to 5 ml 0.9% sodium chloride solution
   b. 20 to 40 kg: 0.5 ml in 3 to 5 ml 0.9% sodium chloride solution
   c. >40 kg: 0.75 ml in 3 to 5 ml 0.9% sodium chloride solution

(Note that this dose schedule is empiric and not based on any documented dose-response curve and may not be entirely appropriate for every patient.) This form of therapy may be repeated on an as needed basis, usually every 2 to 4 hours; however, recurrence of severe symptoms within 30 to 60 minutes of a treatment should alert personnel to the possibility of a failed extubation. Monitor heart rate and ECG closely during the treatment to identify excess sym-

pathetic stimulation (e.g., heart rate >200 beats/min) and dysrhythmias.

5. Insert an endotracheal tube, using an internal diameter one size smaller than the one previously used. This should be done under optimal conditions, preferably in the operating room, so that an atraumatic intubation can be accomplished and laryngoscopy to identify the source of edema can be performed. If a severe edematous process or necrotic laryngeal lesions are identified, tracheotomy may be a preferable route of securing the airway.
6. Although steroids and antihistamines have been recommended for treatment of postintubation croup, their efficacy has not been established either in the animal model or in clinical trials.

Postextubation distress with aphonia

1. Withhold feedings.
2. Administer cool humidified mist with oxygen as needed.
3. Obtain lateral airway roentgenograms; consider tomograms of the larynx.
4. Perform laryngoscopy and bronchoscopy under general anesthesia to identify synechiae or vocal cord malfunction.
5. Surgical correction or tracheotomy, as well as long-term follow-up by an otolaryngologist, may be necessary.

Second attempts at extubation

1. Withhold feedings.
2. Administer cool humidified mist with oxygen if necessary.
3. Elevate head of bed 30 degrees.
4. Administer aerosolized racemic epinephrine to the mouth and nose. The goal of therapy is to precipitate saturated water and medication around the tube to decrease swelling.
5. Give dexamethasone (Decadron), 0.4 mg/kg/dose IV for 4 doses, the first 6 hours before extubation and the second at the time of extubation.

6. An alternative method is to extubate the patient under general anesthesia and allow him to wake up slowly while being carefully observed.

7. Racemic epinephrine treatments as outlined above may be given as needed for hoarseness, retractions, and stridor after extubation.

8. Laryngoscopy and bronchoscopy should be planned if the second attempt at extubation fails or if symptoms suggest the presence of an airway granuloma. Tracheotomy may be necessary while combined medical and surgical management (systemic and/or intralesional steroids, dilation laser surgery) is instituted.

ADDITIONAL READING

Abbott, T.R.: Complications of prolonged nasotracheal intubation in children, Br. J. Anaesth. **40**:347-353, 1968.

Allen, T.H., and Steven, I.M.: Prolonged nasotracheal intubation in infants and children, Br. J. Anaesth. **44**:835-840, 1972.

Applebaum, B.: Tracheal intubation, Philadelphia, 1976, W.B. Saunders, Co.

Bergstrom, J., Moberg, A., and Orell, S.R.: On the pathogenesis of laryngeal injuries following prolonged intubation, Acta Otolaryngol. **55**:342-356, 1962.

Blanc, V.F., and Tremblay, N.A.G.: The complications of tracheal intubation: a new classification with a review of the literature, Anesth. Analg. **53**:202-212, 1974.

Casthely, P., Chalon, J., Ramanathan S., and others: Tracheobronchial cytologic changes during prolonged cannulation, Anesth. Analg. **59**:759-763, 1980.

Chalon, J., Loew, D.A.Y., and Malebranche, J.: Effects of dry anesthetic gases on tracheobronchial ciliated epithelium, Anesthesiology **37**:338-343, 1972.

Debain, J.J., Lebrigand, H., Binet, J.B., and others: Quelques incidents et accidents de l'intubation trachéale prolongée, Ann. Otolaryngol. (Paris) **85**:379-386, 1968.

Donnelly, W.H.: Histopathology of endotracheal intubation, Arch. Pathol. **88**:511-520, 1969.

Farmati, O., Quinn, J.R., and Fennell, R.H.: Exfoliative cytology of the intubated larynx in children, Can. Anaesth. Soc. J. **14**:321-325, 1967.

Goddard, J.E., Phillips, O.C., and March, J.H.: Betamethasone for prophylaxis of postintubation inflammation: a double blind study, Anesth. Analg. **46**:348-353, 1967.

Hazards of prolonged intubation and tracheotomy equipment, editorial, J.A.M.A. **204**:624, 1968.

Hilding, A.C.: Laryngotracheal damage during intracheal anesthesia, Ann. Otol. Rhinol. Laryngol. **80**:565-581, 1971.

Howland, W.S., and Lewis, J.S.: Mechanisms in the development of postintubation granulomas of the larynx, Ann. Otol. Rhinol. Laryngol. **73**:1007-1011, 1964.

Jordan, W.S., Graves, C.H., and Elwyn, R.A.: New therapy for postintubation laryngeal edema and tracheitis in children, J.A.M.A. **212**:585-588, 1970.

Markham, W.G., Blackwood, M.J.A., and Conn, A.W.: Prolonged nasotracheal intubation in infants and children, Can. Anaesth. Soc. J. **14**:11-21, 1967.

Maze, A., and Block E.: Stridor in pediatric patients, Anesthesiology **50**:132-145, 1979.

Orlowski, J.P., Ellis, N.G., Amin, N.P., and others: Complications of airway intrusion in 100 consecutive cases in a pediatric ICU, Crit. Care Med. **8**:324-331, 1980.

Otherson, H.B.: Intubation injuries of the trachea in children: management and prevention, Ann. Surg. **189**:601-606, 1979.

Owen-Thomas, J.B.: A follow-up of children treated by prolonged nasal intubation, Can. Anaesth. Soc. J. **14**:543, 1967.

Papsidero, M.J., and Pashley, N.R.: Acquired stenosis of the upper airway in neonates—an increasing problem, Ann. Otol. Rhinol. Laryngol. **89**:512-514, 1980.

Rasche, R.F.H., and Kuhns, L.R.: Histopathologic changes in airway mucosa of infants after endotracheal intubation, Pediatrics **50**:632-637, 1972.

Stetson, J.B., and Guess, W.L.: Causes of damage to tissues by polymers and elastomers used in fabrication of tracheal devices, Anesthesiology **33**:635-652, 1970.

Stoelting, R.K., and Proctor, J.: Acute laryngeal obstruction after endotracheal anesthesia, J.A.M.A. **206**:1558-1559, 1968.

Waterman, P.M., and Smith, R.B.: Tracheal intubation and pediatric outpatient anesthesia, Eye Ear Nose Throat Mon. **52**:173-177, 1973.

Way, W.L., and Sooy, F.A.: Histological changes produced by endotracheal intubation, Ann. Otol. Rhinol. Laryngol. **74**:799-812, 1965.

30 Croup

FRANCES C. MORRISS

DEFINITION AND PHYSIOLOGY

Croup is a nonspecific designation applied to a clinical syndrome characterized initially by mild elevation of temperature, malaise, rhinitis, and loss of appetite. Physical examination at this time usually reveals injected mucous membranes of the oropharynx, nasopharynx, and ear, mild cervical lymphadenopathy, clear mucoid rhinitis, and the absence of pulmonary findings. After 2 to 3 days, the child develops hoarseness, inspiratory stridor, a typical barking cough, tachypnea, and retractions. This picture usually lasts 3 to 5 days, during which time symptoms may progress or stay relatively unchanged, and is followed by a convalescent period of 2 to 3 days.

There is a significant population of children with recurrent croup (more than 2 episodes). As a group, these children have a male preponderance, an earlier onset of the initial episode, a familial predisposition to allergies, a tendency to develop asthma subsequently, a greater association with airway hyperreactivity (as demonstrated by histamine challenge), and slightly lower than normal flow rates as measured by pulmonary function tests.

There is little evidence for a bacteriologic cause of the syndrome. The most commonly isolated viral agents are parainfluenza 1, 2, and 3, influenza A and B, and respiratory syncytial virus. These types of viral infections are predominantly infections of younger children, generally less than 30 months of age. Influenza and parainfluenza occur in epidemic form during the winter and spring months, with biennial peaks. Respiratory syncytial virus oc-curs endemically and sporadically on a yearly basis and affects infants less than 6 months of age. The most severe spectrum of symptoms occurs with the first infection in young infants, and though reinfection occurs, the disease caused is usually mild. Although all these agents have been implicated as causes of croup, they may also cause bronchiolitis, bronchitis, and pneumonia, and frequently symptoms of several syndromes are present in the same child. Viral agents involve the entire respiratory tract, and the localization of symptoms to any specific portion of the respiratory tract depends on other factors that are probably related to the host rather than to the specific virus.

Less commonly, tracheitis secondary to *Candida*, diphtheria, *Haemophilus influenzae*, pneumococci, streptococci, and/or staphylococci may cause upper airway obstruction indistinguishable from viral laryngotracheobronchitis. In these cases, cultures and direct visualization of the airway are necessary to make the diagnosis.

The pathophysiology of a viral infection helps explain this seeming lack of specificity. Viral agents are intracellular and spread in a contiguous fashion; therefore, infection of any portion of the respiratory membrane implies potential infection of the whole. Localization of symptoms depends on the age of the child and the degree of inflammation. Inflammation initially causes an increase in secretions from the mucous glands of the involved area, with an associated loss of ciliary activity. Nasopharyngeal obstruction caused by thick mucoid secretions leads to mouth breathing and results in the

197

bypassing of the natural humidifying mechanism. Water must then be evaporated from the lower respiratory tract to saturate incoming air. The child is often febrile and has increased water loss and decreased oral intake, all of which tend to produce thick secretions. The presence of thickened secretions leads to frequent episodes of coughing. In addition, there is edema of the mucous membranes of the pharynx, larynx, trachea, and bronchi. Because the airway diameter of the infant is small, any degree of swelling will compromise the lumen, and breathing becomes more difficult. The smallest diameter of the infant airway is at the level of the cricoid, the only complete tracheal cartilage (Fig. 30-1). Swelling in this area is quickly manifested as stridor, which is heard on inspiration because the inspiratory phase of breathing causes further narrowing of the upper respiratory tract. Edema of the vocal cords is manifested as hoarseness. The presence of thickened secretions in an inflamed, irritable trachea with a compromised lumen sets the stage for obstruction and associated signs of increased respiratory work, namely intercostal and substernal retractions associated with use of the accessory muscles of respiration. The increased work of breathing, plus the hypermetabolic state induced by fever, leads to increased oxygen consumption and increased cardiac work. There may be small-airway obstruction, with concomitant atelectasis, alveolar infiltrates, or pulmonary edema. As inflammation increases and tiring occurs, the obstruction may become complete, with carbon dioxide retention, hypoxemia, and ultimately respiratory arrest. Cyanosis is a late sign of respiratory compromise, and significant degrees of hypoxemia and hypercarbia may exist without much change in the vital signs. Increasing tachycardia and tachypnea may be the only clinical correlates of a worsening status.

The few autopsy reports available substantiate the above process of epithelial, mucosal, and submucosal inflammatory changes that are seen in the trachea, bronchi, and bronchioles.

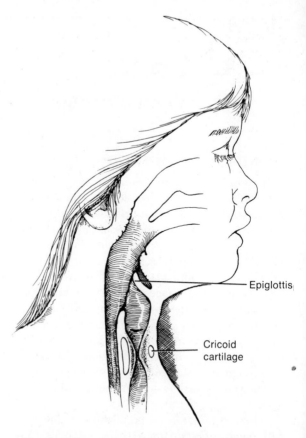

Fig. 30-1. Site of airway narrowing associated with croup. Although the entire respiratory membrane is involved, life-threatening compromise of the tracheal lumen occurs at the level of the cricoid cartilage. Note the normal-size epiglottis.

There may be a crusted exudate along the entire respiratory membrane overlying necrotic mucosa, and hyaline membranes can be found lining the alveoli, with patches of atelectasis.

The child most at risk to develop severe obstruction is:

1. The young infant (<12 months of age), who has a small airway diameter. One millimeter of airway edema can compromise the tracheal lumen by 50%.
2. The child whose history suggests subglottic stenosis or airway hyperreactivity.

Table 30-1. Clinical croup score

	0	1	2
Inspiratory breath sounds	Normal	Harsh with rhonchi	Delayed
Stridor	None	Inspiratory	Inspiratory and expiratory
Cough	None	Hoarse cry	Bark
Retractions and flaring	None	Flaring and suprasternal retractions	As under 1 plus subcostal, intercostal retractions
Cyanosis	None	In air	In 40% O_2

From Downes, J.J., and Raphaely, R.: Pediatric intensive care, Anesthesiology **43**:242-250, 1975.

a. The child with recurrent croup.
b. The child with a history of postintubation croup.
c. The child with a history of previous airway instrumentation and/or ventilation, particularly one with a history of prematurity and airway intervention.
d. The child with congenital stridor.
e. The highly allergic child.
f. The child who has the onset of croup at greater than 3 to 4 years of age.

MONITORING

See also Chapter 4.
1. Close, repeated observation for signs of increasing distress (Table 30-1).
2. Frequent auscultation to check air entry.
3. Chest and lateral neck roentgenograms initially; repeat chest roentgenograms as indicated.
4. Serial arterial blood-gas tensions and pH every 4 to 6 hours, depending on the degree of respiratory distress. Consider placing an arterial catheter, although it is necessary only in a few of the most ill patients.
5. Viscosity and quantity of secretions.

MANAGEMENT
Specific measures

Specific measures are directed at liquefying pulmonary secretions and reducing airway edema to relieve obstruction.
1. Adequate hydration. Give IV fluids at a rate greater than maintenance (usually 1.5 times).

Attempts to rehydrate a patient with respiratory compromise by the oral route only are inappropriate.
2. Humidify inspired gases (cool mist).
3. Discontinue known drying agents such as antihistamines or proprietary preparations containing atropine.
4. Aerosolized racemic epinephrine (see p. 195). This form of therapy may be used on as-needed basis. Because a rebound effect exists, the child must be hospitalized so that close observation can be maintained between treatment periods. Children requiring epinephrine within 30 minutes after receiving a treatment probably have significant obstruction and may need to have the airway instrumented.
5. Antibiotics and steroids are usually not indicated for uncomplicated viral croup.

Supportive measures

1. Continuous close observation.
2. Nothing by mouth.
3. Avoid respiratory depressants and sedatives.
4. Vigorously treat with antipyretics any fever greater than 38.5° C to avoid an increase in respiratory and cardiac work and drying of secretions.
5. Transfuse packed RBCs to increase oxygen-carrying capacity if Hct is less than 30%.
6. Increase inspired oxygen concentration if hypoxemia is present. Administration of oxygen to the air-hungry child will not mask symptoms of obstruction.

Treatment of severe obstruction

1. Early consultation with services skilled in airway maintenance, e.g., intensive care, pulmonary, surgery, and anesthesia, so that a rapid coordinated effort can be made if severe obstruction occurs. A specific protocol for management of severe obstruction is helpful (see Chapter 31).
2. Airway instrumentation.
   a. The decision to place an artificial airway depends on repeated close evaluation by trained observers. Suggested criteria include:
      (1) Marked progressive anxiety.
      (2) Hypoxemia (Pa_{O_2} <50 mm Hg) with supplemental oxygen; cyanosis occurs late.
      (3) Hypercarbia (Pa_{CO_2} >55 mm Hg).
      (4) Fatigue, which may be evidenced by increasing heart and respiratory rates, apneic episodes in small infants, inability to sleep, inability to tolerate any manipulation such as IV placement, and inability to take oral feedings.
      (5) Clinical evidence of progressive, severe obstruction (increasing stridor, increasing retractions, pulmonary edema, poorly heard or absent breath sounds).
   b. Type of airway. The type of airway chosen (endotracheal tube versus tracheostomy tube) depends on the competency of the personnel to perform intubation, tracheostomy, and tube care. The intubator or surgeon must be familiar with the problems of the small child's airway. Either procedure may be complicated by pneumothorax or pneumomediastinum.
      (1) If an endotracheal tube is used, it should not be cuffed and it should be at least one size smaller than the child would normally require (i.e., internal diameter should be 0.5 mm less than usual), preferably of a soft polyvinyl (atraumatic) material that molds to the airway at body temperature.
      (2) If subglottic swelling is so great that only a very small tube (i.e., two or more sizes smaller than expected) can be passed, tracheotomy should be performed immediately. The resistance to breathing through such a small tube will be too great, and it will be impossible to clear pulmonary secretions adequately. Patients can become severely stressed and die even with a patent artificial airway in place if it is too small.
3. Tube management. Remember that children with croup have a high incidence of complications, notably subglottic stenosis after airway intervention.
   a. Humidify gases and provide 2 cm H_2O CPAP.
   b. Suction hourly and as needed.
   c. Perform CPT if atelectasis or infiltrates are present, frequency to be determined by the patient's fatigability.
   d. Restrain the child. Head movement should be minimized by the use of sandbags or restraints. Elevate head of bed 30 degrees.
   e. Mild sedatives should be used to improve tube tolerance. Before giving sedatives, always check to be certain that the patient is not fighting or restless because of hypoxia. (See Chapter 31.)
4. Pulmonary edema may complicate severe airway obstruction; treatment should include diuresis and CPAP or positive-pressure ventilation.

ADDITIONAL READING

Downes, J.J., and Raphaely, R.: Pediatric intensive care, Anesthesiology 43:242-250, 1975.

Eden, A., Kaufman, R.Y., and Yu, R.: Corticosteroids and croup: controlled double blind study, J.A.M.A. 200:403-404, 1967.

Glezen, W.P., and Denny, F.W.: Etiology of acute lower

respiratory disease in children, N. Engl. J. Med. **288:**499-505, 1973.

Gurwitz, D., Corey, M., and Levison, H.: Pulmonary function and bronchial reactivity in children after croup, Am. Rev. Respir. Dis. **122:**95-99, 1980.

James, J.A.: Dexamethasone in croup: a controlled study, Am. J. Dis. Child. **117:**511-516, 1969.

Jones, R.S.: The management of acute croup, Arch. Dis. Child. **47:**661-668, 1972.

Mitchell, D.P.: Skill more crucial than approach in management of croup crises, Hosp. Practice **9:**200-205, 1974.

Mitchell, D.P., and Thomas, R.L.: Secondary airway support in the management of croup, J. Otolaryngol. **9:**419-422, 1980.

Newth, C.J.L., Levinson, H., and Bryan, A.C.: The respiratory status of children with croup, J. Pediatr. **81:**1068-1073, 1972.

Rowe, L.D.: Advances and controversies in the management of supraglottitis and laryngotracheobronchitis, Am. J. Otolaryngol. **1:**235-244, 1980.

Taussig, L., Castro, O., Beaudry, P., and others: Treatment of laryngotracheobronchitis (croup): use of intermittent positive pressure breathing and racemic epinephrine, Am. J. Dis. Child. **129:**790-793, 1975.

Wesley, A., Desai, S., Holloway, R., and others: Nasotracheal intubation in the management of infective croup, S. Afr. Med. J. **46:**839-842, 1972.

Westley, C.R., Cotton, E.K., and Brooks, J.G.: Nebulized racemic epinephrine by IPPB for the treatment of croup, Am. J. Dis. Child. **132:**484-487, 1978.

Zach, M., Erben, A., and Ounsky, A.: Croup, recurrent croup, allergy, and airways hyperactivity, Arch. Dis. Child. **56:**336-341, 1981.

31 Epiglottitis

FRANCES C. MORRISS

DEFINITION AND PHYSIOLOGY

Acute epiglottitis is an inflammation of the soft tissues surrounding the laryngeal outlet; the epiglottic cartilage is the structure most characteristically involved. The majority of cases are caused by *Haemophilus influenzae* type B, although streptococci and staphylococci have been infrequently implicated. The course is characterized by a short prodrome (6 to 10 hours) of high fever (38° to 40° C), sore throat, and malaise, followed by rapid development of dysphagia, inability to swallow and drooling, inability to lie down, dyspnea, and profound respiratory distress. Patients usually appear septic, with facial pallor and a mottled gray undertone to the skin; 50% to 70% of patients have positive blood cultures. Progression to complete respiratory obstruction and hypoxemia secondary to inflammatory edema is the usual situation and was commonly fatal until techniques of airway intervention were developed.

The clinical picture of epiglottitis is so typical and so fulminant that suspicion of the process should mandate immediate action. Lateral neck roentgenograms, which show thickening of the epiglottic tissue and aryepiglottic folds that obliterate the vallecula and pyriform sinuses (Fig. 31-1), confirm the diagnosis. The thickened epiglottic shadow often resembles an adult thumb in size and shape. Pharyngeal examination reveals the epiglottis as a swollen cherry-red mass at the base of the tongue. This means of confirming the diagnosis is *not* recommended unless the examiner is prepared to intubate the patient immediately. The two events most often associated with acute decompensation of respiratory status are examination of the pharynx and placing the child supine for roentgenograms or to perform therapeutic procedures. *Do not place the child in the horizontal position.*

An uncommon but serious complication of upper airway obstruction is pulmonary edema in the absence of fluid overload or cardiac disease. Edema may occur after the airway obstruction has been relieved. The mechanism is increased filtration of fluid across pulmonary capillary walls. Inspiration against a closed or obstructed glottis exaggerates the normally negative transpulmonary pressure; if this greater than normal negative pressure is transmitted to peribronchial and perivascular spaces, it .may disrupt the integrity of the pulmonary capillary bed. Hypoxia may also disrupt capillary membrane integrity. In addition, greater negative transpulmonary pressures enhance right-sided venous return and increase pulmonary perfusion pressures, which may already be elevated secondary to alveolar hypoxia and arterial hypercarbia. Right and left ventricular afterload are increased. During expiration airway pressures become positive, decreasing venous return, and opposing the hydrostatic forces that promote transudation of fluid. An abrupt fall in airway pressure caused by relief of the obstruction (intubation) without concomitant preservation of positive expiratory pressure may produce a sudden increase in venous return, with a shift of blood from the peripheral to the pulmonary vascular beds. The acute increase in pulmonary hydrostatic pressures results in edema formation; the severity depends

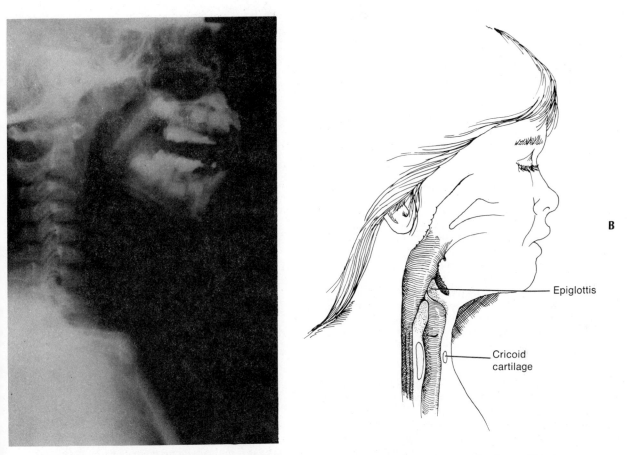

Fig. 31-1. A, Lateral roentgenogram of the neck, showing epiglottic and supraglottic swelling.
B, Site of airway compromise in epiglottis. Note the normal caliber of the airway
at the cricoid cartilage.

on the extent of hypoxic damage to the capillary bed, on the ability of the pulmonary lymphatics to handle large amounts of fluid, and on the increased load on the ventricles. This type of pulmonary edema may be fulminant and life-threatening, and even with prompt therapeutic intervention such edema requires at least 24 hours to clear.

Prognosis is excellent once the respiratory obstruction is treated. Symptomatic epiglottitis is one of the few situations where immediate intervention is mandatory, since only rarely will a child be seen with a swollen cherry-red epi-glottis in the absence of respiratory symptoms. Such a patient may be managed without immediate airway intervention, but provisions must be made for continuous in-hospital observation and immediate intubation should obstructive symptoms appear. In the more usual case, the infection responds promptly to antibiotics and supportive measures once an airway has been established. Although septicemia is common, the incidence of extraepiglottic foci of infection is low. There is a 25% incidence of pneumonia and/or cervical lymphadenitis, and otitis media can also be present. Concurrent arthritis, peri-

PROTOCOL FOR THE TREATMENT OF UPPER AIRWAY OBSTRUCTION
Departments Of Pediatrics, Anesthesiology, and Surgery—Children's Medical Center, Dallas

The following is meant to provide specific, clear-cut recommendations regarding the management of infants and children admitted to Children's Medical Center and Parkland Memorial Hospital with a diagnosis of upper airway obstruction.

1. All children admitted to Children's Medical Center with a diagnosis of upper airway obstruction under emergency situations will be evaluated in the emergency room immediately on arrival by the senior pediatric house officer with the referring physician, who may accompany the patient, depending on the suspected diagnosis.

2. All patients with the suspected diagnosis of acute epiglottitis should be accompanied to the hospital by the referring physician if the initial evaluation occurred at the private office or in another emergency room.

3. On arrival, a clinical assessment must be made as to the severity and emergent nature of the obstruction. If time allows, a history should be taken to rule out other forms of upper airway obstruction that may mimic laryngotracheobronchitis (LTB) and acute epiglottitis.

4. If time allows in the judgment of the senior pediatric house officer and/or the attending physician, x-ray films of the airways should be taken as soon after arrival in the emergency room as possible. An x-ray technician should be immediately available when the patient arrives in the emergency room.

5. The staff surgeon, anesthesiologist, and/or intensivist should be notified that a patient with upper airway obstruction is in the hospital. This does not imply that these individuals must see the patient immediately.

6. If, in the judgment of the primary physician, the patient is stressed and may require an artificial airway, then the staff surgeon, anesthesiologist, and/or intensivist should examine the patient personally. Depending on the severity of the illness, x-ray films may not be possible before direct visualization of the airway, which should be accomplished, if possible, in the operating room.

7. IV solutions should be started in the operating room.

8. Oxygen should be administered in low concentrations immediately on arrival in the emergency room.

9. If a history suggestive of LTB is obtained, after 3 minutes oxygenation in a sitting position the hypopharynx should be visualized by the most senior person present, using either a tongue blade or, preferably, a laryngoscope. Equipment to intubate the patient must be available. If a diagnosis of epiglottitis is obtained historically, then it would be better to await examination in the operating room.

10. If the patient's condition merits immediate attention, consultations should be obtained from the surgical, anesthesia, and/or intensive care staff during the usual operating hours (until 2300, Monday through Friday). In an emergency at night or on weekends, the senior anesthesia resident on call at Parkland Memorial Hospital should be requested to examine and intubate the patient if time has not permitted the attending staff to arrive at the hospital.

11. If intubation can await the arrival of the attending staff, the administration of racemic epinephrine by aerosol or IPPV is indicated.

12. Criteria for admission:
    a. If occurring at rest, any
       (1) Stridor
       (2) Cyanosis
       (3) Retractions
    b. Treatment with racemic epinephrine

13. Suggested criteria for intubation:
    a. Marked, progressive anxiety
    b. Hypoxemia with supplemental oxygen
    c. CO_2 retention
    d. Fatigue
    e. Clinical evidence of progressive severe obstruction

14. Treatment of LTB:
    a. Constant observation
    b. Cool mist
    c. Minimize anxiety
    d. Hydration
    e. Racemic epinephrine by aerosol or IPPV
    f. Oxygen at low concentration

15. Treatment of epiglottitis:
    a. Nasotracheal intubation
    b. Blood and hypopharyngeal cultures
    c. Ampicillin, 150 mg/kg/day IV, and chloramphenicol, 50-75 mg/kg day IV, both given every 6 hours pending culture sensitivities
    d. Observation in the intensive care unit
    e. Proper restraint of the patient

carditis, or meningitis is very unusual.

Because of the urgent nature of the obstructive process, a preset protocol for management is highly recommended (see boxed material). Since the glottic anatomy may be considerably altered secondary to swelling, expert help with intubation should be utilized and a surgeon should be immediately available to perform a tracheotomy, if it is needed. For these reasons, airway intervention is usually performed in an operating room with the patient under general anesthesia. The necessity for a tracheotomy under these circumstances is unusual; most patients are managed quite satisfactorily with the use of a nasotracheal tube.

MONITORING

See also Chapter 4.

Respiratory system

1. Maintain close observation. The patient must not be left alone until the airway is secured, and intubation and resuscitation equipment must accompany the patient at all times. Recent experience suggests that an open airway and adequate ventilation can be maintained easily with positive-pressure ventilation by bag and mask.
2. Obtain a lateral neck roentgenogram if time allows; this should be taken with the patient in the upright position.
3. After intubation:
   a. Obtain a roentgenogram to confirm endotracheal tube position and to check for pulmonary infiltrates and pulmonary edema.
   b. Observe the patient for any signs of increasing obstruction such as retractions, anxiety, struggling.
   c. Arterial blood-gas tensions and pH are usually not necessary if pulmonary edema and pneumonia are absent. A significant alveolar-arterial oxygen gradient in the presence of a normal chest roentgenogram may precede pulmonary edema;

therefore, arterial blood-gas tensions and pH should be obtained in the postintubation period and followed sequentially if abnormal.

Infection

1. Obtain blood cultures initially, and repeat in 24 hours if positive. These are particularly important because of an increasing incidence of ampicillin-resistant *Haemophilus influenzae*. This should be done after the airway is secured.
2. Culture tracheal secretions and/or the epiglottic surface at the time of intubation.
3. Obtain CBC with differential analysis initially, and repeat twice weekly if the patient is receiving chloramphenicol.

MANAGEMENT
Respiratory obstruction

1. *Do not place the patient in the horizontal position.*
2. Increase inspired oxygen concentration.
3. Perform intubation under general anesthesia.
   a. Perform induction with the patient in a sitting position, using an inhalation agent and oxygen. Use of muscle relaxants is usually contraindicated in the presence of severe airway obstruction.
   b. An IV catheter may be placed at this time.
   c. The endotracheal tube should be one size smaller than would normally be used to accommodate mucosal edema. A small leak should be present around the tube with 20 cm H_2O pressure. Secure the airway with an oral endotracheal tube, and then place a nasotracheal tube.
   d. An expert intubator should perform tube placement.
   e. Confirmation of the diagnosis by visualization of the epiglottis and culture of the epiglottic surface is best done at this time.

4. Alternatively, perform intubation using a small (3.2-mm) fiberoptic bronchoscope introduced transnasally.
   a. Study child in the upright position, using 2% lidocaine (Xylocaine) jelly applied to the nares for topical anesthesia.
   b. Once diagnosis is confirmed, pass pre-placed nasotracheal tube over the bronchoscope placed in the trachea.
   c. Pre-extubation airway evaluation may be accomplished by this same method.
   d. The most skilled otolaryngologist available should perform this procedure in the operating room with surgical and anesthesia personnel on standby for intubation by conventional methods and/or tracheostomy if necessary.
5. Administer humidified gas via the endotracheal tube until extubation. Two to four cm of CPAP for several hours may be beneficial in stabilizing hemodynamic changes occurring in the lung as a consequence of relieving airway obstruction.
6. Treat pulmonary edema if present.
   a. Oxygen, CPAP, and mechanical ventilation may be needed to stabilize arterial blood-gas tensions.
   b. Perform frequent suctioning.
   c. Give furosemide (Lasix), 1 mg/kg IV.
   d. Digitalization is not useful.
7. Consider CPT every 6 to 8 hours to prevent atelectasis.

General supportive care

1. Intensive care nursing should continue until extubation. The patient will require respiratory isolation for 12 hours. Proper arm restraints are imperative, since patients usually feel and act markedly better after intubation and 24 hours of treatment. Sedation may occasionally be required. Any one of the following may be used:
   a. Hydroxyzine, 3 mg/kg every 3 to 4 hours PO, IM.
   b. Pentobarbital, 4 to 8 mg/kg every 6 hours PO, IM.
   c. Chloral hydrate, 5 to 10 mg/kg every 6 hours PO.
2. Antibiotics.
   a. Give ampicillin, 150 mg/kg/day IV, and chloramphenicol, 50 to 75 mg/kg/day IV, until antibiotic sensitivities confirm the most appropriate agent.
   b. Duration of therapy is 10 days.
3. Give antipyretics for a temperature greater than 38.5° C. The use of an acetaminophen suppository (1 grain/yr of age) before intubation may decrease tachycardia during anesthesia.
4. Intake.
   a. Give IV fluids (a balanced salt solution) as maintenance for 24 hours or until the patient can swallow.
   b. Clear liquids can be given while the patient is intubated.
5. Use of steroids remains controversial.

Extubation

Because of the immediate marked improvement in symptoms, some authorities recommend extubation in 8 to 10 hours; however, because of the high frequency of positive blood cultures and the lack of data as to how soon the bloodstream is sterilized, 24 hours of antibiotic therapy are recommended before considering extubation. The usual length of intubation is 24 to 36 hours. Other criteria to be satisfied in addition to those mentioned elsewhere (see Chapter 103) are:
1. Return of ability to swallow.
2. Resolution of signs of sepsis.
3. Temperature need not be normal at time of extubation.
4. Evidence of resolution of glottic swelling obtained by direct visualization of the supraglottic tissue with a laryngoscope. The child must be sedated if this is to be done atraumatically. Use sodium thiopental (Pentothal), 2 to 3 mg/kg IV, or diazepam (Valium), 0.1 to 0.2 mg/kg IV. Both agents will provide a short period of sedation.

If these criteria are met, the child can be

extubated once his sedated state has resolved and provided that he has had nothing by mouth for 4 hours. The child should be observed in the PICU for recurrence of obstructive symptoms, although reintubation is highly unlikely. Thereafter, his hospital course may continue on a floor with routine nursing care.

ADDITIONAL READING

Adair, J.C., and Ring, W.: Management of epiglottitis in children, Anesth. Analg. **54**:622-625, 1975.

Battaglia, J.D., and Lockharg, C.H.: Management of acute epiglottitis by nasotracheal intubation, Am. J. Dis. Child. **129**:334-336, 1975.

Galvis, A.G., Stool, S.E., and Bluestone, C.D.: Pulmonary edema following relief of acute upper airway obstruction, Ann. Otol. Rhinol. Laryngol. **89**:124-128, 1980.

Lazoritz, S., Saunders, B.S. and Bason, W.M.: Management of acute epiglottitis, Crit. Care Med. **7**:285-290, 1979.

Margolis, C.Z., Colletti, R.B., and Grundy, G.: Hemophilus influenza type b: the etiologic agent in epiglottitis, J. Pediatr. **87**:322-324, 1975.

Milko, D.A., Marshak, G., and Striker, T.W.: Nasotracheal intubation in treatment of acute epiglottitis, Pediatrics **53**:674-677, 1974.

Molteni, R.A.: Epiglottitis: incidence of extraglottic infection; report of 72 cases and review of literature, Pediatrics **58**:526-531, 1976.

Oh, T.H., and Motoyama, E.K.: Comparison of nasotracheal intubation and tracheostomy in management of acute epiglottitis, Anesthesiology **46**:214-216, 1977.

Rapkin, R.H.: The diagnosis of epiglottitis: simplicity and reliability of radiographs of the neck in the differential diagnosis of the croup syndrome, J. Pediatr. **80**:96-100, 1972.

Szold, P.D., and Glicklich, M.: Children with epiglottitis can be bagged, Clin. Pediatr. **15**:792-793, 1976.

Travis, K.W., Todres, I.D., and Shannon, D.C.: Pulmonary edema associated with croup and epiglottitis, Pediatrics **59**:695-698, 1977.

Vauthy, P.A., and Reddy, R.: Acute upper airway obstruction in infants and children—evaluation by the fiberoptic bronchoscope, Ann. Otol. Rhinol. Laryngol. **89**:417-418, 1980.

32 Apnea

FRANCES C. MORRISS

DEFINITION AND PHYSIOLOGY

Apnea denotes the absence of respiratory activity and has been thought to be the result of a profound CNS insult or depression. The most usual causes in such patients are structural damage to the brainstem (trauma, edema, infection, hemorrhage) or interference with cerebral metabolic function (drug overdose, hypotension, hypoxia, hypoglycemia, etc.). Disorders of peripheral nerves (Guillain-Barré syndrome) or of respiratory musculature may also cause peripheral muscle unresponsiveness to CNS control, functionally mimicking apnea. The management of apnea in these situations requires an artificial airway, institution of adequate assisted ventilation, and treatment of the underlying lesion. Specific techniques are discussed elsewhere (see Chapters 6, 10, 11, 12, 95 and 97).

Changes in the rhythm of breathing, even regularly occurring periods of apnea, are now known to be common during sleep in seemingly healthy persons and may not be a sign of a life-threatening illness. Sleep apnea may be central (i.e., there is no respiratory movement) or obstructive (i.e., respiratory activity occurs but air flow is absent). Sleep apnea is defined as apnea that is less than 10 seconds in duration and occurs fewer than 10 times per night.

The situation in the premature infant is different. Periodicity of respiration is considered normal, and the incidence of clinically significant apneic episodes in otherwise healthy infants is high. Twenty-five percent of infants weighing less than 2,500 g and 84% of those weighing less than 1,000 g exhibit apnea (see Chapter 33).

Control of respiratory activity is located in the pneumotaxic center in the nucleus parabrachialis of the dorsolateral rostral pons. This center monitors the afferent sensory input and alters the rhythmic discharges of the medullary centers responsible for generating efferent impulses to the respiratory musculature. Regulation of respiration depends on:

1. Physical integrity of both the pneumotaxic center and the centers controlling inspiration and expiration.
2. Physiologic integration of these centers.
3. The functional and maturational state of the remainder of the CNS.

Of these three factors, the last two are most significant in understanding neonatal apnea, the assumption being that nonintact respiratory centers are incompatible with life.

Physiologic integration of respiratory centers (Table 32-1)

Efferent activity of the respiratory centers depends on the character and intensity of afferent impulses received, and the preterm infant depends more on afferent input for maintenance of a normal respiratory pattern than does the term infant. A decrease in afferent activity or the presence of inhibitory impulses may result in increased periodicity of breathing or in apnea. Afferent impulses may originate in peripheral sensors, in reflex arcs, or from cortical activity.

Peripheral stimuli known to affect respiration originate in temperature sensors, chemo-receptors, and lung stretch (proprioceptive) receptors. Apnea is increased in a warm environment or when an infant is being warmed. The afferent input from temperature sensors in this instance is probably inhibitory.

Peripheral chemoreceptors for both carbon dioxide and oxygen are probably functional in the neonate. The term newborn infant shows an immediate increase in ventilation when placed in a hypoxic environment and suppression of ventilation when placed in 100% oxygen (i.e., a normal response). However, if he is left in a hypoxic environment, respiratory depression with periodicity progressing to apnea follows the initial increase in minute ventilation. Adults and infants older than 18 days do not exhibit this secondary respiratory depression. This paradoxical response is thought to occur because the central inhibitory effects of hypoxia override the peripheral stimulant effects mediated by the chemoreceptors. The preterm infant placed in 100% oxygen without previously being hypoxic has a biphasic response, with an immediate decrease in ventilation followed by a sustained increase in ventilation. Oxygen will abolish or reduce periodic respiration if such respirations are present. Neonates, both term and preterm, respond to hypercarbia normally (i.e., with an increase in minute ventilation); however, this response is blunted in premature infants and the increase in minute ventilation occurs by an increase in TV rather than in rate. In addition, responsiveness to an increased concentration of carbon dioxide (either exogenous or endogenous) is greater if the infant is normoxic or hyperoxic; this response is decreased in the presence of hypoxia.

Another source of afferent impulses from the periphery is chemical irritant receptors mediated via the vagus and located in the pulmonary ciliary epithelium; under pathologic conditions, release of endogenous chemical irritants (e.g., histamine) may stimulate afferent activity and cause shortening of the expiratory

time and an increase in respiratory rate. Vagal blockade (inhibition of irritant receptors) therefore slows respiration. In addition, the vagus seems also to mediate the normal response to hypercarbia via a carbon dioxide–sensitive sensor other than the carotid body chemoreceptor. In this instance, vagal blockade markedly blunts the normal increase in respiratory rate found with hypercarbia. The sensing mechanism may be pulmonary irritant chemoreceptors.

There are numerous reflexes (normal and abnormal) that influence the rate and pattern of breathing:

1. Stimulation of posterior pharyngeal vagal receptors by suctioning or passage of an NG tube often produces apnea and reflex bradycardia.
2. Hyperinflation of the lung stimulates vagal stretch receptors located between submucosal muscle fibers and prolongs the expiratory phase, thus decreasing respiratory rate (Hering-Breuer reflex).
3. Stimulation of laryngeal chemoreceptors for taste (vagus via the superior laryngeal nerve) with various fluids causes severe apnea and wide swings in systemic arterial blood pressure. Species-specific milk will not elicit this reflex. Therefore, "silent" gastroesophageal reflux (GER) (i.e., no vomiting, choking, or clinical evidence of regurgitation) may present as apnea.
4. Cutaneous or mucocutaneous stimulation in the area of the innervation of the trigeminal nerve (face, nasal mucosa, nasopharynx) with noxious gases, water, saline solution, or cold produces a decrease in the respiratory rate, generation of long respiratory pauses, a decrease in the heart rate, and an increase in systemic arterial blood pressure. Hot and cold stimuli further increase oxygen consumption and contribute to central hypoxic depression.
5. Passive neck flexion, translocation of the mandible posteriorly, or excessive submental pressure may cause the genioglossus mus-

Table 32-1. Factors influencing respiratory instability

Inciting event	Mediated via	Corrective action
Modification of central afferent impulses		
↑ oxygen concentration ↓ carbon dioxide concentration (influenced by sleep)	Carotid body chemoreceptor via glossopharyngeal nerve	Avoid hyperventilation, avoid 100% oxygen
Vagal blockade	Pulmonary vagal irritant chemoreceptors	Avoid cold environment, cold gases, pharyngeal stimulation
↑temperature	Peripheral temperature sensors—multiple cutaneous sensory nerves	Lower environmental temperature to low end of thermal neutral range
Suctioning	Pharyngeal vagal receptors	Avoid pharyngeal stimulation
Inflation of lung	Vagal stretch receptors in pulmonary submucosa	Avoid vigorous assisted ventilation (i.e., greater than normal volumes)
Inhalation of milk, saline solution, glucose	Superior laryngeal nerve taste chemoreceptors at larynx	Close attention to feeding technique
Facial and nasopharyngeal stimulation (cold, fluid, noxious gases)	Trigeminal nerve temperature receptors and chemoreceptors	Close attention to environmental control; avoid nasal stimulation
Airway occlusion	Central hypoxia and respiratory center depression, ? immaturity	Proper head position for resuscitation, feeding, restraint; assure nasal patency; CPAP
REM sleep	↓cortical afferent activity, inhibition of vagal afferents, asynchronous respiratory muscle activity	Cutaneous, vestibular stimulation; CPAP; prone position; theophylline
Drugs	↓cortical afferent activity	Avoid general inhalational anesthesia, respiratory depressants; reverse narcotics
Functional maturational state of central nervous system		
Immaturity	↓ cortical afferents, ↓ central synapses, ↓ concentration of central neurotransmitter, ↓ responsiveness to central carbon dioxide concentration	Growth, theophylline
↓energy substrates Hypoglycemia	Primary respiratory center depression	IV glucose
Hypoxemia (↑ Pao_2 or ↓ oxygen-carrying capacity)		↑ Fio_2 correct pulmonary disorders, keep Hct 40%; theophylline for diaphragmatic fatigue
Electrolyte abnormalities		Correct abnormalities in Na, K, Cl, Ca, Mg
Inadequate cerebral perfusion	Primary respiratory center depression	Correct hypotension and ↑ ICP
↑metabolic demand for energy substrate	Primary respiratory center depression	Correct status epilepticus, hyperpyrexia, sepsis

cle to obstruct functionally the airway at the level of the posterior pharynx. The ability to obstruct the airway of a neonate in such a manner is greatly enhanced by the decreased tone of pharyngeal musculature that occurs with sleep. It has been found that 13% of normal newborns fail to initiate struggling respiratory movements (the normal response) when such airway occlusion occurs. This may be a result of central hypoxic depression or may be the result of disproportionate changes in efferent stimulation to pharyngeal, laryngeal, and inspiratory chest wall muscles such that negative airway pressures generated by contraction of inspiratory muscles are not overcome by contraction of the upper-airway musculature. Such respiratory muscle asynchrony is enhanced during rapid-eye-movement (REM) sleep. At low levels of chemical drive (i.e., hyperoxia and hypocapnia), cranial nerve activity in the larynx and the pharynx may be absent in the presence of significant phrenic nerve activity (i.e., diaphragmatic movement is occurring while upper-airway muscular activity is absent). Subsequent activation of pharyngeal and laryngeal muscles secondary to hypoxia and hypercarbia (i.e., high level of chemical drive) may be inadequate because of the excessive amount of force now needed to reestablish air flow in the obstructed upper airway. Some feeding techniques associated with vigorous tongue movement may also cause intermittent airway occlusion at the oropharyngeal level. It is also well known that infants with abnormal mandibular or midfacial anatomy (e.g., Pierre Robin syndrome, trisomy 21, Apert's syndrome) are at greater risk for developing apnea as a result of airway occlusion during sleep or feeding.

6. In preterm infants the normal suck-swallow pattern seen with oral nipple feeding is associated with early termination of inspiration and a decrease in minute ventilation thought to be secondary to a decrease in sensitivity to carbon dioxide (immature chemorecep-

tors). Term infants compensate for this decrease in respiratory rate by increasing inspiratory drive in order to maintain normal TV and hence avoid hypoxia.

Cortical afferent influences on respiratory regulation include sleep states, drugs, the concentration of central neurotransmitters, and the intensity of cortical traffic in general. The intensity of cortical afferent impulses is reduced in premature infants, who lack dendritic arborization and axodendritic synaptic connections in the respiratory centers. In addition, apneic infants have decreased concentrations of urinary catecholamines, which may reflect a central deficiency of neurotransmitters.

Sleep states, both REM sleep and quiet or slow wave sleep, are known to have profound effects on respiratory control. Normally, during sleep minute ventilation decreases secondary to reduced TV and rate; the tone of skeletal muscles is reduced, with some sparing of diaphragmatic tone, particularly during REM sleep. The relative absence of intercostal muscle tone may cause inward deflection of the rib cage during inspiration, a process that will be accentuated in premature infants, who have physiologically unstable chest walls. Loss of upper airway muscle tone makes obstruction more likely during sleep. Voluntary control of respiration is lost, the effects of environmental stimuli are lost, and control of breathing becomes autonomic. Any condition that produces instability of the autonomic control mechanism will be likely to produce apnea, particularly in premature infants.

There are variable changes to chemical stimuli. During quiet sleep the normal response to an increased concentration of carbon dioxide is blunted (i.e., increasing Pa_{CO_2} causes less of an increase in minute ventilation than would be expected). The response to hypoxia, an increase in minute ventilation, is variable (i.e., blunted in some people, increased in others). Responses to irritant receptor stimulation are blunted; proprioceptor input from muscle spindles seems altered, resulting in more rib cage excursion and less diaphragmatic excursion than in the waking state. Hering-Breuer reflexes may be increased. In premature infants apneic episodes of greater than 6 seconds predominate and persist after the shorter and more frequent apneic episodes seen in REM sleep have resolved.

During REM sleep irregular breathing patterns are common, and a higher incidence of apnea (as well as a higher incidence of low Pa_{O_2} values) is noted in premature infants. Ventilatory responses to chemical stimuli are depressed the same as in quiet sleep; the response to hypoxia is better preserved than the response to hypercarbia. Responses to reflex stimulation of mechanoreceptors vanish; vagal afferent impulses are poorly integrated; cortical afferent impulses seem to be inhibited, causing an enhancement of the oscillatory activity normally seen in the respiratory cycle. Premature infants spend more time in REM sleep than quiet sleep and are thus subject to its inhibitory effects on cortical activity for longer periods of time.

Most drugs capable of central respiratory depression can cause periodic respiration in premature infants, the most striking example being the inhalation agents used for general anesthesia. Eighty percent of infants with a history of prematurity revert to periodic respiratory patterns (and associated apnea) under anesthesia, and this pattern may persist in the postoperative period for several hours. Neonatal depression resulting from maternal narcotic overdose is another example of drug-mediated central respiratory depression causing apnea. Preliminary evidence indicates that phenobarbital, an agent known to disrupt REM sleep, decreases the frequency of apneic episodes. Barbiturates are not a recommended form of therapy, however, unless the infant has a primary seizure disorder.

Functional and maturational state of central nervous system

The maturational status of the premature nervous system can be indirectly surmised from the infant's activity and reflexes; specific examples such as the presence of abnormal reflexes in premature infants, decreased numbers of cortical synapses, possible deficiency in central neurotransmitters, and a more prominent role of REM sleep, have been mentioned above. Undoubtedly, immaturity of central control of respiration plays a large role in the increased incidence of apnea in the premature infant.

Apnea is an extremely common, nonspecific symptom of functional CNS disorders that primarily and directly depress activity of the respiratory centers. The common elements of these disorders are:

1. Decreased delivery of energy substrate (oxygen and glucose) to the CNS secondary to hypoxia, anemia, hypoglycemia, and abnormalities of serum Na, K, Cl, Ca, and Mg.
2. Inadequate cerebral perfusion due to hypotension or intracerebral pathology (increased ICP, infection).
3. Increased demand for energy substrate associated with sepsis, status epilepticus, and hypermetabolic states, including narcotic withdrawal and hyperpyrexia.

Of all of these conditions, hypoxia seems to be the most potent in producing respiratory depression. Not only do primary pulmonary diseases such as hyaline membrane disease and pneumonia cause apnea (usually a sign of a deteriorating state), but less obvious disorders of pulmonary function, such as PDA with pulmonary edema and minimal loss of lung volume, can be associated with irregular respiration or apnea. The mechanism for apnea associated with these less severe disorders is probably intermittent hypoxemia as a result of hypoventilation. Viral pneumonias, especially those caused by respiratory syncytial virus, may present as apnea even in older infants. Blood, urine, and CSF cultures should be obtained as part of the evaluation.

Although apnea is a common event, its occurrence necessitates an investigation for potentially severe and correctable causes. Bradycardia concomitant with apnea requires treatment regardless of the cause. The danger of recurrent apnea lies in the possibility of brain damage from repeated episodes of hypoxia, and therefore detection as well as treatment of apnea is extremely important. For purposes of standardization, apnea will be defined as a pause in breathing for more than 6 seconds (respiratory rate of 10/min) and periodic breathing as two cessations of respiration within 20 seconds. The American Academy of Pediatrics Task Force on Prolonged Apnea defines prolonged apnea as "cessation of breathing for 20 seconds or longer or as a briefer episode associated with bradycardia, cyanosis or pallor."

MONITORING

See also Chapter 4.

1. Monitor respiratory rate continuously via an apnea monitor with a reliable signaling device. The minimal pause in respiration allowable before the alarm is activated should be variable. The standard delay from breath to breath is often 10 to 15 seconds; however, for infants who are consistently bradycardic (heart rate less than 100 beats/min) with this respiratory pause, 5 to 10 seconds may be a better choice. All infants weighing less than 1,800 g should be so monitored. Oscillographic display of respiration may be more useful than a digital display in detecting changes in the volume of each breath. The conditions surrounding any apneic episode should be thoroughly documented (suction, feeding, sleep state, passage of stool, etc.).

2. Measure and record the inspired oxygen concentration (FI_{O_2}) every 4 hours if it is greater than 0.21.

3. Obtain arterial blood-gas tensions and pH initially and as needed. If good correlation is established between direct arterial and transcutaneous oxygen values, constant transcutaneous monitoring may identify periods of significant risk for hypoxia and apnea (e.g., sleep, feeding, CPT) (see Chapter 94).

4. Sleep study prior to discharge may be helpful to identify high-risk infants.

MANAGEMENT
Immediate management

The goal of immediate management of an apneic episode is to restore adequate ventilation. Stimulate the infant gently (flick foot, shake gently) while inspecting the pharynx for regurgitated stomach contents. If any are found, perform gentle pharyngeal suction and empty the stomach. If bradycardia, cyanosis, or pallor accompanies apnea, start artificial ventilation with bag and mask, taking the following precautions:

1. FI_{O_2} should be the same as the infant is currently receiving.
2. If the episode persists in severity, FI_{O_2} may be increased by 0.05 or 0.1.
3. The head should be slightly extended, with the mask placed perpendicularly on the face. Do not apply excessive posterior pressure on the mandible, since this can obstruct the airway. Hold the mandible forward by placing a finger behind the ramus of the mandible and lifting upward. Oral or nasopharyngeal airway may be helpful.
4. Inflate the lungs only enough to raise the chest. Continue until normal respirations and heart rate are restored. (Hyperventilation will suppress respiratory drive.)
5. The rate of assisted ventilation should be about the same as the infant's intrinsic respiratory rate (i.e., 20/min).
6. Try to avoid cold stress. If the infant must be taken from a closed incubator, place him on a warm blanket out of drafts or consider the use of a radiant heat source. Warmed humidified gases should be used.
7. Monitor vital signs frequently during the episode.

Continuing management

Further management of apnea is directed at diagnosing and treating any underlying pathologic process, particularly one of a respiratory nature. Adequacy of substrate (oxygen and glucose) delivery as well as good cerebral perfusion (normal systemic blood pressure for age) must be assured. If no discrete, identifiable cause (pneumonia, hypoglycemia, inhalation of stomach contents, recurrent airway obstruction, etc.) is found, treatment is directed toward avoiding situations known to produce apnea and toward creating situations that increase afferent impulses.

Assuring adequacy of substrate delivery and cerebral perfusion

1. Increase FI_{O_2} only if Pa_{O_2} is less than 60 mm Hg. Although provision of an oxygen-enriched environment will markedly decrease apneic episodes, without arterial or transcutaneous oxygen monitoring, the risk of retrolental fibroplasia may be excessive and so prohibitive in premature infants.
2. Treat any respiratory disorders vigorously. Apnea secondary to loss of lung volume may respond to CPAP alone. Avoid mechanical ventilation unless severe pulmonary disease is present.
3. Treat upper-airway obstruction aggressively. Consider tracheostomy in a symptomatic neonate with facial dysplasia in whom an indwelling NG tube does not relieve or prevent the airway obstruction.
4. Treat sepsis; rule out meningitis.
5. Correct metabolic abnormalities (e.g., acidosis, hypoglycemia, hyponatremia, hypocalcemia).
6. Keep Hct greater than 40% to maintain adequate oxygen-carrying capacity.
7. Correct congestive heart failure by fluid management and ligation of PDA if indicated.
8. Support systemic arterial blood pressure.
9. Provide adequate glucose as $D_{10}W$. Dextrostix should be greater than 90 mg/dl.
10. If appropriate, administer naloxone (Narcan) to reverse any narcotics the infant may have received prenatally.
11. Treat primary seizure disorders with anticonvulsants.

12. Diagnose and treat CNS pathology (e.g., hydrocephalus, hemorrhage).

Avoiding stimulation of reflexes known to be associated with apnea

1. Pay careful attention to suctioning technique.
2. Avoid hyperoxia and hyperinflation of lungs.
3. Avoid cold and other noxious cutaneous stimuli to face and head.
4. Monitor warming procedures carefully. Do not warm infants at a rate greater than 1° C every 30 to 60 minutes.
5. Avoid hyperflexion of the neck, especially with feeding.
6. Assure bilateral patency of nostrils.
7. If the infant chokes excessively with nipple feedings, switch to gavage technique. Be certain to burp the infant well, and prop him upright after feedings to prevent regurgitation. Use of an occluded nipple or pacifier during gavage feedings may prevent airway occlusion by the tongue and subsequent reflex changes in the respiratory cycle.
8. If feeding problems persist, investigate the possibility of gastroesophageal reflux (barium swallow, esophageal pH study).
9. Low Pa_{O_2} associated with feedings in the absence of documented reflux may respond to a decrease in the volume of feedings or a change to continuous drip feedings or to placing the infant in the prone position during sleep.

Increasing afferent stimuli

1. Institute cutaneous and vestibular stimulation; both stroking the extremities (5 minutes out of 15) and placing the infant on an oscillating waterbed have proved effective. Use of music boxes and radios may be helpful.
2. Asynchronous respiratory muscle activity seen with REM sleep becomes more stable in the prone position.
3. Decrease the environmental temperature to the lower end of the neutral thermal range (see Tables 18-1 and 18-2).
4. Institute nasal CPAP, 2 to 4 cm H_2O, if frequent assisted ventilation is still necessary or

if apneic episodes seem related to upper airway obstruction occurring during sleep. Positive airway pressure may stint upper airway and prevent obstruction at the time of inspiration. A minimal reduction in FRC, which may contribute to recurrent apnea, will also be corrected.

5. For refractory apnea, in an effort to avoid mechanical ventilation, some authors recommend the use of theophylline.
   a. Give 2 mg/kg orally every 6 hours, *or*
   b. Give a 5.5 mg/kg IV loading dose followed by 1.1 mg/kg IV every 8 hours.
   c. The therapeutic serum range is 7 to 13 μg/ml.
   d. Only several doses may be required to halt apneic episodes until more conservative measures such as CPAP become effective.
   e. The exact mechanism of action by which xanthines inhibit apnea is unknown, but increased levels of cyclic AMP secondary to inhibition of cyclic nucleotide phosphodiesterase may effect the CNS levels of neurotransmitters. It has recently been shown that theophylline has a direct effect on diaphragmatic muscle, improving contractility, and that infants whose apneic episodes are the result of muscle fatigue show fewer apneic episodes related to fatigue when placed on the agent. Because of a myriad of side effects and the increased possibility of high serum levels secondary to decreased hepatic detoxification, long-term use of theophylline should be reserved for centers that are capable of monitoring serum levels.
   f. Theophylline should never be used to treat apnea associated with well-defined causes (e.g., sepsis, respiratory distress); its use is reserved for infants in whom correctable causes of apnea have been excluded.
6. When no definable cause exists and all other measures fail, endotracheal intubation and assisted ventilation may be instituted.

Posthospitalization management

Follow-up of infants who have recurrent apneic episodes is extremely important, since as a group they have a higher incidence of sudden infant death syndrome (SIDS) (see Chapter 33).

ADDITIONAL READING

American Academy of Pediatrics Task Force on Prolonged Apnea: Prolonged apnea, Pediatrics **61**:651-652, 1978.
Anas, N., Boettrich, C., Hall, B., and Brooks, J.G.: The association of apnea and respiratory syncytial virus infection in infants, J. Pediatr. **101**:65-68, 1982.
Aranda, J.V., Sitar, D.S., Parsons, W.D., and others: Pharmacokinetic aspects of theophylline in premature newborns, N. Engl. J. Med. **295**:413-416, 1976.
Aubier, M., Detroyer, A., Sampson, M., and others: Aminophylline improves diaphragmatic contractility, N. Engl. J. Med. **305**:249-253, 1981.
Cherniack, N.: Respiratory dysrhythmias during sleep, N. Engl. J. Med. **305**:325-330, 1981.
Daily, W.J.R., Klaus, M., and Meyer, H.B.P.: Apnea in premature infants: monitoring, incidence, heart rate changes and an effect of environmental temperature, Pediatrics **43**:510-518, 1969.
Downing, S.E., and Lee, J.C.: Laryngeal chemosensitivity: a possible mechanism for sudden infant death, Pediatrics **55**:640-649, 1975.
Fagenholz, S.A., O'Connell, K., and Shannon, D.C.: Chemoreceptor function and sleep state in apnea, Pediatrics **58**:31-36, 1976.
Fleming, P.J., Bryan, A.C., and Bryan, M.H.: Functional immaturity of pulmonary irritant receptors and apnea in newborn preterm infants, Pediatrics **61**:515-518, 1978.
Gabriel, M., and Albani, M.: Rapid eye movement sleep, apnea and cardiac slowing influenced by phenobarbital administration in the neonate, Pediatrics **60**:426-430, 1977.
Gabriel, M., Albani, M., and Schulte, F.J.: Apnea spells and sleep states in preterm infants, Pediatrics **57**:142-148, 1976.
Gould, J.B., Lee, A.F.S., James, O., and others: The sleep state characteristics of apnea during infancy, Pediatrics **59**:182-194, 1977.
Haddad, G.G., and Mellins, R.B.: The role of airway receptors in the control of respiration in infants: a review, J. Pediatr. **91**:281-286, 1977.
Hoppenbrouwers, T., Hodgman, J., Harper, R.N., and others: Polygraphic studies of normal infants during the first six months of life. III. Incidence of apnea and periodic breathing, Pediatrics **60**:418-425, 1977.
Kattwinkel, J.: Neonatal apnea: pathogenesis and therapy, J. Pediatr. **90**:342-347, 1977.

Kattwinkel, J., Mars, H., Fanaroff, A.A., and others: Urinary biogenic amines in idiopathic apnea of prematurity, J. Pediatr. **88**:1003-1006, 1976.

Kattwinkel, J., Nearman, H.S., Fanaroff, A.A., and others: Apnea of prematurity: comparative therapeutic effects of cutaneous stimulation and nasal continuous positive airway pressure, J. Pediatr. **86**:588-592, 1975.

Konig, H., and Mazzi, E.: Apnea resulting from obstruction of the nares by an eye shield, J. Pediatr. **89**:652-653, 1976.

Korner, A.F., Kraemer, H.C., Haffner, E., and others: Effects of waterbed flotation on premature infants: a pilot study, Pediatrics **56**:361-367, 1975.

Krauss, A.N., Klain, D.B., and Auld, P.M.: Chronic pulmonary insufficiency of prematurity, Pediatrics **55**:55-58, 1975.

Parmalii, A.H., Stern, E., and Harris, M.H.: Maturation of respiration in prematures and young infants, Neuropaediatrie **3**:294, 1972.

Rigatto, H.: Respiratory control and apnea in the newborn infant, Crit. Care Med. **5**:2-9, 1977.

Rigatto, H., Brady, J.P., and Verduzco, R.T.: Chemoreceptor reflexes in preterm infants. I. The effect of gestational and postnatal age on the ventilatory response to inhalation of 100% and 15% oxygen, Pediatrics **55**:604-620, 1975.

Shannon, D.C.: Pathophysiologic mechanisms causing sleep apnea and hypoventilation in infants, Sleep **3**:343-349, 1980.

Shannon, D.C., Gotay, F., Stein, I.M., and others: Prevention of apnea and bradycardia in low–birth weight infants, Pediatrics **55**:589-594, 1975.

Shannon, D.C., Marsland, D.W., Gould, J.B., and others: Central hypoventilation during quiet sleep in two infants, Pediatrics **57**:342-346, 1976.

Shivpuri, C.R., Martin, R.J., Carlo, W.A., and others: Decreased ventilation in preterm infants during oral feeding, J. Pediatr. **103**:285-289, 1983.

Stark, A.R., and Tach, B.T.: Mechanisms of airway obstruction leading to apnea in newborn infants, J. Pediatr. **86**:982-985, 1976.

Tankin, S.: Sudden infant death syndrome: hypothesis of causation, Pediatrics **55**:650-659, 1975.

Uauy, R., Shapiro, D.L., Smith, B., and others: Treatment of severe apnea in prematures with orally administered theophylline, Pediatrics **55**:595-598, 1975.

33 Sudden infant death syndrome and apnea of infancy

JOHN G. BROOKS

DEFINITION AND PHYSIOLOGY
Sudden infant death syndrome

The sudden infant death syndrome (SIDS) is defined as "the sudden death of any infant or young child which is unexpected by history, and in which a thorough postmortem examination fails to demonstrate an adequate cause for death." Infants who experience severe postneonatal apneic episodes (apnea of infancy) may be admitted to intensive care units, and some of them are at increased risk of SIDS.

The incidence of SIDS in the general population is 1.5 to 2/1000 live births, resulting in approximately 7,000 deaths annually in the United States. It is the largest single cause of postneonatal infant mortality. The incidence peaks at 2 to 4 months of age; less than 1% of SIDS deaths occur in the first 2 weeks of life, but 91% occur in the first 6 months of life. SIDS occurs more frequently during the winter months, in lower income families, in males, in low-birth-weight infants (LBW), and in families with a previous SIDS victim. The risk is inversely proportional to the birth weight, with a SIDS rate of 11 per 1,000 live births for infants with a birth weight of 1 to 1.5 kg. The risk of SIDS in siblings who are subsequently born in affected families is approximately 20 per 1,000, and if one member of a twin pair dies of SIDS, the risk for the surviving twin is 42 per 1,000. The death occurs during sleep and is silent. There is frequently a history of a minor upper respiratory infection at the time of the death, but the infection is not thought to cause the death. The immediate cause of death in SIDS has not been discovered, but it is likely that several different mechanisms can produce the same clinical picture, and that in most cases there is a primary respiratory arrest with a secondary cardiac arrest.

In order to establish the diagnosis of SIDS, an autopsy must be performed. Other causes of sudden unexpected infant death which must be excluded, include meningitis, myocarditis, intracranial hemorrhage, and child abuse. Intrathoracic petechiae are frequently seen at postmortem examinations of SIDS victims, but their significance is not clearly understood.

During the past decade, specialized autopsy studies have provided increasing evidence that SIDS victims were not completely normal prior to their unexpected deaths. Specific postmortem findings, all compatible with recurrent or chronic hypoxemia, include hypertrophy of the medial smooth muscle of the pulmonary arterioles, prolonged retention of periadrenal brown fat, increased extramedullary hematopoiesis, and abnormal proliferation of astroglial cells in the reticular formation of the CNS.

This histologic evidence of chronic or subacute premortem abnormalities in SIDS victims has sparked great interest in possible physiologic derangements that might be recognized in living infants to identify them as being at high risk for SIDS so that appropriate preventive measures could be initiated in an attempt to prevent SIDS. Several infants with documented prolonged apneic episodes during sleep have subsequently succumbed to SIDS. Apnea of infancy in some infants may be a nonfatal expression of the same mechanism that is capable of causing SIDS. Although this has not been clearly proven, there is great concern about infants with apnea among both parents and health professionals. Careful study of these affected infants may provide clues to the cause of SIDS.

Apnea of infancy

Apnea of infancy (AI) is defined as "an unexplained and frightening episode of cessation of breathing for 20 seconds or longer, or a shorter respiratory pause associated with bradycardia, cyanosis, or pallor." There is often associated limpness. This definition describes a clinical syndrome, not a specific disease process. Since the initial frightening episode is usually observed by nonmedical personnel only, the aspects of the definition that are most useful are the presence or absence of color change and respiratory movement. Affected infants are at a tenfold to thirtyfold increased risk of SIDS. AI has been referred to as aborted SIDS or near-miss SIDS, but this terminology is undesirable, since it implies a more definite relationship between apneic episodes and SIDS than may be warranted for a given patient, and since it may contribute to some unnecessary confusion and concern in the parents. The parents of most SIDS victims have never noted frightening apnea or cyanosis prior to their infants' deaths, so the SIDS infants who have a history of AI probably represent only a minority of the cases.

Abnormalities of respiratory control that have been reported and confirmed in AI infants include an increased amount of periodic breathing, an abnormal ventilatory response to hypoxia, and a weak ventilatory response to hypercarbia. Some AI infants demonstrate each of these abnormalities, but the majority probably fall within the wide normal ranges for these variables. The apnea that occurs in AI patients who are at least 40 to 42 weeks postconceptional age is central apnea, not obstructive apnea, in the great majority of cases.

Some specific disease processes that may present with an apneic episode in infants are summarized in Table 33-1. Laryngeal chemoreceptor apnea refers to the respiratory pause, usually associated with bradycardia, that can result from stimulation of receptors around the larynx. This reflex, which involves the superior laryngeal branches of the vagus nerves, can presumably be stimulated by small amounts of refluxed gastric contents, as well as by material that is being swallowed. This is a central, not an obstructive, apnea; it is diagnosed by inference, since a temporal relationship between reflux and apnea is only rarely demonstrated. The most common specific cause of AI is a seizure disorder. An abnormal EEG in such a patient does not prove that the initial spell was due to a seizure disorder, since it is equally likely that the asphyxial episode may have caused the EEG abnormality. In addition to generalized sepsis, certain specific respiratory infections, such as respiratory syncytial virus and *Bordetella pertussis*, may predispose infants to apnea. Apnea of prematurity should not be diagnosed in infants older than 38 weeks postconception. However, some infants up to 42

Table 33-1. Causes of apnea/cyanosis episodes in infants

Laryngeal chemoreceptor apnea
Seizure disorder
Infection (e.g., sepsis, respiratory syncytial virus, *Bordetella pertussis*)
Apnea of prematurity
Upper airway obstruction
Breathholding spells
Congenital heart disease (e.g., tetralogy of Fallot)
Cardiac dysrhythmia
Hyponatremia, hypoglycemia, hypocalcemia
Failure of automatic ventilation ("Ondine's Curse")
CNS tumor
Anemia

weeks postconception or even older may demonstrate breathing patterns that, because of marked periodicity, are suggestive of apnea of prematurity; these patterns may be due to delayed maturation of the respiratory center. Upper airway obstruction associated with apneic episodes may be due to masses, cysts, or laryngospasm. Anemia may predispose premature infants to apnea, but probably not until the hemoglobin is less than 8 or 9 g/dl. The diagnosis of breath-holding spells must be made by exclusion and only with great care in young infants.

MONITORING

See also Chapter 4.

All infants admitted to the hospital with AI should have continuous electronic monitoring of heart rate and respiration for the duration of their hospitalization. In infants less than approximately 3 months corrected age, the alarms should be set to indicate a heart rate less than 80 beats per minute and a respiratory pause of 15 seconds or longer. Note that a 15-second pause is not abnormal in a 3-month-old infant, unless it occurs frequently. Any pause over 20 seconds or a shorter one associated with bradycardia, hypoxemia, or marked pallor is abnormal at any age. While most AI infants are stable at the time of admission, occasional infants who have experienced a severe asphyxial episode may require much more extensive intensive care monitoring and support because of cerebral ischemia and cardiorespiratory instability. (See Chapter 10.)

MANAGEMENT
Sudden infant death syndrome

An autopsy must be performed in order to make the diagnosis of SIDS. In most states it is a legal requirement that the coroner be notified of such a death, and it is within the coroner's jurisdiction to insist upon an autopsy.

The unexpected death of a previously healthy infant is an absolutely devastating event for parents, and it is associated with predictable reactions of denial, guilt, anger, and depression. It is desirable to offer informed counseling to affected families, and it is important they be told of the results of the autopsy as soon as possible, hopefully within 24 hours of the death of the infant, to establish the reality of the diagnosis and to decrease their concern that they may have overlooked a treatable illness. It must be stressed to them repeatedly that at this time SIDS is neither predictable nor preventable. Feelings of guilt and anger, as well as behavior problems, are likely to occur in surviving siblings. Parents should be advised as to how to discuss the infant's death with older siblings at an age-appropriate level. Many communities have local chapters of the National SIDS Foundation, which are available as support groups, as well as other resources, such as the Compassionate Friends, Incorporated. Know the available resources in the community and assess them before making referrals. Information about SIDS and the addresses of local chapters can be obtained by calling the National Sudden Infant Death Syndrome Foundation at 301/459-3388.

Apnea of infancy

Hospitalization and initial evaluation. All patients who present acutely after an episode of AI should be hospitalized for observation (resuscitative intervention may be necessary if spells recur), evaluation, education, and counseling. The initial screening evaluation of affected infants is directed toward identifying any specific and treatable disease processes that could have caused the frightening spell and toward identifying any indirect signs of chronic hypoxemia (e.g., right ventricular hypertrophy [RVH] on ECG, polycythemia). The minimum evaluation which should be performed on all such patients includes:

1. CBC and differential.
2. Serum Na, K, Cl, HCO_3, Ca, and glucose.
3. ECG.
4. Chest roentgenogram.

Additional evaluation. Depending on the results of an initial comprehensive history and physical examination, as well as the screening laboratory studies, an appropriate plan for further evaluation should be formulated. Almost every evaluation of the AI patient should include an EEG. Other studies that may be helpful, depending on the particular patient, include barium esophagram, esophageal manometric and pH studies (see Chapter 63), arterial blood-gas tensions and pH in room air and in 100% oxygen, lateral neck roentgenograms, direct laryngoscopy or bronchoscopy, echocardiography, CT scan, CSF cultures, fluorescent antibody studies for RSV or *Bordetella pertussis,* and serology. A 12- or 24-hour cardiorespirogram (pneumogram, i.e., a hard-copy recording of heart rate and respiratory pattern) may be of some use in identifying infants with severe disorders of respiratory control, but it has definite limitations. There are no published, complete, age-adjusted normals for interpreting such studies. Some data exist about the normal ranges for respiratory variables such as percent of periodic breathing or duration of longest pause, but there is no proof that infants who are outside the normal ranges for these variables are at increased risk of SIDS.

Therapy. Whenever a treatable, specific diagnosis can be identified, appropriate medical or surgical intervention should be initiated (e.g., tracheotomy or anticonvulsants). Infants with periodic breathing or respiratory pauses longer than 20 seconds may improve the regularity of their respiratory pattern if they are treated with aminophylline as a respiratory stimulant. A starting dose of 1 to 2 mg/kg every 8 to 12 hours is appropriate. This drug should not be used in any patient suspected of having a seizure disorder, since it may exacerbate that problem. Occasional patients with normal EEG's but histories that are strongly suggestive of seizures may respond to anticonvulsants. Such a trial may be diagnostically as well as therapeutically helpful, since patients with seizure disorders are likely to get better on anti-convulsants, while patients with an inadequate respiratory drive are likely to get worse with such therapy. This type of clinical trial should be conducted in the hospital with continuous cardiorespiratory monitoring.

Electronic home monitoring of infants thought to be at high risk for SIDS is a controversial and unproven intervention. Any one of the following criteria is a reasonable indication for starting such therapy in patients being evaluated for AI:

1. A family history of SIDS or AI.
2. Recurrent apnea requiring intervention.
3. Convincing history of a serious apneic episode associated with definite change of color (to pallor or cyanosis) or limpness.

All of the following criteria must be met before discontinuing home monitoring:

1. At least 6 months of age.
2. At least 2 months without an apneic episode requiring intervention.
3. Must have experienced an upper respiratory tract infection without associated apnea requiring intervention.

A variety of home monitors are available; the most successful at this time is an impedance system in which both heart rate and respiratory pause thresholds can be set.

Any patient discharged with a home monitor must have continuous and immediate access to an appropriate support system, including medical, technical, and psychosocial expertise. Parents and other key caretakers must be instructed in infant CPR before discharge, and they must have the skills reinforced at appropriate intervals. They must also be well instructed in the use and troubleshooting of the monitor system.

Subsequent siblings of SIDS victims

The risk of SIDS in subsequent siblings is at least tenfold greater than in the general population, so they present a difficult problem with management. There are no data about whether any intervention is effective in decreasing the incidence of SIDS in this population. Methods that have been used are administration of aminophylline and use of home monitors. There is no proof that sleep studies are reliable for determining which infants need intervention. Since the risk for the surviving member of a twin pair is 4.2 percent (42 in 1000), it is appropriate to consider hospital admission of the surviving twin and initiation of home monitoring. Hospitalization immediately following the death of the first twin facilitates education of the family about the monitor and CPR.

Premature infants

While the incidence of SIDS is increased among prematurly born infants, it is not possible to identify those premature infants who are at particularly high risk.

ADDITIONAL READING
Sudden infant death syndrome

Naeye, R.L.: Sudden infant death, Sci. Am. **242:**56-62, 1980.

Peterson, D.R., Chinn, N.M., and Fisher, L.D.: The sudden infant death syndrome: repetitions in families, J. Pediatr. **97:**265-267, 1980.

Shannon, D.C.: The sudden infant death syndrome, Clin. Chest Med. **1:**327-337, 1980.

Valdes-Dapena, M.A.: Sudden infant death syndrome: a review of the medical literature, 1974-1979, Pediatrics **66:**597-613, 1980.

Apnea of infancy

American Academy of Pediatrics Task Force on Prolonged Apnea: Prolonged apnea, Pediatrics **61:**651-652, 1978.

Anas, N.A., Boettrich, C., and Brooks, J.G.: The association of apnea and respiratory syncytial virus infection in infants, J. Pediatr. **101:**65-68, 1982.

Downing, S.E., and Lee, J.C.: Laryngeal chemosensitivity: a possible mechanism for sudden infant death, Pediatrics **55:**640-649, 1979.

Favorito, J., Orchardo Pernice, J.M., and Ruggiero, P.: Apnea monitoring to prevent SIDS, Am. J. Nurs., January 1979, pp. 101-104.

Herbst, J.J., Book, L.S., and Bray, P.F.: Gastroesophageal reflux in the "near-miss" sudden infant death syndrome, J. Pediatr. **92:**73-75, 1978.

Kelly, D.H., Shannon, D.C., and O'Connell, K.: Care of infants with near-miss sudden infant death syndrome, Pediatrics **61:**511-514, 1978.

34 Hyaline membrane disease

DANIEL L. LEVIN

DEFINITION AND PHYSIOLOGY

Hyaline membrane disease is a clinical condition associated with an immature lung and characterized by alveolar collapse and the resulting abnormalities of pulmonary gas exchange. Because of their small size, alveoli in the preterm infant (75 μ in the preterm infant versus 100 μ in the full-term infant and 200 μ in the adult) are difficult to inflate and once open tend to collapse and remain atelectatic. These problems are partially due to the lack of an adequate amount of surface-active material at the air-liquid interface of the alveolus. Inadequate surface-active material results in high surface tensions, especially at end-expiration, a condition that promotes alveolar collapse and sustained atelectasis. There is some evidence that the inadequate amount of surface-active material may not be due to a decreased production of the material but to the presence of inhibitor substances in the alveolar-tracheal fluid of infants (and animals) with hyaline membrane disease. There is a definite gender difference in infants with hyaline membrane disease with male infants being more susceptible. Differences in the response of male versus female premature lambs to identical replacement therapy with exogenous surface active material (exosurf) suggest that males may have more of the inhibitor substance than females.

The force necessary to maintain a patent alveolus is expressed by Laplace's law, which describes the force necessary to keep a sphere open: $P = 2ST/r$, where P = distending pressure, ST = surface tension, and r = radius of the alveolus (Fig. 34-1). The premature infant with an immature lung has a small alveolar radius and a high air-liquid surface tension, both of which necessitate a high intra-alveolar pressure to keep the alveolus open. The preterm infant's chest cage is poorly suited to meet this task because of decreased muscle mass and strength, both of which reduce the infant's ability to develop negative intrathoracic pressure during inhalation, and because of pliable ribs, which increase compliance and allow partial collapse of the thoracic cavity with diaphragmatic contraction and at end-expiration. Both a lack of adequate intrathoracic pressure and increased chest wall compliance promote atelectasis.

Because TV is decreased secondary to alveolar atelectasis, respiratory rate increases in an effort to maintain a normal minute ventilation. Although the minute ventilation is increased, a great proportion of the increase results in increased dead space ventilation, so that alveolar ventilation is decreased. The lung compliance is decreased, and airway resistance is increased. All of these factors result in increased work of breathing. The infant attempts to develop large negative intrathoracic pressures in order to inflate the lungs more efficiently, and these efforts are expressed by the clinical finding of retractions. To overcome the tendency of the alveoli to collapse at end-expiration, the infant partially closes the glottis, thus increasing airway pressure; this is manifested clinically as grunting. The increased work of breathing, in association with poor caloric intake, cold stress, and hypoxia, which are commonly present in stressed premature infants,

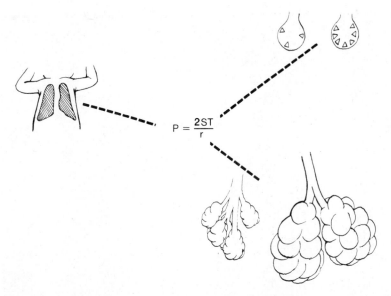

Fig. 34-1. Laplace's law and hyaline membrane disease. The preterm infant has a weak chest wall and cannot develop adequate pressure *(P)*. He also has a small alveolar radius *(r)* and deficient surface-active material, with a high air-liquid surface tension *(ST)*.

results in rapidly developing fatigue.

Cyanosis is a prominent finding in patients with hyaline membrane disease. Hypoventilation, abnormal distribution of ventilation and pulmonary blood flow due to atelectasis, and extrapulmonary right-to-left (R → L) shunting via the foramen ovale and the ductus arteriosus can all contribute to cyanosis.

Asphyxia (elevated Pa_{CO_2}, decreased Pa_{O_2}, decreased blood pH, and elevated blood potassium concentration) and shock (decreased arterial and central venous blood pressure, decreased capillary filling, hypothermia, and oliguria) are frequently diagnosed in patients with hyaline membrane disease. It is debatable whether these findings are the result of hyaline membrane disease with atelectasis or whether in some patients asphyxia and shock contribute to the development of hyaline membrane disease. Both situations probably occur. Patients who have decreased availability of surface-active material, hypoproteinemia, and moderate hyaline membrane disease and who do not receive appropriate ventilatory support develop atelectasis and increased lung water and become progressively hypoxemic and fatigued, developing respiratory failure, asphyxia, and shock. Other patients, who have relatively good stores and availability of surface-active material and who would have had a mild or insignificant clinical course of hyaline membrane disease become asphyxiated or hypotensive and thus develop pulmonary ischemia, injuring type II alveolar cells that produce surface-active material; these patients may develop severe hyaline membrane disease. There are some suggestions that pulmonary ischemia may be important in the development of hyaline membrane disease not only during the intrapartum and immediate postpartum periods but also in utero.

Regardless of whether asphyxia and shock are primary or secondary events, the decrease in cardiac output results in a redistribution of organ blood flow and vasoconstriction, manifested by pallor, pulmonary and peripheral edema, ileus, hemolysis, jaundice, and DIC.

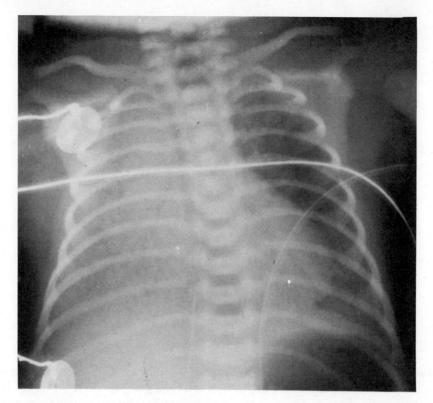

Fig. 34-2. Chest roentgenogram of baby with hyaline membrane disease, on the first day of life. Note the reticulogranular pattern, which is asymmetrical (right worse than left), and the general loss of lung volume.

As a result of atelectasis and increased lung water, the chest roentgenogram will show air bronchograms superimposed on a reticulogranular pattern that is usually diffuse but may be asymmetrical or localized (Fig. 34-2). The application of positive pressure by CPAP or by IMV and PEEP will change the appearance of the roentgenograms.

The disease is self-limiting. The patient's condition will deteriorate for 48 hours and start to improve by 72 hours as production of or availability of surface-active material increases. Improvement is often heralded by the onset of diuresis, which begins at 24 to 36 hours of life, lasts for 64 to 72 hours, and precedes the improvement in ventilation by approximately 50 hours. Forced diuresis with furosemide cannot initiate the diuresis, which indicates that it may be related to a pulmonary capillary leak and/or to increased antidiuretic hormone (ADH) levels or to renal dysfunction in these infants. Delayed onset of this diuresis is related to the occurrence of chronic lung disease in these infants. Delayed diuresis and fluid retention may result in a hemodynamically significant PDA, which is frequently found in premature infants who develop chronic lung disease or, alternatively, the chronic lung disease may be the result of the PDA. It is difficult if not impossible to judge the presence of a hemodynamically significant PDA in premature infants with significant respiratory disease by the usual clinical criteria.

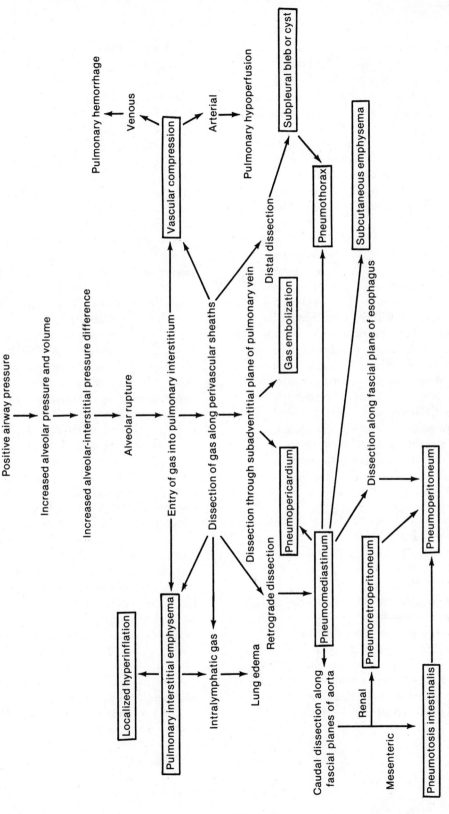

Fig. 34-3. Positive airway pressure and pulmonary air leaks. (From Perkin, R.M., and Levin, D.L.: Adverse effects of positive-pressure ventilation in children. In Gregory, G.A., editor: Respiratory failure in the child, New York, 1981, Churchill Livingstone.)

Studies utilizing prophylactic early (2 to 3 days of age) closure of the PDA in small preterm infants (<1000 g) with respiratory distress, either by surgery or indomethacin, have shown a decrease in the incidence of chronic lung disease in the treated infants.

A prolonged course is usually associated with pulmonary ischemia, exposure of the lung to high oxygen concentrations, positive-pressure breathing, and increased lung water, all of which may cause lung damage and chronic lung disease.

Other complications of both the disease and its therapy include pulmonary air leaks (pulmonary interstitial emphysema, pneumothorax, pneumomediastinum, pneumopericardium, pneumoperitoneum (Fig. 34-3), PDA with congestive heart failure, intraventricular hemorrhage, secondary infection, multiple metabolic derangements, and retrolental fibroplasia. Retrolental fibroplasia is thought to be due to the exposure of the immature retinal blood vessels to oxygen tensions higher than can be tolerated. The vessels constrict, causing ischemia peripherally. Eventually proliferation of new vessels and retinal detachment occur, resulting in serious visual impairment or blindness. There is some evidence that hypoxia subsequent to the hyperoxic episode is important in the pathogenesis.

MONITORING

See also Chapter 4.

Respiratory system

1. Record the color of the skin, nail beds, and mucous membranes every 2 hours.
2. Note the presence of retractions and the character of breath sounds every 2 hours.
3. Assess the effort the infant is making to breathe (e.g., distressed, working hard).
4. Record the quantity and character of oral, pharyngeal, and tracheal secretions frequently.

5. Measure arterial blood-gas tensions and pH.
   a. Make an initial determination on all infants with any respiratory abnormality. This may be done using either a transcutaneous oxygen (Ptc_{O_2}) monitor or an intra-arterial blood sample. Carefully note the inspired oxygen concentration and sampling site (e.g., $FI_{O_2} = 0.4$, right radial artery). The results of the initial determination can be used in conjunction with the clinical picture to assess the need for further sampling. In most cases, infants who are placed on oxygen or who require ventilatory assistance need repetitive determinations of arterial blood-gas tensions and pH during the acute phase of the illness (2 to 4 days). This is usually most suitably done via an indwelling arterial catheter in order to obtain Pa_{CO_2} and pH_a values as well as Pa_{O_2} and to continuously monitor systemic arterial blood pressure. This method is usually supplemented by continuous Ptc_{O_2} monitoring in order to avoid excessive periods of hyperoxia and hypoxia and to decrease the risks of retrolental fibroplasia and chronic lung disease (see Chapter 94).
   b. Sampling should be done every 2 hours as well as 10 minutes after any respiratory support change, during the acute phase of the illness (usually 2 to 4 days) except in those infants who are mildly ill (requiring less than 30% oxygen with minimal chest roentgenogram findings). The rate of sampling can be decreased during the recovery phase when stability has been clearly demonstrated. It is unwise to decrease the rate of sampling prematurely unless Ptc_{O_2} is being utilized, since this may increase the patient's risk for hyperoxemia or hypoxemia and will tend to prolong the duration of intubation and mechanical ventilation, both of which carry significant risk.

c. When a patient is recovering from an acute course of hyaline membrane disease, is stable, and is receiving 40% oxygen or less, remove the indwelling arterial catheter and monitor the patient by the Ptc_{O_2} technique until the patient no longer requires supplemental oxygen. Obtain individual arterial blood samples only if the infant's condition deteriorates or if a question arises about the accuracy of other methods of assessment.

Hematologic system

1. Repeat WBC counts if infection is diagnosed, and repeat platelet counts if infection or bleeding is a concern (Chapters 20 and 41).
2. Obtain PT, PTT, fibrinogen, and fibrin split product determinations if DIC is being considered (see Chapter 20).

Neurologic system

1. Observe infant for signs of intracranial hemorrhage (decrease in Hct, blood pressure, or activity; seizures; increase in head size or ICP).
2. Obtain head sonogram initially at 2 to 3 days or when signs appear. Obtain serial sonograms to document increased size of hemorrhage or ventricles or the occurrence of a new hemorrhage.
3. Obtain routine funduscopic examinations by the same examiner for retrolental fibroplasia, starting at 3 to 4 weeks of age.
4. Use of Ptc_{O_2} monitoring may decrease the severity of retrolental fibroplasia by decreasing the number and duration of hyperoxic and hypoxic episodes.

MANAGEMENT

Although clinicians agree on the need to keep stressed infants in a neutral thermal environment and to prevent hypoglycemia, it is fair to state that there is almost no general agreement on the other aspects of management of patients with hyaline membrane disease. This section presents one way in which such patients may be managed.

Renal-metabolic system

1. Maintain Dextrostix readings between 45 and 90 mg/dl with IV glucose. This may require glucose at a rate of 250 to 350 mg/kg/hr (10% glucose in water at 60 to 80 ml/kg/24 hr). Nutritional intake via the gastrointestinal tract is usually not possible during the first 2 days and is limited thereafter in severely ill or unstable patients. Small gavage feedings (2 to 3 ml/kg every 2 to 3 hours) of half-strength formula can be introduced on the third day of life in stable patients. Patients who weight less than 1200 grams and those with severe lung disease will probably benefit from continuous NG feedings rather than intermittent bolus NG feedings, which distend the stomach, elevate the diaphragm, and decrease lung volume, all of which may cause intrapulmonary shunting and hypoxemia. This is true even in patients with endotracheal tubes as long as their cardiovascular-respiratory status is reasonably stable and gastric reflux is not a problem. Paralyzed patients can receive enteral feedings.
2. Maintain a body temperature of 36.5° to 37.2° C. The neutral thermal environment (temperature and humidity at which heat loss is minimal and metabolic demands and oxygen consumption are lowest) varies with the size and age of the patient (see Tables 18-1 and 18-2).
3. Fluid management is controversial. Excessive fluid administration may contribute to a deterioration of the ventilatory status secondary to pulmonary edema and to the development of congestive heart failure from PDA. Conversely, hypotension in association with hypovolemia is thought to occur commonly in patients with hyaline mem-

brane disease and to contribute to pulmonary ischemia, therefore making the hyaline membrane disease worse. Begin fluid administration at 60 to 80 ml/kg/24 hr; add 20% of maintenance requirements for infants in radiant warmers and 10% for infants under phototherapy lights. Electrolytes are not given on the first day of life, but sodium, 3 to 4 mEq/kg/24 hr, and potassium and chloride, 1 to 2 mEq/kg/24 hr, are given thereafter. Maintenance calcium gluconate at 200 mg/kg/24 hr is given on the first day and increased if the serum calcium level is less than 7.5 mg/dl (see Chapter 16). Serum phosphate should be checked before any IV phosphate is given. Urine output is maintained at more than 2 ml/kg/hr with a specific gravity less than 1.010.

4. Furosemide, 1 mg/kg IV, is useful to promote diuresis if excessive fluid administration leads to edema or if congestive heart failure is present. It may be especially useful in conjunction with the administration of blood products. It probably cannot force an early diuresis. Furosemide should not be given more frequently than every 12 hrs during the first 3 weeks of life.

5. Microscopic hematuria with proteinuria, glycosuria, and inappropriately high urine pH is commonly seen in babies who have been asphyxiated or who are hypotensive. These findings probably reflect acute tubular damage. Usually no specific treatment other than that directed at the initial cause is necessary. Some patients do continue to lose significant urinary bicarbonate and may develop metabolic acidosis after the initial period of hypotension and hypoxia is resolved and in the absence of evidence of sepsis. Frequently these patients require slow, cautious infusion of bicarbonate, 1 mEq/kg IV over 1 to 2 hours, to replace renal losses until tubular function returns. Monitor fluid volume and serum sodium status closely.

Respiratory system

Supplemental oxygen. Give supplemental oxygen to maintain Pa_{O_2} between 50 and 70 mm Hg. If Pa_{O_2} is less than 50 mm Hg in 60% to 80% oxygen, intubate patient and place him on CPAP. Initially use a pressure of 4 to 6 cm H_2O and sequentially increase the oxygen concentration to 100% if Pa_{O_2} is still less than 50 mm Hg. Increase CPAP to 8 cm H_2O and then to 10 cm H_2O if Pa_{O_2} remains less than 50 mm Hg on 100% oxygen. Avoid CPAP greater than 10 cm H_2O, since this may be associated with pulmonary air leaks and decreased cardiac output. If Pa_{O_2} is less than 50 mm Hg with 100% oxygen and with CPAP of 10 cm H_2O, institute IMV (see below).

Indications for IMV with PEEP

1. Pa_{CO_2} is greater than 50 mm Hg (acutely).
2. The patient is apneic on CPAP.
3. Pa_{O_2} is less than 50 mm Hg with 100% oxygen and CPAP of 10 cm H_2O.

Methods of IMV and PEEP

1. *Use the lowest pressures possible. Barotrauma to the lungs is probably a major factor in the pathogenesis of chronic lung disease.*
2. Generally, a pressure-limited, time-cycled mechanical ventilator with a constant flow of gas between mechanical positive pressure breaths is used. This allows the spontaneously breathing patient to breathe at whatever TV he can generate (normal = 6 cc/kg/breath) between machine breaths.
3. Pa_{O_2} increases with increasing mean airway pressure. The greatest change in Pa_{O_2} for a change in mean airway pressure occurs with the use of PEEP (or CPAP), the next greatest with peak inspiratory pressure, and the least with prolonged inspiratory: expiratory (I : E) ratios.
4. Preterm infants with hyaline membrane disease may be better ventilated in the prone than in the supine position.
5. Start with a peak pressure of 18 to 20 cm H_2O and a PEEP of 4 to 10 cm H_2O.

6. Use an I:E ratio of 1:1 or less. This requires high inspiratory gas flows.
7. Assess adequacy of TV by chest wall movement and auscultation of breath sounds. Assess adequacy of alveolar ventilation by carbon dioxide elimination.
8. Use the slowest rate possible to maintain Pa_{CO_2} between 35 and 45 mm Hg (e.g., start at 10 to 15 breaths/min). It is preferable to use rapid respiratory rates rather than high peak inflating pressures to achieve a normal Pa_{CO_2}.
9. If carbon dioxide retention is still present and/or the infant's spontaneous respiratory efforts seem to interfere with the mechanical ventilator, sedation (morphine sulfate, 0.1 mg/kg IV every 4 hours as needed) or paralysis (d-tubocurarine, 0.5 mg/kg IV as needed, or pancuronium [Pavulon], 0.1 mg/kg IV as needed) may be used to improve the efficiency of the mechanical ventilator and to increase chest wall compliance. Use of muscle relaxants in these infants decreases the time that they are hyperoxic or hypoxic and may improve oxygenation by improving the distribution of ventilation. Infants treated with muscle relaxants are able to be removed from supplemental oxygen sooner and have fewer elevations of ICP than infants who are not given muscle relaxants. There is a decreased chance of pulmonary air leaks due to the use of high inflating pressures and struggling. An acute increase in ventilation rate will be necessary after the patient has been paralyzed. If these maneuvers are not successful, higher peak inspiratory pressures may be used. Always check the mechanical ventilator to make certain that the infant is not rebreathing carbon dioxide when a persistent elevation of Pa_{CO_2} occurs.
10. High-frequency ventilation (200 to 300 breaths/min or more) is now being tested for use in these infants. It may provide adequate alveolar ventilation and better oxygenation with less risk of barotrauma to the lungs.
11. When lung compliance has improved but PEEP or CPAP has not been appropriately decreased, overdistention of the lungs may occur and may result in carbon dioxide retention. Under these circumstances, decreasing PEEP or CPAP may decrease Pa_{CO_2}. When lung function has improved, excessive PEEP or CPAP increases the risk for pulmonary interstitial emphysema and pulmonary air leaks.
12. As the patient improves, withdraw respiratory support in a cautious, orderly fashion, documenting the patient's arterial blood-gas tensions and pH after each step. Ptc_{O_2} monitoring can decrease but not eliminate the need for arterial blood-gas sampling during this phase. Reverse or discontinue paralyzing agents and sedatives before mechanical ventilation is discontinued.
    a. Oxygenation.
       (1) Decrease the oxygen concentration to less than 60%. If Pa_{O_2} is between 70 and 100 mm Hg, decrease the oxygen by 5%; if Pa_{O_2} is between 100 and 150 mm Hg, decrease the oxygen by 10%; if Pa_{O_2} is greater than 150 mm Hg, decrease the oxygen by 15%.
       (2) Decrease CPAP by 2 cm H_2O not more frequently than every 2 to 4 hours until a level of 2 cm H_2O is reached. Be careful to maintain the Pa_{O_2} between 50 and 70 mm Hg during this process. Do not decrease CPAP too rapidly, or massive atelectasis may occur and then more pressure will be required to reinflate the lung than was required for the previously beneficial level of CPAP.
    b. Alveolar ventilation.
       (1) If high pressures have been used, decrease the peak pressure until it is

at 20 cm H_2O, keeping Pa_{CO_2} between 35 and 45 mm Hg. Very small infants (<1200 g) with increased thoracic compliance may be overventilated (Pa_{CO_2} <35 mm Hg) at inflating pressures of 20 cm H_2O; 14 to 16 cm H_2O may be more reasonable. Overdistention as well as hypocarbia may cause apnea.

(2) Decrease the respiratory rate (usually 2 to 4 breaths/min approximately every 2 hours), keeping Pa_{CO_2} between 35 and 45 mm Hg.

(3) Some adjustments in oxygen concentration (up or down) may be made concurrently during the weaning process in order to keep Pa_{O_2} between 50 and 70 mm Hg. During the recovery phase of uncomplicated hyaline membrane disease, it is probably better to have a patient in 70% or 80% oxygen and ready for extubation rather than, for example, on a mechanical ventilator at 20 cm H_2O peak pressure and 6 cm H_2O PEEP, a rate of 20 breaths/min, and 25% oxygen. During the healing phase, higher inspired oxygen concentrations (with Pa_{O_2} between 50 and 70 mm Hg) are less of a risk to the patient than excessive ventilating pressures and an artificial airway.

(4) Small, ill, poorly nourished infants may have difficulty providing the muscular work of breathing when mechanical ventilation is decreased. Diaphragmatic muscular fatigue may be particularly important during this phase of treatment and may precede apnea, which is frequently observed during this phase.

(5) When the patient is on 2 cm H_2O of CPAP and at whatever oxygen concentration is necessary to maintain Pa_{O_2} between 50 and 70 mm Hg, he may be considered for extubation (see Chapter 103). In patients with uncomplicated hyaline membrane disease, the inspired oxygen concentration usually does not need to be increased when they are extubated.

(6) Extreme care must be taken to maintain a patent airway. Endotracheal tubes should be suctioned every hour (see Chapter 100).

(7) Pulmonary air leaks are a frequent complication of hyaline membrane disease, especially when it is treated with positive-pressure ventilation (see Fig. 34-3). Treatment of such leaks must be prompt (see Chapter 102).

12. CPT is essential to remove pulmonary secretions and prevent large areas of atelectasis and pneumonia. It should be performed at least every 4 to 6 hours (see Chapter 99) and continued postextubation since atelectasis, especially of right upper lobe, is a common late problem.

13. Patients usually require several days of oxygen therapy after extubation. They are still recovering from their disease process during this period.

Cardiovascular system

1. Heart rate.
   a. Bradycardia is usually associated with hypoxemia. This may be due to the basic disease process but is frequently due to mechanical complications. Evaluate the position and patency of the endotracheal tube and check for accidental disconnection of the oxygen source and pulmonary air leaks. Bradycardia may also be a preterminal finding in association with an intraventricular hemorrhage (IVH). Treat bradycardia with manual bag and mask ventilation while the equipment is being checked. Use the same $F_{I_{O_2}}$ that was being used with mechanical ventilation.
   b. Tachycardia is commonly due to hyper-

volemia secondary to excessive fluid administration or congestive heart failure. Fluid restriction and administration of furosemide, 1 mg/kg IV once or twice every 24 hours, may be used to treat these conditions. Tachycardia may also be due to hypovolemia associated with poor capillary filling, decreased urine output, and hypotension. In this case, increased fluid administration is the treatment of choice (see Chapter 16).

2. Evaluate arterial blood pressure in conjunction with signs of adequate peripheral perfusion (capillary filling, pulses, urine output, and metabolic acidosis). There is a range of normal (see Appendix C). Treatment of low blood pressure in patients who do not exhibit any signs of abnormal perfusion is usually unnecessary. Overtreatment with fluid may be harmful. In addition, during the first few hours of life, retained lung water (as much as 30 ml/kg) may still be available to the patient. If the patient receives volume expansion and then absorbs this lung water, he may become hypervolemic and develop increased LAP and pulmonary edema. This will decrease lung compliance and impair oxygenation and ventilation. When patients are obviously hypovolemic (e.g., bleeding) or in shock and adequate ventilation does not alleviate the situation, volume replacement is indicated (see Chapter 14).

3. Remember that patients on mechanical ventilators can develop pulmonary air leaks with tension pneumothorax and/or tension pneumopericardium and that shock may be due to these mechanical factors.

Hematologic system

1. Provide patients in respiratory distress with an adequate oxygen-carrying capacity (see Chapter 12). Maintain Hct at approximately 40% to 45%.
2. Thrombocytopenia is usually due to infection and/or shock with DIC. Treatment is

most appropriately directed at the initial cause (see Chapter 20).

Gastrointestinal system

1. Necrotizing enterocolitis is a major problem in small, stressed infants (see Chapter 57).
2. Remember that infants who are paralyzed cannot swallow and therefore their gastrointestinal tract, evaluated by abdominal roentgenogram, will have an absent gas pattern. The frequency of stools will be significantly decreased.
3. Prolonged mechanical ventilation should prompt the institution of a parenteral feeding regimen (see Chapter 111).

Nervous system

1. Ventriculomegaly may be treated initially with repetitive draining of CSF via lumbar puncture but may require ventriculoperitoneal shunts in some patients.
2. The antioxidant vitamin E when given prophylactically, 100 mg/kg/day PO in two divided doses, started early in the infant's course, may decrease the severity if not the incidence of retrolental fibroplasia.

ADDITIONAL READING

Barr, R.A., Bailey, P.E., Summers, J., and Cassidy, G.: Relation between arterial blood pressure and blood volume and effect of infused albumin in sick preterm infants, Pediatrics **60:**282-289, 1977.

Bell, E.F., Gray, J.C., Weinstein, M.R., and Oh, W.: The effects of thermal environment on heat balance and insensible water loss in low-birth-weight infants, J. Pediatr. **96:**452-459, 1980.

Bell, E.F., Neidich, G.A., Cashore, W.J., and Oh, W.: Combined effect of radiant warmer and phototherapy on insensible water loss in low-birth-weight infants, J. Pediatr. **94:**810-813, 1979.

Bell, E.F., Weinstein, M.R., and Oh, W.: Heat balance in premature infants: comparative effects of convectively heated incubator and radiant warmer, with and without plastic heat shield, J. Pediatr. **96:**460-465, 1980.

Bland, R.D., Kim, M.H., Light, M.J., and Woodson, J.L.: High-frequency mechanical ventilation of low-birth-weight infants with respiratory failure from hyaline membrane disease: 92% survival, Pediatr. Res. **11:**531, 1977.

Boros, S.J., and Campbell, K.: A comparison of the effects

of high frequency–low tidal volume and low frequency–high tidal volume mechanical ventilation, J. Pediatr. **97**:108-112, 1980.

Boros, S.J., Matalon, S.V., Ewald, R., and others: The effect of independent variations in inspiratory-expiratory ratio and end expiratory pressure during mechanical ventilation in hyaline membrane disease: the significance of mean airway pressure, J. Pediatr. **91**:794-798, 1977.

Clyman, R.I., Heymann, M.A., and Clements, J.A.: Sex differences in the response to surfactant replacement therapy, Clin. Res. **30**:141A, 1982.

Crone, R.K., and Favorito, R.N.: The effects of pancuronium bromide on infants with hyaline membrane disease. J. Pediatr. **97**:991-993, 1980.

Finer, N.N., and Tomney, P.M.: Controlled evaluation of muscle relaxation in the ventilated neonate, Pediatrics **67**:641-646, 1981.

Fox, W.W., Berman, L.S., Dinwiddie, R., and Shaffer, T.H.: Tracheal extubation of the neonate at 2 to 3 cm H_2O continuous positive airway pressure, Pediatrics **59**:257-261, 1977.

Gluck, L., and Kulovich, M.U.: Fetal lung development: current concepts, Pediatr. Clin. North Am. **20**:367-379, 1973.

Gregory, G.A.: Respiratory care of newborn infants, Pediatr. Clin. North Am. **19**:311-324, 1971.

Gregory, G.A., Kitterman, J.A., Phibbs, R.H., and others: Treatment of the idiopathic respiratory-distress syndrome with continuous positive airway pressure, N. Engl. J. Med. **284**:1333-1340, 1971.

Hallman, M., Scheinder, H., Ikegami, M., and Jobe, A.H.: Comparison of two natural surfactants, Clin. Res. **30**: 142A, 1982.

Hutchinson, A.A., Ross, K.R., and Russel, G.: The effect of posture on ventilation and lung mechanics in preterm and light-for-date infants, Pediatrics **64**:429-432, 1979.

Ikegami, M., Jacobs, H., and Jobe, A.: Inhibition of surfactant function in the respiratory distress syndrome (RDS), Clin. Res. **30**:143A, 1982.

Knight, P.J., and Abdenour, G.: Pneumoperitoneum in the ventilated neonate: respiratory or gastrointestinal origin? J. Pediatr. **98**:972-974, 1981.

Langman, C.B., Engle, W.D., Baumgart, S., and others: The diuretic phase of respiratory distress syndrome and its relationship to oxygenation, J. Pediatr. **98**:462-466, 1981.

Mahoney, L., Carnero, V., Brett, C., and others: Prophylactic indomethacin therapy for patent ductus arteriosus, Clin. Res. **30**:144A, 1982.

Muller, N., Volgyesi, G., Eng, P., and others: The consequences of diaphragmatic muscle fatigue in the newborn infant, J. Pediatr. **98**:793-797, 1979.

Ogata, E.S., Gregory, G.A., Kitterman, J.A., and others:

Pneumothorax in the respiratory distress syndrome: incidence and effect on vital signs, blood gases, and pH, Pediatrics **58**:177-183, 1976.

Peterson, R.G., Simmons, M.A., Rumack, B.H., and others: Pharmacology of furosemide in the premature newborn infant, J. Pediatr. **97**:139-143, 1980.

Phelps, D.L., and Rosenbaum, A.L.: Effect of hypoxemia on recovery from oxygen induced retinopathy in the kitten model, Clin. Res. **30**:146A, 1982.

Phibbs, R.H.: Supportive care of the premature and sick newborn infant. In Rudolph, A.M., editor: Pediatrics, ed. 16, New York, 1977, Appleton-Century-Crofts.

Pohjavuori, M., and Fyhrquist, F.: Hemodynamic significance of vasopressin in the newborn infant, J. Pediatr. **97**:462-465, 1980.

Pollitzer, M.J., Shaw, D.G., Reynolds, E.O.R., and Thomas, R.M.: Pancuronium during mechanical ventilation speeds recovery of lungs of infants with hyaline membrane disease, Lancet **1**(8216):346-348, Feb. 14, 1981.

Sniderman, S.H., Riedel, P.A., Bert, M.D., and others: Influence of transcutaneous oxygen ($TcPO_2$) monitoring and other factors on incidence of retrolental fibroplasia (RLF), Clin. Res. **30**:148A, 1982.

Spitzer, A.R., Fox, W.W., and Delivoria-Papadopoulos, M.: Maximal diuresis—a factor in predicting recovery from respiratory distress syndrome and the development of bronchopulmonary dysplasia, J. Pediatr. **98**:476-479, 1981.

Stark, A.R., Bascom, R., and Frantz, I.V., III: Muscle relaxation in mechanically ventilated infants, J. Pediatr. **94**:439-443, 1979.

Stevenson, J.G.: Fluid administration in the association of patent ductus arteriosus complicating respiratory distress syndrome, J. Pediatr. **90**:257-261, 1977.

Stewart, A.R., Finer, N.N., and Peters, K.L.: Effects of alterations of inspiratory and expiratory pressures and inspiratory/expiratory ratios on mean airway pressure, blood gases, and intracranial pressure, Pediatrics **67**:474-481, 1981.

Stocks, J., and Godfrey, S.: The role of artificial ventilation, oxygen, and CPAP in the pathogenesis of lung damage in neonates: assessment by serial measurements of lung function, Pediatrics **57**:352-362, 1976.

Tooley, W.H.: Hyaline membrane disease. In Rudolph, A.M., editor: Pediatrics, ed. 16, New York, 1977, Appleton-Century-Crofts.

Valdes-Cruz, L.M., and Ludell, G.G.: Specificity and accuracy of echocardiographic and clinical criteria for diagnosis of patent ductus arteriosus in fluid-restricted infants, J. Pediatr. **98**:298-301, 1981.

Yeager, A.S., Grumet, F.C., Hafleigh, E.B., and others: Prevention of transfusion-acquired cytomegalovirus infection in newborn infants, J. Pediatr. **98**:281-287, 1981.

35 Meconium inhalation syndrome

DANIEL L. LEVIN

DEFINITION AND PHYSIOLOGY

Meconium is a breakdown product of digested amniotic fluid, fetal hair, squamous epithelial cells, and gastrointestinal secretions. Fetal asphyxia and other forms of intrauterine stress cause increased gastrointestinal motility and evacuation of meconium from the colon into the amniotic fluid. During normal fetal breathing and the gasping that is associated with asphyxia, the mixture of amniotic fluid and meconium is inhaled into the fetal trachea. If the fetus is born at this time and begins air breathing, the thick meconium is moved distally into the smaller airways and alveoli, causing an uneven obstruction and preventing a normal flow of air to and from gas-exchanging surfaces. This causes respiratory distress due to mismatching of ventilation and perfusion and decreased lung compliance. Because of the decreased lung compliance, the infant begins to make increased respiratory efforts to create greater negative intrathoracic pressures and improve the flow of gas into the lungs. Expiratory grunting, tachypnea, and retractions similar to those seen in infants with hyaline membrane disease are present. Early in the course, infants usually hyperventilate, and Pa_{CO_2} is lower than normal. Later, in severe cases, alveolar hypoventilation may be detected by hypercarbia. Hypoxia may be present early in the course of the disease, and it progresses rapidly in severely affected infants. Pulmonary vascular resistance is elevated because of hypoxemia, acidemia, and hyperinflation of the lungs. Hypoventilation and intrapulmonary, atrial, and ductus arteriosus $R \rightarrow L$ shunting all contribute to systemic hypoxemia manifested clinically as cyanosis. Air trapping secondary to obstructions of multiple small airways by meconium results in overdistention of portions of the lung and contributes to a high incidence of pulmonary air leaks (pneumothorax, pneumomediastinum). Respiratory failure occurs in the most severe cases. Some of the adverse effects of meconium may be due to direct chemical irritation.

The chest roentgenogram shows patchy infiltrates of uneven distribution and increased lung fluid, which clears during the first 24 hours (see Fig. 35-1). Pulmonary air leaks are common. Occasionally the infiltrates completely clear during the first 24 hours; however, the infant remains persistently cyanotic. Many of these infants have evidence of $R \rightarrow L$ shunting at the level of the atrial septum and/or the ductus arteriosus. They may be considered to have persistent pulmonary hypertension of the newborn in association with meconium inhalation syndrome. It is not clear whether there is a cause-and-effect relationship between the two or whether they are concomitant disease states (see Chapter 39). Some infants have an extensive abnormal distribution of excessive smooth muscle in pulmonary arteries, which probably existed prior to delivery. Although it is not unusual for sick infants to have thrombocytopenia, there seems to be a significant association between inhalation syndromes,

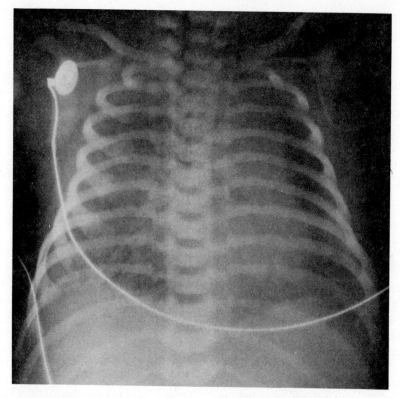

Fig. 35-1. Chest roentgenogram of infant with meconium inhalation syndrome, taken on the first day of life. Note the patchy, uneven distribution of the infiltrates.

thrombocytopenia, and persistent pulmonary hypertension. Many infants who have this association are unresponsive to pulmonary vasodilation therapy (tolazoline HCl) and eventually die. At autopsy they have diffuse pulmonary microthrombi, which appear to be platelet plugs, in the vessels throughout the lungs. The intraluminal obstruction could be caused by inhaled material (meconium or amniotic fluid), causing platelet clumping with intraluminal obstruction, which would explain the lack of increase in systemic oxygenation with vasodilator therapy. In addition, the platelet clumping may cause release of vasoconstrictors such as thromboxane A_2.

Most infants improve within 24 to 48 hours. Some demonstrate persistent tachypnea with respiratory alkalosis even after Pa_{O_2} and chest roentgenograms are normal. This may be because of continued stimulation of irritant receptors in the small airways by foreign material for several days.

MONITORING

See also Chapter 4.

Respiratory system

1. Note respiratory efforts and retractions.
2. Auscultate the chest every hour to check for bilateral breath sounds.
3. Measure arterial blood-gas tensions and pH.
   a. Obtain an initial sample in all infants with persistent signs of distress (note sampling site, e.g., right radial artery).
   b. Use an indwelling arterial catheter in infants with:

(1) Hypoxemia requiring more than 40% oxygen to maintain Pa_{O_2} at greater than 50 mm Hg.

(2) Hypercarbia with Pa_{CO_2} greater than 50 mm Hg (usually requires mechanical ventilation).

(3) Tension pneumothorax.

(4) Unstable cardiovascular system.

c. In infants who are sick enough to require an indwelling arterial catheter, obtain at least one set of simultaneous Pa_{O_2} samples from preductus and postductus arteriosus sites (see Chapter 39). A difference of 10 mm Hg or greater in oxygen tension (higher preductus) indicates significant R → L shunting.

d. In infants requiring an indwelling arterial catheter, measure blood-gas tensions and pH every 2 to 3 hours during the acute phase of the disease (24 to 48 hours).

4. Repeat chest roentgenograms when there are any signs of deterioration (sudden hypoxemia, hypercarbia, hypotension, bradycardia), since there is a high risk of pulmonary air leaks.

Cardiovascular system

1. In patients in whom persistent pulmonary hypertension is suspected and who are severely affected (require hyperventilation and/or vasodilator therapy), insert a 4-French, double-lumen pulmonary artery catheter to measure pulmonary arterial blood pressure.

Other systems

1. Serum Mg in infants with persistent hypoxemia and pulmonary hypertension.

2. Platelet count, PT, and PTT in patients in shock (see Chapter 20).

MANAGEMENT
Respiratory system

In delivery room

1. If the infant is delivered with thick meconium in the mouth, rapidly suction the mouth and pharynx. Immediately intubate the patient and, using your mouth (with face mask in place) or a Delee Trap, suction the trachea directly through the endotracheal tube. This should be accomplished before the onset of the infant's respiratory activity.

2. Repeat tracheal suctioning until no meconium is aspirated.

3. When no further meconium is obtained, gently inflate the lungs with 20 cm H_2O of pressure and 60% to 80% oxygen. Continue until the infant's color is good and he is spontaneously breathing.

4. Extubate.

Outside delivery room

1. If the patient shows only minimal signs of persistent respiratory difficulty (e.g., tachypnea, cyanosis requiring oxygen, excessive secretions), he can be moved to an intermediate-care facility and given chest percussion, postural drainage, humidified gas, and oxygen if necessary. These infants are usually stable within a few hours.

2. If the infant is in respiratory distress or persistently hypoxemic, admit him to the PICU.

a. Give oxygen to maintain Pa_{O_2} between 50 and 70 mm Hg. If persistent pulmonary hypertension is documented, keep Pa_{O_2} greater than 100 mm Hg but no more than this if the infant is preterm.

b. Intubate the patient if:
(1) Pa_{O_2} is less than 50 mm Hg in 80% oxygen.
(2) Pa_{CO_2} is greater than 50 mm Hg.
(3) The patient is apneic.

c. Usually these patients need mechanical ventilation, not CPAP alone. Because of peripheral air trapping with overinflation of some areas of the lung, attempt to keep the inflating pressures and constant end-pressures low (see Chapter 34) to decrease the risk of pulmonary air leaks and to avoid impairing pulmonary capillary blood flow (see Fig. 35-2). However, because of the decreased lung compliance, this may not be possible, and high ven-

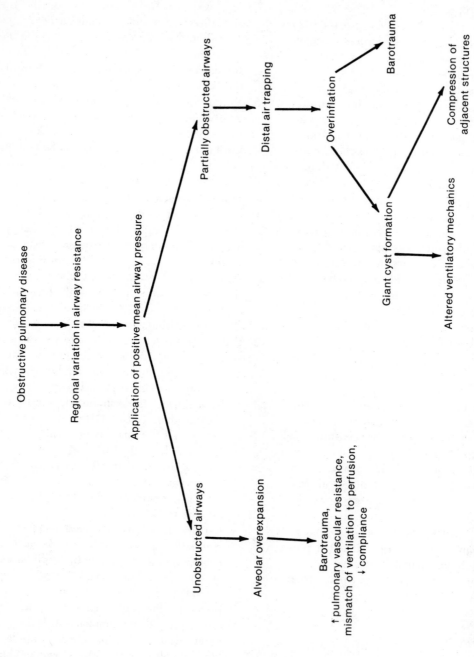

Fig. 35-2. Application of positive airway pressure in patients with obstructive pulmonary disease results in different physiologic events in different areas of the lungs. (From Perkin, R.M., and Levin, D.L.: Adverse effects of positive-pressure ventilation in children. In Gregory, G.A., editor: Respiratory failure in the child, New York, 1981, Churchill Livingstone.)

tilatory pressures may be required.

d. Patients with R → L shunting at the level of the atrial septum and/or the ductus arteriosus, either with or without persistent pulmonary infiltrates, may benefit from tolazoline (Priscoline), a vasodilator, if the main pathophysiologic abnormality is pulmonary vasospasm. The method of administration of this drug is detailed in Chapter 39.

e. Administration of prostaglandin E_1 (PGE_1), a vasodilator, has been tried unsuccessfully in a few infants who, it was determined at autopsy, had severe morphologic abnormalities of the pulmonary vascular bed, which probably occurred in utero. PGI_2 has also been tried in these infants without much success.

f. Give vigorous chest percussion and postural drainage every 2 to 3 hours (see Chapter 99).

g. Relieve tension pneumothoraces promptly (see Chapter 102).

Cardiovascular system

1. Bradycardia is usually associated with hypoxemia due to either the disease process itself or mechanical malfunctions. Check the position and patency of the endotracheal tube and assure the delivery of oxygen. Tension pneumothorax or pneumopericardium with cardiac tamponade may also be a cause of bradycardia.
2. Tachycardia may be due to hypoxemia or hypovolemia. If the patient remains tachycardic once hypoxemia is relieved, check capillary filling, urinary output, and metabolic component of serum pH for signs of hypovolemia and poor peripheral perfusion.
3. Systemic hypertension is associated with asphyxia and will improve after relief of asphyxia. Hypotension may be caused by hypovolemia or cardiac tamponade due to tension pneumothorax.
4. Pulmonary arterial hypertension may be re-

lieved by the interventions described in Chapter 39, but can be refractory to all therapeutic attempts.

Renal-metabolic system

1. Patients are frequently stressed, cold, hypoglycemic, and hypocalcemic. Wipe the patient's skin to remove amniotic fluid, the presence of which increases heat loss by evaporation. Provide an adequate heat source.
2. Start an IV infusion of glucose at 250 to 350 mg/kg/hr to maintain Dextrostix reading between 45 and 90 mg/dl.
3. Give calcium gluconate, 200 mg/kg/24 hr IV, for maintenance, and increase the dose if the serum calcium level is less than 7.5 mg/dl.
4. Give fluids to provide liquefaction of pulmonary secretions and to attain a urinary output of greater than 2 ml/kg/hr and a urine specific gravity of less than 1.010. This usually requires 80 to 100 ml/kg/24 hr, plus 20% of maintenance requirements for infants under radiant warmers. In some cases more fluids may be required. However, too much fluid may be detrimental, causing hypervolemia, increased LAP, and pulmonary edema, thereby worsening lung function.
5. Maintain serum electrolytes at normal levels.
6. Asphyxiated, stressed infants may become hypomagnesemic. In documented cases of hypomagnesemia (<1.2 mg/100 ml), give magnesium (0.8 mEq/kg/24 hr IV in three divided doses). Give it slowly over 1 hour. Alternatively, administration of enteral antacids may cause hypermagnesemia and systemic hypotension.

Hematologic system

1. Provide a good oxygen-carrying capacity. Maintain Hct at greater than 45%.
2. DIC may develop in association with shock (see Chapter 20).

ADDITIONAL READING

Fox, W.W., Gewitz, M.H., Dinwiddie, R., and others: Pulmonary hypertension in perinatal aspiration syndromes, Pediatrics 59:205-211, 1977.

Gooding, G.A., and Gregory, G.A.: Roentgenographic analysis of meconium aspiration of the newborn, Radiology 100:131-135, 1971.

Gregory, G.A.: Meconium aspiration. In Rudolph, A.M., editor: Pediatrics, ed. 16, New York, 1977, Appleton-Century-Crofts.

Gregory, G.A., Gooding, C.A., Phibbs, R.H., and Tooley, W.H.: Meconium aspiration in infants: a prospective study, J. Pediatr. 85:848-852, 1974.

Levin, D.L., and Gregory, G.A.: The effect of tolazoline on right-to-left shunting via a patent ductus arteriosus in meconium aspiration syndrome, Crit. Care Med. 4:304-307, 1976.

Levin, D.L., Weinberg, A.G., and Perkin, R.M.: Pulmonary microthrombi syndrome in newborn infants with unresponsive persistent pulmonary hypertension, J. Pediatr. 101:299-303, 1983.

Murphy, J.D., Rabinovitch, M., Goldstein, J.D., and Reid, L.M.: The structural basis of persistent pulmonary hypertension of the newborn infant, J. Pediatr. 98:962-967, 1981.

Segall, M.L., Goetzman, B.W., and Shick, J.B.: Thrombocytopenia and pulmonary hypertension in the perinatal aspiration syndromes, J. Pediatr. 96:727-730, 1980.

Truog, W.F., Lyrene, R.K., Standhaert, T.A., and others: Effects of PEEP and tolazoline infusion on respiratory and inert gas exchange in experimental meconium aspiration, J. Pediatr. 100:284-290, 1982.

Vidyasagar, D., Yeh, T.F., Harris, V., and Pildes, R.S.: Assisted ventilation in infants with meconium aspiration syndrome, Pediatrics 56:208-213, 1975.

36 Neonatal asphyxia

DANIEL L. LEVIN

DEFINITION AND PHYSIOLOGY

Asphyxia is defined as a lack of oxygen. During the anoxic or severely hypoxic state, aerobic metabolism converts to anaerobic metabolism, increasing lactic acid and decreasing carbon dioxide production. The metabolism of lactic acid in the liver and the elimination of carbon dioxide from the lungs during the period of anoxia are concomitantly impaired, causing further depression of pH. Hydrogen ions move into cells, which then release potassium, causing hyperkalemia. The major physiologic consequence of asphyxia is CNS depression. The initial response is an increase in respiratory effort, both in rate and depth. This is called primary hyperpnea and is followed by a period of apnea called primary apnea. After approximately 1 minute, rhythmic gasping begins. This continues for several minutes, with the gasps eventually becoming weaker and ending in secondary apnea.

Neonatal asphyxia is associated with many intrapartum events (Table 36-1). Many newborns with intrapartum asphyxia are thought to be hypovolemic, since during asphyxia the fetus becomes hypertensive, a circumstance that favors blood flow from the fetus into the placenta. If delivery occurs at this point, a significantly increased residual placental blood volume may exist, and the newborn may be hypovolemic. During the first few hours and days of life, asphyxia may be caused by CNS depression due to trauma, hemorrhage, drugs, or infections; airway obstruction; congenital lung abnormalities; pulmonary parenchymal disorders such as hyaline membrane disease and inhala-

tion or infectious pneumonia; pulmonary air leaks; congenital heart disease with poor cardiac output; sepsis; and hemorrhage.

Periventricular hemorrhage is a major and probably a common sequela of neonatal asphyxia. In addition, anoxic encephalopathy, seizures, myocardopathy with shock, nephropathy, hypoglycemia, hypocalcemia, hypomagnesemia, and capillary damage leading to peripheral and pulmonary edema can occur secondary to neonatal asphyxia.

MONITORING

See also Chapter 4.

Immediate newborn period

The assessment of neonatal asphyxia at the moment of birth is aided by use of the Apgar score (Table 36-2). Five findings (A, appearance or color; P, pulse rate; G, grimace or reflex irritability; A, activity or muscle tone; and R, respiratory rate and effort) are scored 0, 1, or 2 at 1 and 5 minutes as indicated in the table. A score of 8 or more at 1 minute is associated with excellent survival, and a score of 4 or less at 1 minute is usually associated with severe problems or death.

After immediate newborn period

Cardiorespiratory system

Measure arterial blood-gas tensions and pH initially and every 15 to 20 minutes until the immediate life-threatening situation is stabilized. Repeat every 2 hours during continued acute illness and 10 minutes after every therapeutic intervention.

239

Table 36-1. Disorders that commonly cause intrapartum asphyxia

Maternal conditions

Diabetes

Hypertension

Toxemia

Maternal treatment with reserpine, lithium, magnesium, ethyl alcohol, β-adrenergic drugs

Abnormal estriol levels

Anemia (hemoglobin less than 10 g/dl)

Blood group isoimmunization with high levels of bilirubin present in amniotic fluid

Abruptio placenta

Placenta previa

Antepartum hemorrhage

Previous prenatal death

Narcotic, barbiturate, tranquilizer, or psychedelic drug use

Ethyl alcohol intoxication

Conditions of labor and delivery

Forceps delivery other than low elective

Vacuum extraction delivery

Breech or other abnormal presentation and delivery

Cesarean section

Prolonged second stage of labor

Prolapsed umbilical cord

Maternal hypotension

Sedative or analgesic drugs given intravenously within 1 hour of delivery or intramuscularly within 2 hours of delivery

Fetal conditions

Multiple births

Polyhydramnios

Meconium-stained amniotic fluid

Abnormal heart rate or rhythm

Acidosis (fetal scalp capillary blood)

Decreased rate of growth (uterine size)

Premature delivery

Amniotic fluid surfactant test negative or intermediate within 24 hours of delivery

From Gregory, G.A.: Cardiopulmonary care of the newborn infant at birth. In Rudolph, A.M., editor: Pediatrics, ed. 16, New York, 1977, Appleton-Century-Crofts.

Table 36-2. Apgar score

Observation	Normal	Score		
		0	1	2
A, appearance or color	Pink with effective ventilation, acrocyanosis	Blue, pale	Pink body with acrocyanosis	Pink
P, pulse	120-160 beats/min	Absent	<100/min	>100/min
G, grimace or reflex irritability	Grimace, cough, or sneeze with nasal catheter	Absent	Grimace	Cough or sneeze
A, activity or muscle tone	Movement of all extremities	Limp	Some flexion of extremities	Active motion
R, respiratory effort	Gasp at birth, with deep efforts by 30 seconds and regular respirations of 30-60/min by 90 min	Absent	Slow, irregular	Good, crying

Measure systemic arterial blood pressure (see Appendix C, Table C-1).

Renal-metabolic system

1. Serum Ca and Mg levels immediately and every 12 to 24 hours.
2. BUN and serum creatinine level initially. Repeat if renal dysfunction is suspected.

MANAGEMENT

Management is directed primarily at correcting the asphyxia by provision of oxygen and ventilation, reversing its consequences (acidosis, hypovolemia, hyperkalemia), and correcting any associated disorders that are contributing to the episode. In addition, every effort must be made to diagnose and treat the specific underlying disorder responsible for the asphyxial episode.

Respiratory support

1. Clear airway of secretions. Be careful. Deep pharyngeal suctioning may cause vagal stimulation and bradycardia.
2. Supply oxygen and alveolar ventilation. In the spontaneously and effectively breathing infant (Apgar score of 5 or greater at 1 minute), this may be done by directing oxygen to the nose and mouth. Use 60% to 80% humidified oxygen. If the infant is moderately asphyxiated (Apgar score of 3 or 4 at 1 minute), use a face mask and anesthesia bag and manually assist ventilation. If this does not improve the infant's condition (Apgar score of 5 or more at 5 minutes) or if the infant is severely asphyxiated (Apgar score of 0 to 2 at 1 minute), orally intubate the infant quickly, give him 2 to 5 breaths with 30 to 40 cm H_2O pressure, and then continue to assist ventilation using 20 cm H_2O of pressure.
3. Continue oxygen administration and assisted ventilation until the infant is pink, vigorous, and spontaneously breathing. Slowly withdraw assisted ventilation and supplemental oxygen. Once the infant is spontaneously breathing and pink and the heart rate and blood pressure are stable for several minutes after supplemental oxygen and assisted ventilation have been withdrawn and no or a small amount of secretions are being aspirated from the endotracheal tube, the tube may be removed. Rapid withdrawal of support may result in a return of the original asphyxiated state.
4. Stimulation may be beneficial. Clearing the airway, giving oxygen to the nose, and gently slapping the heels will help mildly asphyxiated infants. Do not turn the infant upside down and slap the buttocks. This is very traumatic.
5. For respiratory acidosis, see below.

Cardiovascular system

1. The use of bicarbonate and volume expanders in neonatal asphyxia has been questioned because hyperosmolar fluids may cause intracranial hemorrhage and volume expanders may result in hypervolemia, left atrial distention, and pulmonary edema. This last situation may be partially due to the wide range of normal systemic arterial blood pressures in newborn infants of different gestational ages, postnatal ages, and body weights (see Appendix C, Table C-1) and in part due to the myocardial dysfunction seen in some infants with asphyxia.
2. Acidosis.
   a. Respiratory acidosis (elevated Pa_{CO_2}) is best treated with assisted ventilation, which increases cardiac output and delivery of oxygen to the tissues, decreases lactic acid production, and improves circulation and carbon dioxide elimination. At a pH of 7.10 or greater, ventilation alone will usually correct the acidosis. If a component of metabolic acidosis (base deficit) or severe respiratory acidosis (pH of approximately 7.10 or less) persists after 10 to 15 minutes of adequate ventilation, give sodium bicarbonate for a one-fourth correction of the metabolic compo-

nent of acidosis, ¼ (0.6 × body weight [kg] × base deficit), undiluted, at a rate of 1 mEq/kg/min. With extremely low pH values (less than 7.10), pulmonary vasoconstriction may be so great that pulmonary blood flow is inadequate to deliver carbon dioxide to the lungs for elimination. Sodium bicarbonate, 1 to 2 mEq/kg given at a rate of 1 mEq/kg/min, or a one-fourth correction of the base deficit, if it is known, may be used to raise the pH, promote pulmonary vasodilation, and increase pulmonary blood flow. Adequate alveolar ventilation must be maintained during sodium bicarbonate administration to eliminate efficiently carbon dioxide as soon as pulmonary blood flow increases or Pa_{CO_2} will rise and compound the acidosis. Excessive correction of acidosis, resulting in alkalosis, is dangerous and causes depression of cardiac output. Therefore, the effect of assisted ventilation and administration of alkali must be carefully documented. A pH of 7.35 to 7.45 is ideal.

b. Metabolic acidosis (base deficit less than −5 mEq/L) is usually associated with respiratory acidosis, as discussed above, or with inadequate cardiac output secondary to myocardial depression or hypovolemia. All metabolic factors that adversely affect myocardial performance should be treated, including correction of cold stress, hypoglycemia, and hypocalcemia. If the patient is thought to be hypovolemic as assessed by systemic arterial blood pressure measurement, degree of peripheral vasoconstriction with poor capillary filling, and low CVP (<3 cm H_2O at end-expiration), treat with:
 (1) Whole blood, 10 ml/kg, or
 (2) Plasma or Plasmanate, 10 ml/kg, or
 (3) 25% albumin, 1 g (4 ml)/kg, or
 (4) 5% albumin, 10 ml/kg, or
 (5) 0.9% sodium chloride solution, 10 ml/kg.

c. These volume-expanding agents may be repeated as long as the measured CVP does not become greater than 10 cm H_2O.

d. Patients who have a normal CVP while exhibiting peripheral vasoconstriction may become hypotensive after hypoxia and acidosis are treated and vasodilation occurs. Be prepared to give these patients volume expanders at this point (see above).

e. Do not treat the measured blood pressure; *treat the patient.* Always evaluate the entire situation, including degree of peripheral vasoconstriction (capillary filling), color, degree of metabolic acidosis, and urine output.

f. The above measures will usually restore the circulation in patients with neonatal asphyxia. If, however, cardiac output is still impaired after these measures and/or if the CVP is elevated, the use of an inotropic agent such as dopamine or isoproterenol may be considered (see Chapter 14).

3. The treatment of hypovolemia is presented above, in the discussion of metabolic acidosis.

4. Perform cardiac massage when the heart rate is less than 100 beats/min or peripheral pulses cannot be palpated (see Chapter 5). During cardiac massage, observe the electronic display of systemic blood pressure recorded via the arterial catheter and blood pressure transducer. Attempt to develop systolic blood pressures that are normal for age.

Renal-metabolic system

1. Provide IV glucose to maintain Dextrostix at 45 to 90 mg/dl. Asphyxiated infants become hypoglycemic and need vigorous glucose administration.

2. Give calcium chloride, 0.25 ml/kg, preferably via a centrally placed catheter, during

the acute anoxic episode, because this form of calcium contains the maximum amount of ionized calcium. Calcium gluconate must be metabolized in the liver before ionized calcium is available. After the acute episode, use 200 mg/kg or more of calcium gluconate per 24 hours if the serum calcium level is less than 7.5 mg/dl.

3. Serum magnesium level may be low. Give magnesium sulfate, 0.8 mEq/24 hr IV, in three divided doses each over 1 hour for a serum magnesium level <1.2 mEq/L.
4. Provide potassium, 2 mEq/kg/24 hr, once a patient is urinating. Renal tubular function is often impaired in these patients (vasomotor nephropathy) and potassium should be withheld if this is the case.
5. Dry the infant's skin, especially the newborn, to prevent heat loss (see Chapter 18) and place him a heat-giving environment.
6. Minimal acceptable urine output is 0.5 ml/kg/hr.

Central nervous system

1. Relief of asphyxia usually improves the neurologic status.
2. Prolonged asphyxia may result in intracranial hemorrhage (see Chapter 24), seizures (see Chapter 9), or generalized CNS depression.

Other systems

Management of other specific complications of neonatal asphyxia, such as necrotizing enterocolitis, congestive heart failure, seizures, DIC, and renal failure, is discussed elsewhere.

ADDITIONAL READING

Apgar, V.: A proposal for a new method of evaluation of the newborn infant, Anesth. Analg. 32:260-267, 1953.

Bland, R.D., Clark, T.L., and Harden, L.B.: Rapid infusion of sodium bicarbonate and albumin into high-risk premature infants soon after birth: a controlled, prospective trial, Am. J. Obstet. Gynecol. 124:263-267, 1976.

Cabal, L.A., Devaskar, U., Siassi, B., and others: Cardiogenic shock associated with perinatal asphyxia in preterm infants, J. Pediatr. 96:705-710, 1980.

Corbet, A.J., Adams, J.M., Kenny, J.D., and others: Controlled trial of bicarbonate therapy in high-risk premature newborn infants, J. Pediatr. 91:771-776, 1977.

Donnelly, W.H., Bucciarelli, R.L., and Nelson, R.M.: Ischemic papillary muscle necrosis in stressed newborn infants, J. Pediatr. 96:295-300, 1980.

Finberg, L.: The relationship of intravenous infusions and intracranial hemorrhage: a commentary, J. Pediatr. 91:777-778, 1977.

Gregory, G.A.: Cardiopulmonary care of the newborn infant at birth. In Rudolph, A.M., editor: Pediatrics, ed. 16, New York, 1977, Appleton-Century-Crofts.

Guyton, A.C.: Metabolism of carbohydrates and formation of adenosine triphosphate. In Guyton, A.C., editor: Textbook of medical physiology, ed. 3, Philadelphia, 1966, W.B. Saunders Co.

James, L.S.: Emergencies in the delivery room. In Behrman, R.E., editor: Neonatal-perinatal medicine: diseases of the fetus and infant, ed. 2, St. Louis, 1977, The C.V. Mosby Co.

Robertson, N.R.C., and Hawat, P.: Hypernatremia as a cause of intracranial hemorrhage, Arch. Dis. Child. 50:938-942, 1975.

Versmold, H.T., Kitterman, J.A., Phibbs, R.H., and others: Aortic blood pressure during the first 12 hours of life in infants with birth weight 610 to 4,200 grams, Pediatrics 67:607-613, 1981.

Volpe, J.J.: Neonatal periventricular hemorrhage: past, present, and future, J. Pediatr. 92:693-696, 1978.

Wigglesworth, J.S., Keith, I.H., Girling, D.J., and others: Hyaline membrane disease, alkali and intraventricular hemorrhage, Arch. Dis. Child. 51:775-762, 1976.

37 Cyanotic congenital heart disease

EDGAR A. NEWFELD

DEFINITION AND PHYSIOLOGY

Cyanosis is the clinical sign of systemic arterial unsaturation and is a blue or purplish coloration best seen in the mucous membranes (such as in the mouth), in the tongue and lips, and in the nail beds. It can be caused by cyanotic congenital cardiac defects and also by a variety of noncardiac causes. Central cyanosis exists when unsaturated blood is delivered to the aorta, and it results from anatomic right-to-left (R → L) shunts (heart defects) or physiologic R → L shunts, i.e., pulmonary disease. With central cyanosis, the arterial blood oxygen saturation and Pa_{O_2} are lower than normal. In contrast, peripheral cyanosis is caused by pooling of unsaturated blood in the extremities and is often related to poor systemic circulation or exposure to cold. In this circumstance, the aortic blood is normally saturated and has a normal Pa_{O_2}. In newborns, hypoglycemia, hypocalcemia, and sepsis can cause cyanosis by causing apnea and hypoventilation and also by producing low cardiac output with shock. Increased ICP secondary to hemorrhage, trauma, tumor, or infection can cause cyanosis by the same mechanism.

Chronic systemic arterial unsaturation has a profoundly unfavorable effect on the body. In a newborn it can cause metabolic acidosis secondary to lactic acid production from anaerobic metabolism. In an older child it causes growth failure, especially in muscular development. A R → L shunt also increases the risk of brain abscess and cerebrovascular thrombosis.

MONITORING

See also Chapter 4.

A cyanotic newborn should have laboratory tests to rule out noncardiac causes of cyanosis, specifically serum glucose, calcium, hematocrit, and temperature determinations. Sepsis should be ruled out in cases where it represents a reasonable possibility. Smear a drop of the patient's blood on a glass slide and expose it to 100% oxygen to see if it turns red, thus excluding the diagnosis of methemoglobinemia. A complete history of the pregnancy and birth will help in deciding whether the cyanosis may be the result of noncardiac causes. A careful complete physical examination with an emphasis on the cardiovascular system should follow the history.

Physical examination

See specific cardiac defects below.

Laboratory tests

All cyanotic newborns (and most older children) should have certain laboratory tests:
1. Chest roentgenogram. Determines heart size and shape and the pulmonary vascular markings and excludes pulmonary disease.
2. ECG. Rules out dysrhythmias and helps distinguish certain types of cardiac defects.
3. Echocardiogram. Can help in several important diagnoses, especially hypoplastic left heart syndrome.
4. Arterial blood-gas tensions and pH. Determine the severity of cyanosis, whether acidosis is present, and whether there is pulmo-

nary dysfunction, indicated by elevated Pa_{CO_2}. Repeat these in a high-oxygen environment when pulmonary disease is a possibility. In patient with cyanotic congenital heart disease, it is usually impossible to increase Pa_{O_2} more than 10 to 15 mm Hg when the patient is placed in an FI_{O_2} of 1.0, but with pulmonary disease, an increase of more than 25 mm Hg is common.

5. Hemoglobin and hematocrit. Neonatal polycythemia with a Hb level of 20 to 25 g/dl and a Hct greater than 65% may mimic cyanotic heart disease and can be associated with cardiorespiratory symptoms, such as tachypnea and congestive heart failure (see Chapter 38).

6. Cardiac catheterization. This is the definitive diagnostic test and should be done in all patients with cyanotic heart disease to establish the exact anatomic diagnosis. In a newborn, catheterization should be done as soon as possible, since rapid clinical deterioration is not uncommon at this age and emergency surgery may be needed.

DIAGNOSIS AND MANAGEMENT OF SPECIFIC CARDIAC DEFECTS

Patients with a R → L cardiac shunt may have diminished pulmonary blood flow caused by some form of obstruction of the pulmonary arterial blood flow. Increased pulmonary blood flow may be present as a result of the mixing of systemic and pulmonary venous blood without pulmonary arterial obstruction. The pulmonary blood flow pattern is often well demonstrated on a chest roentgenogram and, therefore, is a convenient way of classifying cyanotic congenital cardiac defects.

In general, patients with diminished pulmonary blood flow are not in congestive heart failure and may not need digoxin or diuretics. Initial treatment should include correction of any metabolic acidosis, oxygen, and prompt diagnostic cardiac catheterization. Patients with increased pulmonary blood flow may be in congestive heart failure, and although prompt diagnosis is important, they may benefit from digitalization and diuretics, as well as oxygen and correction of acidosis, before cardiac catheterization. Improvement in cardiac output may lessen the risk of catheterization and help to clarify the clinical diagnosis. A strong diagnostic impression before study will enhance the yield of cardiac catheterization.

Lesions with diminished pulmonary blood flow

Tetralogy of Fallot

Pathophysiology. The defects consist of a large ventricular septal defect (VSD), infundibular and usually valvar pulmonary stenosis (70%), and some degree of aortic overriding of the VSD. The pulmonic stenosis obstructs blood flow to the lungs, and there is a R → L shunt through the VSD.

History. Cyanosis is usually not evident at birth. It begins within the first few months of life and may occur in spells characterized by marked increase in cyanosis, irritability, and tachypnea followed by limpness and/or sleep or loss of consciousness. In the older child there may be squatting when fatigue occurs.

Physical examination. Mild to moderate cyanosis and clubbing of fingers and toes, a systolic ejection murmur at the mid left sternal border, and a right ventricular cardiac impulse are typical. The second heart sound (S_2) may be single.

Laboratory tests. The chest roentgenogram may show a boot-shaped heart and decreased pulmonary vascular markings, and a right aortic arch (found in 30% to 40% of patients) may also be visualized (Fig. 37-1). The ECG reveals right axis deviation (RAD) and right ventricular hypertrophy (RVH). An echocardiogram can show the aorta overriding the septum.

Cardiac catheterization. The angiographic appearance is characteristic.

Treatment. Either a systemic-pulmonary arterial shunt operation or intracardiac repair

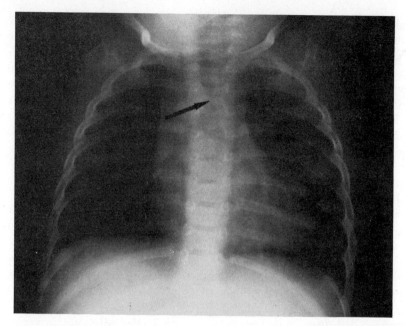

Fig. 37-1. Chest roentgenogram of a young infant with tetralogy of Fallot. Note decreased pulmonary vascular markings and the right aortic arch indenting the trachea on the right side *(arrow).*

as a primary procedure is indicated (as an emergency in the presence of severe spells), depending on the suitability of the anatomy.

Pulmonary atresia with VSD (pseudotruncus)

Pathophysiology. The defect consists of complete atresia of the right ventricular outflow tract and/or pulmonary valve, a large VSD, and pulmonary blood flow supplied by a PDA and/ or bronchial collateral vessels. There is usually diminished pulmonary blood flow, which often depends on a small PDA, and a large R → L shunt through the VSD.

History. Cyanosis is noted soon after or at birth, except for rare cases with large pulmonary blood flow via collateral vessels.

Physical examination. Cyanosis, a right ventricular impulse, a continuous murmur at the base or in the back, an ejection click due to a dilated aorta, and a single S_2 are typical. Pulse pressure may be increased in intensity if the PDA is large.

Laboratory tests. The chest roentgenogram shows a boot-shaped heart and diminished pulmonary vascular markings, and there may be a right aortic arch. The ECG reveals RAD and RVH. The echocardiogram may show the aorta overriding the ventricular septum.

Cardiac catheterization. Angiography reveals pulmonary atresia, collateral circulation to the lungs, and a R → L shunt through the VSD.

Treatment. This lesion usually requires a systemic-pulmonary arterial shunt operation in infancy, often as an emergency. Prostaglandin E_1 (PGE_1), 0.05 μg/kg/min, infused in the aorta near the ductus orifice can maintain its patency, increase Pa_{O_2}, and improve the patient's condition while awaiting surgery. Corrective surgery using a valved Dacron conduit is usually deferred until the patient is older.

Pulmonary atresia without VSD

Pathophysiology. The right ventricular cavity is usually hypoplastic and has a thick muscular wall. The pulmonary valve is atretic, and pulmonary blood flow is supplied by a PDA. A large R → L atrial shunt is present.

History. Cyanosis is present from birth, and

rapid deterioration is common when the PDA shunt diminishes.

Physical examination. Marked cyanosis is typical. There is often no murmur or a faint continuous murmur of a PDA and a single S_2.

Laboratory tests. The chest roentgenogram reveals little if any cardiomegaly as well as markedly diminished pulmonary blood flow. The ECG can reveal normal or left axis deviation (LAD), atrial hypertrophy, and left ventricular hypertrophy (LVH) for age, with absent or diminished right ventricular forces. The echocardiogram may show a small right ventricular cavity.

Cardiac catheterization. The right ventricular angiogram is diagnostic.

Treatment. Emergency cardiac catheterization is indicated. This should be followed by surgery consisting of a pulmonary valvotomy to establish blood flow through the right ventricle and a systemic-pulmonary arterial shunt procedure.

Critical pulmonary valve stenosis

Pathophysiology. The pathophysiology is similar to that of pulmonary atresia without a VSD (see above). This is especially true if the right ventricular cavity is hypoplastic. The right ventricle may be dilated if congestive heart failure is present. Pulmonary blood flow is minimal from the right ventricle through a stenotic valve, and circulation to the lungs occurs primarily through a PDA.

History. Cyanosis is noted soon after birth. As newborns, these babies are often large by weight. If right heart failure is present, they may manifest abnormal respiratory signs.

Physical examination. Cyanosis, a right ventricular impulse, a systolic ejection murmur usually present from birth, and a single or split S_2 with a very soft pulmonic component are the typical findings. A continuous murmur of a PDA may be present. Hepatomegaly and peripheral edema occur when right ventricular failure is present.

Laboratory tests. The chest roentgenogram reveals diminished pulmonary vascular markings and either a normal-size heart or globular cardiomegaly. The ECG reveals RAD and severe RVH when the right ventricular cavity is dilated or absent right ventricular forces when it is hypoplastic, as in pulmonary atresia. Right atrial hypertrophy (RAH) is common.

Cardiac catheterization. The right ventricular angiogram is diagnostic. No attempt should be made to enter the pulmonary artery, since the catheter may totally obstruct the valve orifice, causing cardiac arrest.

Treatment. Emergency pulmonary valvotomy is indicated if the right ventricular cavity is adequate; if the right ventricular cavity and tricuspid valve are hypoplastic, a systemic-pulmonary arterial shunt operation should be performed, as in pulmonary atresia (see above).

Tricuspid atresia

Pathophysiology. The tricuspid orifice is atretic, and all systemic venous blood shunts from right to left through an ASD. The hypoplastic right ventricle fills via a VSD, which can be small, medium, or (rarely) large. Pulmonary blood flow is diminished if either the VSD or a tiny right ventricular cavity obstructs pulmonary blood flow. A PDA is often present.

History. Cyanosis is present at birth or soon thereafter. Rapid clinical deterioration can occur if the PDA closes, and this is not uncommon.

Physical examination. Cyanosis and a murmur caused by a VSD and/or a PDA are present. A single S_2 or one with a soft pulmonic component is heard.

Laboratory tests. The ECG reveals LAD, RAH, and LVH for age, with diminished right ventricular forces. This type of ECG in a cyanotic infant should suggest the diagnosis. The chest roentgenogram reveals diminished pulmonary blood flow and a normal-size heart. Echocardiography reveals a hypoplastic right ventricle and no tricuspid valve.

Cardiac catheterization. A right atrial angiogram is diagnostic, and balloon atrial septostomy should be performed.

Treatment. A systemic-pulmonary arterial

shunt operation should be performed, often as an emergency procedure if the PDA is closing.

Ebstein's anomaly of the tricuspid valve

Pathophysiology. There is downward displacement of the tricuspid valve into the right ventricular cavity, resulting in a tricuspid insufficiency of a variable degree. A R → L atrial shunt is present, and pulmonary blood flow is thereby diminished. Severe congestive heart failure can result from the tricuspid regurgitation, accentuated in the newborn period because of the normally high pulmonary vascular resistance.

History. The patient can have cyanosis at birth or after several months. When tricuspid regurgitation is severe, the infant has severe congestive heart failure in the neonatal period.

Physical examination. A triple or quadruple gallop rhythm is typically heard at the left sternal border and is associated with a blowing regurgitant systolic murmur and occasionally a diastolic murmur as well. Hepatomegaly and

peripheral edema can be present, and cyanosis and clubbing are common.

Laboratory tests. The chest roentgenogram shows marked cardiomegaly, with a large right atrium, and diminished pulmonary blood flow (Fig. 37-2). The ECG reveals RAD, RAH, and occasionally mild RVH. Complete right bundle-branch block is seen occasionally.

Cardiac catheterization. A right atrial angiogram may be diagnostic, and a PDA may be present.

Treatment. This is the only cyanotic lesion with diminished pulmonary blood flow for which digitalization and diuretic therapy may be useful. No early surgical therapy is indicated, and since this lesion can be confused with pulmonary atresia or severe pulmonary stenosis, for which surgery is necessary, an accurate diagnosis is essential.

Other lesions. There are other complex lesions associated with diminished pulmonary blood flow because severe pulmonic stenosis or

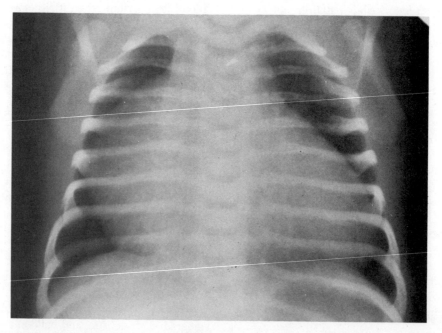

Fig. 37-2. Chest roentgenogram of a 3-day-old infant with Ebstein's malformation of the tricuspid valve. Massive cardiomegaly and decreased pulmonary vascular markings are significant features.

atresia is part of the complex. Treatment usually requires a systemic-pulmonary arterial shunt operation if cyanosis is severe. Complete discussions of these complex lesions can be found in standard textbooks of pediatric cardiology.

Lesions with increased pulmonary blood flow

Complete transposition of the great vessels
Pathophysiology. The aorta arises completely from the right ventricle, and the pulmonary artery arises completely from the left ventricle. The unsaturated systemic venous blood reenters the systemic arterial circulation, and the saturated pulmonary venous blood reenters the pulmonary arterial circulation. Life is sustained by some degree of intracardiac mixing of the two circulations via the foramen ovale, a PDA, or a VSD if present. When there is inadequate mixing (i.e., inadequate flow of unsaturated blood to the lungs and saturated blood to the body), cyanosis and progressive metabolic acidosis lead to deterioration and death, usually within the first few days or weeks of life.

History. Cyanosis is present from birth, and when mixing is poor it is marked, progressive, and unaffected by the administration of oxygen.

Physical examination. Marked cyanosis, tachypnea, a right ventricular impulse, a single loud S_2, and often the absence of any murmur are found. However, except for cyanosis and tachypnea, some infants may appear remarkably normal during the first few days of life.

Laboratory tests. The chest roentgenogram reveals, classically, an egg-shaped heart with increased pulmonary blood flow (Fig. 37-3), but it may be deceptively normal in appearance in the newborn. The ECG reveals RAD and RVH but may also be considered normal for a newborn. Pa_{O_2} is usually less than 40 mm Hg unless a VSD or PDA is present but rarely it may be elevated. Echocardiography can be helpful.

Cardiac catheterization. Angiograms are diagnostic, and all infants with complete trans-

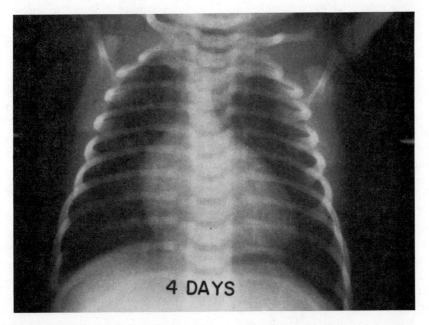

Fig. 37-3. Chest roentgenogram of a newborn with complete transposition of the great vessels. Note cardiomegaly, with "egg on end"–shaped heart and increased pulmonary vascular markings.

position of the great vessels should have a balloon atrial septostomy.

Treatment. Balloon atrial septostomy often provides adequate palliation by creating good "mixing" at the atrial level. Digitalization may be indicated, and metabolic acidosis should be diagnosed and corrected. If clinical signs suggest that palliation is inadequate, recatheterization and possible surgery (either palliative or corrective) are indicated.

Total anomalous pulmonary venous drainage

Pathophysiology. Instead of draining normally to the left atrium, the pulmonary veins come together to form a common pulmonary vein that then drains to one of several different sites leading back to the right atrium. The common sites of drainage include the left vertical vein (which empties into the innominate vein), the coronary sinus, the superior vena cava (directly), the right atrium (directly), the portal venous system (subdiaphragmatically), and also a combination of sites (mixed type). The pulmonary venous drainage may be obstructed anywhere along its pathway back to the heart. There is complete mixing of the systemic venous and pulmonary venous blood, with a R → L atrial shunt that supplies the left ventricle and hence the systemic circulation. If significant pulmonary venous obstruction occurs, this results in marked pulmonary venous congestion, pulmonary venous hypertension, and pulmonary arterial hypertension, which often may be to suprasystemic levels. When no pulmonary venous obstruction is present, there is a marked increase in pulmonary blood flow. Congestive heart failure is common with or without pulmonary venous obstruction.

History. The presence of tachypnea and cyanosis soon after birth (in patients with pulmonary venous obstruction) makes this lesion easily confused with respiratory distress of pulmonary origin.

Physical examination. Cyanosis, dyspnea, a hyperdynamic right ventricular impulse, a gallop rhythm, a loud S_2 that may be single, and occasionally systolic and diastolic flow murmers are found in the typical case. A markedly enlarged and firm liver is found when pulmonary venous obstruction is present, particularly in the subdiaphragmatic type of drainage. Pulmonary rales may be present, and peripheral pulses are normal or diminished when severe heart failure is present.

Laboratory tests. The chest roentgenogram may be typical if drainage is obstructed, and it shows markedly increased pulmonary venous markings and normal cardiac size (Fig. 37-4). Without obstruction of drainage there is cardiomegaly and active pulmonary vascular congestion. The ECG reveals RAD, RAH, and severe RVH. The echocardiogram may show the common pulmonary vein behind the left atrium. Abdominal sonography may demonstrate dilated veins in the liver as well as a dilated common pulmonary vein in the abdomen in patients with anomalous pulmonary venous return below the diaphragm.

Cardiac catheterization. A pulmonary arterial angiogram is diagnostic, showing the pulmonary venous drainage to abnormal sites. Severe pulmonary arterial hypertension is common, and a PDA should be looked for, since the surgeon needs to ligate it before cardiopulmonary bypass.

Treatment. Digitalization, diuretics, oxygen, and even assisted ventilation may be necessary as supportive therapy; surgical correction is the definitive treatment and should be done as soon as possible when venous obstruction is present.

Hypoplastic left heart syndrome

Pathophysiology. In the common form, aortic and/or mitral valve atresia and a diminutive slitlike left ventricular cavity are present. When a VSD is present with mitral atresia, the left ventricle may not be as hypoplastic and the aortic valve may not be atretic. Blood returning via the pulmonary veins to the left atrium must traverse the foramen ovale to the right atrium, and therefore the systemic circulation depends

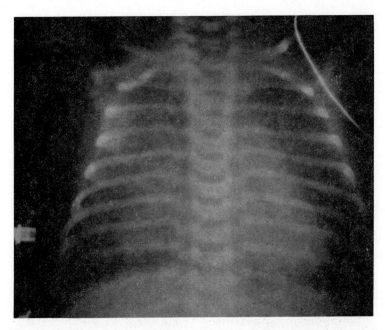

Fig. 37-4. Chest roentgenogram of a 5-day-old infant with obstructed total anomalous pulmonary venous drainage to the portal vein, with marked pulmonary venous congestion. Note similarity to the roentgenographic appearance of hyaline membrane disease.

on the right ventricle and a R → L shunt through the PDA. As the pulmonary vascular resistance falls and the PDA begins to close (usually within the first few hours or days of life), the systemic output falls, leading to severe metabolic acidosis and death.

History. The baby is usually thought to be normal at birth, and signs of cardiorespiratory distress and congestive heart failure usually begin within the first 48 hours of life.

Physical examination. The typical findings include tachypnea, slight cyanosis, a markedly hyperdynamic precordium, and markedly diminished peripheral pulses. A characteristic ashen color and mottling of the skin occur when cardiac output falls. A systolic precordial murmur may be present, S_2 is loud and single, and a gallop rhythm is commonly heard. The liver is markedly enlarged and firm.

Laboratory tests. The chest roentgenogram shows cardiomegaly and increased pulmonary

vascular markings, with both arterial and venous congestion. The ECG shows RAD, RAH, and severe RVH with little or no left ventricular potential. ST-segment and T-wave changes may be present, especially if metabolic acidosis has begun. The echocardiogram can be diagnostic, showing a large right ventricular cavity and a tiny left ventricular cavity, with an absent or hypoplastic mitral and/or aortic valve (see Chapter 93).

Cardiac catheterization. This is usually not necessary when the clinical findings and echocardiogram are diagnostic, but it may be required to rule out other lesions when the findings are atypical. A single-frame aortogram using an umbilical arterial catheter with the tip at the level of ductus arteriosus can be diagnostic (Fig. 37-5).

Treatment. A new radical form of surgery is being proposed and some success has been reported, but it remains controversial and by no

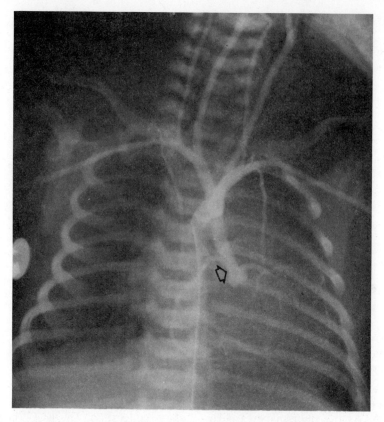

Fig. 37-5. Single-frame aortogram using umbilical arterial catheter with tip at the level of the ductus arteriosus. Note the tiny ascending aorta (arrow).

means universally accepted. Usually death occurs from falling systemic output within the first few days or weeks of life. Digitalization, diuretics, and oxygen may temporarily improve the congestive heart failure but only for a short time. Extensive supportive care should be avoided, since it only delays the inevitable outcome.

Persistent common truncus arteriosus

Pathophysiology. There is a single arterial trunk arising from the heart from which the systemic and pulmonary arteries originate. A large VSD is present, situated below the orifice of the common trunk, so that the right and left ventricles empty directly into it. Pulmonary blood flow is usually markedly increased, producing congestive heart failure within the first few weeks of life.

History. The baby is often thought to be normal at birth but develops congestive heart failure after a few days of life. Cyanosis is minimal.

Physical examination. Mild cyanosis, often not clinically obvious, a hyperdynamic precordium, bounding peripheral pulses, a systolic or continuous (to and fro) murmur, and gallop rhythm may be present in the typical case. S_2 is often, but not always, single, and a systolic ejection click is commonly heard.

Laboratory tests. The chest roentgenogram shows cardiomegaly, increased pulmonary blood flow, and occasionally a right aortic arch. The ECG shows combined ventricular hypertrophy, with prominent precordial voltages and RAD. The echocardiogram may show a single, large, arterial trunk overriding the interventricular septum.

Cardiac catheterization. Angiography, with injection of contrast material directly into the arterial trunk, is necessary to define the anatomy and to differentiate this lesion from aorticopulmonary window.

Treatment. Digitalis and diuretics should be given for the congestive heart failure. If the failure is unremitting, bilateral pulmonary artery banding should be performed in infancy to lower distal pulmonary arterial blood pressures and to decrease the excessive pulmonary blood flow. Later in childhood a corrective procedure using a valved conduit to function as a main pulmonary artery is performed. Recently, primary corrective surgery has been successfully performed in early infancy and may replace pulmonary artery banding as the procedure of choice.

ADDITIONAL READING

Barrett-Boyes, B.G., and Neutze, M.J.: Primary repair of tetralogy of Fallot in infancy using profound hypothermia with circulatory arrest and limited cardiopulmonary bypass, Ann. Surg. **178:**406-411, 1973.

Batton, D.G., Maisels, M.J., Fripp, R.R., and Heald, J.I.: Arterial hyperoxia in a newborn infant with transposition of the great vessels, J. Pediatr. **100:**300-302, 1982.

Bonchek, L.I., Starr, A., Sunderland, C.O., and Menashe, V.D.: Natural history of tetralogy of Fallot in infancy, Circulation **48:**392-397, 1973.

Cole, R.B., Muster, A.J., Lev, M., and Paul, M.H.: Pulmonary atresia with intact ventricular septum, Am. J. Cardiol. **21:**23-31, 1968.

Delisle, G., Ando, M., Calder, A.L., and others: Total anomalous pulmonary venous connection: report of 93 autopsied cases with emphasis on diagnostic and surgical considerations, Am. Heart J. **91:**99-122, 1976.

Freed, M.D., Rosenthal, A., Bernhard, W.F., and others: Critical pulmonary stenosis with diminutive right ventricle in neonates, Circulation **48:**875-881, 1973.

Levin, D.L., Paul, M.H., Muster, A.J., and others: d-Transposition of the great vessels in the neonate, Arch. Intern. Med. **137:**1421-1425, 1977.

Mair, D.D., and Ritter, D.G.: Truncus arteriosus. In Moss, A.J., Adams, F.H., and Emmanuoilides, G.C., editors: Heart disease in infants, children and adolescents, ed. 2, Baltimore, 1977, The Williams & Wilkins Co.

Nadas, A.S., and Fyler, D.C.: Pediatric cardiology, Philadelphia, 1972, W.B. Saunders Co.

Newfeld, E.A., Cole, R.B., and Paul, M.H.: Ebstein's malformation of the tricuspid valve in the neonate, Am. J. Cardiol. **19:**727-731, 1967.

Olley, P.M., Coceani, F., and Bodach, E.: E-type prostaglandins: a new emergency therapy for certain cyanotic congenital heart malformations, Circulation **53:**728-731, 1976.

Paul, M.H.: d-Transposition of the great arteries. In Moss, A.J., Adams, F.H., and Emmanuoilides, G.C., editors: Heart disease in infants, children and adolescents, ed. 2, Baltimore, 1977, The Williams & Wilkins Co.

Rosenthal, A.: Tricuspid atresia. In Moss, A.J., Adams, F.H., and Emmanuoilides, G.C., editors: Heart disease in infants, children and adolescents, ed. 2, Baltimore, 1977, The Williams & Wilkins Co.

Rudolph, A.M.: Congenital diseases of the heart, Chicago, 1974, Year Book Medical Publishers, Inc.

Sinha, S.N., Rusnak, S.L., Sommers, H.M., and others: Hypoplastic left ventricle syndrome, Am. J. Cardiol. **21:**166-173, 1968.

Van Praagh, R., Ando, M., and Dungan, W.T.: Anatomic types of tricuspid atresia: clinical and developmental implications, Circulation **44:**111-115, 1971.

Van Praagh, R., Van Praagh, S., Nebesar, R.A., and others: Tetralogy of Fallot: underdevelopment of the pulmonary infundibulum and its sequelae, Am. J. Cardiol. **26:**25-33, 1970.

38 Neonatal polycythemia

DANIEL L. LEVIN

DEFINITION AND PHYSIOLOGY

Polycythemia is defined as a greater than normal hematocrit of free-flowing venous blood. For the newborn, various hematocrit levels from 63% to 75% have been stated as the upper limit of normal. Capillary (heel or finger stick) hematocrit is greater than both peripheral vein hematocrit and umbilical vein (central) hematocrit, but no consistent relationship exists so that the peripheral or central venous hematocrit can be predicted by the capillary hematocrit. There is a weak correlation between peripheral and central hematocrit, with the later being the lower value.

An increase in hematocrit contributes to an increase in blood viscosity. Blood viscosity is also influenced by shear rate during flow (shear rates increase with increased flow). At low flow, shear rates are decreased and viscosity is increased (Fig. 38-1). RBCs tend to clump at low flow and this increases viscosity. In one study 80% of neonates with an umbilical vein hematocrit greater than or equal to 63% had increased blood viscosity and 94% of infants with an umbilical vein hematocrit of less than or equal to 63% had a normal blood viscosity.

With an increase in viscosity there is an increase in systemic and pulmonary vascular resistances and a decrease in tissue perfusion. Cardiac output decreases, and renal blood flow is reduced. With increasing pulmonary vascular resistance there is R → L shunting of blood at the level of the atrial septum and the ductus arteriosus. The increase in the oxygen-carrying capacity of the blood secondary to an elevated hematocrit is not enough to compensate for the de-

creased tissue perfusion, decreased cardiac output, and R → L shunting, so that the delivery of oxygen to the tissues is decreased. The increased pulmonary vascular resistance and hypoxemia also result in increased pulmonary arterial blood pressure. Tissue hypoxia occurs throughout the body, with adverse metabolic effects in many organs, including the brain, myocardium, kidney, liver, and bowel. Increased viscosity and RBC clumping lead to sludging of cells in the microcirculation and ultimately to thrombosis in diffuse vascular beds.

Polycythemia may be caused by chronic intrauterine fetal hypoxemia, as seen in small for gestational age infants; infants of toxemic mothers; infants of diabetic mothers; infants with twin-twin, maternal-twin, and large placental-fetal transfusions; and infants with trisomy 21, trisomy D, adrenal hyperplasia, or alpha-chain hemoglobinopathies.

Normally, at birth an infant receives a placental transfusion of 5 to 20 ml/kg. Over 2 to 6 hours, the plasma volume decreases (via the kidneys) and hematocrit rises. Rarely, signs of a large transfusion with congestive heart failure are present at birth. These infants should have a large blood volume with an increased plasma volume and a normal hematocrit and viscosity. After the initial few hours in these infants and earlier in infants with intrauterine causes of polycythemia, there is a normal plasma volume but increased blood volume and RBC volume with an increasing hematocrit.

Polycythemic infants may be plethoric or cyanotic and exhibit respiratory distress. It

254

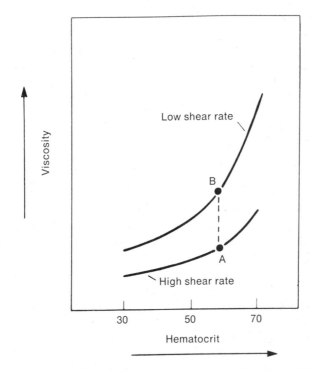

Fig. 38-1. Effects of hematocrit and shear rate on blood viscosity. The dotted line between *A* and *B* illustrates the increase in viscosity that would occur in flowing blood with a hematocrit of 60% if flow changed from a high to a low rate. (From Phibbs, R.H.: Neonatal polycythemia. In Rudolph, A.M., editor: Pediatrics, ed. 16, New York, 1977, Appleton-Century-Crofts.)

may be difficult to distinguish this condition from respiratory disease or congenital heart disease, and polycythemia may coexist with either of these. CNS abnormalities include an abnormal cry, tremulousness, agitation or depression, poor feeding, and convulsions. There is some concern that infants with convulsions may have residual brain damage with or without a permanent seizure disorder. Renal manifestations include enlarged kidneys, hematuria, oliguria, anuria, and renal vein thrombosis. Polycythemia may contribute to the development of necrotizing enterocolitis. Hypoglycemia and hypocalcemia are frequently present and may further depress cardiac output and decrease peripheral blood flow. As excess RBCs are destroyed, bilirubin is produced, and hyperbilirubinemia may result.

MONITORING

See also Chapter 4.

Hematologic system

1. In an ideal setting, all newborns should have a capillary hematocrit performed at 2 to 4 hours of age. This is a screening test.
2. If the capillary hematocrit is greater than 65%, perform a free-flowing venous hematocrit.
3. Hematocrits may fall below this level (65%) in patients with polycythemia if sludging has occurred.
4. Obtain platelet counts, since platelets may decrease with RBC sludging.
5. Ideally, whole blood viscosity and blood and plasma volume should be measured, but these are rarely available.

Cardiorespiratory system

1. Measure arterial blood-gas tensions and pH before and after partial exchange transfusion.
2. Simultaneous Pa_{O_2} determinations from pre-ductus and postductus arteriosus sites are helpful in determining if cyanosis is due in part to $R \rightarrow L$ shunting through a PDA (see Chapter 39).
3. Echocardiography can be used to demonstrate increased pulmonary vascular resistance by prolonged right pre-ejection period/right ventricular ejection time (RPEP/RVET) ratios that fall after an exchange transfusion or serially over the first few days of life as the hematocrit falls.
4. Obtain chest roentgenogram and repeat if abnormal.
5. Obtain a full 12-lead ECG.

Renal-metabolic system

1. Monitor serum bilirubin level (late rise at 2 to 4 days).
2. Check urine for blood.
3. Measure urine output carefully.

Central nervous system

1. Watch for seizures.
2. Evaluate level of activity (crying, sucking, muscle tone, tremulousness, agitation or depression) every 4 hours.
3. Evaluate success of oral feedings (i.e., volume of intake, residuals, abdominal girth).

MANAGEMENT

Management is controversial. Some authors recommend lowering the hematocrit in all polycythemic babies, and others recommend waiting for abnormal signs. Since abnormalities are related to blood viscosity and flow and these are rarely measured, the venous hematocrit is used clinically to determine which patients are at risk. If all babies with free-flowing venous hematocrits greater than a certain level (e.g., 65%) are treated, the risks of unnecessary treatment for some must be weighed against the risks of

late treatment for others. The major risk of late treatment may be permanent residual CNS abnormalities.

Once the decision to treat these infants is made, proceed as follows.

Hematologic system

Hypervolemia with congestive heart failure

1. Rarely, this occurs in the first few hours of life.
2. Slowly remove 10 ml/kg blood by means of phlebotomy.
3. Continue to measure Hct, since polycythemia may still occur later (after 2 to 6 hours).

Polycythemia with hypervolemia

1. Perform a partial exchange transfusion using albumin, 4 g/dl (mix 16 ml of albumin [25 g/dl] with 84 ml of 0.9% sodium chloride solution), to isovolumically decrease RBC mass. FFP may be substituted for 25% albumin.
2. Decrease the Hct to 50% or 55% by using the following formula to determine the volume to be exchanged:

$$V = \frac{Hct_i - Hct_f \times \text{Body weight (kg)} \times 90 \text{ ml/kg}}{Hct_i}$$

where:

   V = volume to be exchanged
   Hct_i = initial hematocrit
   Hct_f = final hematocrit
   90 ml = blood volume per kg body weight

3. Use the same routes in the suggested order of preference as for exchange transfusion (see Chapter 107).
4. Push the albumin, 4 g/dl, and withdraw whole blood in 5-ml aliquots.
5. After the partial exchange transfusion is completed, slowly decrease the blood volume by 10 ml/kg.

Polycythemia with normovolemia

1. Do not use simple phlebotomy in these patients. With a normal blood volume, phlebotomy will decrease cardiac output and

peripheral blood flow, resulting in a decrease in shear rate and an increase in viscosity.

2. Perform an exchange transfusion with albumin, 4 g/100 ml, as outlined above.
3. Do not decrease the blood volume after the exchange. There is some evidence that attempts at isovolumic exchange transfusion actually result in a decrease in blood volume as well as in RBC volume and in an increase in plasma volume.

Cardiorespiratory system

1. Place the patient on supplemental oxygen if hypoxemia is present.
2. Tachypnea, tachycardia, and cyanosis are usually relieved after treatment of polycythemia and/or hypervolemia.
3. Polycythemia can coexist with serious congenital heart disease and pulmonary disease. If the patient does not improve, investigate these possibilities further.

Renal-metabolic system

1. Maintain a normal body temperature.
2. Maintain Dextrostix readings between 45 and 90 mg/dl with IV glucose.
3. Use calcium gluconate, 100 mg/kg IV slow push, to treat a serum calcium level less than 7.5 mg/dl.
4. If blood is present in the urine, monitor urine output, BUN, and serum creatinine levels, and kidney size closely. Sonography may be helpful to document a kidney felt to be enlarged on the basis of palpation (i.e., due to renal vein thrombosis).
5. If blood is present in the stools, measure abdominal girth serially, check for gastric residual, and obtain abdominal roentgenograms serially (see Chapter 57).
6. Measure serum bilirubin levels until safe levels are demonstrated (see Chapter 64).

Central nervous system

1. After exchange transfusion, treat seizures with oxygen, calcium, and glucose as indicated.
2. Give phenobarbital, 10 mg/kg IV loading dose followed by 5 mg/kg/day in three divided doses, if the above measures do not eliminate the seizures.
3. Obtain a follow-up neurologic evaluation.

ADDITIONAL READING

Brans, Y.W., Shannon, D.L., and Ramamurthy, R.S.: Neonatal polycythemia. II. Plasma, blood, and red cell volume estimates in relation to hematocrit levels and quality of intrauterine growth, Pediatrics 68:175-182, 1981.

Fouron, J.C., and Hebert, F.: Circulatory effects of hematocrit variations in normovolemic newborn lambs, J. Pediatr. 82:995-1003, 1973.

Gatti, R.A., Muster, A.J., Cole, R.B., and Paul, M.H.: Neonatal polycythemia with transient cyanosis and cardiorespiratory abnormalities, J. Pediatr. 69:1063-1072, 1966.

Geierman, C., Young, G., and Pyk, W.: Echocardiographic study of pulmonary vascular resistance (PVR) in polycythemia neonates, Pediatr. Res. 12:381, 1978.

Gross, G.P., Hathaway, W.E., and McGaughey, H.R.: Hyperviscosity in the neonate, J. Pediatr. 82:1004-1012, 1973.

Hakanson, D.O., and Oh, W.: Necrotizing enterocolitis and hyperviscosity in the newborn infant, J. Pediatr. 90:458-461, 1977.

Herson, V.C., Raye, J.R., Rowe, J.C., and Phillips, A.F.: Acute renal failure associated with polycythemia in a neonate, J. Pediatr. 100:137-139, 1982.

LeBlanc, M.H., Kotagal, U.R., and Leonard, I.K.: The physiologic effects of hypervolemic polycythemia in newborn dogs, Pediatr. Res. 14:457, 1980.

Phibbs, R.H.: Neonatal polycythemia. In Rudolph, A.M., editor: Pediatrics, ed. 16, New York, 1977, Appleton-Century-Crofts.

Ramamurthy, R.S., and Brans, Y.W.: Neonatal polycythemia. I. Criteria for diagnosis and treatment, Pediatrics 68:168-174, 1981.

Stevens, K., and Wirth, F.H.: Incidence of neonatal hyperviscosity at sea level, J. Pediatr. 97:118-119, 1980.

39 Persistent pulmonary hypertension of the newborn

DANIEL L. LEVIN

DEFINITION AND PHYSIOLOGY

Persistent pulmonary hypertension of the newborn (PPHN) is a condition in which pulmonary vascular resistance remains at the fetal level and therefore pulmonary arterial blood pressure will be similar to systemic arterial blood pressure. PPHN may be associated with diseases of known cause and pathogenesis, e.g., CNS abnormalities that cause hypoventilation; infection, particularly group B β-hemolytic streptococcal pneumonia; polycythemia; upper airway obstruction, e.g., micrognathia; pulmonary parenchymal disorders, e.g., retained fetal lung fluid, hyaline membrane disease, meconium inhalation syndrome; congenital lung disorders, e.g., diaphragmatic hernia and hypoplastic lungs; and congenital heart disease, e.g., VSD. Another form of persistent pulmonary hypertension that is not associated with any of these known mechanisms, has been described and variously referred to as persistent fetal circulation, persistent pulmonary vascular obstruction, progressive pulmonary hypertension, persistent fetal cardiopulmonary circulatory pathway, and persistent transitional circulation. The following discussion refers to this type of idiopathic PPHN.

Infants with PPHN are usually full-term, although some are preterm, and many have a history of prenatal or intrapartum stress or a positive maternal obstetric history. Shortly after birth, these infants are cyanotic, tachypneic, or in some cases apneic, and may have a systolic murmur. Hypoxemia, hypercarbia, acidemia, hypoglycemia, and hypocalcemia are characteristic.

Simultaneous Pa_{O_2} samples or Ptc_{O_2} measurements from preductus arteriosus (temporal or right radial arteries) and postductus arteriosus (abdominal aorta) sites are helpful in diagnosis if there is a large R $\rightarrow$ L shunt through the ductus arteriosus (Fig. 39-1). In some patients, R $\rightarrow$ L shunting at the level of the atrial septum is so great that the small volume of well-oxygenated blood returning to the left atrium from the pulmonary veins is rapidly diluted with poorly oxygenated blood so that ascending aortic blood is also unsaturated. In other patients, the ductus arteriosus may be prematurely closed in utero. In both of these cases, one would not expect to see a significant difference (>10 mm Hg O_2 tension) between preductus and postductus arteriosus blood samples. Echocardiography showing abnormal right ventricular and pulmonary artery size, abnormal right ventricular systolic time intervals (RVSTI) or RPEP/RVET, and abnormal pulmonic valve motion may be helpful in diagnosis and may actually be able to predict deterioration in patients 1 to 5 hours prior to its occurrence. Cardiac catheterization and cineangiography reveal anatomically normal hearts with poor ventricular function; mitral, tricuspid, and/or pulmonic valve insufficiency; and R $\rightarrow$ L shunts at the atrial septum and/or the ductus arteriosus (Fig. 39-2). Catheterization and cineangiography should be performed when anatomic congenital heart disease cannot be

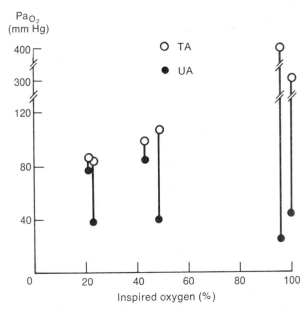

Fig. 39-1. Difference in temporal *(TA)* and abdominal aortic *(UA)* Pa_{O_2} samples obtained simultaneously. Sets are from six infants. Note the increasing oxygen difference with increasing inspired oxygen concentration.

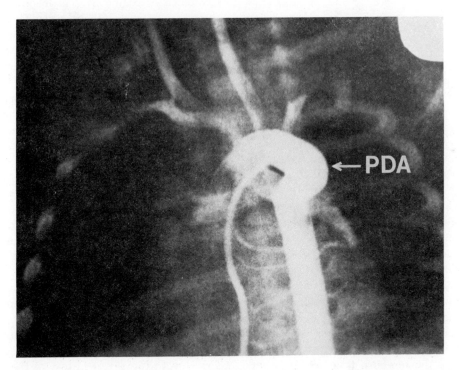

Fig. 39-2. Pulmonary angiogram in infant with persistent pulmonary hypertension and massive R → L shunt via PDA.

Table 39-1. Possible causes of PPHN

1. Intrauterine increase in pulmonary arterial smooth muscle
   a. Genetically determined
   b. Secondary to chronic intrauterine stress and fetal pulmonary arterial hypertension
   c. Intrauterine constriction of the ductus arteriosus (e.g., with diaphragmatic hernia, pharmacologic agents)
2. Decrease in total number of pulmonary arterial resistance vessels (decreased cross-sectional area of pulmonary vascular bed) either in actual number or due to intraluminal occlusion of vessels by thrombi or emboli
3. Alteration in levels of vasoactive agents
   a. Increased availability of pulmonary vasoconstrictors before or after birth (e.g., angiotensin II, TXA_2, $PGF_{2\alpha}$)
   b. Decreased availability of vasodilators before or after birth (e.g., bradykinin, PGE_2, PGI_2)
4. Main pulmonary artery distention

excluded by noninvasive means or when an infant with PPHN does not respond as expected to conventional medical management. Chest roentgenograms show well-expanded lung fields with or without a suggestion of pulmonary venous congestion; cardiomegaly is common.

The cause is unknown, and the entity should probably be considered a syndrome with multiple pathogenic mechanisms (Table 39-1).

Some mechanisms may be related to maternal ingestion of medication, such as prostaglandin synthetase–inhibitors (e.g., salicylate, indomethacin, naproxen), which can cross the placenta, decrease prostaglandin levels, and thereby allow the ductus arteriosus (Fig. 39-3) and the pulmonary resistance vessels to constrict, physiologically (Fig. 39-4) and morphologically altering the pulmonary vascular bed. This mechanism may also result in myocardial ischemia (Fig. 39-5) and transient tricuspid insufficiency of the newborn (Fig. 39-6). Other

drugs or their metabolites taken by pregnant women, for example, hydantoin, may cross the placenta and either the drug or its metabolites may cause fetal pulmonary hypertension by a direct effect on pulmonary vasculature. A decrease in the cross-sectional area of the pulmonary vascular bed may be due to a lack of normal development in the number of pulmonary resistance vessels, either as an isolated event or in association with other lesions, such as congenital diaphragmatic hernia. It may also occur from intraluminal occlusion of pulmonary resistance vessels in the perinatal period due to thrombi, which are possibly platelet plugs. Many circulatory vasoactive agents affect the pulmonary vascular bed both in utero and after birth, and alterations in the normal balance of these agents may affect pulmonary vascular tone. These agents may exert their effect on the pulmonary vascular smooth muscle via the endothelial cells. Endothelial cells may have an obligatory role in the relaxation of smooth muscles since relaxation by acetylcholine requires the presence of endothelial cells. The ability of the endothelial cell to carry out its normal function can be altered by exposing it to an hypoxic environment. Elevations of pulmonary arterial blood pressure can be elicited by distention of the main pulmonary artery via a sympathetically mediated reflex. This mechanism may play a role in pulmonary vasoconstriction and can increase the amount of pulmonary vascular smooth muscle occurring in utero, secondary to constriction of the ductus arteriosus.

Infants with a transient imbalance of circulating vasoactive agents would be expected to have a short course, whereas those with excessive pulmonary arterial smooth muscle may be ill for several days until the muscles relax and the muscle mass decreases (Fig. 39-7). Some infants with both an increase in the amount of medial wall smooth muscle and peripheral extension of the muscle into small arteries that are not normally muscularized may not be able to overcome the limitations of pulmonary blood flow due to the severe extent of the morpho-

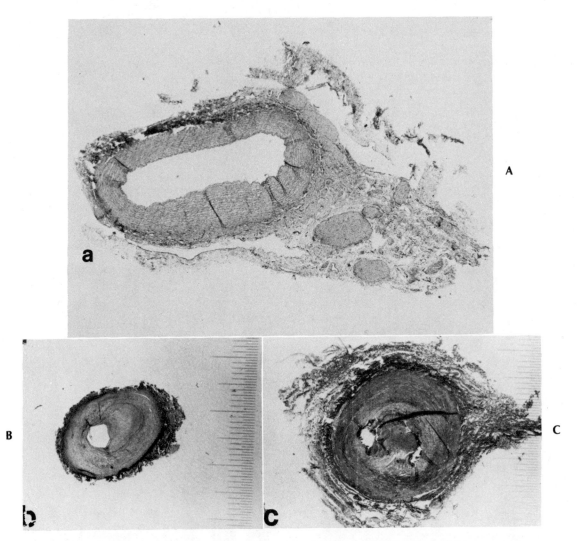

Fig. 39-3. A, Ductus arteriosus of a normal newborn. **B,** Photomicrograph (10×) of ductus arteriosus of patient exposed in utero to salicylates. The ductus arteriosus is 1.9 mm at its greatest external diameter. Note the pinpoint lumen (0.4 mm). **C,** Photomicrograph (10×) of ductus arteriosus of patient with normal heart who died at 6 weeks of age. The maximum external diameter is 2.7 mm. Note the similarity in the fibrosis of the lumen and the small size of the ductus arteriosus in the study patient as compared to this patient. (From Levin, D.L., Fixler, D.E., Morriss, F.C., and Tyson, J.: Morphologic analysis of the pulmonary vascular bed in infants exposed in utero to prostaglandin synthetase inhibitors, J. Pediatr. **92:**478-483, 1978.)

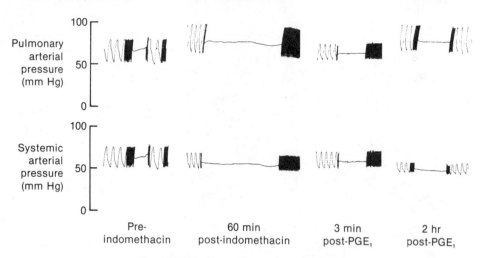

Pulmonary arterial pressure (mm Hg)

Systemic arterial pressure (mm Hg)

Pre-indomethacin   60 min post-indomethacin   3 min post-PGE₁   2 hr post-PGE₁

Fig. 39-4. For legend see opposite page.

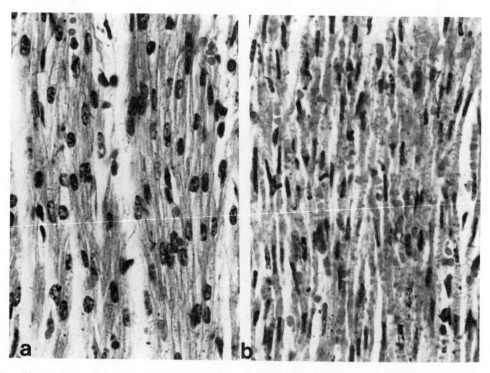

Fig. 39-5. Photomicrographs of sections from the tricuspid valve posterior papillary muscle from a control fetus *(a)* and from a fetus with intrauterine constriction of the ductus arteriosus due to indomethacin *(b)*. Note the loss of cross striations, fragmentation of the sarcoplasm, and nuclear pyknosis in the study fetus. (From Levin, D.L., Mills, L.J., Weinberg, A.G., and others: Hemodynamic, pulmonary vascular and myocardial abnormalities secondary to pharmacologic constriction of the fetal ductus arteriosus, Circulation **60:**360-364, 1979. Reproduced by permission of the American Heart Association, Inc.)

Fig. 39-4. Fetal pulmonary and systemic arterial blood pressures (minus intra-amniotic pressure) obtained from continuous, simultaneous recordings in one fetus before and 60 minutes after maternal administration of indomethacin, 3 minutes after 1 dose of 5 μg of PGE$_1$ into the fetal inferior vena cava, and 2 hours later. Note the pulmonary-systemic arterial blood pressure differences which are due to pulmonary arterial hypertension. (From Levin, D.L., Mills, L.J., Weinberg, A.G., and others: Constriction of the fetal ductus arteriosus after administration of indomethacin to the pregnant ewe, J. Pediatr. **94:**647-650, 1979.)

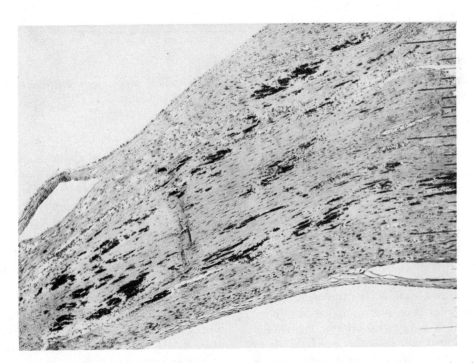

Fig. 39-6. Photomicrograph (25×) of histologic specimen from the posterior papillary muscle of the tricuspid valve in a patient exposed in utero to salicylates. The irregular, dark-staining areas are calcium. The absence of active inflammation indicates that this is an old lesion. (From Levin, D.L., Fixler, D.E., Morriss, F.C., and Tyson, J.: Morphologic analysis of the pulmonary vascular bed in infants exposed in utero to prostaglandin synthetase inhibitors, J. Pediatr. **92:**478-483, 1978.

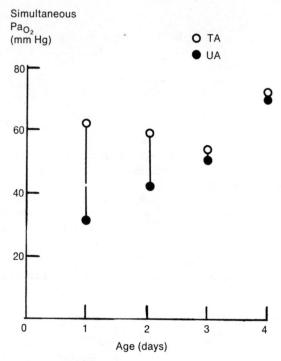

Fig. 39-7. Simultaneous preductus and postductus arteriosus blood oxygen tensions from one infant during the first 4 days of life. Note the disappearance of the R → L shunt.

logic abnormalities. Those with a small pulmonary vascular bed may have a prolonged course or never improve.

MONITORING

See also Chapter 4.

Measure arterial blood-gas tensions and pH.

1. An initial determination should be made on all infants with any respiratory abnormality or cyanosis. Carefully note the inspired oxygen concentration and sampling site (e.g., $FI_{O_2} = 0.4$, right radial artery). The results of the initial determination can be used in conjunction with the clinical picture to assess the need for further sampling. In most cases, infants with PPHN are very unstable and deteriorate rapidly and therefore need repetitive arterial blood-gas tension and pH

determinations during the acute phase of the illness (2 to 4 days). This is most suitably done via an indwelling arterial catheter (see Chapter 87), supplemented by continuous Ptc_{O_2} measurements either proximal to the flow of ductus arteriosus blood into the aorta (right upper quadrant) or in both preductus and postductus arteriosus sites. In some infants with extreme differences in preductus and postductus arteriosus blood oxygen tensions, indwelling arterial catheters or one catheter and one Ptc_{O_2} monitor may be needed in two sites (e.g., right radial artery and posterior tibial artery or abdominal aorta via an umbilical artery or lower body by Ptc_{O_2}).

2. Sampling should be done every hour as well as 10 minutes after every respiratory sup-

port change during the acute phase of the illness (usually 2 to 4 days). The rate of sampling can be decreased during the recovery phase when stability has been clearly demonstrated. It is unwise, however, to decrease the rate of sampling prematurely, since this may increase the patient's risk of hypoxemia and result in massive pulmonary vasoconstriction, acute right ventricular dilation, in adequate systemic output, severe hypoxemia, and death.

3. When a patient is recovering from PPHN and is on 30% oxygen or less, remove the indwelling arterial catheter and assess the patient by Ptc_{O_2} measurements. Take samples by individual arterial punctures if the patient deteriorates or questions of accuracy arise.

MANAGEMENT
Respiratory system

1. Maintain preductus arteriosus blood samples as with:
   a. Pa_{O_2} between 100 and 125 mm Hg (in full-term infants) to provide a margin of safety for unexpected dips in Pa_{O_2}.
   b. Pa_{CO_2} between 20 and 25 mm Hg. Hyperventilation can increase systemic oxygenation and lower pulmonary arterial blood pressure. There are no known long-term side effects of this therapy.
   c. pH greater than 7.30 and less than 7.60. A respiratory alkalosis may improve systemic oxygenation. Tolazoline HCl can cause gastric hypersecretion, and because of loss of HCl, patients can develop a significant metabolic alkalosis, which can complicate respiratory alkalosis. Metabolic alkalosis must be diagnosed and treated by decreasing tolazoline HCl and replacing potassium chloride losses. Cimetidine probably should not be used (H_2 blocker), and antacids can cause hypermagnesemia.
   d. Base deficit between −5 and +5

2. Take the following steps successively to achieve the above values:
   a. Increase the ambient oxygen to 100%.
   b. Intubate the patient if Pa_{O_2} is less than 60 mm Hg in 60% oxygen.
   c. Use CPAP, starting at 4 cm H_2O and then increasing by 2 cm H_2O successively to 10 cm H_2O if Pa_{O_2} does not increase to 100 mm Hg. Rapidly decrease the CPAP if it does not improve oxygenation.
   d. Institute mechanical ventilation using peak inspiratory pressures starting at 20 cm H_2O. One may have to increase inflation pressures up to 40 to 60 cm H_2O or more to move the patient's chest visibly or to identify breath sounds by auscultation (i.e., achieve an adequate TV).
   e. Use respiratory rates starting at 20 breaths/min and advance to 80 to 100 breaths/min, increasing by 10 breaths/min.
   f. Use an I:E ratio of 1:1 or less at high gas flow rates.
   g. Paralyze the patient with tubocurarine, 0.5 mg/kg IV, or pancuronium (Pavulon), 0.1 mg/kg IV. Repeat after any movement (usually diaphragmatic) is observed. Carefully document movement before the next dose is given.
   h. Use a test dose of tolazoline (Priscoline), 1 mg/kg (total dose) in four divided doses, 0.25 mg/kg/dose, every minute for 4 minutes. Administer this into a vein on the head or upper extremity or via a central venous or right atrial catheter. *One must continuously display systemic arterial blood pressure when using this drug, which is a systemic as well as a pulmonary vasodilator.* There is a great deal of controversy concerning the use of tolazoline HCl since it does not seem to work in many patients and may cause many side effects such as hypotension and hemorrhage. However, tolazoline

seems to be a direct pulmonary vasodilator under hypoxic conditions and an indirect pulmonary vasodilator under normoxic conditions and with its use the effects of hyperventilation and respiratory alkalosis are enhanced. The drug works in many patients and in many of those in whom it does not work, pathologic anatomic reasons are often found to explain why it would not have been expected to work (e.g., undiagnosed congenital heart disease, decreased number of pulmonary resistance vessels, diffuse pulmonary microthrombi). Amongst survivors treated with tolazoline HCl, there seems to be little evidence of late morbidity that can be attributed to the use of the drug itself.

i. Measure Pa_{O_2} at 0, 5, 10, and 15 minutes after test dose. If Pa_{O_2} increases more than 15 mm Hg, start tolazoline at 2 mg/kg/hr IV infusion. *Do not interrupt the infusion.* This may be increased to as much as 10 mg/kg/hr to provide adequate oxygenation, although this is very dangerous, since hypotension, anuria, and bleeding may occur.

j. Monitor all secretions (endotracheal, NG, stool) and urine for blood. If the patient becomes oliguric or anuric, a dopamine infusion, 5 to 15 μg/kg/min IV, and furosemide, 1 mg/kg IV every 12 hours, may be used to restore urine output.

k. Administer tolazoline for at least 24 hours while decreasing inspired oxygen, peak inspiratory pressures, and respiratory rates but maintaining the arterial blood-gas tensions indicated above.

l. If the therapeutic maneuvers up to this point are not successful, consider using exogenous prostaglandins. PGE_1 has been tried but was not satisfactory. PGI_2 was successfully used in one patient but was unsatisfactory in subsequent trials.

PGD_2 may be a selective pulmonary as opposed to a systemic vasodilator during the first few days of life. As of this writing it has not been used in human infants.

m. After 24 hours of tolazoline if improvement has been indicated by the ability to decrease oxygen, peak inspiratory pressure, and respiratory rates, try decreasing tolazoline by one fourth the dose. Measure arterial blood-gas tensions and pH at least at 15, 60, and 120 minutes after the decrease. Do not decrease the tolazoline by a rate greater than one fourth the original dose every 8 hours. The patient may deteriorate after 4 to 6 hours and require the previously established tolazoline dose. If this occurs, wait 24 hours before decreasing the tolazoline again.

n. After the patient is no longer receiving tolazoline, discontinue the muscle relaxant.

o. Decrease the inspired oxygen sequentially by 1% to 2% until 40% is reached.

p. Decrease the peak inspiratory pressure sequentially by 2 to 4 cm H_2O to 20 cm H_2O.

q. Decrease PEEP sequentially in 2-cm H_2O steps to 2 to 4 cm H_2.

r. Decrease the respiratory rate to zero.

s. Extubate (see Chapter 103).

t. Keep arterial blood gas tensions and pH at recommended levels throughout the process of withdrawing ventilation and pharmacologic support.

Cardiovascular system

1. Ensure an adequate circulating blood volume, especially before use of vasodilators. Give 0.9% sodium chloride solution, 10 ml/kg IV push, repetitively until systemic arterial blood pressure, capillary filling, and urine output are adequate.

2. If total serum protein levels are less than 5 mg/dl, given albumin (1 g/kg) or FFP (10

ml/kg) IV until systemic arterial blood pressure, capillary filling, and urine output are adequate.

Hematologic system

1. Ensure an adequate oxygen-carrying capacity. The Hct should be approximately 45%.
2. Bleeding may occur, especially from the gastric mucosa, if tolazoline is used. Try to discontinue tolazoline at the first sign of bleeding. If the patient's oxygenation deteriorates, restart the tolazoline. If DIC is present, treat accordingly (see Chapter 20). Maintain current type and crossmatch during the period the tolazoline infusion is being used.

Gastrointestinal system

See Hematologic system above.

Renal-metabolic system

1. Maintain Dextrostix between 45 and 90 mg/dl. These patients are frequently hypoglycemic.
2. Maintain normal body temperatures (36.5° to 37.2° C). Cooling the blood increases pulmonary vascular resistance.
3. Maintain serum Na, K, Cl, Ca, and Mg within normal limits. (Patients are frequently hypocalcemic and hypomagnesemic.) Give calcium gluconate, 200 mg/kg/24 hr, as maintenance and more if the serum calcium level is less than 7.5 mg/dl. Give magnesium sulfate, 0.8 mEq/kg/24 hr in three divided doses slowly IV over 1 hour, if the serum magnesium level is less than 1.2 mg/dl.
4. It is important to ensure urine output of at least 0.5 ml/kg/hr.

ADDITIONAL READING

Adams, J.M., Hyde, W.H., Proceanoy, R.S., and Rudolph, A.J.: Hypochloremic metabolic alkalosis following tolazoline-induced gastric hypersecretion, Pediatrics 66:298-300, 1980.

Baylen, B.G., Emmanouildes, G.C., Jusatsch, C.E., and others: Main pulmonary artery distention: a potential mechanism for acute pulmonary hypertension in the human newborn infant, J. Pediatr. 96:540-544, 1980.

Boyle, R.J., and Oh, W.: Transcutaneous Po₂ monitoring in infants with persistent fetal circulation who are receiving tolazoline therapy, Pediatr. 62:605-607, 1978.

Brett, C., Dekle, M., Leonard, C.H., and others: Developmental follow-up of hyperventilated neonates: preliminary observations, Pediatrics 68:588-591, 1981.

Bucciarelli, R.L., Egan, E.A., Gessner, I.H. and Eitzman, D.V.: Persistence of fetal cardiopulmonary circulation: one manifestation of transient tachypnea of the newborn, Pediatrics 58:192-197, 1976.

Cohen, R.S., Stevenson, D.K., Malachowski, N., and others: Late morbidity among survivors of respiratory failure treated with tolazoline, J. Pediatr. 97:644-647, 1980.

Donnelly, W.H., Bucciarelli, R.L., and Nelson, R.M.: Ischemic papillary muscle necrosis in stressed newborn infants, J. Pediatr. 96:295-300, 1980.

Drummond, W.H., Gregory, G.A., Heymann, M.A., and Phibbs, R.H.: The independent effects of hyperventilation, tolazoline, and dopamine on infants with persistent pulmonary hypertension, J. Pediatr. 98:603-611, 1981.

Fox, W.W., Gewitz, M.H., Dinwiddie, R., and others: Pulmonary hypertension in the perinatal aspiration syndromes, Pediatrics 59:205-211, 1977.

Gersony, W.M., Duc, G.V., and Sinclair, J.C.: "PFC" syndrome (persistence of the fetal circulation), Circulation 40(Suppl. III):111, 1969.

Harker, L.C., Kirkpatrick, S.E., Friedman, W.F., and Bloor, C.M.: Effects of indomethacin on fetal rat lungs: a possible cause of persistent fetal circulation (PFC), Pediatr. Res. 15:147-151, 1981.

Haworth, S.G.: Normal structural and functional adaptation to extrauterine life, J. Pediatr. 98:915-918, 1981.

Humphrey, M., Kennon, S., and Pramanik, A.K.: Hypermagnesemia from antacid administration in a newborn infant, J. Pediatr. 98:313-314, 1981.

Levin, D.L.: Effects of inhibition of prostaglandin synthesis on fetal development, oxygenation, and the fetal circulation, Semin. Parinatol. 4:35-44, 1980.

Levin, D.L.: Idiopathic persistent pulmonary hypertension of the newborn. In Rudolph, A.M., editor: Pediatrics, ed. 16, New York, 1977, Appleton-Century-Crofts.

Levin, D.L.: Morphologic analysis of the pulmonary vascular bed in congenital left-sided diaphragmatic hernia, J. Pediatr. 92:805-809, 1978.

Levin, D.L., Cates, L., Newfeld, E.A., and others: Persistence of the fetal cardiopulmonary circulatory pathway: survival of an infant after a prolonged course, Pediatrics 56:58-64, 1975.

Levin, D.L., Fixler, D.E., Morriss, F.C., and Tyson, J.: Morphologic analysis of the pulmonary vascular bed in infants exposed in utero to prostaglandin synthetase inhibitors, J. Pediatr. **92:**478-483, 1978.

Levin, D.L., and Gregory, G.A.: The effect of tolazoline on right-to-left shunting via a patent ductus arteriosus in meconium aspiration syndrome, Crit. Care Med. **4:**304-307, 1976.

Levin, D.L., Heymann, M.A., Kitterman, J.A., and others: Persistent pulmonary hypertension of the newborn infant, J. Pediatr. **89:**626-630, 1976.

Levin, D.L., Hyman, A.I., Heymann, M.A., and Rudolph, A.M.: Fetal hypertension and the development of increased pulmonary vascular smooth muscle: a possible mechanism for persistent pulmonary hypertension of the newborn infant, J. Pediatr. **92:**265-269, 1978.

Levin, D.L., Mills, L.J., Parkey, M., and others: Constriction of the fetal ductus arteriosus after administration of indomethacin to the pregnant ewe, J. Pediatr. **94:**647-650, 1979.

Levin, D.L., Mills, L.J., Weinberg, A.G., and others: Hemodynamic, pulmonary vascular, and myocardial abnormalities secondary to pharmacologic constriction of the fetal ductus arteriosus: a possible mechanism for persistent pulmonary hypertension and transient tricuspid insufficiency in the newborn infant, Circulation **60:**360-364, 1979.

Levin, D.L., Weinberg, A.G., and Perkin, R.M.: Pulmonary microthrombic syndrome in newborn infants with unresponsive persistent pulmonary hypertension, J. Pediatr. **102:**299-303, 1983.

Lock, J.E., Coceani, F., and Olley, P.M.: Direct and indirect pulmonary vascular effects of tolazoline in the newborn lamb, J. Pediatr. **95:**600-605, 1979.

Lock, J.E., Olley, P.M., Coceani, F., and others: Use of prostacyclin in persistent fetal circulation, Lancet **1:**1343, June 23, 1979.

Murphy, J.D., Rabinowitch, M., Goldstein, J.D., and Reid, L.M.: The structural basis of persistent pulmonary hypertension of the newborn infant, J. Pediatr. **98:**962-967, 1981.

Riggs, T., Hirshfeld, S., Fanaroff, A., and others: Persistence of fetal circulation syndrome: an echocardiographic study, J. Pediatr. **91:**626-631, 1977.

Rowe, R.D.: Abnormal pulmonary vasoconstriction in the newborn, Pediatrics **59:**318-321, 1977.

Rudolph, A.M.: High pulmonary vascular resistance after birth I. Pathophysiologic considerations and etiologic classification, Clin. Pediatr. **19:**585-590, 1980.

Setzer, E., Ermocilla, R., Tonkin, I., and others: Papillary muscle necrosis in a neonatal autopsy population: incidence and associated clinical manifestations, J. Pediatr. **96:**289-294, 1980.

Soifer, S.J., Morin, F.C., and Heymann, M.A.: Developmental changes in the effect of prostaglandin D_2 on the pulmonary circulation in the newborn lamb, J. Pediatr. **100:**458-463, 1982.

Truog, W.E., Feusner, J.H, and Baker, D.L.: Association of hemorrhagic disease and the syndrome of persistent fetal circulation with the fetal hydantoin syndrome, J. Pediatr. **96:**112-114, 1980.

Valdes-Cruz, L.M., Dudell, G.G., and Ferrara, A.: Utility of M-mode echocardiography for early identification of infants with persistent pulmonary hypertension of the newborn, Pediatrics **68:**515-525, 1981.

Wilkinson, A.R., Aynsley-Green, A., and Mitchell, M.D.: Persistent pulmonary hypertension and abnormal prostaglandin E levels in preterm infants after maternal treatment with naproxen, Arch. Dis. Child. **54:**942-945, 1979.

Yeh, T.F., and Lilien, L.D.: Altered lung mechanics in neonates with persistent fetal circulation syndrome, Crit. Care Med. **9:**83-84, 1981.

40 Infection

Special pediatric intensive care considerations and isolation techniques

DANIEL L. LEVIN
PATTI DUER

PHYSIOLOGY

Patients in intensive care units are particularly prone to acquiring secondary infections because (1) there are usually many patients in one area, (2) the volume of air per patient is small and cannot be changed frequently without creating annoying drafts, (3) they are compromised hosts (e.g., small babies, immunosuppressed patients), (4) they are receiving broad-spectrum antibiotics that select for resistant organisms, and (5) they have many invasive devices (e.g., arterial and venous catheters, endotracheal tubes, chest tubes, bladder catheters, intracranial drains, and ICP catheters). In addition, many patients are admitted to a PICU because they have an infectious disease that has made them unstable or vulnerable (e.g., meningococcemia, encephalitis with coma, sepsis with shock).

MONITORING

See also Chapter 4.

The following routines are observed for all patients admitted to the PICU:

1. In a unit where there is a mixture of medical and surgical patients and older children and neonates, one should obtain survey cultures from all patients at the time of admission. This is not necessary in a unit where separation of these types and ages of patients is possible.

2. Survey cultures are repeated every other week to identify possible sources of nosocomial infection.

3. Cultures are obtained from the rectum, nose, endotracheal or tracheostomy tube (when secretions appear abnormal), umbilical cord, and any suspicious wound or drainage site.

MANAGEMENT
General principles

1. A minimum of 70 square feet per patient should be provided. This is enough for an adult-size hospital bed, and the space around each patient would therefore increase when cribs and incubators are used.

2. Sinks should be provided at all entrances and in all patient areas. Everyone entering the unit must wash hands and wear either a clean gown or scrub clothes.

3. Aerosol cans containing a hexachlorophene, alcohol, or chlorhexidine foam should be placed at every patient's bedside. Everyone should be required to wash hands with this foam before and after touching each patient.

4. Each patient should be provided with his own stethoscope, blood pressure cuff, etc., so that equipment is not moved from patient to patient.

5. All equipment that is in contact with or contains water (e.g., ventilator tubing, IV tub-

269

ing, suction bottles) should be changed every 24 to 48 hours.

Isolation

Initiation of isolation precautions

1. A separate room is required for each patient who needs isolation. The door to this room must remain closed at all times. Each isolation room should have an adjacent anteroom for personnel to wash hands and to gown.
2. The air in the isolation rooms should be in negative balance in relation to the air in the hallways so that air moves into these rooms and not the reverse. Air in the isolation room should be changed completely every hour, and all air leaving the room should go directly out of the hospital.
3. Each patient should be supplied with the equipment needed for 24 hours of care. An isolated patient's supplies are for his use only.

Maintenance of isolation

1. Each room must have separate containers for linen and trash. These containers should be emptied at least every 8 hours. Contaminated linen and trash should be double-bagged and labeled appropriately.
2. Contaminated excreta should be either disposed of in an isolated sewage system or double-bagged (e.g., an infant's diaper).
3. Rubber and plastic reusable items must be double-bagged and gas sterilized. Steam sterilization is used for glass and metal items.
4. All patient specimens (e.g., blood, urine, spinal fluid) are contaminated and must be labeled as such.
5. Hands must be washed before and after patient contact. The appropriate attire (gowns, masks, and/or gloves) must be worn before entering the room and discarded before leaving the room.

Types of isolation

Strict. The following precautions are necessary:
1. Protective gowns.
2. Gloves for patient contact.
3. Masks.
4. Careful hand-washing with attention to proper disposal of items contaminated by use on the patient.

Respiratory. The following precautions are necessary:
1. Protective gowns.
2. Masks.
3. Careful hand-washing with attention to proper disposal of items contaminated by respiratory tract secretions.

Wound and skin. The following precautions are necessary:
1. Protective gowns.
2. Gloves when direct contact with the infected area is required.
3. Careful hand-washing with attention to proper disposal of items that come in contact with the infected area (e.g., linens, dressings, gloves).

Enteric. The following precautions are necessary:
1. Protective gowns.
2. Gloves when patient care requires contact with the patient's excreta.
3. Careful hand-washing and proper disposal of excreta. When the patient's infection is in the bloodstream (e.g., hepatitis), precautions must be taken for disposal of equipment (such as needles) that comes in contact with the blood.

Termination of isolation

1. All disposable patient-care supplies should be discarded.
2. Permanent equipment such as monitors, infusion pumps, and beds should be cleaned with a germicidal agent (e.g., Amphyl).
3. Housekeeping personnel should clean the room according to a protocol. This may be followed by the use of an ultraviolet light.

Patients to be isolated

1. Draining or purulent wounds require isolation until resolution or negative culture (e.g., septic hip after open drainage, incisional abscess).

2. *Pseudomonas* colonization (defined as a predominant culture of *Pseudomonas* organisms from stool, tracheal secretions, or other body sites) requires isolation or at least separation from other patients. The presence of light growth of *Pseudomonas* mixed with other organisms does not necessitate isolation.
3. Enteropathogenic *Escherichia coli*, *Shigella* sp., or *Salmonella* sp. in stool require isolation until stool culture reverts to normal flora.
4. Colonization with *Staphylococcus aureus* does not require isolation per se. If secretions are purulent (i.e., if the child is symptomatic) or if the strain belongs to one of the known pathogenic phage types (e.g., group 1 52/52A/79/80), the patient should be isolated until the organism is eliminated by appropriate therapy.
5. Positive blood cultures and/or sepsis alone need not require isolation.
6. Meningitis or epiglottitis patients need to be isolated during the first 12 hours of appropriate antibiotic therapy because of concomitant carriage of organisms in the nasopharynx.
7. Special cases (unusual organisms, immunosuppressed host, osteomyelitis, pulmonary abscess, viral illnesses) require consultation with the infectious disease service or the hospital infection control nurse.
8. In the event of epidemic nosocomial colonization and disease in the PICU, more stringent isolation procedures will be required than those outlined above.
9. Questions regarding isolation often arise with a number of nontransmissible conditions. The following is a partial list of illnesses that do *not* require isolation:
   a. Viral encephalitis.
   b. Rocky Mountain spotted fever.
   c. Primary tuberculosis.
   d. Tularemia (if no open drainage).
   e. Stevens-Johnson syndrome.
   f. Tetanus.
   g. Toxoplasmosis.
   h. Reye's syndrome.
   i. Peritonitis.

Reverse isolation

Reverse isolation is indicated for patients who are immunosuppressed or unusually susceptible to infection (e.g., burn patients).

Initiation of reverse isolation precautions
1. A private room is necessary for the patient who requires reverse isolation.
2. A laminar flow system is ideal. This system circulates filtered air along parallel lines, which helps to prevent bacterial contamination of the air. If a laminar system is not available, air filters in the room should be changed between patients.
3. The door to this room must remain closed at all times.
4. Each reverse isolation room should have an adjacent anteroom for personnel to gown and wash hands.
5. The room must be thoroughly cleaned with a germicidal agent before the patient's entry. An ultraviolet light must be used to prepare an aseptic environment for the patient.

Maintenance of reverse isolation
1. All articles must be sterilized before patient contact.
2. Sterile linen must be used.
3. Gloves, masks, gowns, and hats must be worn by all personnel entering the room.
4. Hands must be thoroughly washed before patient contact.

Prevention of employee infection

Accidental needle sticks and/or exposure to infected blood and body secretions occur frequently in the PICU setting. In consideration for the health and welfare of the employees, the infection control department is notified immediately at the time of the incident and proper prophylactic measures for the employee are taken based on the patient's condition and diagnosis.
1. Hepatitis B or Hepatitis non A-non B: if the status of the patient is unknown, blood is

drawn for Hepatitis B surface antigen (HbsAg) determination on the patient and Hepatitis B surface antibody (HbsAb) on the employee, and the employee receives appropriate prophylactic treatment based on the test results.

2. Meningococcal disease: Considering the degree of intimacy and/or type of exposure of the employee and the length of the antibiotic treatment that the patient has received, penicillin or rifampin is prescribed for the employee.

3. Other communicable diseases (e.g., pertussis, diphtheria, rabies, pneumonic plague, bacterial sepsis): Appropriate antibiotic therapy is provided for the employee.

ADDITIONAL READING

LaForce, F.M., and Eickhoff, T.C.: The role of infection in critical care, Anesthesiology 47:195-202, 1977.
Sanford, J.P.: Infection control in critical care units, Crit. Care Med. 2:211-216, 1974.

41 Sepsis

J. PATRICK HIEBER

DEFINITION AND PHYSIOLOGY

The term sepsis connotes a constellation of signs and symptoms associated with the presence of an infectious agent in the bloodstream: bacteremia, viremia, fungemia, or rickettsemia. Such infections may be transient or persistent, and they may be clinically silent for hours to days (rarely for weeks) before they cause the patient to become septic. Manifestations of this clinical problem are protean and include those summarized in Table 41-1. Age is an important variable to be taken into account when evaluating these patients. For example, the septic neonate will often manifest subtle lethargy, feeding difficulties, hypothermia, and hypoglycemia, whereas the older patient may be expected to have confusion, generalized seizures, coma, hyperthermia, and rigors in many instances. Many of the signs and symptoms have complex causes; for example, tachypnea may be due to associated pneumonia, hypoxia, respiratory compensation for metabolic acidosis, and/or CNS dysfunction. Most symptoms are related to shock syndrome and may be viewed as effects of circulatory failure.

The mechanisms whereby infectious organisms produce the complex pathophysiology of sepsis are largely unknown, but those that have been identified or suspected are listed in Table 41-2. In the case of gram-negative bacteremia, elaboration of endotoxin is a proven cause of decreasing cardiac output and increasing capillary permeability. Vasculitis may also be induced by localization of the organisms in the endothelium or by toxins, which may also have deleterious effects on distant organ systems (CNS, hepatic, renal). It is intriguing that the metabolic and immune responses of the host may be fundamental to the disease manifestations as well as to the eventual eradication of the organism.

LABORATORY EVALUATION

After the clinical diagnosis is appreciated, culture and Gram stains of blood, CSF, urine, and other affected sites before therapy are the primary methods of documenting a bacterial cause. When positive, counterimmunoelectro-

Table 41-1. Manifestations of sepsis

Alteration in level of consciousness
Seizures
Tachypnea, tachycardia
Temperature and blood pressure instability
Inadequate peripheral circulation
Skin rashes—petechial, ecchymotic, pustular
Ileus
Decreased urine flow
Hypoglycemia, hypocalcemia
Disseminated intravascular coagulation

Table 41-2. Mechanisms of sepsis

Endotoxin
Vasculitis
  Organism in endothelium (virus, rickettsia)
  Toxins (staphylococcal α-toxin, streptococcal hemolytic and erythrogenic toxins)
Host response
  Hypoglycemia, hypocalcemia
  T-cell (causes hepatocyte destruction in type B hepatitis)
  Antigen-antibody complexes (serum sickness, glomerulonephritis)

phoresis (CIE) may provide a specific diagnosis within a few hours. The usefulness of the WBC count and differential analysis has been improved by the recent observation that a patient with an absolute polymorphonuclear leukocyte count $\geq 10,000/mm^3$ and/or an absolute band-form count $\geq 500/mm^3$ has an 80% chance of having a bacteremia. Cultures for fungi should be attempted but may be negative at the same time that clinical response to therapy and serologic studies document a fungal etiologic role. Tissue culture and serology are standard methods of viral diagnosis, but often results return too slowly to be clinically useful. Recent applications of tissue staining (Tzanck test) and electronic microscopy to skin lesions and of immunofluorescent staining to nasopharyngeal secretions indicate that prompt, specific diagnosis of viral disease will become available to the clinician in the near future. Rickettsial disease is an area where the laboratory is of minimal help in early diagnosis; typical history and findings on physical examination in association with thrombocytopenia and hyponatremia often demand therapy long before confirmatory serology is available.

MONITORING

See also Chapter 4.

Infection

1. Cultures and Gram stains of blood, CSF, urine, and other affected sites before therapy and repeat any positive cultures until negative results are obtained.
2. Repeat cultures 24 to 36 hours after discontinuing therapy.
3. Erythrocyte sedimentation rate (ESR) serially until normal.
4. WBC count and differential analysis serially until normal.

Cardiorespiratory system

1. A widening pulse pressure may be indicative of vasodilation as a result of endotoxin-induced release of vasoactive substances. Narrowed pulse pressure or pulsus paradoxus may be associated with a significant pericardial effusion.
2. Measure Pa_{O_2}, Pa_{CO_2}, and pH every 2 hours. Metabolic acidosis is frequently observed in septic patients.

Hematologic system

1. Obtain platelet count.
2. If oozing, petechiae, thrombosis, or other evidence of abnormal clotting occurs, screen for DIC (see Chapter 20) by examining a blood smear and measuring PT and PTT.

Other systems

Observe for the potential complication of ISADH (see Chapter 51).

MANAGEMENT

Only rarely are the specific etiologic agent and its antimicrobial sensitivities known at the initiation of therapy. Therefore, drugs are chosen to cover the most likely pathogens (Table 41-3). Typically, neonates receive ampicillin and an aminoglycoside, patients 6 weeks to 6 years of age receive ampicillin and chloramphenicol, and older patients receive penicillin alone. The choice of which aminoglycoside to use depends on the current antimicrobial sensitivity patterns of each hospital. When the patient is immunocompromised, regardless of age, combinations of gentamicin with either carbenicillin or cephalothin are often used to provide coverage against staphylococci and *Pseudomonas* organisms. Chloramphenicol may be used alone in the case of penicillin hypersensitivity. As soon as the organism is identified and its sensitivities determined, antimicrobial therapy should be tailored to provide maximum bacterial killing with minimal toxicity, in the narrowest possible spectrum. The dosages employed depend on the patient's age and renal and hepatic function and on knowledge of the drug's pharmacology, so that therapeutic concentra-

Table 41-3. Common causative agents of sepsis

Organism	Usual patient age	Clinical clues	Drug(s) of choice
E. coli and other enterics	Neonate	Immunocompromised older patients, steroids, malignancy, indwelling catheters, sickle hemoglobinopathies	Aminoglycoside: kanamycin or gentamicin
Group B streptococci	Neonate	Older patients with diabetes; pregnancy; cirrhosis; malignancy	Ampicillin and aminoglycoside in neonate; penicillin in older patient
Group D streptococci and *Listeria monocytogenes*	Neonate	Older patients with diabetes; pregnancy; cirrhosis; malignancy	Ampicillin and aminoglycoside
Haemophilus influenzae	6 wk–6 yr	Asplenia, buccal cellulitis, arthritis, epiglottitis, meningitis	Chloramphenicol until known to be ampicillin-sensitive or cefamandole if CNS infection is excluded
Pneumococci, meningococci, group A streptococci	6 wk–adult	Asplenia, decreased immunoglobulins	Penicillin
Staphylococci	All ages	Furuncles, osteomyelitis, arthritis, postoperative state, indwelling foreign bodies, deep-tissue abscess	Methicillin or nafcillin until proved penicillin-sensitive
Viruses	All ages	Congenital infection syndrome (cytomegalovirus, rubella), season of year, immunocompromised host, vesicular rash, encephalitis with temporal lobe localization	Herpes simplex: adenine arabinoside, 15 mg/kg as 12-hr IV infusion daily × 10 days. Experimental drug may be efficacious if started early in course of encephalitis.
Rickettsiae	Children–adults	Tick exposure, spring-summer-fall, conjunctivitis with centripetal rash	Chloramphenicol or tetra-tetracycline

tions are achieved at the sites of infection (Table 41-4). Steroids are often mentioned as being useful in restoring capillary integrity and improving cardiac output in the septic patient. Most of the data are anecdotal and uncontrolled. Studies in patients with meningococcemia show that most patients have normal to increased levels of endogenous steroids and that massive dosages of steroids do not significantly affect the clinical outcome. These facts, in conjunction with the myriad of adverse side effects associated with steroid usage, including decreased host defenses against infection (decreased chemotaxis, phagocytosis, and delayed hypersensitivity), argue strongly against the use of steroids for sepsis in all but the most unusual settings.

Effective therapy will clear the blood of or-

Table 41-4. Antibiotics commonly used for sepsis—daily dosages (IM or IV)

Drug	0-7 days of age	>7 days of age	Toxicity and remarks	Suggested routine evaluation for potential toxicities
Penicillin G	100,000-150,000 units/kg/day* divided q8-12h	150,000-250,000 units/ kg/day (maximum 20 million units/ day) divided q4-8h	When treating meningitis, use the higher dosages and shorter intervals noted, to provide maximum concentrations of drug in CSF	Biweekly Hb and Hct, weekly serum potassium
Ampicillin	100 mg/kg/day divided q12h	150-200 mg/kg/day (maximum 10-14 g/ day) divided q6-8h		
			Rarely may cause hemolytic anemia and hypokalemia	
Kanamycin	15-20 mg/kg/day divided q12h	20-30 mg/kg/day divided q8-12h		
			Monitor for nephrotoxicity and ototoxicity during prolonged therapy; reduced dosage necessary in the presence of decreased renal function	Biweekly urinalysis, BUN, and serum creatinine; creatinine clearance if these values become abnormal
Gentamicin	5 mg/kg/day divided q12h	7.5 mg/kg/day (6 mg/kg/day in patients over age 2 yr) divided q8h		
Cefamandole	Not used	50-150 mg/kg/day divided q4-6h	Unreliable CNS penetration	
Chloramphenicol	25 mg/kg once daily	25-50 mg/kg/day divided q12-24h (50-100 mg/kg/day divided q6h in patients over 3 mo of age)	IV only; observe for Gray syndrome and bone marrow suppression; avoid when liver dysfunction present	Weekly CBC and platelet count
Tetracycline	Not used	25-50 mg/kg/day divided q6h (as a 2-hr infusion) in patients over 2 mo of age	Stains teeth and bones in patients <6-7 yr of age; avoid when liver dysfunction present	
Nafcillin	Not used	50-100 mg/kg/day divided q6h in patients >1 mo of age	Avoid when liver dysfunction present	

Data from Nelson, J.D.: Pocketbook of pediatric antimicrobial therapy, ed. 4, Dallas, 1980, published by author.
*Note: When ranges of dosages and intervals are stated, the smaller dosages and lower intervals are intended for infants weighing less than 2000 g.

Table 41-4. Antibiotics commonly used for sepsis—daily dosages (IM or IV)—cont'd

Drug	0-7 days of age	>7 days of age	Toxicity and remakrs	Suggested routine evaluation for potential toxicities
Methicillin	50-75 mg/kg/day divided q8-12h	100-150 mg/kg/day divided q6-8h (100-200 mg/kg/day divided q6h in patients >1 mo of age)	Monitor for cystitis and nephrotoxicity	Biweekly urinalysis, BUN, and serum creatinine
Carbenicillin	200 mg/kg/day divided q12h	300-400 mg/kg/day divided q6-8h	Combine with aminoglycoside for synergy against pseudomonas; rarely may cause hypokalemia	Weekly serum potassium

ganisms promptly, and persistence of bacteremia should prompt a search for occult sites of infection (indwelling catheters, deep tissue abscesses) as well as a thorough review of the current therapy (dosage, route and frequency of administration, sensitivity of the organism). Serial assessment of renal and hepatic function, temperature, CBC, and sedimentation rate is essential for the early diagnosis of drug toxicity and provides the basis for adjustments in dosage. In the absence of severe underlying disease or secondary foci of infection, therapy is continued for 3 to 5 days beyond the point when the trend of most clinical and laboratory factors is toward normal, usually a total of 7 to 10 days. A major exception to this rule is rickettsial disease, in which 14 to 21 days of therapy is considered the minimum.

Supportive and specific therapy for the associated problems of shock, acute renal failure, and DIC are discussed in Chapters 14, 17, and 20, respectively.

42 Toxic shock syndrome

JANE D. SIEGEL

DEFINITION AND PHYSIOLOGY

Toxic shock syndrome was first described in children ages 8 to 17 years, in 1978. During the next 18 months, more than 100 suspected cases of toxic shock syndrome were reported to the Centers for Disease Control (CDC) in Atlanta. Although the clinical features of these later cases were similar to those in the cases originally described, 95% of affected individuals were young women in the first 5 days of their menstrual period. Toxin-producing strains of *Staphylococcus aureus* were isolated from the mucosal surfaces of the majority of both groups of patients. Retrospective analysis has shown that the earliest cases that meet the strict definition of toxic shock syndrome occurred in 1972. However, a literature review suggests that severe cases of staphylococcal scarlet fever reported in 1927 may have been, in reality, the first cases of toxic shock syndrome. As a result of intensive surveillance and investigation of affected patients identified during the past 3 years, the epidemiology, clinical manifestations, and pathogenesis of toxic shock syndrome have been well described.

Toxic shock syndrome is predominantly a disease of women of childbearing age, with 80% of cases occurring in women less than 30 years of age. Men account for 2.5% of all cases. The usual age of reported cases varies from 6 to 61 years, but we have encountered a confirmed case in a two-year-old boy. Toxic shock syndrome has also been reported to occur in adults within the first 5 days following surgery.

The case definition of toxic shock syndrome that has been adopted by the CDC is presented in Table 42-1. These patients often present with a 1 to 2 day history of fever greater than 38.5° C, sore throat, myalgias, vomiting, and watery diarrhea. They typically develop a diffuse, blanching rash that has a characteristic sunburn appearance and that is mainly truncal in distribution, with accentuation in the inguinal and axillary folds as well as in areas of pressure. Indurative edema of the palms and soles may develop. Desquamation of the involved skin and of the palms and soles occurs during the second week of illness. A vaginal discharge may be observed. Hypotension occurs during the first 48 to 72 hours of illness and may be severe and prolonged due to massive vasodilatation and rapid movement of serum proteins and fluid from the intravascular to the extravascular compartment. The multisystem involvement may be a reflection of the rapid onset of hypotension and decreased organ perfusion or the result of the action of a toxin on multiple target organs. Diffuse vasculitis has been observed in skin biopsies and postmortem specimens. Acute renal failure results from both prerenal impairment and intrinsic renal disease. Late sequelae include a reversible hair and nail loss, vocal cord paralysis, and a peripheral neuropathy.

In most patients initial laboratory findings reveal a leukocytosis with a high proportion of immature neutrophils. Other findings include thrombocytopenia, hyponatremia, hypocalcemia, evidence of hepatic and renal dysfunction, elevated CPK, and myoglobinuria. CSF is usually normal but rarely may show a pleocytosis of less than 100 cells/μl with normal glucose and protein.

There is a recurrence rate of approximately 30% in menstruating females. These women

Table 42-1. Case definition of toxic shock syndrome

Fever: temperature $\geq 38.5°$ C
Rash: diffuse macular erythroderma (sunburn appearance)
Desquamation of palms and soles 1 to 2 weeks after onset of illness
Hypotension: systemic arterial systolic blood pressure ≤ 90 mm Hg for adults or below fifth percentile by
    age for children less than 16 years of age; drop in systemic arterial diastolic blood pressure ≥ 15 mm Hg
    from lying to sitting (orthostatic syncope)
Multisystem involvement—three or more of the following:
    Gastrointestinal: vomiting or diarrhea at onset of illness
    Muscular: severe myalgia or CPK level at least twice the upper limit of normal for laboratory
    Mucous membrane: vaginal, oropharyngeal, or conjunctival hyperemia
    Renal: BUN or creatinine at least twice the upper limit of normal for laboratory or urinary sediment
        with ≥ 5 white cells per high power field in the absence of urinary tract infection
    Hepatic: total bilirubin, SGOT, or SGPT at least twice the upper limit of normal for laboratory
    Hematologic: platelets $\leq 100,000/\mu l$
    Central nervous system: disorientation or alterations in consciousness without focal neurologic signs
        when fever and hypotension are absent
Negative results on the following tests, if obtained:
    Blood, throat, CSF cultures
    Rise in titer to Rocky Mountain spotted fever, leptospirosis, or rubeola

Adapted from Shands, K.N., Schmid, G.P., Dan, B.B., and others: N. Engl. J. Med. **303:**1436-1442, 1980.

usually experience recurrences within a month or two of the initial episode, but an interval of a year or more has been documented. The recurrences are usually milder than the initial episode, but have been on occasion more severe, with some patients requiring multiple intensive care unit admissions. The maximum number of reported recurrences is five. Failure to eradicate the toxin-producing staphylococcus and to produce antibody to the toxin during convalescence increase the risk of recurrence. The overall case fatality rate for toxic shock syndrome is 7.8%.

The differential diagnosis of staphylococcal toxic shock syndrome includes bacterial septicemia, Kawasaki disease, staphylococcal scalded skin syndrome, scarlet fever, Rocky Mountain spotted fever, leptospirosis, rubeola, Stevens-Johnson syndrome, viral hepatitis, Legionnaire's disease, and hemolytic-uremic syndrome.

Staphylococcus aureus has been clearly implicated as the etiologic agent of toxic shock syn-

drome. This pathogen has been isolated from at least one mucosal surface or from a sequestered collection of pus (abscess, empyema) in the majority of patients who have been cultured prior to the initiation of antimicrobial therapy. Blood cultures, however, are sterile in 95% of cases. *Staphylococcus aureus* has been isolated from vaginal cultures in 96% of women with toxic shock syndrome, but in only 10% of matched controls. Ninety-two percent of isolates from patients are resistant to penicillin as compared to 57% of isolates from controls. A previously undescribed toxin has been isolated from patient strains and characterized, and it is believed to be responsible for the production of the clinical manifestations of toxic shock syndrome. The clinical diagnosis of probable cases is now confirmed by the isolation of *Staphylococcus aureus* from a mucosal surface or collection of pus and by identification of this toxin. Measurement of antibody to the toxin in acute and convalescent sera further supports the diagnosis. The pathogenic staphylococci are eradicated from all sites within 72 hours of therapy with a β-lactamase–resistant antistaphylococcal drug.

The use of tampons has been associated with a significantly increased risk of developing toxic shock syndrome. However, the association with one particular brand has not been upheld. Tampons may act either as a vehicle for the introduction and perpetuation of the offending pathogen or as a local irritant, causing cervicovaginal ulcerations that permit systemic invasion of the locally produced toxin.

MONITORING

See also Chapter 4.

Infection

1. Cultures of blood, all mucosal surfaces (nasopharynx; conjunctiva; trachea, if intubation performed; rectum; vagina), and stool, if diarrhea is present.
2. Any strain of *Staphylococcus aureus* that is isolated should be sent to the state laboratory, which will send it to the CDC for toxin testing.
3. Appropriate cultures and serologic tests should be obtained to exclude other diagnostic possibilities, as indicated in individual patients.
4. WBC count and differential.
5. Body temperature.

Cardiorespiratory system

See Septic shock, p. 72.

Hematologic system

See Septic shock, p. 73.

Renal-metabolic system

See Septic shock, p. 73.

MANAGEMENT
Infection

1. Remove tampons and irrigate vagina with sterile saline.

2. Drain abscess or empyema.
3. Administer a β-lactamase–resistant antistaphylococcal drug such as nafcillin, 150 mg/kg/day divided every 6 hours, or vancomycin, 40 mg/kg/day divided every 6 hours, for 10 days. Antistaphylococcal antibiotics reduce the recurrence rate in young women who have menstrually related illnesses. If the drug is given early in the acute illness, the clinical course may be shortened.

Cardiorespiratory system

See Septic shock, pp. 73-88.

Renal-metabolic system

See Septic shock, pp. 73-88.

ADDITIONAL READING

Centers for Disease Control: Toxic shock syndrome—United States, 1970-1980, Morbid. Mortal. Weekly Rep. 30:25-33, 1981.

Chesney, P.J., Davis, J.P., Purdy, W.K., and others: Clinical manifestations of toxic shock syndrome, J.A.M.A. 246:741-748, 1981.

Davis, J.P., Chesney, P.J., Wand, P.J., and others: Toxic-shock syndrome: epidemiologic features, recurrence, risk factors and prevention, N. Engl. J. Med. 303:1429-1435, 1980.

Schlievert, P.M., Shands, K.N., Dan, B.B., and others: Identification and characterization of an exotoxin from *Staphylococcus aureus* associated with toxic-shock syndrome, J. Infect. Dis. 143:509-515, 1981.

Shands, K.N., Schmid, G.P., Dan, B.B., and others: Toxic shock syndrome in menstruating women, N. Engl. J. Med. 303:1436-1442, 1980.

Todd, J., and Fishaut, M.: Toxic-shock syndrome associated with phage group I staphylococci, Lancet 2:1116-1118, 1978.

Tofte, R.W., and Williams, D.N.: Toxic shock syndrome: clinical and laboratory features in 15 patients, Ann. Intern. Med. 94:149-156, 1981.

Turner, G.R., Jackson, M.A., and Levin, D.L.: Toxic shock syndrome in a 23-month-old male infant, J. Pediatr. Infect. Dis. 2:314-316, 1983.

43 Encephalitis/meningitis

J. PATRICK HIEBER

DEFINITION AND PHYSIOLOGY

CNS infections may be manifested primarily by signs and symptoms of meningeal inflammation (fever, headache, nuchal rigidity) or of CNS dysfunction (altered consciousness, seizures, sensory-motor or autonomic disturbances), termed meningitis and encephalitis, respectively. Most often, the patient with CNS infection will have a mixed syndrome of meningoencephalitis. Although fungi, rickettsiae, and parasites may produce CNS infections, bacteria and viruses are by far the most common causes. The principal route by which these organisms gain access to the meninges and the CNS is hematogenous dissemination from a distant site of infection or colonization (e.g., of the nasopharynx). Less commonly, operative contamination, contiguous spread from a parameningeal focus (otitis media, sinusitis, etc.), or arthropod vectors are responsible. Thus, the major causes of bacterial meningitis classified according to age and underlying diseases are identical to those of bacterial sepsis (see Table 41-3). *Mycobacterium tuberculosis* must be added to complete this list. The pathogens commonly responsible for encephalitis/aseptic meningitis in this country are summarized in Table 43-1. The vast majority of presumed viral CNS infections (negative bacterial and fungal studies) are without a specific identifiable pathogen in the routine diagnostic laboratory.

The incidence of viremia and bacteremia is far greater than that of CNS infections. The mechanisms underlying the predilection of certain organisms to localize in the CNS are just beginning to be elucidated. One important variable is the antigenic characteristics of the bacterial capsule. For example, *Escherichia coli* and group B streptococci account for over 70% of all bacterial meningitis in neonates; surprisingly, the K1 serotype of *E. coli* (out of 100 K types) and the type III strain of group B streptococci (out of five types) account for 90% of all such episodes. Furthermore, the polysaccharide antigens of these two organisms are similar to antigens on the surface of pneumococci,

Table 43-1. Cases of encephalitis/aseptic meningitis in the United States (1974)

Category and causes	Percent of total
Enteroviral (echo, Coxsackie, polio)	6.0
Associated with childhood infections	2.0
Mumps	
Chickenpox	
Measles	
Other agents	3.9
California encephalitis	
Adenovirus	
Mycobacterium pneumoniae	
Herpes simplex	
Herpes zoster	
Lymphocytic choriomeningitis	
Viral-unspecified	
Indeterminate	88.1
Complex	
Associated with non-CNS enteroviral isolate	
Associated with other non-CNS isolate	
Unknown	
TOTAL	100.0

meningococci, and *Haemophilus influenzae*, the prime causes of meningitis in older patients.

The signs and symptoms noted above are provoked by cellular damage and death and the resulting inflammatory response (cerebritis) provoked by the proliferating organisms and their toxins. In addition, transient neurologic dysfunction and/or permanent sequelae may be due to several factors, including vasculitis, thrombosis, infarction, subdural effusion/empyema, and postinflammatory hydrocephalus.

CLINICAL AND LABORATORY EVALUATION

The history should emphasize exposure to infectious diseases such as tuberculosis, meningococcemia, and viral infections. While performing the physical examination, one should be attentive to the neurologic status of the patient and to dermatologic clues of the etiologic agent; e.g., petechiae progressing to purpura

fulminans strongly suggest meningococcemia. A diligent search for other less obvious sites of infection (pericardium, lungs, bones, and joints) seeded during the bacteremia should be made by examination and chest roentgenogram. Blood should be drawn for culture, and an aliquot of serum may be saved to be paired with a convalescent specimen when a nonbacterial cause is likely.

CSF examination is the major diagnostic test. If multiple signs of increased ICP are noted (bulging fontanelle, widened sutures, retinal hemorrhages or papilledema, irregular respiration, decreased heart rate, and increased systemic arterial blood pressure), LP should be done in consultation with a neurosurgeon to minimize the chances of herniation. In all cases, the needle should have a stylet and be of a narrow gauge (23G). It is important to realize that the normal CSF values in the neonate are considerably different from those in patients more than 6 months old (Table 43-2). Most patients are easily classified as having either bacterial or viral disease (Table 43-3). However, pretreatment of bacterial cases with antibiotics and the early polymorphonuclear cellular predominance

Table 43-2. Normal values for CSF examination

	Neonates		Patients >6 mo of age
	Preterm	Term	
WBC/mm³			
Mean	9	8	0
±2 SD	0-25	0-22	0-4
PMNs* (%)	57	61	0
Protein (mg/dl)			
Mean	115	90	<40
Range	65-150	20-170	
Glucose (mg/dl)			
Mean	50	52	>40
Range	24-63	34-119	
CSF/blood glucose (%)			
Mean	74	81	50
Range	55-150	44-248	40-60

Adapted from Sarff, L.D., Platt, L.H., and McCracken, G.H., Jr.: Cerebrospinal fluid evaluation in neonates: comparison of high-risk infants with and without meningitis, J. Pediatr. **88:**473-477, 1976.
*Polymorphonuclear leukocyte.

Table 43-3. CSF characteristics in encephalitis/meningitis

Setting	Range of WBC count (cells/mm³)
Acute bacterial	500 or greater
Acute bacterial pretreated with antibiotics	500 or greater
M. tuberculosis	10-350
Aseptic (presumed viral)	50-500 (rarely >1,000) (herpes may be hemorrhagic)

*Polymorphonuclear leukocyte.

and low CSF glucose values seen in some viral cases may produce confusing intermediate values. In these cases, special examinations of the CSF by CIE or latex agglutination for the detection of bacterial antigens or analysis of CSF for the presence of endotoxin or increased concentrations of LDH will often permit a firm diagnosis of bacterial cause. Negative results, however, do not rule out a bacterial cause.

MONITORING

See also Chapter 4.

Infection

1. CBC with differential analysis initially and serially thereafter until normal.
2. Platelet count initially and serially thereafter until normal.
3. CSF (see Management, pp. 283-285).

Neurologic system

1. Repeated neurologic examinations should be performed by the nurse according to a specific protocol (see Chapters 6 and 10) and recorded every hour on a neurologic examination flow sheet.

2. In children less than 2 years of age, daily measurement of head circumference is especially important because of the incidence of hydrocephalus after severe infection.
3. Observe closely for seizure activity.
4. Because of the frequency of ISADH syndrome (see Chapter 51), it may be helpful to measure initially spot urine Na, K, and osmolality with simultaneous serum Na, K, and osmolality.

MANAGEMENT

Initial antibiotic therapy should be given to all patients with meningoencephalitis, except those with a clearly aseptic (nonbacterial) process. In most cases, therapy is directed against the most likely bacterial pathogens based on the patient's age and underlying problems (see Table 41-3): ampicillin and an aminoglycoside from birth to 6 weeks, ampicillin and chloramphenicol from 6 weeks to 6 years, and penicillin alone for older patients. Because of the occasional Gram-variable appearance of organisms and the more frequent misinterpretation of Gram stains, it is most conservative to narrow the spectrum after culture and/or CIE provide

Differential count	CSF:blood glucose (%)	CSF protein (mg/dl)	Gram stain	Culture
PMN* predominance (monocytosis may be seen with *Listeria*)	<40	>100	Positive	Positive
PMN predominance	<40	>100	May be negative (especially meningococcus)	
Lymphocyte predominance (PMNs early)	<30	300 or greater	Negative (acid-fast stain of pellicle may be positive)	Positive
Lymphocyte predominance (PMNs early)	>40 (may be <40 early)	<100	Negative	Occasionally positive for virus

a specific etiologic diagnosis (see Table 41-3). The penicillins and aminoglycosides penetrate the CSF relatively poorly; therefore, it is important to use the higher dosages and shorter intervals noted in Table 41-4 for each group.

Over the past few years it has been recognized that 10% to 15% of *H. influenzae* strains are ampicillin-resistant by virtue of their ability to produce β-lactamase. Therefore, chloramphenicol has been added to the initial therapy of the age group from 6 weeks to 6 years, in which *H. influenzae* is the major bacterial pathogen. Ampicillin is also used initially to provide bactericidal activity against the other major pathogens and to provide protection against the recently reported (rare) strains of chloramphenicol-resistant *H. influenzae*. Testing of the strain for β-lactamase production soon after plate isolation usually provides a basis for discontinuation of the chloramphenicol on the second day of therapy. In cases due to β-lactamase–positive strains, continued therapy with chloramphenicol alone increases the risk of hematologic toxicity. The serious, often permanent, aplastic reaction known to occur after approximately one in 50,000 exposures is idiosyncratic, non–dose related, and totally unpredictable. In contrast, serial monitoring of CBC and platelet count is helpful in detecting the more common, transient, dose-related bone marrow suppression that rarely necessitates premature discontinuation of the drug.

A repeat LP should be performed 24 to 36 hours after the initiation of therapy. Persisting (or worsening) abnormalities of CSF cell count, glucose, and protein are commonly seen at this point, but effective antibiotic therapy will have rendered the Gram stain and culture negative in most cases (Table 43-3). Persistence of enteric organisms for several days is common, but persistence of other organisms occurs less commonly. Delayed sterilization should prompt a search for correctable factors, including review of the drug(s) in relation to the sensitivities of the organism as well as dosage and route of administration; also search for a sequestered parameningeal focus of infection, such as sinusitis, otitis media, subdural empyema, or ventriculitis. Subdural empyema may be treated by operative drainage or repeated needle aspiration until sterile and dry. Therapy for ventriculitis (positive Gram stain and culture; >100 WBCs/mm^3) is still evolving. Currently, daily intraventricular instillation (via indwelling reservoir or needle) of gentamicin until ventricular fluid culture is sterile is being evaluated. Conflicting reports in the literature on the efficacy and potential toxicity of this approach have led to the recent trials of newer antibiotics, such as moxalactam. Such aggressive therapy is being studied because previous studies have shown that the neurologic sequelae of meningitis are well correlated with the length of time required to achieve CSF sterilization. The currently recommended drugs and duration of therapy for the major age groups and pathogens are summarized in Table 43-4.

Patients with bacterial meningitis may be removed from isolation 12 hours after onset of therapy. Most patients are afebrile after 4 to 5 days of therapy; the differential diagnosis of prolonged fever includes the complications noted above as well as thrombophlebitis, nosocomial infection (upper respiratory tract, urinary tract, etc.), and drug fever. The question of whether an LP should be performed at the end of therapy is a controversial one. When the patient's hospital course has been uncomplicated, CSF examination may be omitted. When a final LP is deemed prudent, one must interpret the results cautiously to avoid unnecessary prolongation of therapy; several recent studies have shown that up to 25% of patients in whom therapy is stopped without subsequent relapse may have one or more abnormalities in CSF values.

Prophylactic antibiotic therapy is recommended for those intimately exposed to a confirmed case of meningococcal disease. Unless the organism is known to be sulfa-sensitive, rifampin is the drug of choice, 20 mg/kg/day

Table 43-4. Therapy for bacterial meningoencephalitis

Setting	Usual duration of positive CSF cultures	Recommended drug(s) and duration of therapy	Remarks
Neonate with enteric meningitis (rarely older patients)	3-4 days	Ampicillin and aminoglycoside for 21 days from date of first sterile culture	Both drugs continued in order to take advantage of potential synergistic killing
Neonate with group B streptococcus, *Listeria monocytogenes*, enterococcus	<36 hr	Ampicillin and aminoglycoside for 14 days from date of first sterile culture	
H. influenzae	<36 hr	Ampicillin and chloramphenicol initially; then either one (depending on sensitivities) for a total of 10-14 days	During last 5 days of therapy ampicillin may be given IM and chloramphenicol PO
Pneumococcus, streptococcus, meningococcus	<24 hr	Penicillin G for 7 (meningococcus) to 14 (streptococcus, pneumococcus) days	
M. tuberculosis	Not applicable	Isoniazid, 20 mg/kg/day PO or IM divided q12-24h, *and* rifampin, 20 mg/kg/day divided q12-24h × 18-24 mo, *and* streptomycin, 30 mg/kg/day IM divided q12h	Change streptomycin to 2 times weekly after 2-3 weeks; continue 6-8 weeks total; PAS may be substituted for rifampin after 2-3 months if cost is a problem

orally in divided doses every 12 to 24 hours (600 mg) for 3 to 5 days. Children less than 2 years of age with intimate (family or day care center) exposure to invasive *H. influenzae* type B disease are also candidates for rifampin prophylaxis. Since public health policy is still evolving on this subject, each case must be considered individually.

Therapy for the viral meningoencephalitides is generally supportive, since specific antiviral therapy is unavailable for most cases. If a brain biopsy diagnosis of herpes simplex can be made before the patient is in deep coma, therapy with adenosine arabinoside has been shown to decrease mortality and neurologic sequelae (see Table 41-3). Decisions on the need for and the duration of isolation depend on the mode of spread of the particular virus involved.

General supportive therapy for patients with meningoencephalitis (regardless of cause)

includes attention to temperature regulation, seizures, and fluid electrolyte balance. The last area is especially important in light of the common occurrence of cerebral edema and ISADH syndrome. In general, fluids are given initially at a rate sufficient to provide adequate circulation and to maintain the urine specific gravity in the range of 1.010 to 1.015, i.e., about two-thirds maintenance. In most cases, steroids have been shown to be of no benefit; an exception to this rule has been demonstrated in tuberculous meningitis, in which steroids have been shown to decrease mortality but to have no effect on neurologic sequelae.

ADDITIONAL READING

Chartrand, S.A., and Cho, C.T.: Persistent pleocytosis in bacterial meningitis, J. Pediatr. **88:**424-426, 1976.

Cox, F., Trincher, R., Rissing, J.P., and others: Rifampin prophylaxis for contacts of *Haemophilus influenzae* type B disease, J.A.M.A. **245:**1043-1045, 1981.

Feigin, R.D., Wong, M., Shackelford, P., and others: Countercurrent immunoelectrophoresis of urine as well as of CSF and blood for diagnosis of bacterial meningitis, J. Pediatr. **89:**773-775, 1976.

McCracken, G.H., Jr.: Rapid identification of specific etiology in meningitis, J. Pediatr. **88:**706-708, 1976.

McCracken, G.H., Jr., Mize, S.G., and Threlkeld, N.: Intraventricular gentamicin therapy in gram-negative bacillary meningitis of infancy, report of the Second Neonatal Meningitis Cooperative Study Group, Lancet **1:**787-791, 1980.

Migeon, C.J., Kenny, F.M., Hung, W., and Voorhess, M.L.: Study of adrenal function in children with meningitis, Pediatrics **40:**163-183, 1967.

Pickering, L.K., Ericsson, C.D., Ruiz-Palacious, G., and others: Intraventricular and parenteral gentamicin therapy for ventriculitis in children, Am. J. Dis. Child. **132:** 480-483, 1978.

Schaad, U.B., McCracken, G.H., Jr., Threlkeld, N., and Thomas, M.L.: Clinical evaluation of a new broad-spectrum oxa-beta-lactam antibiotic, moxalactam, in neonates and infants, J. Pediatr. **98:**129-136, 1981.

Stiehm, E.R., and Damrosch, D.S.: Factors in the prognosis of meningococcal infection, J. Pediatr. **68:**457-467, 1966.

Swartz, M.N.: Intraventricular use of aminoglycosides in the treatment of gram-negative bacillary meningitis: conflicting views, editorial, J. Infect. Dis. **143:**293-295, 1981.

44 Peritonitis

J. PATRICK HIEBER
WILLIAM DAMMERT

DEFINITION AND PHYSIOLOGY

Inflammation of the serous peritoneal lining may be due to bacterial infection and/or chemical irritation. A classification of bacterial peritonitis by primary and secondary types is given in Table 44-1.

Primary peritonitis may rarely occur in the absence of underlying disease at any age, but more commonly it is seen at the extremes of life and in association with nephrosis, ascites, or cirrhosis. The majority of cases are due to pneumococci or streptococci, although *Haemophilus influenzae* and gram-negative enteric organisms have been isolated occasionally. These infections are almost always monomicrobial; this fact and the high incidence of associated bacteremia form the basis for the presumption that the organisms arrive at the peritoneum via a hematogenous route.

In contrast, secondary peritonitis is due to leakage of bowel contents into the abdominal cavity. Both chemical irritation (from meconium, feces, bile, gastric and pancreatic secretions, food, or talcum powder) and bacterial infection are etiologically important. The bacterial flora of the gastrointestinal tract is a complex mixture of aerobic and anaerobic organisms; thus, leakage of this material often results in a polymicrobial infection. Currently, it is believed that no single organism is the primary pathogen but that the components interact in a complex synergistic enhancement of one another. Animal experiments suggest that the aerobic enteric organisms are primarily responsible for early toxicity, peritoneal inflammation, and death, whereas the anaerobes are responsible for late abscess formation. *Bacteroides fragilis* is a particularly common anaerobic isolate.

Patients may have large fluid deficits due to decreased intake, vomiting, fever, and accumulation of fluid and protein in the bowel and peritoneal cavity similar to burn patients. Stress and hypovolemia may result in shock, hypothermia, hypoglycemia, and DIC.

MONITORING

See also Chapter 4.

Abdomen

1. Examine the abdomen every 2 to 4 hours for guarding, rebound, involuntary spasm of abdominal wall musculature, tenderness, and anterior wall cellulitis.
2. Measure abdominal girth every 2 to 4 hours.
3. Note vomiting or diarrhea.
4. Obtain abdominal roentgenogram (lateral or upright view) to check for ileus and signs of peritoneal fluid or perforation with extraluminal free air. Check for calcification, obstructions, and foreign bodies.
5. If surgery is not imminent (perforation), perform diagnostic paracentesis (see Chapter 109) to obtain fluid for Gram stain, cell count, and aerobic and anaerobic culture.

Renal-metabolic system

1. Obtain serum Na, K, Cl, osmolality, and creatinine and BUN and TSP initially and once every 24 hours.

Table 44-1. Bacterial peritonitis

	Associated conditions	Bacterial pathogens	Drug(s) of choice
Primary	Nephrosis Cirrhosis Ascites Neonates	Usually monomicrobial: Pneumococcus Streptococcus Rarely *H. influenzae, E. coli,* or other enterics	Penicillin (plus an aminoglycoside if organism unknown)
Secondary	Leakage of bowel con- tents secondary to: Abdominal trauma Surgery Appendicitis Bowel obstruction	Usually polymicrobial: 2-3 aerobic enterics (*E. coli,* *Klebsiella, Proteus,* etc.) *plus* 3 or more anaerobes (*Bacte-* *roides fragilis, Fusobacteri-* *um, Clostridium,* etc.)	Aminoglycoside *plus* Carbenicillin/ticarcillin or cefoxitin (alternatives for anaerobic or- ganisms: chloramphenicol, clin- damycin, metronidazole)

2. Obtain serum amylase initially; repeat if abnormal.
3. With excessive losses from the gastrointestinal tract (NG, ileostomy, stool, etc.), measure Na and K content of drainage fluid.

MANAGEMENT
Abdomen

1. Use an NG tube to decompress the stomach.
2. Select the proper antibiotics.
   a. Penicillin G is the drug of choice in the initial therapy for primary peritonitis; an aminoglycoside may be added initially if the Gram stain of peritoneal fluid does not reveal gram-positive cocci. No surgical drainage of the abdomen is necessary.
   b. Secondary peritonitis always requires combined antibiotic therapy. The aminoglycosides are the drugs of choice for the gram-negative, aerobic component of the infection (see Table 41-4). The drug of choice for the anaerobic component is less clear, since *B. fragilis* is often resistant to penicillin yet remains a major pathogen in intra-abdominal sepsis. Chloramphenicol, clindamycin, and metronidazole are all highly effective against *B. fragilis* and the other anaer-

obes but have been associated with rare side effects, including bone marrow depression and/or aplasia, pseudomembranous colitis, and potential carcinogenicity, respectively. Thus, they should be used in children when no alternative exists. The semisynthetic penicillins, carbenicillin and ticarcillin, are highly effective against the gamut of anaerobes, including *B. fragilis*. Similar coverage is provided by cefoxitin. These three drugs have less potential toxicity than the other available drugs and thus are the drug of choice in this setting.

3. In addition to antimicrobial therapy, secondary peritonitis requires surgical intervention for evacuation of foreign material and drainage of purulent material as well as reinstitution of the integrity of the bowel wall. All the major classes of antibiotics have been shown to diffuse readily into peritoneal fluid; therefore, intraperitoneal instillation is unnecessary.

Renal-metabolic system

1. Control temperature to minimize cardiorespiratory distress and oxygen and glucose consumption. Use a cooling blanket or

sponge bath with tepid water for hyperthermia and a radiant warmer for hypothermia.
2. Adjust electrolyte content of fluids and give calcium to correct documented abnormalities.
3. Patients may require 1½ to 3 times maintenance fluids because of ongoing losses. Not all fluid losses can be measured because fluid moves into sequestered sites. Assess the circulating blood volume (systemic arterial blood pressure, pulse rate, urine output). Maintain urine output at a minimum of 1 ml/kg/hr. Treat shock with volume replacement (see Hypovolemic shock, p. 74).
4. Maintain Dextrostix at more than 90 mg/dl.
5. Frequent doses of FFP, 10 ml/kg over 30 to 60 minutes, may be required to maintain TSP greater than 5.0 mg/dl.

Cardiorespiratory system

1. Tachycardia may be due to fever and infection but also may reflect hypovolemia.

2. Maintain a normal systemic arterial blood pressure for age.
3. Maintain CVP between 5 and 10 mm Hg.
4. Patients in shock may require intubation and assisted mechanical ventilation until stabilized (see Chapter 14).

Hematologic system

1. Patients may have anemia, which can seriously compromise their ability to tolerate stress. Maintain Hct at more than 35%.
2. DIC is frequently found in patients with peritonitis (see Chapter 20).

ADDITIONAL READING

Fowler, R.: Primary peritonitis: changing aspects 1956-1970, Aust. Paediatr. J. 7:73-83, 1971.
Gedring, D.N., Hall, W.H., and Schierl, E.A.: Antibiotic concentrations in ascitic fluid of patients with ascites and bacterial peritonitis, Ann. Intern. Med. 86:708-713, 1977.
Nichols, R.L.: Intraabdominal sepsis: characterization and treatment, J. Infect. Dis. 135[Suppl.]:S54-S57, 1977.

45 Acute suppurative bone and joint disease

J. PATRICK HIEBER

DEFINITION AND PHYSIOLOGY

Acute hematogenous dissemination is the primary route by which bacteria gain access to the bones and joints; much less commonly, penetrating trauma or spread from contiguous infection is responsible. The mechanisms whereby organisms localize at these sites are uncertain, although preceding minor trauma and the sluggish circulation of the metaphyseal-end arteries are often cited as explanations. In addition to the signs and symptoms of bacteremia (see Chapter 41), the localized infection will produce edema, joint tenderness and effusion, and decreased range of motion in the involved bone and/or joint. The bacteremia may occasionally seed other sites simultaneously (lungs, CNS, kidneys, other bones/joints), which may escape initial detection because of distraction caused by the major presenting complaint.

As noted previously (see Chapter 41), the age and state of the patient are clinically helpful when considering the most likely etiologic agents (Table 45-1). It is important to note the common occurrence of *Staphylococcus aureus* in all age groups and of *Salmonella* and other enteric organisms in compromised hosts, especially those with decreased splenic function, such as patients with sickle hemoglobinopathies.

LABORATORY EVALUATION

Early in the course of disease, roentgenograms may reveal only deep soft-tissue swelling, whereas demineralization, sclerosis, and perios-

teal reaction may be noted later. Radionuclide scans may be helpful early if the plain roentgenograms are not diagnostic. The WBC count is often elevated, and the differential count is shifted to the left in septic arthritis but may be unremarkable in osteomyelitis. The blood culture is often positive and the ESR elevated in both conditions. Sickle hemoglobinopathy should be ruled out when appropriate. BUN, creatinine, and urinalysis are helpful in the diagnosis of occult renal infection and serve as a baseline for later monitoring for renal toxicity due to prolonged antibiotic therapy, especially with methicillin and the aminoglycosides.

After the initial evaluation has ruled out trauma and superficial cellulitis, the prime diagnostic test is aspiration of the involved bone and/or joint. Bones are tapped at the point of maximal tenderness with a large-bore (20-gauge or larger) steel spinal or bone marrow needle (aluminum will bend) and aspirated while the needle is passing through the soft tissue and subperiosteal spaces. All joints except the hip may be safely tapped on the ward using regular needles; hip aspirates are best obtained under fluoroscopic control. If no fluid is obtained, Hypaque arthrography should be done to be certain the joint space was entered. The blood and/or pus obtained should be Gram stained and sent for culture, and the laboratory should be alerted to save the pathogen recovered for future serum inhibition and bactericidal testing. An LP should be performed routinely in neonates with bone and/or joint infections and in

Table 45-1. Acute suppurative bone and joint disease: common etiologic agents

Setting	Osteomyelitis	Arthritis	Initial therapy
Neonate	Staphylococci, streptococci, gonococci, E. coli, and other enterics (osteomyelitis and/or arthritis)		Methicillin plus an aminoglycoside
Infants and children	Staphylococci, H. influenzae (rare)		Nafcillin* or cefamandole†
		H. influenzae, staphylococci, pneumococci, streptococci, gonococci	Cefamandole or chloramphenicol if <2 yr, chloramphenicol plus nafcillin if >2 yr, nafcillin alone if >6 yr
Compromised host	Consider gram-negative enterics, especially salmonellae, in cases involving decreased splenic function (osteomyelitis and/or arthritis)		Add gentamicin

*Vancomycin (50 mg/kg/day divided q6h IV) or cephalothin (75-125 mg/kg/day divided q6h IV) may be used in a patient with penicillin allergy.
†Cefamandole (50-150 mg/kg/day divided q6h IV) should be used only when CNS infection has been excluded.

older infants and children with arthritis to rule out clinically inapparent meningitis.

MONITORING

See also Chapter 4.

Infection

1. WBC count with differential analysis daily until stable.
2. Serial ESR rates until normal.
3. Serial roentgenograms of the involved area until healed.

Other

1. Arterial blood-gas tensions and pH initially and every 2 hours if shock is present.
2. BUN and creatinine twice weekly if patient is taking nephrotoxic drugs.

MANAGEMENT

After culture has been obtained, antimicrobial therapy is begun based on the Gram-stain morphology or CIE results from the aspirated fluid: gram-positive cocci in clusters indicate staphylococci; gram-positive cocci in pairs or chains indicate pneumococci or other streptococci; gram-negative rods are usually enterics; gram-negative pleomorphic rods are usually H. influenzae; gram-negative diplococci indicate gonococci or meningococci (see Tables 41-3 and 41-4). If the Gram stain is not diagnostic, therapy with an antibiotic(s) covering the broader range of potential pathogens is initiated (Table 45-1) and continued until firm identification of a specific pathogen allows the choice of definitive therapy. If purulent material is obtained by subperiosteal or intraosseous aspiration, surgical drainage of the osteomyelitis should be performed as soon as possible. If only bloody fluid is obtained, medical therapy alone should be initiated, and the patient should be reevaluated frequently as to the need for surgery. In the case of arthritis, all joints except the hip (and possibly the shoulder) may be treated by daily aspiration until the cell count and volume of fluid are greatly diminished, usually 2 to 4 days. Immediate surgical drainage is indicated when the hip is involved in view of its tenuous blood supply and the difficulty in complete evacuation of pus by needle aspiration. Rarely, surgical drainage of other joints is necessitated by prolonged effusion. All major antimicrobial agents (except amphotericin B) penetrate the joint and synovial fluid quite well; thus, routine instillation of drugs into the joint space is unnecessary and may produce a chemical synovitis.

Blood cultures should be repeated daily until negative. Bacteremia that persists after 24 to 36 hours of therapy raises the possibility of the presence of one or more sites of occult infection, which should be aggressively searched for (chest roentgenogram, skeletal survey, echocardiogram, radionuclide scans, intravenous pyelogram, etc.) and surgically drained if possible.

For the usual patient, a good clinical response to therapy, as indicated by decreasing fever, WBC counts, and ESR and by lack of roentgenographic progression, allows a change from parenteral to oral antibiotics (Table 45-2) after approximately 5 to 7 days of therapy. The oral phase of therapy demands that the patient be able to reliably take and retain the drug and that the serum bactericidal activity be documented to be in the therapeutic range ($\geq 1:8$ for staphylococci, *Pseudomonas*, coliform bacteria; $\geq 1:32$ for others) 1 hour after an oral dose. Thus, in the majority of cases a change to oral therapy requires continued hospitalization but at least allows discontinuation of the painful and hazardous IV route. Passive range of motion exercises should be begun as soon as the acute pain and swelling subside in order to prevent contractures; when the lower extremity is involved, full weight-bearing should be avoided for a minimum of 6 weeks.

The duration of antibiotic therapy is a function of the causative organism and the response to therapy. For infections due to highly susceptible organisms such as pneumococci, other streptococci, and *H. influenzae,* 10 days of therapy is usually sufficient. Gonococcal infections in adults have been treated successfully with 3 days of penicillin therapy; the necessary duration in children is probably no greater. Staphylococcal infections are treated for 21 days unless good surgical drainage is not obtained or if the clinical response is slow. In these cases, a careful search for disseminated occult foci is crucial, and a minimum of 4 to 6 weeks of therapy is

Table 45-2. Oral antibiotic therapy for acute suppurative bone and joint disease*

Organisms	Drugs
Penicillin-susceptible staphylococci, streptococci (including pneumococci, gonococci)	Penicillin V, 100 mg/kg/24 hr in 4 doses
Staphylococcus aureus, penicillin-resistant	Dicloxacillin, 150 mg/kg/24 hr in 4 doses, *or* cephalexin, 150 mg/kg/24 hr in 4 doses
H. influenzae, β-lactamase–positive; Salmonella	Cefaclor, 150 mg/kg/24 hr in 3 doses, *or* chloramphenicol, 50-75 mg/kg/24 hr in 4 doses
H. influenzae, β-lactamase–negative; Salmonella	Ampicillin, 150 mg/kg/24 hr in 4 doses, *or* amoxicillin, 100 mg/kg/24 hr in 4 doses
Coliform bacteria	Ampicillin or cephalexin (if susceptible) in dosages given above

*Note: In the hospital and monitoring serum bactericidal titers.

recommended. Patients are discharged when they are clinically improved (afebrile, WBC count and ESR normal, no pain or tenderness) and when antibiotic therapy is complete. An exception to the latter criterion is in chronic or complicated cases in which prolonged oral outpatient therapy is planned. Long-term follow-up is essential so that joint dysfunction and growth disturbances of long bones may be discovered and treated as soon as possible.

ADDITIONAL READING

Nelson, J.D.: Oral antibiotic therapy for serious infections in hospitalized patients, J. Pediatr. **92:**175-176, 1978.

Nelson, J.D., Howard, J.B. and Shelton, S.: Oral antibiotic therapy for skeletal infections of children. I. Antibiotic concentrations in suppurative synovial fluid, J. Pediatr. **92:**131-134, 1978.

Tetzlaff, T.R., Howard, J.B., McCracken, G.H., Jr., and others: Antibiotic concentrations in pus and bone of children with osteomyelitis, J. Pediatr. **92:**135-140, 1978.

46 Sickle cell crisis

GEORGE R. BUCHANAN

DEFINITION AND PHYSIOLOGY

Children with sickle cell anemia and related hemoglobinopathies (sickle hemoglobin C [SC] disease and S-beta thalassemia) have chronic hemolytic anemia periodically interrupted by episodes of acute crisis. The most frequent type of crisis is the vaso-occlusive, or painful, crisis, believed to be secondary to ischemia and infarction of bone, bone marrow, or other organs following blockage of capillaries by rigid, nondeformable sickle cells. These episodes, frequently triggered by hypoxia, acidosis, hypothermia, or infection, occur with extremely variable frequency and severity from patient to patient and in any one patient over time. Some children, particularly those with SC disease and S-beta thalassemia, have them only rarely. Most crises can be managed at home, in the emergency room, or in the nonintensive care hospital setting by nonspecific measures such as vigorous hydration, analgesics, and correction of predisposing factors.

However, there are other acute crises that may disrupt the steady state, lead to life-threatening complications, and require intensive care. These include the following.

Bacterial septicemia and/or meningitis

Patients with homozygous sickle cell anemia have a markedly increased risk of septicemia and meningitis, particularly from *Streptococcus pneumoniae*, but also from *Haemophilus influenzae* and enteric pathogens. These serious infections occur most frequently in the child between 9 months and 4 years of age and are thought to be primarily due to impaired splenic function. The risk of infection is much less pronounced in the child with SC disease or S-beta thalassemia.

Aplastic crisis

Brief periods of decreased RBC production secondary to viral infection may lead to life-threatening anemia in a child whose circulating RBCs have a markedly shortened life span. Hemolytic crises, i.e., accelerated hemolysis rather than decreased red cell production as a cause of a decreasing hematocrit, are less common; they may be secondary to glucose-6-phosphate dehydrogenase deficiency or other disorders. Most children with sickle cell anemia chronically maintain a hemoglobin level of 7 to 9 g/dl.

Splenic sequestration crisis

Unexplained acute engorgement of the splenic sinuses with blood may result in massive splenomegaly, shock, and severe anemia, often with a fatal outcome. The patient, by sequestering as much as one half of his blood volume in his spleen, essentially "bleeds into his spleen." This complication may be recurrent and most commonly occurs in patients who already have some splenomegaly, e.g., children with SC disease, S-beta thalassemia, or sickle cell anemia who are less than 4 years old.

Organ-related sickling

Sickling can occur suddenly within the capillary bed or by occlusion of the main arterial blood supply of one or more organs, leading to syndromes of stroke, pulmonary infarction, extreme jaundice and hepatic enlargement, gross hematuria, and bone infarction. Such patients are often seriously ill and may be left with chronic or permanent deficits due to extensive irreversible infarction.

MONITORING

See also Chapter 4.

Critically ill patients with sickle cell anemia need to have careful attention paid to numerous variables.

Hematologic system

1. Hct and Hb every day.
2. Reticulocyte count every day or every other day.
3. Total and differential WBC count every other day. Patients with sickle cell anemia have a mild leukocytosis and a normal differential count in the steady state. Although the WBC count may increase with vaso-occlusive crises, a shift to the left usually means bacterial infection.

Other systems

1. Assess hydration every 2 hours.
2. Monitor temperature every hour and every 30 minutes if less than 36° C or more than 38° C.
3. Determine if localizing signs or an altered level of consciousness are present, possibly indicating a stroke.

MANAGEMENT

Individual severe crisis situations are managed as follows.

Severe vaso-occlusive crisis

1. Elimination of triggering events, if present. Use antibiotics and/or antipyretics for infection, alkali for acidosis, and supplemental oxygen for hypoxemia.

2. Fluid replacement. Give fluids at a rate 1½ to 2 times maintenance to correct any deficits and to dilute the patient's sickled cells.
3. Analgesia. Administer aspirin or acetaminophen, codeine, meperidine or morphine (depending on severity) frequently. A continuous IV infusion of meperidine or repetitive subcutaneous injections of morphine are often necessary to alleviate pain.
4. Packed RBC transfusions. Exchange or modified exchange transfusion has been advocated before surgery and potentially dangerous diagnostic tests (e.g., arteriography) in an attempt to stop the sickling process. Firm data are lacking in many circumstances, but this form of therapy may be of benefit to patients with stroke, massive pulmonary infarction, or severe, intractable, recurrent crises. Simple transfusions to increase the hematocrit are usually not indicated unless the hemoglobin level is markedly below the value of the steady state and the patient is having symptoms of anemia. In such circumstances, packed RBCs should be administered extremely slowly (see Chapter 106).

Aplastic crisis

Packed RBC transfusions (usually 5 to 7 ml/kg over 3 to 4 hours) should be given to increase the hematocrit to 18% to 20%, and the child should have frequent determinations of hematocrit and reticulocytes until his own bone marrow resumes active production of red cells.

Sequestration crisis

Whole blood or volume expanders and packed RBCs must be quickly administered if the patient is hypovolemic secondary to sequestration of blood in the spleen. Subsequent packed RBC transfusions (see above and Chapter 106 for doses) and close observation are then required until the spleen is reduced in size and the hematocrit stabilizes several days later.

Such crises can occur very rapidly, and the child requires close nursing care and observation until he is hemodynamically stable.

Serious bacterial infection

Serious bacterial infection is managed in patients with sickle cell disease in a similar fashion as in children without hemoglobinopathy (see Chapter 41). The patient's hydration, temperature, and blood pH and oxygen tension must be maintained in the normal range to prevent further sickling.

ADDITIONAL READING

Charache, S.: The treatment of sickle cell anemia, Arch. Intern. Med. **133:**698-705, 1974.

Pearson, H.A., and Diamond, I.K.: Sickle cell disease crises and their management. In Smith, C.A., editor: The critically ill child: diagnosis and management, ed. 2, Philadelphia, 1977, W.B. Saunders Co.

Schwartz, E., editor: Hemoglobinopathies in children, Littleton, Mass., 1980, PSG Publishing Co., Inc.

Davis, J.R., Vichinsky, E.P., and Lubin, B.H.: Current treatment of sickle cell disease. In Current Problems in Pediatrics, vol. 10, no. 12, Chicago, 1980, Year Book Medical Publishers, Inc., pp. 1-64.

Keeley, K., and Buchanan, G.R.: Acute infarction of long bones in children with sickle cell anemia, J. Pediatr. **101:**170-175, 1982.

47 Hemolytic-uremic syndrome

RONALD J. HOGG
GEORGE R. BUCHANAN

DEFINITION AND PHYSIOLOGY

The hemolytic-uremic syndrome is a disorder of uncertain cause characterized by hemolytic anemia, thrombocytopenia, and renal failure. The severity of each of these components of the syndrome varies considerably, but in general the intensive care patient will show severe manifestations of all three. This entity is one of the most common causes of acute renal failure and acquired hemolytic anemia in infants and children in many parts of the world.

Many infectious organisms have been suggested as etiologic agents in this disorder, with Coxsackie viruses being the most frequently isolated. However, it is apparent from the various studies that no specific etiologic agent can be incriminated in the majority of patients. The pathogenesis of the syndrome is also obscure. The basic lesion appears to involve a thrombotic microangiopathic process affecting the renal microvasculature. Whether the initiation of the angiopathy depends on immunologic mechanisms or a primary thrombotic process cannot be established with certainty at present, although the prevailing view appears to favor the concept that microvascular thrombosis is a secondary phenomenon. The mechanism by which the microangiopathy produces the characteristic clinical and laboratory abnormalities of the syndrome can be stated with more confidence, although once again disparate views exist on this subject. It would appear that passage through abnormally narrowed glomerular capillaries inflicts mechanical trauma on erythrocytes and platelets with the result that the life span of these elements is sharply curtailed. The areas of platelet destruction and/or deposition have been examined by injecting radioisotope-tagged platelets and observing the sites where maximal counts occurred. By this means it was shown that there is no significant platelet deposition in the kidneys. These studies were performed in situations where the syndrome was already clinically apparent, and hence it is possible that platelet deposition in the kidney may have occurred before the time of study.

The mechanical fragmentation of erythrocytes leads to a shortened life span of these cells and results in the presence of schistocytes, burr cells, and helmet cells on the peripheral blood smear. The hemolytic anemia may be rapidly progressive, as evidenced by the dramatic decrease in hemoglobin levels in many patients. Most children are able to mount a moderate reticulocyte response, with the result that 5% to 20% reticulocytes may be present along with nucleated RBCs in the peripheral smear.

The degree of renal failure is determined by the extent of glomerular capillary obstruction. In the most severe cases, renal blood flow and glomerular filtration rate are greatly reduced, and widespread cortical necrosis may develop. In some patients, however, absent renal perfusion as shown by renal scan may be followed by eventual recovery of renal function. Often associated with the renal ischemia is a severe degree of systemic hypertension. High levels of plasma renin activity have been demonstrated in such patients, suggesting that increased vasomotor activity may be more important than fluid overload in the pathogenesis of the hypertension seen in hemolytic-uremic syndrome.

The role of local or disseminated intravascular coagulation in the hemolytic-uremic syndrome is also controversial. PT and PTT are normal, and fibrin degradation products are only slightly increased in the majority of cases. The consensus at this time is that fibrin thrombi do not play a primary role in the microangiopathy.

Two other organ systems are also often severely affected in patients with hemolytic-uremic syndrome: the gastrointestinal tract and the CNS. Once again the pathophysiology underlying these derangements is obscure. Hemolytic-uremic syndrome usually occurs in infants and young children, the majority of whom have a prodomal illness that is indistinguishable from acute gastroenteritis. The severity of gastrointestinal involvement is variable, with some patients developing bloody diarrhea associated with abdominal pain. This may be so dramatic that the clinical picture mimics ulcerative colitis. The correct diagnosis may be further confused by the fact that barium enema and sigmoidoscopy may also be compatible with ulcerative colitis. However, rectal biopsy shows only edema and submucosal hemorrhage. The diagnosis becomes apparent when oliguria and pallor develop and when a peripheral blood smear shows the characteristic picture of fragmented erythrocytes and thrombocytopenia. Before this time there may be a considerable delay in diagnosis.

The neurologic manifestations of hemolytic-uremic syndrome often lead to the initial requirement for intensive care management. The severity of the disturbance is extremely variable, and there does not appear to be a constant relationship between the impairment of renal and neurologic function. Thus, one patient may develop status epilepticus, decerebrate posturing, hemiparesis, etc. in the absence of severe serum electrolyte disturbances or markedly elevated levels of arterial blood pressure, whereas another patient will show only minimal signs of neurologic irritation despite prolonged anuria and systemic hypertension. It would appear, therefore, that another factor must be responsible for the extent of the neurologic impairment in some patients. Unlike the situation with thrombotic thrombocytopenic purpura, it is usually not possible to demonstrate microvascular damage in the brain of a patient with hemolytic-uremic syndrome. The lack of a close correlation between the variables presently measured and the neurologic disturbances seen in some patients has prompted a number of nephrologists to initiate dialysis in those patients with severe neurologic signs before other clinical and laboratory findings appeared to warrant such a measure. Excellent results have been obtained with this approach, even in children who had severe neurologic complications that were resistant to anticonvulsant therapy.

As a result of the system failures discussed above, it is apparent that patients with hemolytic-uremic syndrome may have a diversity of clinical problems. The biochemical and cardiovascular complications attendant upon acute renal failure are discussed in Chapter 17, and a chapter on the technique and complications of acute peritoneal dialysis (Chapter 110) is also included.

MONITORING

See also Chapter 4.

The monitoring necessary in the serial evaluation of patients with hemolytic-uremic syndrome concerns the functions of those organ systems involved, with emphasis placed on the problems caused by renal failure and the hematologic manifestations. Monitoring information in acute renal failure is discussed in Chapter 17. The hematologic manifestations should be monitored as follows:

1. Check Hct every 24 hours with examination of the peripheral blood smear to evaluate

RBC morphology. Initially it may be necessary to check the Hb level and Hct every 8 to 12 hours because of rapid hemolysis.
2. Evaluate coagulation initially to exclude the diagnosis of DIC (PT, PTT, fibrin split products, and fibrinogen).
3. Obtain platelet count every 24 hours.
4. Exclude other causes of acute acquired hemolytic anemia by direct Coombs' test and glucose-6-phosphate dehydrogenase screening studies if there is any doubt about the correct diagnosis.

MANAGEMENT

The management of hemolytic-uremic syndrome usually requires a multidisciplinary approach.

Basic disease process

There are many opinions regarding the optimal treatment of this disease, reflecting the diversity of views of the nature of the basic disease process. Investigators who believe that primary glomerular endothelial damage and platelet adherence thereto initiate the disease process have claimed that agents that inhibit platelet function, notably aspirin, dipyridamole, and sulfinpyrazone, represent the most logical form of therapy. Isolated anecdotal experience with these drugs in hemolytic-uremic syndrome and the related disorder, thrombotic thrombocytopenic purpura, has been reported, but there is no indication for routine use of these agents at the present time.

Plasma transfusions, plasmaphoresis, and plasma exchanges are being increasingly used in thrombotic thrombocytopenic purpura, and dramatic successes have been reported. However, the rationale for these modalities remains obscure and firm data regarding plasma therapy in hemolytic-uremic syndrome are lacking.

Extensive experience has been accumulated in various parts of the world on the use of heparin in hemolytic-uremic syndrome. The reports that have emerged are almost impossible to evaluate because of the tremendous heterogeneity of the patient populations studied. At the present time it would appear that anticoagulation does not offer any additional benefit to patients in whom the complications of the disease process are treated appropriately. The same comment applies to the use of thrombolytic drugs such as streptokinase, although the experience with these agents is more limited.

Systemic complications

Treatment of systemic complications is by far the most important aspect of management.

The hematologic complications are managed by transfusion of packed red cells when the patient becomes symptomatic of anemia or when the hematocrit falls to less than 20%. These transfusions should be given extremely slowly (e.g., 3 to 5 ml/kg over several hours) if the child is hypertensive or volume overloaded. The blood should be as fresh as possible to reduce the potassium load delivered to a patient in whom hyperkalemia is a constant threat. Even if the above precautions are adhered to, it is important to measure the serum potassium levels soon after blood administration.

Platelet transfusions are rarely required, since bleeding symptoms are usually not severe, and such transfusions are of little benefit in most cases because of shortened platelet survival time. In addition, transfused platelets are of potential harm, since they may contribute to platelet plugging in the renal microvasculature. Transfusions of platelets should therefore be administered only if the platelet count is less than 10,000/mm^3 and significant hemorrhage is occurring or if peritoneal dialysis is to be instituted.

Treatment of the complications of acute renal failure is discussed in Chapter 17.

Gastrointestinal disturbances are often the initial management problems. As stated previously, there are some patients in whom severe rectal bleeding may dominate the initial presentation. The majority of such patients respond to medical management consisting of close attention to disturbances of fluid and acid-base balance. However, significant infarction of the bowel may occur and necessitate surgical intervention in extreme cases.

The management of neurologic problems with early dialysis has been discussed above.

The final part of treatment concerns the long-term management. Most patients achieve complete recovery from this disorder despite the presence of anuria for 2 to 3 weeks in many cases. The mortality in severe cases has been reduced to approximately 10% to 25% in most large centers. The major long-term complication is hypertension, the incidence of which varies from 10% to 50% in different areas. Most large studies contain one or two patients in whom recurrent attacks or familial involvement occurs. The incidence of such problems appears to be low, but their existence should be remembered in the counseling of parents.

ADDITIONAL READING

Case Records of the Massachusetts General Hospital, Case 12-1981, N. Engl. J. Med. **304:**715-722, 1981.

Gianantonio, C.A., Vitacco, M., Mendilaharzu, F., and others: The hemolytic-uremic syndrome, Nephron **11:**74-192, 1973.

Kaplan, B.S., Thomson, P.D., and Chadarevian, J.P.: The hemolytic-uremic syndrome, Pediatr. Clin. North Am. **23:**761-777, 1976.

Sorrenti, L.Y., and Lewy, P.R.: The hemolytic-uremic syndrome, Am. J. Dis. Child. **132:**59-62, 1978.

Tune, B.M., Leavitt, T.J., and Gribble, T.J.: The hemolytic-uremic syndrome in California: a review of 28 non-heparinized cases with long-term follow-up, J. Pediatr. **82:**304-310, 1973.

48 Diabetic ketoacidosis

JOHN J. CHIPMAN
JAMES F. MARKS

DEFINITION AND PHYSIOLOGY

Impending or present coma and cardiovascular instability are late signs in a cascade of interrelated pathophysiologic events occurring in the patient with severe diabetic ketoacidosis (DKA). Successful management of these patients is based on an understanding of these events.

The sine qua non of diabetes mellitus is the absolute or relative lack of insulin. Inappropriately high glucagon secretion may also contribute to the marked endogenous hyperglycemia. The exact molecular or biochemical cause of the insulin and glucagon defects remains unknown. However, several known pathophysiologic events occur in DKA: (1) hyperglycemia, (2) hyperosmolality, (3) dehydration and electrolyte imbalance, and (4) ketoacidosis and buffer depletion.

Hyperglycemia is the consequence of increased glycogen breakdown, increased gluconeogenesis, and decreased peripheral utilization. When glycogen stores become inadequate, metabolic pathways shift in the direction of increased lipolysis, gluconeogenesis, and ketogenesis to meet energy needs. The serum may gradually become lipemic because of the mobilized lipids, acidosis worsens because of increased production of acetoacetic and β-hydroxybutyric acid, and ammonium ion production increases. A predictable downhill course follows without the intervention of exogenous insulin, fluids, electrolytes, and glucose substrate.

Significant dehydration results from the hyperglycemic osmotic diuresis. This is worsened because of the vomiting associated with ketoacidosis. Ketones are also readily excreted, taking with them sodium and potassium in increased amounts. Dehydration worsens, the glomerular filtration rate falls, and signs of prerenal azotemia and shock may appear. Severe DKA is usually associated with a loss of 100 ml water, 8 mEq Na, 6 mEq Cl, and 6 to 10 mEq K per kg of usual body weight.

Correction of the metabolic acidosis occurs within the blood buffer system and from CNS stimulation to increase alveolar ventilation. The buffer system, as indicated below, shifts to the right to remove the excess hydrogen ion:

$$\text{Ketone acid} + HCO_3^- \rightarrow \text{Ketone salt} +$$
$$H_2CO_3 \rightarrow CO_2 + H_2O$$

Because of differences in CO_2 and HCO_3^- diffusion rates across the blood-brain barrier, the CNS respiratory drive lags behind the changes in blood pH. During the recovery phase, the patient may become alkalotic because of a continued increase in alveolar ventilation due to this delay.

Hyperosmolality, acidosis, contracted vascular volume, and decreased oxygen consumption all contribute to the diabetic coma. Furthermore, the cause of the coma may not be clear initially. Children with diabetes mellitus may also be comatose because of hypoglycemia or nonketotic hyperosmolality, although the latter state is rare. Drug ingestion may cloud the picture in a toddler or adolescent, and infection may contribute to the acidosis, the respiratory distress, or refractoriness to insulin therapy. A chief complaint of abdominal pain before more obvious signs of DKA are present is not uncommon and may delay appropriate therapy. A knowledge of precipitating events is essential for successful management of DKA. A successful outcome depends on frequent monitoring and management changes consistent with clinical and metabolic changes.

MONITORING

See also Chapter 4.

Initial assessment

1. History and physical examination. Note the previous weight, precipitating events, and details of the physical state of the patient. Include examination for candidiasis of genital mucous membranes.
2. To confirm the diagnosis, check the urine yourself for sugar (4+) and acetone (usually large) using Ketodiastik and Acetest tablets. Capillary glucose value is usually greater than 250 mg/dl as determined with Dextrostix, Chemstrip bG, or Visidex Strips.

Renal-metabolic system

1. Obtain CBC with differential WBC count, serum glucose and acetone, BUN, and blood pH (note the source, venous or arterial).
2. Obtain appropriate cultures (blood, urine, and throat) if indicated.
3. Establish urine collection.
4. Check capillary glucose hourly.
5. Check urine every hour for volume, sugar, and acetone.
6. Check serum acetone every 2 to 4 hours until it clears.
7. Measure serum glucose and venous pH every 2 hours until stable, then serum glucose every 4 hours.
8. Measure serum electrolytes and osmolality at 4 and 8 hours after the start of therapy (and every 4 hours stable).

9. Measure serum PO_4 and Ca if treating with potassium phosphate at 0, 4, 6, and 8 hours or until normal.

Cardiorespiratory system

1. Vital signs. Check systemic arterial blood pressure hourly until ketoacidosis resolves and more often if the patient is in shock.
2. Check ECG lead II rhythm strip every 4 hours while potassium is being given IV in 40 mEq/L concentrations. If the patient is receiving potassium and is oliguric or if he is receiving more than 40 mEq of potassium per liter, check the cardiac monitor every 15 to 30 minutes until it is possible to reduce the potassium given to less than 40 mEq/L, based on an increase in serum potassium to 3 mEq/L or greater and normal T waves on ECG.

Neurologic system

1. Determine level of consciousness (see Chapter 6) every 1 to 2 hours until stable. Check fundi every 1 to 2 hours in any comatose or stuporous patient until symptoms resolve. A decreased level of consciousness in the course of therapy mandates immediate evaluation for cerebral edema and treatment if signs of edema are found.

Other systems

Keep flow sheet current and readily available (Fig. 48-1). Vital signs, mental status, serum glucose, acetone, electrolytes; CO_2, pH, BUN, urine sugar and acetone determination (SAD), intake and output, insulin doses, and potassium and bicarbonate therapy should be included.

MANAGEMENT
Fluid and electrolyte therapy

If the patient is in shock, 0.9% sodium chloride or lactated Ringer's solution, 20 to 30 ml/ kg, is required for the first 1 to 2 hours to stabilize the systemic arterial blood pressure. To

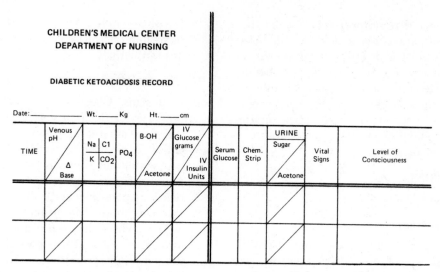

CHILDREN'S MEDICAL CENTER
DEPARTMENT OF NURSING

DIABETIC KETOACIDOSIS RECORD

Date:_____   Wt.____Kg   Ht.____cm

TIME	Venous pH / Δ / Base	Na / K	Cl / CO2	PO4	B-OH / Acetone	IV Glucose grams / IV Insulin Units	Serum Glucose	Chem. Strip	URINE Sugar / Acetone	Vital Signs	Level of Consciousness

Fig. 48-1. The DKA flow sheet is attached to the PICU flow sheet (Fig. 4-1) in order to allow for complete tabulation and proper correlation of the intake and output record with the information on this sheet. *B-OH, β*-Hydroxybutyric acid.

avoid fluid overload and cerebral edema, the amount of sodium given initially should be subtracted from the calculation of total sodium needs.

After shock is corrected or if the patient is not in shock, calculate fluid requirements: 1½ to 2 times normal maintenance fluids for increased insensible losses and ongoing losses in addition to replacement for 10% dehydration. Add maintenance and replacement requirements and give 50% over the first 8 to 12 hours and 50% over the remaining 24 to 36 hours (see Chapter 16).

The initial fluids should be isotonic rather than hypotonic to minimize possibility of cerebral edema. To estimate the degree of hypertonicity in the absence of significant hyperlipemia, the following formula (by Katz) is useful:

Corrected serum Na = Measured $(Na)_s$ +
$$[(Plasma\ glucose - 100) \times 0.016]$$

Because serum glucose decreases more rapidly than serum ketones, enough glucose should

be added to fluid therapy to maintain the blood glucose level at 250 to 300 mg/dl until blood is free of ketones. Usually 3 to 4 g of glucose per unit of insulin given will stabilize blood glucose concentrations.

Add potassium phosphate, 20 mEq/L, to the initial fluids (monitor for hyperkalemia). When renal function is normal, potassium should be increased to 30 to 40 mEq/L (half as potassium chloride and half as potassium phosphate, monitor serum potassium and ECG). After 6 to 8 hours this may be decreased to 20 to 30 mEq/L if the serum potassium returns to and stabilizes in the normal range. To avoid hypocalcemia due to hyperphosphatemia, potassium phosphate should be changed to potassium chloride after 6 to 8 hours.

Fluid therapy must be adjusted to the clinical course of the patient in response to meticulous monitoring.

Bicarbonate therapy

At low pH values (pH < 7.15), ventilation and left ventricular systolic blood pressure are depressed. To protect the patient from these untoward effects, the severely acidotic patient should receive an infusion of sodium bicarbonate, 1.5 to 2.0 mEq/kg, given over 20 to 30 minutes with the initial fluids. This avoids a theoretical worsening of acidosis due to dilution of an already low buffer system at the time of volume expansion. It also adds to the buffer system until ketone production falls behind ketone oxidation, which is an endogenous source of bicarbonate.

Insulin therapy: low-dose constant-infusion method

1. Start with regular insulin, 0.1 unit/kg IV push (optional).
2. After the initial IV dose, start a continuous IV infusion of regular insulin at a dose of 0.1 unit/kg/hr. Fifty units of regular insulin may be diluted in 250 ml 0.9% sodium chloride solution. Give the insulin by IV under the control of a calibrated, linear infusion pump, to ensure infusion at a constant rate. Prepare a fresh solution every 8 hours.
3. If 2 to 4 hours after beginning insulin therapy the blood glucose level has not fallen 50 mg/dl/hr, increase the insulin infusion to 0.2 unit/kg/hr. Beware of glucose falling too rapidly (>100 mg/dl/hr).
4. Stop the constant infusion as soon as serum acetone is undetectable and change immediately to a sliding scale as shown below, giving insulin every 4 to 6 hours or 30 minutes before meals and at midnight if the patient is eating. Sliding scale is calculated as follows:
   a. Basal regular insulin requirements:
      New diabetic: 0.5-0.75 unit/kg body weight/24 hr.
      Old diabetic: previous dosage or 0.75-1 unit/kg/24 hr.
      This total dose is divided giving $3/10$ for breakfast, $1/5$ for lunch, $1/5$ to $3/10$ for dinner, and $1/10$ each for any afternoon snack, bedtime snack and midnight, if necessary.

   b. To this sliding scale 1 unit regular insulin is added for each 30 to 50 mg/dl change in blood glucose above the 150 mg/dl level before each meal.
   c. If acetone clears at a time when a meal is not planned, one may:
      (1) continue infusion at one-half the previous rate (≤0.05 units/kg) and provide 3 to 4 g glucose/unit insulin given, until the next meal, *or*
      (2) give 0.05 to 0.1 unit/kg regular insulin subcutaneously (SC) and continue IV glucose as above until eating commences. CAUTION: One should probably delay cessation of infusion until 30 minutes after first dose of subcutaneous insulin.

COMPLICATIONS
Cerebral edema

It is known that cerebral edema and uncal herniation are present in some patients with DKA who die in spite of improving biochemical values. Similar findings have been reproduced in animal experiments by a rapid decrease in blood glucose from a hyperosmolar state, and this mechanism may be the cause of death in some diabetic patients. Other mechanisms that have been implicated but not confirmed include rapid administration of fluid, rapid correction of acidosis with alkali, and excessive hypophosphatemia. Since the ranges of safety in clinical variables are unknown, the emphasis must be placed on close observation of the patient's management and response.

Hypokalemia or hyperkalemia

Regardless of the serum potassium level, patients with severe DKA have marked intracellular losses of potassium. As insulin improves glucose transport across membranes, potassium moves intracellularly with the glucose. This event along with an expanding extracellular fluid volume and correction of the acidosis can lead to marked hypokalemia. In contrast, potassium replacement therapy that is too vigorous or given while the patient still has poor renal perfusion can lead to hyperkalemia. The ECG must therefore be monitored closely in patients with severe DKA.

Rebound from low-dose infusions

Because IV insulin has a short half-life (less than 5 minutes), subcutaneous insulin therapy should begin 30 minutes before the infusion is stopped. Otherwise, a rebound of increasing serum glucose should be expected.

ADDITIONAL READING

Alberti, K.G.M.M., and Hockaday, T.D.R.: Diabetic coma: a reappraisal after five years, Clin. Endocrinol. Metabol. 6:424-455, 1977.

Dell, B.: Diabetic ketoacidosis. In Winters, R.W., editor: The body fluids in pediatrics, Boston, 1973, Little, Brown & Co.

Drash, A.L.: The treatment of diabetic ketoacidosis, J. Pediatr. 91:858-860, 1977.

Drop, S.L.S., Duval-Arnold, B.J.M., Gober, A.E., and others: Low-dose intravenous insulin infusion versus subcutaneous insulin injection: a controlled comparative study of diabetic ketoacidosis, Pediatrics 59:733-738, 1977.

Duck, S.C., and Kohler, E.: Cerebral edema in diabetic ketoacidosis, J. Pediatr. 98:674-676, 1981.

Foster, D.W., and McGarry, J.D.: The metabolic derangements and treatment of diabetic ketoacidosis, N. Engl. J. Med. 309:159-169, 1983.

Katz, M.M.: Hyperglycemia-induced hyponatremia: calculation of expected serum sodium depression, N. Engl. J. Med. 289:843, 1973.

Kaufman, I.A., Keller, M.A., and Nyhan, W.L.: Diabetic ketosis and acidosis: the continuous infusion of low doses of insulin, J. Pediatr. 87:846-848, 1975.

Kaye, R.: Diabetic ketoacidosis: the bicarbonate controversy, J. Pediatr. 87:156-159, 1975.

Kreisberg, R.A.: Diabetic ketoacidosis: new concepts and trends in pathogenesis and treatment, Ann. Intern. Med. 88:681-695, 1978.

Lightner, E.S., Kappy, M.S., and Revsin, B.: Low-dose intravenous insulin infusion in patients with diabetic ketoacidosis: biochemical effects in children, Pediatrics 60:681-688, 1977.

McGarry, J.D., and Foster, D.W.: Hormonal control of ketogenesis, Arch. Intern. Med. 137:495-501, 1977.

Perkin, R.M., and Marks, J.F.: Low-dose continuous intravenous insulin infusion in childhood diabetic ketoacidosis, Clin. Pediatr. 18:540-548, 1979.

Rosenbloom, A.L., Riley, W.J., Weber, F.T., and others: Cerebral edema complicating diabetic ketoacidosis in childhood, J. Pediatr. 96:357-361, 1980.

Tamborlane, W.V., Jr., and Genel, M.: Discordant correction of hyperglycemia and ketoacidosis with low-dose insulin infusion, Pediatrics 61:125-127, 1978.

Unger, R., Raskin, P., Srikant, C.B., and Orci, L.: Glucagon and the a-cell, Recent Prog. Horm. Res. 33:477-517, 1977.

Winters, R.W.: Physiology of acid-base disorders. In Winters, R.W., editor: The body fluids in pediatrics, Boston, 1973, Little, Brown & Co.

49 Acute adrenocortical insufficiency

JAMES F. MARKS

DEFINITION AND PHYSIOLOGY

Distress secondary to acute insufficiency of adrenocortical function is occasionally seen in the pediatric patient. By far the most common cause in the infant and young child is the salt-losing form of congenital adrenal hyperplasia, absence of the enzyme 21-hydroxylase. Less common causes are congenital adrenal hypoplasia, acute infection, hemorrhage into the adrenal glands, inadequate replacement of adrenocorticosteroids after surgery for removal of adrenal tumors, and inappropriate tapering of steroids in patients who have been receiving long-term steroid therapy. In the older child, all of these causes still pertain, but one does see a few individuals with acute adrenocortical failure who have idiopathic Addison's disease, usually associated with other endocrinopathies, most likely on an autoimmune basis.

The mechanism for salt depletion in the 21-hydroxylase deficiency type of congenital adrenal hyperplasia is at least twofold. First, there is a deficiency in production of both hydrocortisone and aldosterone. Second, there can also be production of metabolites, such as 17-hydroxy-progesterone and progesterone, that competitively inhibit the action of aldosterone at its distal tubular site in the kidney. These hormonal abnormalities may result in hyperkalemia, hyponatremia, azotemia, acidosis, and disorders of carbohydrate metabolism and hypoglycemia.

The typical infant with the salt-losing form of congenital adrenal hyperplasia is dehydrated and has signs of acute and chronic hypovolemia with or without peripheral vascular collapse. Female infants with this disease have ambiguous (masculinized) external genitalia secondary to excessive androgen production associated with pituitary feedback stimulation of the adrenal cortex. However, male infants have normal external genitalia. Even 31 years after the initial description of therapy for this condition, two thirds of the patients seen are female, a finding that suggests that roughly half of the male infants with congenital adrenal hyperplasia are being missed. Since approximately two thirds of these babies have the salt-losing form, presumably a significant number are still dying undiagnosed in infancy, even though Wilkins and his colleagues described the appropriate diagnostic and therapeutic measures in 1950.

The onset of acute adrenal symptoms typically occurs in the second week of life, although infants with this condition may decompensate as early as 3 days of age and as late as 1 month. One infant with acute adrenal insufficiency and congenital adrenal hyperplasia was first seen at 2 months of age.

MONITORING

See also Chapter 4.

Renal-metabolic system

1. Record temperature every 2 hours. Patients are frequently hypothermic.

305

2. Obtain serum Na, K, Cl, and Ca initially; repeat immediately and then every 4 to 6 hours until stable. Then repeat once each day. Elevated K and low Na values are classic findings.

Cardiorespiratory system

1. Continuously monitor ECG. Hyperkalemia causes serious dysrhythmias.
2. Obtain arterial blood-gas tensions and pH every 2 hours until normal.

Endocrine system

1. Institute 24-hour urine collection for measurement of ketosteroids and pregnanetriol. It is unusual to have sufficient time to do this before initiation of treatment, since infants are frequently in shock.
2. Obtain blood for 17-hydroxyprogesterone and plasma renin testing. There is no overlap between normal and affected babies in level of 17-hydroxyprogesterone in the blood. Plasma renin levels are elevated.

MANAGEMENT
Renal-metabolic system

1. Maintain body temperature in a neutral thermal environment to minimize oxygen consumption (see Chapter 18).
2. Maintain Dextrostix readings at greater than 45 mg/dl.
3. Correct hypovolemia, hyponatremia, and hyperkalemia.
   a. Use 0.9% sodium chloride solution with 5% glucose, 20 ml/kg IV over 20 minutes, to correct shock (see Chapter 14).
   b. Continue 0.9% sodium chloride solution with 5% glucose at one-third maintenance and 10% replacement for the first 8 hours (see Chapter 16).
   c. Reassess the patient at 4 and 8 hours to determine if 10% replacement will be adequate, and adjust infusion.
   d. Continue 0.9% sodium chloride solution

if necessary with 5% glucose until the serum sodium level is ≥135 mEq/L; then change to 0.45% sodium chloride solution with 5% glucose.
   e. Do not add potassium to IV fluids during the first 24 hours.
   f. If there are signs on ECG of cardiotoxicity due to hyperkalemia, treat with sodium polystyrene sulfonate (Kayexalate) (see Chapter 17).
   g. Use sodium bicarbonate, 1 mEq/kg at a rate of 1 mEq/kg/min IV, for signs of cardiotoxicity until an effect from sodium polystyrene sulfonate (Kayexalate) is seen. Repeat as necessary for ventricular dysrhythmias (see Chapter 5). NOTE: A large number of babies who have high serum potassium concentrations have relatively minor ECG changes.
   h. After the acute episode is controlled, usually on the second day of therapy, continue 0.45% sodium chloride solution with 5% glucose at maintenance rates.
   i. After control is achieved, add potassium as indicated by serum potassium determinations (do not add potassium unless serum potassium level is less than 3.0 mEq/L). Usually, the institution of oral feedings will allow adequate potassium intake without resorting to IV potassium.

Endocrine system

Endocrine management is directed toward replacement of missing adrenal corticosteroid moieties; once adequate levels are established, the volume, mineral, and carbohydrate abnormalities will also be corrected. Until endocrine replacement is complete, the frequency of monitoring should not be decreased.

Glucocorticoid replacement

1. As an initial dose of glucocorticoid, give hydrocortisone hemisuccinate (Solu-Cortef) by IV push: 25 mg to infants less than 6 months

of age, 50 mg to children 6 months to 6 years of age, and 100 mg to children more than 6 years of age.

2. Give cortisone acetate, 60 mg/m² IM, at the same time as a repository source of glucocorticoid 6 to 9 hours later. The half-life of cortisone acetate is 24 hours, and duration of action is 2 to 3 days.

3. Give one-third to one-half the initial dose of hydrocortisone hemisuccinate every 3 hours for three doses, at which time the cortisone acetate should be absorbed and acting. The half-life of IV hydrocortisone hemisuccinate is 60 to 90 minutes, and duration of action is approximately 4 hours.

4. On the second day, give cortisone acetate, 30 mg/m² IM. Continue this for 2 more days and then switch to oral hydrocortisone, 16 to 24 mg/m² in two to four daily doses.

Mineralocorticoid replacement

1. Mineralocorticoid must be given either IM or orally, the currently available forms in the United States. Give aqueous deoxycorticosterone acetate (DOCA), 1 mg IM initially in a newborn and 2 to 5 mg IM in an older child.

2. On the second day of therapy, give 1 mg of DOCA IM.

3. Long-term therapy should be with fludrocortisone acetate (Florinef), 0.05 to 0.2 mg/day orally.

Salt therapy

Once oral feedings are begun, usually on the third day, add sodium chloride, 1.5 to 3 g/day, to the infant's feedings; the amount in each feeding is determined by dividing the total amount by the number of feedings to evenly distribute the salt throughout the day.

Perioperative

1. Give cortisone acetate, 60 mg/m² IM, 12 hours before the operation. This will produce a high steroid level just before and during anesthesia, which are times of maximal stress normally associated with high levels of circulating steroid.

2. Give cortisone acetate, 30 mg/m² IM, with the preoperative medications. This will produce a peak steroid level during the postoperative period.

3. Correct serum electrolyte and fluid imbalances vigorously. Give 0.9% sodium chloride solution with 5% glucose rather than lactated Ringer's solution during the operation.

4. Postoperatively give 0.45% sodium chloride solution with 5% glucose if serum electrolytes remain normal.

5. For minor procedures, add 50 mg of hydrocortisone hemisuccinate to the intraoperative IV fluids.

6. For progressively more complicated cases (higher anticipated stress situation), increase the dose of glucocorticoids. The dose should be at least 30 to 60 mg hydrocortisone or its equivalent per m² IV every 3 to 4 hours.

7. Continue cortisone acetate, 30 mg/m² IM every 24 hours, until the infant can take oral steroids.

8. For mineralocorticoid replacement, give aqueous desoxycorticosterone acetate (DOCA), 1 mg per 0.1 mg fludrocortisone acetate (Florinef) taken, normally every 24 hours. Continue until the child is taking oral steroids.

9. Frequently reassess the patient for signs and symptoms of adrenal insufficiency and increase replacement dosage of glucocorticoid and mineralocorticoid if necessary. Perioperatively, closely monitor Na, K, Cl, osmolality, and glucose as well as clinical signs pertaining to volume status and cardiac function.

ADDITIONAL READING

Hughes, I.A., and Winter, J.S.D.: The application of a serum 170H-progesterone radioimmunoassay to the diagnosis and management of congenital adrenal hyperplasia, J. Pediatr. 88:766-773, 1976.

Janoski, A.: Naturally occurring adrenal steroids with salt-losing properties: relationship to congenital adrenal hyperplasia. In Lee, P.A., Plotnick, L.P., Kowarski, A.A., and Migeon, C.J., editors: Congenital adrenal hyperplasia, Baltimore, 1977, University Park Press.

New, M.I., Miller, B., and Peterson, R.E.: Aldosterone excretion in normal children and in children with adrenal hyperplasia, J. Clin. Invest. **45:**412-428, 1966.

Rosler, A., Levine, L.S., Schneider, B., and others: The interrelationship of sodium balance, plasma renin activity and ACTH in congenital adrenal hyperplasia, J. Clin. Endocrinol. Metab. **45:**500-512, 1977.

Wilkins, L., Lewis, R.A., Klein, R., and Rosenberg, E.: Suppression of adrenal secretions by cortisone in case of congenital adrenal hyperplasia: preliminary report, Bull. Johns Hopkins Hosp. **86:**249, 1950.

50 Thyrotoxic crisis

JAMES F. MARKS

DEFINITION AND PHYSIOLOGY

Hyperthyroidism in children is uncommon. In approximately 2% of the cases of thyrotoxicosis the onset occurs before 15 years of age. The most common cause in children is Grave's disease (diffuse toxic goiter); the thyrotoxic phase of Hashimoto's thyroiditis is the second most common cause. The many rare and uncommon types of hyperthyroidism seen in adults (toxic nodular goiter, pituitary TSH-secreting adenoma, hyperthyroidism secondary to hydatidiform mole or choriocarcinoma) are virtually unknown in the pediatric age group.

Hyperthyroidism is characterized by an excess of circulating thyroid hormone, and the physiologic effects are related to this excess. Thyrotoxic crisis (thyroid storm) represents an acute exaggeration of the signs and symptoms of hyperthyroidism such that life-threatening organ system involvement (particularly cardiac and CNS) may result. This situation cannot be differentiated from hyperthyroidism by laboratory studies but must be diagnosed on the basis of clinical manifestations that can be extremely variable. Thyroid storm should be suspected in any patient exhibiting a hypermetabolic state of unknown cause. The signs and symptoms seen are extreme tachycardia, tachypnea, cardiac failure with hypotension, profound hyperthermia (40° to 42° C), nausea, vomiting and diarrhea to the point of dehydration, delirium, acute psychotic behavior, and coma. Untreated thyroid storm can be fatal. On rare occasions one may see apathetic thyrotoxic crisis, in which the patient may be extremely lethargic rather than obviously agitated. The precipitating events that usually occur in a patient who is either undiagnosed or incompletely treated include inappropriately timed surgery, abrupt withdrawal of antithyroid medication, acute severe infection, acute trauma, and the presence of other acute organ dysfunction, such as DKA.

The most common modes of therapy for hyperthyroidism include destruction of the thyroid gland by surgery or radioactive ^{131}I, pharmacologic suppression of synthesis or release of thyroid hormone, and counteraction of related autonomic nervous system manifestations.

MONITORING

See also Chapter 4.

Metabolic system

1. Measure serum thyroxine, triiodothyronine, and thyroid stimulating hormone (TSH) initially, and repeat as needed until a steady state has been reached.
2. Pay particular attention to temperature (see Chapter 18).

MANAGEMENT

Management of thyrotoxic crisis is aimed at diagnosis and treatment of any underlying illness or precipitating factor, general organ system support, reduction in the production and secretion of thyroid hormone, and diminution of its metabolic effects.

Diagnosis and treatment of underlying disorders

1. Cancel surgery.
2. Check medication history for noncompliance.

3. Obtain appropriate cultures and start antibiotic therapy.

General supportive therapy

See also Chapters 6, 13, 16, and 18.
1. Aspirin is contraindicated in control of fever.
2. Fluid replacement should be parenteral.

Blocking of synthesis and release of thyroid hormone

1. Use propylthiouracil in massive doses up to 1.2 g/24 hr (15 mg/kg in three to four doses) orally or via NG tube to block synthesis. Propylthiouracil will also inhibit extrathyroidal (peripheral) conversion of thyroxine to triiodothyronine (the most active form of thyroid hormone).
2. One hour after the above, give a form of sodium or potassium iodide that blocks release of preformed hormone: Lugol's solution (USP), 500 mg orally every 6 hours, or sodium iodide, 500 mg as a constant IV infusion over 8 hours.

Treatment of physiologic effects of increased thyroid hormone level

1. Institute beta blockade with propranolol (Inderal).
   a. Give a loading dose of 1 to 3 mg IV in increments of 0.5 mg every 1 minute. Discontinue propranolol when HR is normal for age or maximum dose is given.
   b. Give a maintenance dose of 1 to 2 mg/kg/24 hr orally, divided into three to four doses (i.e., every 6 to 8 hours).
   c. Propranolol is contraindicated in patients with limited cardiac reserve, heart block, atrial flutter, or bronchial asthma. Propranolol masks the symptoms of hypoglycemia, and diabetics must have monitoring of serum glucose levels.
   d. Symptomatic bradycardia can be reversed with atropine, 0.01 mg/kg IV or SC.
2. Corticosteroids are thought to block peripheral conversion of thyroxin to triiodothyronine and have been reported to increase survival.
   a. Give prednisone, 2 mg/kg/24 hr orally, or
   b. Give hydrocortisone, 3 to 7 mg/kg IV every 4 to 6 hours.

ADDITIONAL READING

Mackin, J.F., Conary, J.J., and Pittman, C.S.: Thyroid storm and its treatment, N. Engl. J. Med. **291:**1396-1398, 1974.

Mukhtar, E.D., Smith, B.R., Pyle, G.A., and others: Relation of thyroid-stimulating immunoglobulins to thyroid function and effects of surgery, radioiodine, and antithyroid drugs, Lancet **1:**713-715, 1975.

Toft, A.D., Irvine, W.J., and Hunter, W.M.: A comparison of plasma TSH levels in patients with diffuse and nodular non-toxic goiter, J. Clin. Endocrinol. Metab. **42:**973-976, 1976.

Turner, J.G., Brownlee, B.E., Sadler, W.A., and others: An evaluation of lithium as an adjunct to carbinazole treatment in acute thyrotoxicosis, Acta Endocrinol. (Kbh) **83:**86-92, 1976.

Volpe, R.: Thyrotoxicosis. In Oppenheimer, J.H., editor: Thyroid today, vol. 1, Evanston, Ill., 1977, Ethical Communications, Inc.

Williams, R.H., editor: Textbook of endocrinology, ed. 6, Philadelphia, 1981, W.B. Saunders Co., pp. 117-248.

51 Inappropriate secretion of antidiuretic hormone

JAMES F. MARKS

DEFINITION AND PHYSIOLOGY

Antidiuretic hormone (ADH or vasopressin) is normally excreted in response to a rise in plasma tonicity and volume depletion. When ADH release occurs in the absence of hypertonicity and volume depletion and with unimpaired renal and adrenal function, the syndrome of inappropriate secretion of antidiuretic hormone (ISADH) is said to occur. Under such circumstances, serum sodium and chloride levels and serum osmolality are less than normal, frequently low enough to produce neurologic symptoms of water intoxication, such as confusion, stupor, coma, and seizures. Urinary osmolality, specific gravity, and sodium are increased. An interesting secondary feature of this condition is increased urinary sodium loss, which likely contributes to the development and prolongation of the hypotonicity. Urinary volume is reduced.

In adults, ISADH may occur on a chronic basis associated with tumors such as bronchogenic carcinoma. It may occur in the pediatric age group as the so-called interphase response in children who are undergoing neurosurgery. This transient phenomenon is mentioned in the discussion of diabetes insipidus (Chapter 52). The most common form of ISADH syndrome in childhood is acute and frequently self-limited. Head injury may sometimes give rise to rupture of the pituitary stalk with a transient period of ISADH. Meningitis, encephalitis, brain abscess, subarachnoid hemorrhage, and the Guillain-Barré syndrome have been described as producing the disorder of ISADH.

A number of circumstances occur in which hyponatremic syndromes may mimic ISADH. Addison's disease is one of these. Myxedema and hypopituitarism are entities in which ISADH has also been suspected. However, the cause in myxedema is more likely reduced kidney perfusion rather than excess secretion of vasopressin. Other entities that may mimic ISADH are a postanesthetic apparently inappropriate vasopressin release, cardiac failure, and hypoproteinemia of various etiologic types, although in such syndromes it has not been proved that vasopressin is present in inappropriately large amounts. One significant difference between such children and those with classic ISADH is their tendency to conserve rather than lose sodium. With the development of sensitive and accurate radioimmunoassays for vasopressin, it is probable that many of these borderline areas will be studied in sufficient depth to more precisely establish the pathogenesis. This discussion is restricted to the classic type of ISADH.

MONITORING

See also Chapter 4.

1. Obtain simultaneous serum and urine Na, K, Cl, and osmolalities initially and every 4 to 6 hours.
2. Measure serum ADH levels if available.

MANAGEMENT

1. The basis of therapy is fluid restriction. Reduce fluid intake by 25%.
2. Reevaluate in 4 to 6 hours. If there is no improvement, decrease fluids to 50% maintenance. Further restriction to 30% or 35% maintenance fluids may occasionally be necessary.
3. Increase fluids when serum Na, K, Cl, and osmolality return to normal and neurologic abnormalities have improved.
4. If seizures are present, 5% hypertonic saline solution, 3 mEq/kg, may be given. Half of this amount should be given over 15 minutes and the remainder over 2 hours. The long-term benefit of hypertonic saline solution without concomitant fluid restriction is minimal.
5. Lithium carbonate and demethoxytetracycline have been used in chronic states of ISADH but are not indicated in the acute, self-limited state.

ADDITIONAL READING

Baker, R.S., Hurley, R.M., and Feldman, W.: Treatment of recurrent syndromes of inappropriate secretions of antidiuretic hormones with lithium, J. Pediatr. 90:480-481, 1977.

Crawford, J.D., and Bode, H.H.: Disorders of the posterior pituitary in children. In Gardner, L.I., editor: Endocrine and genetic disorders of childhood and adolescence, ed. 2, Philadelphia, 1975, W.B. Saunders Co., pp. 151-153.

52 Central diabetes insipidus

JAMES F. MARKS

DEFINITION AND PHYSIOLOGY

Diabetes insipidus is due to the failure of synthesis and/or release of vasopressin from the hypothalamus or posterior pituitary; in the absence of vasopressin the distal nephron is unable to concentrate urine. As a result, polyuria and polydipsia occur. In a basal nonstressed state, most children more than 3 to 4 years of age are able to keep their water requirements balanced by massive fluid intake. Obviously, the children seen in the PICU because of factors such as altered consciousness or stress will be unable to meet these needs.

Diabetes insipidus is encountered in the PICU in two groups of patients. The first group is composed of children who have undergone neurosurgical procedures, some of whom will have had diabetes insipidus before surgery and many of whom will develop diabetes insipidus postoperatively. The largest category of patients in this group is children who have had surgery for craniopharyngioma. The second group is made up of children who have diabetes insipidus after trauma or CNS infection.

The biphasic or triphasic, postoperative clinical course characteristic of children who have normal urine-concentrating abilities preoperatively begins with polyuria hours after surgery. This brisk hyposthenuric polyuria lasts 2 to 3 days followed by a 2- to 3-day period in which there is apparent absorption of residual vasopressin. Subsequently, there will usually be onset of permanent diabetes insipidus. Patients with diabetes insipidus in the postoperative period may void as much as 200 to 300 ml of urine per m^2 per hour and may go into hypovolemic shock.

MONITORING

See also Chapter 4.

Renal-metabolic system

1. Record intake and output every hour or half-hour if urine volume is excessive or if the patient is hemodynamically unstable.
2. Obtain simultaneous serum and urine Na, K, Cl, and osmolalities initially and every hour until stable.
3. Determine urine specific gravity every hour.
4. Obtain urine SAD every 4 hours.

Neuroendocrine system

Diagnose the specific cause.

MANAGEMENT
Renal-metabolic system

1. Give 0.45% sodium chloride solution in 2.5% dextrose, 20 ml/kg IV, over 20 minutes initially to correct shock.
2. Do not depend on fluid administration to stabilize the patient. Until a response to vasopressin is documented, the volume of fluids administered must equal that lost as urine. Once shock is corrected, use solutions with sodium at 10 to 15 mEq/L until the vasopressin is working. Once concentration of urine occurs (specific gravity >1.010), the rate of IV infusion may be decreased (see Neuroendocrine system below).

3. Intravenous glucose administration should be such that urinary glucose determinations are 0 to +1.

Neuroendocrine system

1. Give short-acting aqueous vasopressin (Pitressin) by constant IV infusion.
2. Give 15 mU/hr. Dilute to a standard preparation as 2 mU/ml. Note that vasopressin comes as 20 units/ml; meticulous technique for proper dilution must be followed.
3. Note the response in urine volume every 15 minutes and in serum and urine Na, K, Cl, and osmolality every hour. If there is not a substantial decrease in urine volume and increase in urine osmolality and specific gravity within ½ to 1 hour, increase the infusion to 30 mU/hr. Continue sequential increases in vasopressin dose until the urine volume and concentration are normal (output 1 ml/kg/hr, specific gravity >1.010, serum osmolality 280 to 300 mOsm/ml). This is usually accomplished at a dose between 15 and 60 mU/hr. For infants, start with 2 mU/hr. Increase the infusion by 2 mU/hr at ½- to 1-hour intervals until urine volume and con-

centration are normal. This is usually accomplished at a dose between 2 and 8 mU/hr.
4. Because any increase in the solute load (food, hypertonic solutions, glucose, etc.) presented to the kidneys for excretion will increase obligatory urine output, the patient should be NPO until diabetes insipidus is under control.
5. Maintain this dose until:
   a. The initial phase of diabetes insipidus stops, *or*
   b. The patient is able to take one of the nasal preparations of vasopressin analogs. (DDAVP, which has recently been released for use by the FDA, is the preferred treatment.)

ADDITIONAL READING

Crawford, J.D., and Bode, H.H.: Disorders of the posterior pituitary in children. In Gardner, L.I., editor: Endocrine and genetic disorders of childhood and adolescence, ed. 2, Philadelphia, 1975, W.B. Saunders Co., pp. 138-145.
Hogg, R.J., and Balfe, J.W.: Defective cyclic AMP generation following pit infusion in girls with nephrogenic diabetes insipidus, Pediatr. Res. 11:551, 1977.

ANESTHESIA AND SURGERY

53 Anesthesia

Perioperative principles

FRANCES C. MORRISS

DEFINITION AND PHYSIOLOGY
General principles

The task of the anesthesiologist is to render the patient capable of tolerating painful and traumatic physical invasion without harmful alteration of physiologic homeostasis. This goal is accomplished by administering potent pharmacologic agents, by either inhalational or intravenous technique, or by utilizing locally acting agents to anesthetize the spinal cord or major nerve plexuses.

In order to plan for the safe and rational use of an anesthetic agent, the following points should be considered:

1. Requirements necessary to accomplish the surgical procedure.
2. Patient's state of health.
3. Patient or parent preference in regard to the type of anesthetic agents or techniques to be used.
4. Anesthesiologist's preference for agents and techniques.

Surgical requirements. To be adequately, easily, and rapidly performed, most surgery requires of the patient amnesia, analgesia, muscle relaxation, and elimination of autonomic reflex activity in varying degrees. Other considerations may include patient position (e.g., prone versus supine, sitting), necessity for specialized techniques (e.g., induced hypotension, cardiopulmonary bypass), amount of blood loss expected, pharmacologic agents that may be used by the surgeon (e.g., antibiotics, injectable epinephrine, methyl methacrylate), and discharge status (e.g., outpatient versus inpatient). Satisfaction of surgical needs will provide the surgeon with a quiet operative field and a physiologically stable patient.

Emergency procedures undertaken on an unprepared patient or procedures performed on high-risk patients, as defined by the American Society of Anesthesiologists classification system, require specialized techniques both in administering the anesthetic and in monitoring its effects intraoperatively. Anesthesiologists consider the unprepared patient to have a full stomach, regardless of the history detailing the time of last oral intake, and thus to be at high risk for inhalation of stomach contents, particularly when airway protective reflexes are lost during the induction of anesthesia (at the time patient becomes unconscious). To minimize this risk the following measures are taken:

1. Preoxygenation with 100% oxygen for 3 minutes to increase oxygen stored in the lungs so that a short period of apnea will not result in hypoxia. Note that the younger the patient, the shorter this safe time period will be because of the higher metabolic rate and hence higher consumption of oxygen.
2. Pretreatment (i.e., before induction of anesthesia) with atropine to increase the opening pressure of the gastroesophageal sphincter and with a small dose of a nondepolarizing muscle relaxant to prevent muscle fasciculations associated with the use of succinylcholine. Fasciculations, which occur in patients older than age 6 to 8 years, increase

315

intra-abdominal pressure and thereby increase the possibility of forceful or passive stomach emptying. Preoperative gastric emptying with an NG tube may be helpful, but the presence of an NG tube does *not* preclude the possibility of inhalation of stomach contents. An antacid such as Maalox may also be given to raise the gastric pH above 2.5 and hence to minimize the pulmonary lesion should it occur.

3. Rapid-sequence IV induction of anesthesia with an agent that induces unconsciousness within seconds (e.g., thiopental, ketamine) and a depolarizing muscle relaxant (succinylcholine) that causes paralysis within 30 seconds. Thus the airway may be secured and stabilized quickly; hypoxia will be avoided if intubation occurs within 1 to 2 minutes.

4. Avoid positive pressure ventilation (which would force air into the stomach) until the airway is protected by an endotracheal tube. After age 8 to 10 years the tube should possess an inflatable cuff so that the airway may be sealed more effectively against passive regurgitation. Remember that once anesthesia is induced, airway protective reflexes remain obtunded or absent until the patient awakens fully.

5. Cricoid pressure applied at the time of loss of consciousness to occlude the esophagus and prevent passive regurgitation. Since the cricoid is the only complete tracheal ring, pressure applied perpendicularly over it will cause esophageal occlusion without airway compromise and may make visualization of the larynx easier. Pressure should be maintained until intubation occurs.

These procedures may be bypassed by intubating the patient awake so that protective reflexes are preserved or by utilizing a regional anesthetic technique that does not require intubation. Unfortunately, these practices require patient cooperation and are not appropriate for young children. Neonates, however, because of the high risk of airway obstruction and the expected difficult intubation, are usually intubated awake.

Patient health status. An anesthetic agent given a patient must be compatible with any health problems he may have. The relative risk of surgery may be estimated from the American Society of Anesthesiologists physical status classification that follows:

Class 1: The patient has no organic, physiologic, biochemical or psychiatric disturbance. The pathologic process for which operation is to be performed is localized and does not entail a systemic disturbance.

Class 2: Mild to moderate systemic disturbance caused either by the condition to be treated surgically or by other physiologic processes. . . . Some might choose to list the extremes of age here.

Class 3: Severe systemic disturbance or disease from whatever cause, even though it may not be possible to define the degree of disability with finality.

Class 4: Indicative of the patient with severe systemic disorders that are already life threatening, not always correctable by operation.

Class 5: The moribund patient who has little chance of survival but is submitted to surgery in desperation.

Emergency operation (E): Any patient in one of the classes listed previously who is operated upon as an emergency is considered to be in poorer physical condition.

The higher the physical status class, the greater the risk of morbidity and/or mortality. Numerous studies have shown that anesthetic difficulties encountered in Class 1 or 2 patients are generally the result of mishap, carelessness, or neglect; patients in higher classes encounter problems related to their disease processes and experience greater numbers of cardiac arrests under anesthesia. Patients under the age of 12 months or over 70 years also experience greater risk for cardiac arrest intraoperatively.

Most anesthetic agents have specific contraindications (see Table 53-1) and a careful preoperative history and physical examination must

Table 53-1. Potential harmful effects of anesthetic agents

Agent	Potentially harmful associated effects
Inhalational	
Halothane (Fluothane)	Myocardial depression, dose-related sensitization of myocardium to endogenous or exogenous catecholamines
	Hypercarbia with spontaneous ventilation (decreased TV)
	Trigger agent for malignant hyperpyrexia
	Shivering
	Allergic hepatic reaction
Enflurane (Ethrane)	Shivering
	Vasodilation
	Increased airway irritability, especially with inhalation induction
	Lowers threshold for seizures in presence of hypocarbia
Isoflurane (Forane)	Vasodilation (hypotension)
	Shivering
	Tachycardia
Nitrous oxide and oxygen	Myocardial depression
	Equilibrates with nitrogen in closed air spaces (pneumothorax, gastrointestinal tract) and increases in volume
Intravenous	
Induction agents	
Ketamine	Increased airway secretions
	Increased ICP and intraocular pressure
	Increased heart rate and blood pressure
	Obtundation of protective airway reflexes without respiratory depression
	Postoperative hallucinations
Diazepam (Valium)	Thrombophlebitis
	Prolonged postoperative drowsiness
Thiopental (Pentothal)	Myocardial depression
	Histamine release usually expressed as bronchospasm, swelling and erythema along course of vein, rash
	No analgesia
Narcotics	Respiratory depression, apnea, nausea, and vomiting
Morphine	Hypotension, especially associated with hypovolemia
	Histamine release
	Spasm of sphinctor of Oddi
Meperidine (Demerol)	Hypotension
	Hypertension
Fentanyl	Chest wall rigidity
Muscle relaxants	Paralysis of respiratory muscles
Succinylcholine	Fasciculations
	Dysrhythmias, bradycardia, potassium release, especially from damaged muscles
	Increased intraocular pressure
	Trigger agent for malignant hyperpyrexia
	Myoglobinuria
	Masseter spasm
d-Tubocurarine	Histamine release (bronchospasm, hypotension, rash)
Pancuronium (Pavulon)	Tachycardia
Metocurine (Metubine)	None

be done to detect dysfunction of major organ systems, potentially harmful drug interactions, allergies, chemical imbalances, and familial disposition to anesthetic-related difficulties (e.g., malignant hyperpyrexia, atypical pseudocholinesterase levels). Particular attention must be given to cardiorespiratory function, which is generally depressed by anesthetics, and to those systems (renal, hepatic) that detoxify and eliminate drugs. Chronic conditions such as diabetes mellitis or seizure disorders that may interfere with or worsen during surgery are evaluated to determine optimal perioperative management. Careful review of laboratory data is necessary, and previously undetected problems such as hypokalemia or anemia must be explored and corrected prior to surgery.

In emergency situations every effort should be made to correct metabolic aberrations and to stabilize vital signs so that the patient undergoes the procedure in as good a physical condition as is possible. Highly unstable patients are often placed in the PICU for insertion of IV catheters, invasive monitoring devices, and endotracheal tubes while the operating room is being readied. Complete stabilization is not always possible, but marked improvement in physiologic variables such as pulse rate, systemic arterial blood pressure, peripheral perfusion, temperature, and oxygenation can occur and increase the probability of a trouble-free anesthetic and surgical intervention.

For elective surgery a patient should be in as optimal physical, psychological, and chemical condition as possible, even if achieving this state means delaying surgery for specialty consultation, pulmonary toilet, transfusion, or correction of metabolic abnormality. Particularly in Class 1 or 2 patients, the greatest risk of untoward events is anesthetic not surgical, and adequate preparation is mandatory.

Patient and physician preference. Personal preferences of the patient or his parents should be considered if the agents or techniques requested are not contraindicated by the patient's state of health or the surgeon's requirements.

Usually patient comfort and safety can be combined in a single technique. The anesthesiologist should not utilize an agent or technique with which he is not thoroughly familiar, particularly in the critically ill patient or an emergency situation. When the patient's preference is to be superseded, a careful explanation of the reasons, risks, and benefits of the procedures in question, will usually allay his (or the parent's) anxiety and ensure better cooperation.

Components of anesthesia

After considering the above factors, the anesthetic may be divided into its component parts and appropriate drugs and methods can be chosen to accomplish specific purposes.

Premedication and preoperative preparation. The better acquainted the patient and his parents are with what is going to occur, the calmer and more cooperative they will be. Allaying parental anxiety will often promote calmer and more appropriate handling of a young child or an infant than sedation will. Young children should be given as detailed an account of the upcoming events as they can assimilate; frightening or painful processes should be explained as well. Children accept many unpleasant procedures if they understand them. Under no circumstances should a child be told an untruth in the mistaken belief that he is being spared anxiety; the procedure will be more traumatic because it was not expected. Sedatives, anticholinergics, and analgesics may be given prior to surgery for amnesia, drying of secretions (helpful in the young child who will have inhalation induction), or pain relief (helpful for transporting the child with a fracture or painful injury). Careful attention must be paid to how long young infants are without fluid and calories, in order to avoid dehydration and hypoglycemia. For infants 4 hours is a sufficient period to remain without intake and still ensure an empty stomach. Routine daily medications such as anticonvulsants, digitalis, insulin, bronchodilators, or steroid maintenance therapy should not be withheld.

Choice of regional versus general anesthesia. Regional anesthesia is used infrequently in children, and therefore this discussion will highlight general anesthetic techniques.

Induction of anesthesia. Inhalation of a potent vaporized anesthetic mixed with nitrous oxide (N_2O) and oxygen provides a nontraumatic method of induction for infants, while standard IV induction is used more commonly for older children. Rapid IV induction technique is appropriate for the high-risk or unprepared patient with a full stomach. Inability to start an IV infusion preoperatively is insufficient reason to change the induction technique if an IV induction is the safest route; the surgeon can provide intravascular access via a cutdown. In the critically ill patient most monitoring modes should be established prior to induction since this period is one of great physiologic change and is statistically associated with a large number of problems, particularly hypotension and dysrhythmias.

Airway management and ventilation. Intubation is indicated whenever protection of the airway is needed (e.g., full stomach, Trendelenburg position), the possibility of airway obstruction exists (e.g., prone position, sharing the airway with the surgeon, abnormal airway or facial anatomy), or control of ventilation is necessary (e.g., thoracotomy, paralysis to relax muscles for high abdominal incisions). The decision to control ventilation implies use of muscle relaxants and artificial ventilation controlled either by hand (preferred in infants in order to be able to appreciate changes in lung compliance) or by mechanical ventilator. If respiration is not controlled, the patient may breathe spontaneously via the tube. For cases where intubation is unnecessary, the patient will usually breathe spontaneously and airway management consists of preventing obstruction (jaw thrust, oral airway, head in sniffing position) while administering anesthetic gas or oxygen via a mask.

Maintenance of anesthesia. Adequate depth of anesthesia is maintained throughout the operation by inhalational or intravenous agents.

With the inhalational method a single potent agent (halothane, enflurane, isoflurane) administered with a nitrous oxide–oxygen or air-oxygen mixture satisfies all requirements and has the additional advantage of being easily adjusted to changing requirements in regard to depth of anesthesia. Rapid changes in the blood concentration of the agent are made simply by changing the alveolar concentration of the drug, and this is done by increasing or decreasing the inhaled concentration of anesthetic. The second technique, which uses intravenous agents, is called balanced anesthesia because each surgical requirement is satisfied by a different agent. Narcotics are given for pain relief, muscle relaxants for relaxation, and a neuroleptic agent (e.g., Innovar, ketamine) or an amnestic (e.g., diazepam) for amnesia. Balanced anesthesia usually includes the use of nitrous oxide and oxygen via an endotracheal tube or mask. Obtundation of reflexes occurs when an adequate depth of anesthesia is achieved with the combination therapy described above. It is more difficult to alter the depth of balanced anesthesia since most drugs must be metabolized, bound, or in some way altered before their pharmacologic effects can be changed.

Fluids. Fluid management may also be divided into components. The patient receives his basic hourly maintenance fluids calculated in the usual way (see Chapter 16) plus some portion of the deficit accrued while he was NPO. For short cases one third to one half of the deficit may be given; for long cases all of it will be replaced. Extra fluid losses occurring the night prior to surgery (e.g., from fever, extensive bowel preparation, diarrhea) should be anticipated and corrected preoperatively with IV replacement. In addition, intraoperative fluid losses should be replaced. Intraoperative losses are difficult to measure directly because they often consist of third-space losses; that is, evaporative losses from the surface of exposed bowel or tissue or sequestered losses secondary to large tissue dissections. They have been measured indirectly with radioactive labeled ions and found to be maximal (on the order of 8 to 10 ml/kg/hr) for bowel, retroperitoneal, or pelvic surgery and to have salt content losses approximating plasma. For noninvasive surgery (endoscopic, ophthalmic, otic, dental) fluid losses are minimal and need not be considered. Maintenance solutions may be either D_5 0.25% sodium chloride solution or D_4 modified lactated Ringer's solution. Third-space losses are replaced by the crystalloid equivalent of plasma (0.9% sodium chloride solution, Ringer's lactate). Blood losses less than 10% to 15% of the circulating blood volume are replaced with crystalloid with at least 1 to 1½ ml for each ml lost. Greater blood losses are replaced ml for ml with whole blood or packed RBCs reconstituted with 0.9% sodium chloride solution or plasma to the volume of whole blood. If excessive protein-containing fluids are lost (e.g., ascitic fluid), FFP or 5% albumin solution may be given. These protein-containing solutions are often used to replace volume when rapid blood loss is encountered and no blood for transfusion is available; in fact, protein-containing solutions are preferred in neonates or in children with poor cardiac reserve because smaller total volumes can be given to support the failing circulation. Adequacy of the patient's fluid status is constantly reassessed throughout the operation by monitoring of vital signs, urine output, peripheral perfusion, CVP, and other variables as indicated.

Most patients receiving an anesthetic have high blood sugars secondary to low metabolic utilization of glucose as a result of decreased muscle activity and perhaps, with inhalation agents, peripheral interference with glucose uptake. However, infants less than 2 years of age or debilitated patients are rarely given non–glucose-containing solutions. The signs and symptoms of hypoglycemia are masked by deep anesthesia and the developing CNS is particularly vulnerable to lack of glucose. Patients requiring constant fluid infusions for drug administration (catecholamines, insulin, vasopressin) or parenteral alimentation receive

them as a part of their intraoperative fluids through a second IV, though often the drug infusion concentration may need to be increased in order to decrease the volume administered.

Special techniques. Induced hypotension, endoscopy (shared airway), cardiopulmonary bypass, and other special techniques may be necessary to accomplish specific surgical goals and these techniques usually require a high degree of skill for proper use. Administration of an anesthetic to a neonate or a premature infant less than 6 months of age also requires a high degree of skill as well as a specialized knowledge of pediatrics. It should not be undertaken lightly or by an anesthesiologist who is not experienced in dealing with such children. Planning the anesthesia for these patients must take into consideration their unique physiology:

1. Increased susceptibility to heat loss, particularly in the cold environment (18°-22° C) of the operating room (OR) (see Chapters 85 and 86).
2. Airway anatomy which predisposes the patients to difficult intubation, obstruction, and postintubation croup (see Table 53-2 and Chapter 95).
3. Increased metabolic requirement for calories and energy substrate.

Table 53-2. Neonatal airway anatomy affecting intubation

1. Short neck
2. Relative macroglossia
3. Narrow, easily obstructed nasal passages
4. Cephalad and anterior larynx, with long axis directed inferiorly and anteriorly (secondary to apposition of hyoid bone and thyroid cartilage)
5. Long, U-shaped, stiff epiglottis protruding at 45-degree angle
6. Narrowest diameter of airway at cricoid cartilage (below vocal cords)
7. Relatively narrow diameter of all airways
8. Short (4-cm) trachea
9. Obligate nose breather

Table 53-3. Factors affecting anesthetic requirements in neonates and infants less than 2 years

| Agent | Altered anesthetic requirements (as compared to adults) | | Change in technique |
	Neonate	Infant <2 yr	
Inhalation agents	Higher minimal alveolar concentration needed to achieve surgical anesthesia	Same as neonate	Higher concentration of agent needed; therefore margin of safety between effective and toxic dose is less
	More rapid rise in anesthetic blood levels due to high cardiac output	More rapid than in adults but less rapid than in neonates	Shorter period of induction; greater fall in blood pressure, particularly if administered via positive pressure ventilation
	More rapid pulmonary excretion	Same as neonate	More rapid emergence
Relaxants			
Succinylcholine (Anectine)	Larger volume of distribution for drug	Same as neonate	Higher dose required to produce paralysis
	Decreased levels of pseudocholinesterase	Normal levels	Usually not significant; phase II block more likely
		20% incidence of myoglobinuria after single dose	
d-Tubocarine	Large variation in effective dose	Not significant	Titrate dose to degree of relaxation needed
	Early depression of ventilation		Must be able to manage airway immediately
Pancuronium (Pavulon)	Minimal elevation in heart rate (cardiac muscle is already working at almost maximal efficiency)	Same as neonate	None
Metocurine (Metubine)	None	None	None
Intravenous anesthetics			
Narcotics	Increased sensitivity to respiratory depression and early onset of apnea, especially in premature infants	None	Narcotic premedication contraindicated in children <1 year, must be able to manage airway
Ketamine (Ketamine)	Efficacy is questionable	Decreased incidence of bad dreams	Wider use for short procedures
Diazepam (Valium)	Preservative agent toxic especially in premature infants	None	Contraindicated in neonates
Barbiturates	Increased sensitivity to respiratory depression and early apnea in premature infants	None	Barbiturate premedication contraindicated in children <6 months old

4. Decreased cardiac reserve.
5. Transitional circulation that may include R → L shunts at the atrial level or a PDA and pulmonary arterial hypertension (see Chapter 39).
6. Increased susceptibility of premature retina to oxygen toxicity.
7. Immature CNS and presence of immature reflexes and of abnormal respiratory control (see Chapters 32 and 33).
8. Decreased pulmonary reserve, different pulmonary mechanics from older children.
9. Technical problems related to small size of patient (e.g., adequate vascular access, need for lightweight equipment, need for different anesthesia circuits, need for oxygen-air blends on anesthesia machines).
10. Reactions to anesthetic agents that differ from those of adults (see Table 53-3).

Termination of the anesthetic. The patient should experience a smooth emergence to consciousness without a major change in vital signs. Not only are anesthetic agents (particularly inhalational ones) withdrawn but muscle relaxants are pharmacologically reversed and the endotracheal tube removed at the end of surgery. In some instances if the patient is unstable or has had extensive or prolonged surgery, reversal and extubation are withheld and controlled ventilation is continued into the postoperative period. Critically ill patients return to the PICU directly so that stabilization and intensive nursing care can occur as soon as possible. All other patients go to the recovery room, where close observation and frequent checking of vital signs by experienced nursing personnel will identify early any potential problems. Such problems are usually related either to the surgery itself or to the anesthetic agents or techniques used.

MONITORING

1. Central to ensuring a stable, reactive patient in the recovery period is meticulous attention to detail and frequent monitoring of physiologic variables. Anesthesia alters the patient's protective reflexes, including his ability to verbally alert anyone to his problems, and the anesthesiologist must assume the protective function. Changes in the stability of major organ systems must be recognized early (or anticipated) and corrected. The more information the anesthesiologist has, the more appropriate the intervention can be. In addition, familiarity with specific surgical situations and procedures is essential in anticipating problems such as extra fluid or blood losses, periods of excessive surgical stimulation, or the potential for air embolus, seizures, or peripheral nerve damage. The more invasive the surgery, the longer the procedure, or the more unstable the patient, the more extensive the monitoring. All procedures and modes of monitoring outlined in this text can easily be used in the OR; indications for need are the same.

2. Routine OR monitoring includes continuous ECG, continuous auscultation of heart and breath sounds via a precordial or esophageal stethoscope, frequent (every 5 minutes) indirect blood pressure determinations, continuous rectal or nasopharyngeal temperature determination, and continuous observation by the anesthesiologist of color, peripheral perfusion, and reflex activity.

3. Other monitoring modes frequently used include continuous intra-arterial systemic blood pressure determination; CVP; ICP; pulmonary artery catheter for pulmonary systolic, diastolic, and wedge pressures and thermodilution cardiac output; continuous urine output; expired oxygen saturation; and degree of muscle relaxation, as measured by nerve stimulator. A meticulous record of these variables, correlated with anesthetic drug administration and surgical events, allows the anesthesiologist to keep the patient adequately anesthetized and physiologically stable. Intraoperative monitoring is continued uninterrupted in the postoperative period until major organ system stability is ensured.

ROLE OF ANESTHESIOLOGIST

The anesthesiologist is the patient's advocate intraoperatively. He or she must ensure that all anesthesia equipment is functioning properly; that positioning is anatomically uncompromising; that fluids, blood products, and drugs, including nonanesthetics such as antibiotics, are compatible with each other and the patient's state; that the surgeon is aware of unsatisfactory or dangerous situations such as hyperthermia, unstable vital signs, excessive blood loss, or prolonged tourniquet time. The anesthesiologist must remain vigilant and ensure that the patient comes to surgery in the best possible condition and returns to that condition as soon after surgery as possible. For complex procedures or derangements in physiology, preoperative anesthetic planning must include discussion with the surgeon about surgical requirements, expectations, and probable outcome.

MANAGEMENT OF SPECIFIC POSTOPERATIVE PROBLEMS
Airway problems

The most common postoperative airway problems are postintubation croup (see Chapter 29) and obstruction, usually related to oversedation and/or incomplete reversal of nondepolarizing muscle relaxants. The longer the procedure, the more likely the patient is to suffer respiratory depression from oversedation. Narcotic anesthetics can be reversed with IV naloxone (Narcan) titrated in small doses until the patient's respiratory rate and TV have increased and the patient is responsive. Nonnarcotic depressants such as barbiturates, phenothiazine, or diazepam have no antidote and must be metabolized before their effects wear off. Inhalation anesthetics after prolonged exposure are stored in fatty tissue, which then becomes a depot for the agent as alveolar and blood concentrations decrease. Sufficient time must be allotted to allow reequilibration and excretion of such stores. The patient remains

drowsy for several hours and may hypoventilate, particularly if narcotics are given for relief of pain or if hypothermia retards the natural drug elimination process. The patient who is extubated while overly sedated may have respiratory insufficiency secondary to central hypoventilation or as a result of upper airway obstruction from relaxed pharyngeal musculature. In addition, protective airway reflexes may be absent or obtunded.

The patient with inadequately reversed muscle relaxant will exhibit signs of air hunger, poor air movement by auscultation, floppy muscle tone, and incoordinated, semipurposeful movements, often attributed to uncooperativeness. Muscle tone at this point is inadequate to sustain the work of breathing. Older children will be unable to sustain a head lift off the bed, to sustain a good hand grasp for more than 10 seconds, or to generate an adequate TV or inspiratory pressure. (FVC is a more sensitive measure than TV for specific measurement.) Specific testing with a nerve stimulator will reveal diminished muscle twitch height (in response to a specific stimulus), which becomes more marked after repeated single stimuli. In response to tetanic stimulation (rapid rate of stimulation) a rapid decline in strength of response is seen; the twitch following cessation of tetanic stimulation is increased (posttetanic facilitation). These criteria apply only to a block secondary to nondepolarizing muscle relaxants.

Regardless of the source (oversedation, airway obstruction, poorly reversed neuromuscular block), respiratory distress should be treated immediately with increased ambient oxygen, bag-and-mask ventilation, assurance of an open airway, and, if needed, reintubation with mechanical ventilation. Once the airway is stabilized, diagnosis and appropriate therapy may be accomplished.

The nondepolarizing muscle relaxants (d-tubocurarine, metocurine, pancuronium) block the action of the neurotransmitter acetylcholine by occupying its specific receptor sites in muscle membrane. With acetylcholine access prevented, local muscle membrane depolarization does not occur and end plate potential never reaches the threshold value for muscle depolarization and contraction. The relaxant-receptor interaction is competitive, and in the presence of excessive acetylcholine, relaxant will be displaced from the receptor, allowing depolarization and contraction to occur once again. This is the means by which the pharmacologic action of muscle relaxants is reversed; anticholinesterases are agents that block enzymatic breakdown of acetylcholine and thus provide an excess of transmitter, which is needed to displace relaxant occupying the receptor site. The bond between the relaxant and the receptor cannot be disrupted for a period of about 30 to 40 minutes after the relaxant has been given; thereafter reversal agents can be given. Since the muscle relaxant is still metabolically active and physically present, reparalysis (recurarization) can occur. Factors that favor incomplete reversal of block are overdose of relaxant (excess relaxant is available to interact with unoccupied muscle receptor sites), end plate receptor loss of sensitivity to acetylcholine (e.g., primary muscle disease such as myasthenia gravis), or depolarization block already existing in muscle (presence of excess depolarizing agent, such as succinylcholine or acetylcholine). Excessive drug may be present because of actual drug overdose, inability to metabolize the relaxant, or large stores of protein-bound unmetabolized agent. This last situation may be seen with renal failure where serum-binding protein may be elevated and the drug cannot be excreted via the kidneys.

Factors that favor recurarization after the initial block has been reversed and that potentiate the action of relaxants and lead to unintentional overdose are:

1. Hyperthermia, which potentiates block (hypothermia antagonizes block even though metabolic breakdown is slowed).
2. Presence of agents with weak membrane-depolarizing capacities (aminoglycoside antibiotics, propranolol, quinidine, procainamide, diphenylhydantoin).
3. Electrolyte imbalances that may affect the repolarization-depolarization process in muscle membrane (hypokalemia, hyperkalemia, hypocalcemia, hypermagnesemia, hyponatremia, acidosis, lithium).
4. Abnormal muscle membrane per se (primary muscle disease such as myasthenia gravis or muscular dystrophy, wasting disease, and secondary muscle disease caused by lower motor neuron lesions). Such diseases may also cause abnormal responses, such as spasm, when muscle relaxants are given.
5. Administration of drugs that displace muscle relaxants from plasma or tissue protein-binding sites and thus increase the concentration of free, active agent.

The treatment for inadequate reversal of relaxant is to promptly reestablish an airway; usually an endotracheal tube and assisted or controlled ventilation are necessary to prevent hypoxia and hypercarbia. Reversal agents may be repeated if nondepolarizing relaxants (d-tubocurarine, pancuronium, metocurine) were used to produce block, 20 or more minutes have elapsed since the initial reversal, and conditions known to potentiate block have been eliminated or diagnosed. The patient should not be given narcotic agents simultaneously with agents to reverse neuromuscular block, since even with adequate reversal of block hypoxia and hypercarbia may occur if central respiratory depression is present. The usual anticholinesterases used are pyridiostigmine, 0.14 mg/kg, or neostigmine, 0.04 mg/kg IV push, accompanied by glycopyrrolate, 0.006 mg/kg, or atropine, 0.01 mg IV push, to prevent the muscarinic (vagal-stimulating) effects that accompany anticholinesterase administration. Otherwise bradycardia, bronchorrhea, and excessive salivation may occur. If adequate ventilation is not reestablished, mechanical ventilation should be continued until return of adequate strength is documented and arterial blood-gas and pH values are normal with spontaneous (unassisted) respiration. Then the patient may be safely extubated.

Hypotension

See also Chapters 14 and 54.

The most usual cause of hypotension in the immediate recovery period is hypovolemia, either relative and secondary to vasodilation, usually drug induced, or absolute and secondary to loss of circulating blood volume. Loss of circulating volume may be related to inadequate replacement of fluid and/or blood intraoperatively or to active hemorrhage occurring postoperatively. In any of the above situations administer fluid (i.e., 10 to 20 ml/kg of Ringer's lactate, 0.9% sodium chloride solution, or 5% albumin) while diagnostic tests are being done. Hemorrhage is generally secondary to inadequate surgical hemostasis, but bleeding diathesis should be investigated, especially if anticoagulants or large-volume transfusions have been given. Relative hypovolemia may be caused by transfusion reaction, drug-induced vasodilation, or residual autonomic blockade accompanying spinal or epidural anesthesia. Chlorpromazine (Thorazine), narcotics, droperidol (Inapsine), and barbiturates are all potent vasodilators. In patients with suspected hypovolemia who need analgesia, narcotic agents should be given in small, repeated IV doses while frequent systemic arterial blood pressure determinations are made; otherwise large drops in blood pressure may occur.

Hypothermia

During prolonged exposure to a cold environment, abnormally low temperatures are common in small children because of their poor ability to conserve and generate heat. Most operating rooms have an ambient temperature between 18°-21° C. Hypothermia increases caloric expenditure, causes hypoglycemia and

apnea in neonates, prolongs drug half-life by decreasing the rate of metabolic reactions in general, promotes shivering and increased oxygen consumption in older children, and retards recovery from general anesthesia. Measurement of core temperature on admission to the recovery room should be routine and passive external warming procedures should be begun immediately if abnormal temperature is documented. Warmed, humidified oxygen should be given and narcotics withheld until core temperature is above 36° C. Dextrostix should be checked in neonates and fluids adjusted if hypoglycemia is documented. Hypothermic patients are usually not extubated because of a high incidence of respiratory instability and the increased work of breathing; if they have been extubated, respiratory support may have to be reinstituted. Estimation of peripheral perfusion and color are difficult in a hypothermic patient; arterial blood gas tensions and pH should be obtained if any doubt exists.

Vomiting

Vomiting, a common postoperative problem, is multifactorial in etiology. Many drugs, such as narcotics and inhalational anesthetics, produce nausea and emesis. Surgery on the gastrointestinal tract is associated with ileus, and the patient in such a case will usually have an NG tube. Surgery on ears or extraocular muscles may adversely affect the semicircular canals and induce vomiting. Swallowing blood after dental procedures or gastric distension from air may induce vomiting. Patients with a history of motion sickness also seem prone to emesis. Regardless of the etiology, emesis is generally innocuous if protective airway reflexes are present; this cannot be assumed to be true in the immediate postoperative period. Patients with a high probability of emesis (e.g., tonsillectomy, strabismus correction) should be placed in a lateral, head-down position, with an emesis basin and suction nearby so that vomitus may be quickly removed from the airway. Persistent vomiting not associated with gastrointestinal surgery can be treated with antiemetics as soon as the patient is alert and can gag and swallow. Fluids must be adjusted to accommodate extra losses. Ambulatory surgical patients should be watched for longer periods than usual, and they may be sent home with antiemetics (one or two doses) if follow-up within 24 hours can be assured.

ADDITIONAL READING

Barash, P.G., Ganz, S., Katz, J.D., and others: Ventricular function in children during anesthesia: an echocardiographic evaluation, Anesthesiology 49:79-85, 1978.

Bennett, E.J.: Fluids for anesthesia and surgery in the newborn and the infant, Springfield, Ill., 1975, Charles C Thomas, Publisher.

Bennett, E.J., Kanchan, P.P., and Grundy, E.M.: Neonatal temperature and surgery, Anesthesiology 46:303-304, 1977.

Betts, E.K., Downes, J.J., Schaffer, D.B., and others: Retrolental fibroplasia and oxygen administration during general anesthesia, Anesthesiology 47:518-520, 1977.

Cook, D.R., and Fischer, C.G.: Neuromuscular blocking effects of succinylcholine in infants and children, Anesthesiology 42:662-665, 1975.

Cook, C.D., and Motoyama, E.K.: Respiratory physiology. In Smith, R.M., editor: Anesthesia for infants and children, ed. 4, St. Louis, 1980, The C.V. Mosby Co., pp. 32-73.

Eckenhoff, J.E.: Some anatomic considerations of the infant larynx influencing endotracheal anesthesia, Anesthesiology 12:401-410, 1951.

Furman, E.B., Roman, D.G., Lemmer, L.A.S., and others: Specific therapy in water, electrolyte and blood-volume replacement during pediatric surgery, Anesthesiology 42:187-203, 1975.

Goudsouzian, N.G., Dorlon, J.V., Savarese, J.J., and others: Re-evaluation of dosage and duration of action of d-tubocurarine in the pediatric age group, Anesthesiology 43:416-424, 1975.

Goudsouzian, N.G., Liu, L.M.P., and Savarese, J.J.: Metocurine in infants and children: neuromuscular and clinical effects, Anesthesiology 49:266-269, 1978.

Goudsouzian, N.G., Ryan, J.E., and Savarese, J.J.: Neuromuscular effects of pancuronium in infants and children, Anesthesiology 41:95-98, 1974.

Nicodemus, H.F., Nassiri-Rahimi, C., Bachman, L., and others: Median effective doses (ED50) of halothane in adults and children, Anesthesiology 31:344-348, 1969.

Nugent, S.K., Lavavuso, R., and Rogers, M.C.: Pharmacology and use of muscle relaxants in infants and children, J. Pediatr. 94:481-487, 1979.

Rackow, H., and Salanitre, E.: Modern concepts in pediatric anesthesiology, Anesthesiology 30:208-234, 1969.

Rashad, K.F., and Benson, D.W.: Role of humidity in prevention of hypothermia in infants and children, Anesth. Analg. 46:712-714, 1967.

Relton, J.E.S., Brett, B.A., and Steward, D.J.: Malignant hyperpyrexia, Br. J. Anaesth. 45:269-276, 1973.

Salem, M.R., Bennett, E.J., Schweiss, J.F., and others: Cardiac arrest related to anesthesia: contributing factors in infants and children, J.A.M.A. 233:238-246, 1975.

Salem, M.R., Wong, A.Y., and Collins, V.J.: The pediatric patient with a full stomach, Anesthesiology 39:435-440, 1973.

Salem, M.R., Wong, A.Y., Mani, M., and others: Premedicant drugs and gastric juice pH and volume in pediatric patients, Anesthesiology 44:216-219, 1976.

Schell, N.B., Karelitz, S., and Epstein, B.S.: Radiographic study of gastric emptying in premature infants, J. Pediatr. 62:342-347, 1963.

Smith, P.C., and Smith, N.T.: Anaesthetic management of a very premature infant, Br. J. Anaesth. 44:736-737, 1972.

Stehling, L.C., and Zauder, H.L., editors: Anesthetic implication of congenital anomalies in children, New York, 1980, Appleton-Century-Crofts.

Steward, D.J.: Manual of pediatric anesthesia, The Hospital for Sick Children, Toronto, Canada, New York, 1979, Churchill Livingstone.

Steward, D.J.: A simplified scoring system for the postoperative recovery room, Can. Anaesth. Soc. J. 22:111-115, 1975.

Steward, D.J., and Creighton, R.E.: The uptake and excretion of nitrous oxide in the newborn, Can. Anaesth. Soc. J. 25:215-217, 1978.

54 Cardiothoracic surgery
Perioperative principles

LAWRENCE J. MILLS
EDGAR A. NEWFELD
DEBRA A. SAYLES

The successful correction of cardiac defects in infants and children requires the close cooperation of all disciplines caring for the patient. The significance of errors in management is inversely proportional to the size of the child, so that near perfection in technique is required at all phases of the patient's care if success is to be achieved in children less than 1 year of age.

The mainstay of precise, expeditious surgery is accurate preoperative anatomic and physiologic diagnosis. The cardiologist must have an intimate knowledge of the surgical procedures in order to obtain the information crucial to the surgeon. Surgeons are greatly hampered if they are required to search for additional lesions or if they find residual shunts or obstructions after the planned repair has been accomplished. Preoperative preparation is quite important. Congestive heart failure should be aggressively treated with digitalis and furosemide, and respiratory failure should be treated even if this requires assisted ventilation. Metabolic acidosis (pH <7.20) should be corrected with sodium bicarbonate, improvement of cardiac output, and oxygenation if possible. Surgical intervention should not be delayed in favor of protracted medical therapy unless prompt and clearly defined improvement occurs during the immediate preoperative period. Unfortunately, in many instances significant improvement cannot be made preoperatively, and the patient must undergo the operation in a less than optimal physiologic state.

Palliative operations are generally performed without the use of cardiopulmonary bypass. These procedures increase pulmonary blood flow (Blalock-Taussig operation, Waterston shunt, Glenn procedure), reduce pulmonary blood flow (pulmonary artery banding), or increase mixing within the heart (Rashkind balloon atrial septostomy, Blalock-Hanlon operation). Other procedures that can be accomplished without resorting to cardiopulmonary bypass are closure of a PDA, resection of a coarctation of the aorta, and relief of pulmonary stenosis.

More complex intracardiac lesions require the use of extracorporeal circulation. The pump-oxygenator combined with a high efficiency heat exchanger allows protection of the myocardium as well as other tissue (e.g., kidney, brain) during the intracardiac repair. Standard cardiopulmonary bypass utilizes venous drainage from the superior and inferior vena cavae and systemic arterial return to the ascending aorta or, less commonly, the femoral artery. Hypothermia (20° to 32° C) is commonly employed to permit reduced bypass flows and increased myocardial protection during periods of aortic cross-clamping. Most lesions can be repaired under these conditions.

For smaller children, accurate repair is facilitated by the technique of profound hypothermia and total circulatory arrest. Midline sternotomy and vessel cannulation are then performed, and the patient is rapidly cooled to 15°

C while on cardiopulmonary bypass. Bypass is then terminated, the patient's blood drained into the bypass reservoir, and the venous return cannula removed to provide dry, quiet, unobstructed access to the heart. Once the surgical repair has been accomplished, bypass is resumed and the patient rewarmed. The limits of hypothermic circulatory arrest have not been clearly defined, but up to 60 minutes appears to be well tolerated by the patient.

Careful and accurate monitoring of a number of physiologic variables is essential to the intraoperative management and is equally crucial in the early postoperative period. The methods and importance of monitoring in various clinical situations are discussed below.

MONITORING

See also Chapter 4.

ECG

The rate of recording observations ranges from as often as every 5 minutes initially to every 2 to 4 hours once the patient's condition is stable. Full 12-lead diagnostic tracings should be made immediately after surgery and whenever a change in rhythm or configuration occurs in a single-lead monitor trace (see Chapter 82). Routine ECG monitoring should never be interrupted in this group of patients.

Temperature, pulse, and respiration

The rate of rewarming is a guide to the adequacy of cardiac output. Hyperthermia may occur early in the postoperative course and should be rapidly treated to reduce excessive systemic oxygen requirements and increased myocardial work. Bradycardia is often the first sign of acute hypoxemia or may represent cardiac conduction system injury leading to varying degrees of heart block. Bradycardia is an emergency situation that demands immediate treatment. Since it is most often related to hypoxemia, first check for adequacy of ventilation, institute manual ventilation with oxygen, and then obtain a full ECG to determine if heart block is present.

Systemic arterial blood pressure (P_{sa})

Considerable information can be obtained from the form of the pressure tracing, from pulse pressure, and from the location of the dicrotic notch. Cuff blood pressures are often difficult to obtain in a cold patient and when significant peripheral vasoconstriction is present. If vasoactive drugs are being administered by constant IV infusion, intra-arterial pressure monitoring is mandatory, since minute-to-minute adjustments of medications are often necessary. (See Chapters 83 and 87 for more information.)

Right- and left-sided filling pressures (preload)

The major hazard associated with the left atrial pressure (LAP) catheter is gas or particulate embolism via the catheter into the systemic circulation (coronary, brain). Use of infusion pumps, Intraflow systems, and careful nursing have eliminated these complications (see Chapters 84, 87, and 90). Blood oxygen samples from the LAP catheter can be used to differentiate intrapulmonary from residual intracardiac right-to-left shunts. Measurement of LAP provides the most accurate guide to colloid replacement and is the earliest indication of hypovolemia. In combination with measurement of the cardiac output, LAP provides an excellent index of left ventricular performance (see Chapters 88 and 90).

Pulmonary arterial blood pressure (PAP)

A pulmonary artery catheter is placed at the time of surgery in patients who have elevated pulmonary vascular resistance preoperatively or elevated pulmonary arterial blood pressure after surgical repair (see Chapter 88). In such patients the pulmonary vascular bed is often extremely reactive, and pulmonary vascular resistance increases with hypoxemia, changes in alveolar oxygen concentration, and/or metabolic acidosis. Monitoring of PAP may be crucial during weaning from mechanical ventilation or during reduction of the inspired oxygen concentration. Normally, pulmonary vascular resistance is 20% of the systemic vascular resistance. Elevations in PAP to greater than 60% of P_{sa} are dangerous and should be reversed if possible. Blood oxygen samples from the pulmonary arterial catheter provide mixed venous blood and, when compared to right atrial blood oxygen samples, can detect residual $L \rightarrow R$ shunts.

Epicardial pacing and diagnostic wires

After surgical repair, temporary removable epicardial pacing wires are sutured to the right ventricle or right atrium whenever there is concern about the maintenance of sinus rhythm in the postoperative period. Operations performed in the vicinity of the atrioventricular node or the bundle of His are always accompanied by the placement of pacing wires. These procedures are closure of VSD, repair of the atrioventricular canal, correction of Ebstein's anomaly, correction of truncus arteriosus, Mustard's operation, repair of a primum-type atrial septal defect, and correction of tetralogy of Fallot. In addition, if preoperative conduction disturbances exist, temporary wires are attached at the time of surgery.

Atrial wires may be used for atrial pacing or sequential atrioventricular pacing. Recordings from the atrial wires provide excellent tracings that can discriminate between supraventricular dysrhythmias and ventricular tachydysrhythmias.

Care must be exercised to avoid contact of pacing wires with electrical equipment, by wrapping them in nonconductive material, since tiny currents delivered directly to the myocardium via pacing wires can induce ventricular fibrillation.

Mediastinal and chest tubes

See also Chapter 102.

Plastic drainage tubes are placed to collect blood and serous drainage from the mediastinum or pleural spaces. These tubes are placed to water-seal drainage to prevent air from being sucked into the chest cavity during inspiration. Water suction of 20 cm can be safely applied to the water-seal bottle to facilitate drainage. Stripping of tubes is done frequently in the immediate postoperative period to remove clots, maintain the patency of the tubes, and ensure continued evacuation of blood and fluid from the mediastinum or pleural spaces.

Removal of chest tubes requires precautions to avoid entry of air into the pleural spaces. Because the chest wall is quite thin in infants, it is a good practice to preplace a purse-string suture around the tube entry site and tie the suture as the tube is removed. This technique is superior to the use of a bulky petroleum-jelly gauze dressing to seal the incision.

Chest tubes are removed when drainage becomes serous in nature and minimal in volume. In children, drainage usually ceases in 36 to 48 hours. If intracardiac blood pressure monitoring catheters have been inserted directly through the myocardium, chest tubes should remain in place until the catheters have been removed. This precaution is not necessary for temporary epicardial pacing wires.

Chest tube drainage should be recorded every hour for the first 8 hours. After this, unless unusual drainage occurs, recording once each shift is sufficient until the tubes are removed.

Urinary output

In all cases in which cardiopulmonary bypass is utilized, a bladder catheter is inserted preoperatively in the operating room. Postoperatively, urinary output can be used as an indirect guide to cardiac output (normal is >1 ml/kg/hr).

Chest roentgenogram

A chest roentgenogram is obtained immediately after the patient's arrival in the recovery area. Specific findings must be noted:
1. Position of the tip of the endotracheal tube.
2. Location of intracardiac catheters.
3. Position of chest tubes and location of the most proximal fenestra.
4. Search for lobar collapse, pneumothorax, or hemothorax.
5. Evaluation of pulmonary vascular markings as signs of fluid overload or areas of pulmonary hypoperfusion.

Chest roentgenograms are repeated every morning as long as the patient is in the PICU. Additional films are required after manipulation of the endotracheal tube and removal of chest tubes or transmyocardial catheters (e.g., pulmonary arterial, LAP). Obtain a chest roentgenogram whenever an unexplained change occurs in arterial blood gas tensions or pulmonary compliance.

Echocardiograms

Previously, the diagnosis of pericardial effusions and chronic postoperative tamponade has been difficult. However, the echocardiogram can identify pericardial accumulations and residual shunts with a high degree of accuracy (see Chapter 93).

Blood studies

Since anesthesia, cardiopulmonary bypass, hypothermia, and various intraoperative medications can all produce significant alteration in the acid-base status and serum electrolytes, careful monitoring of these variables should be done in the operating room, where every attempt is made to correct abnormalities. Arterial blood-gas tensions, pH, and serum Na, K, Cl, and Ca are always obtained in the immediate postoperative period and again within several hours. In unstable patients or those with documented abnormalities in these variables,

repeat determinations are indicated as frequently as every few hours. In patients undergoing intracardiac repair, clotting studies (PT, PTT, and platelet count) should be performed during the immediate postoperative period and repeated frequently until normal.

DETECTION AND MANAGEMENT OF SPECIFIC POSTOPERATIVE PROBLEMS
Low cardiac output

Monitoring. In infants and children, the major determinant of survival after cardiac surgery is adequate cardiac performance and not the incidence of sudden unexpected complications. Cardiac performance, or cardiac output, can be assessed clinically by observing indirect signs, or it can be measured directly.

Indirect signs. Indirect signs of low cardiac output are the signs of poor organ perfusion. They are manifested as cool and pale extremities (skin), oliguria (renal), stupor and other neurologic dysfunction (CNS), and the signs of shock, including the possible development of DIC (see Chapter 14). The variables usually monitored are P_{sa}, LAP, CVP, urinary output, and the metabolic component of pH. Problems of preload, or inadequate left ventricular filling, are manifested by low LAP (should be 10 to 14 mm Hg) in the presence of a normal or decreasing P_{sa}. Abnormal afterload, or increased impedance to left ventricular emptying, is manifested by an adequate or high LAP and a high P_{sa} with signs of low cardiac output. Under these circumstances, systemic vascular resistance is greater than normal (see Chapter 14).

Direct measurement. Cardiac output can be measured in the postoperative period using the dye dilution or the thermal dilution method. The dye dilution technique utilizes indocyanine green (0.625 mg/dl for patients who weigh less than 10 kg, 1.25 mg/dl for patients who weigh between 10 and 20 kg), with the indicator rapidly injected into the right atrium or pulmonary artery and sampled from blood continuously withdrawn from a peripheral systemic arterial catheter through a cuvette densitometer. Cardiac output is determined using an adaptation of the Hamilton-Stewart formula.

The thermal dilution technique utilizes injection of 0.9% sodium chloride solution (either cold or at room temperature) into the right atrium while the temperature of the blood is continuously measured by a thermistor-tipped catheter in the pulmonary artery. This latter method has the advantage of allowing repeated measurements without the need for blood withdrawal (see Chapter 91). Direct measurements of cardiac output taken serially during the early postoperative hours can facilitate the early detection of deteriorating cardiac performance. A cardiac index (cardiac output per m²) of less than 2.0 L/min/m² is associated with a high incidence of postoperative mortality, and if serial measurements suggest a trend of progressively falling values, specific therapeutic measures should be instituted.

Management. When cardiac output is low, specific contributing factors, such as excessive bleeding, cardiac tamponade, and electrolyte or acid-base abnormalities, should be diagnosed and treated. If the heart rate is less than 80 to 90 beats/min, it should be increased to 120 to 140 beats/min in young infants and to 90 to 110 beats/min in older children by either atrial or ventricular electrical pacing. Once these specific factors have been identified and treated, the cardiac output should be reassessed clinically or remeasured directly.

Hypovolemia (inadequate preload). When the cardiac index is less than 2.5 L/min/m² and the P_{sa} and LAP are low, whole blood (if hemoglobin is greater than 15 g/dl, use Plasmanate or FFP) is infused to elevate LAP to 10 to 14 mm Hg. If cardiac output and P_{sa} are still low, an inotropic agent such as dopamine, isoproterenol, or epinephrine should be given (see Chapter 14 for doses and administration).

Impedance to left ventricular emptying (increased afterload). When the left atrial and systemic arterial mean blood pressures are elevated and the measured cardiac index is still less than 3.0 L/min/m², a peripheral vasodilator such as nitroprusside, phentolamine, or nitroglycerine should be given (see Chapter 14 for doses and administration). LAP must be carefully monitored during infusion of vasodilators, since sudden peripheral vasodilatation may rapidly increase the need for volume administration in most patients, and whole blood, packed RBCs, or plasma may be needed in conjunction with this form of therapy.

Postoperative hemorrhage

Postoperative hemorrhage is defined as chest tube drainage greater than 3 ml/kg/hr that persists for more than 3 consecutive hours. Causes of excessive bleeding fall into two categories: surgical bleeding or coagulopathy.

The cause of surgical bleeding is inadequate hemostasis at the time of chest closure. All possible sites have been implicated at one time or another. Cardiac suture lines, cannulation sites, pericardial edges, the sternal periosteum, sites of sternal wires or sutures, exit points of chest tubes, monitoring catheters, and pacing wires are the usual sites, and all must be examined if reexploration is performed.

The most common cause of postoperative hemorrhage is failure to restore normal coagulation after cardiopulmonary bypass. The routine heparin protocol consists of 3 mg/kg given at the time of cannulation, with one quarter of this dose administered for each hour of bypass time thereafter. After decannulation, protamine sulfate, 5 mg/kg, is given. Because of the empiric dosages and the partial dissociation of the heparin-protamine complex, inadequate reversal may occur. In addition, platelet function may be impaired along with dilutional reduction of plasma coagulation factors. Fibrinolysis may contribute to bleeding alone or in addition to the above factors. Use of activated clotting time as a measure of both adequate anticoagulation while on bypass and adequate protamine reversal has proven helpful in reducing bleeding related to induced coagulopathy.

Diagnosis and management. Early determination of a coagulation profile is essential. PT, PTT, TT, platelet count, activated clotting time, and observation of the clotting process in a plain glass tube compose the basic minimal profile. These determinations preferably should not be drawn from a catheter in which a solution containing heparin is running.

Coagulopathy
1. Heparin excess.
   a. Laboratory tests.
      (1) PT mildly prolonged.
      (2) PTT markedly prolonged.
      (3) TT markedly prolonged and not corrected by 1:1 dilution with fresh plasma.
      (4) Clot forms slowly (longer than 8 to 10 minutes) and appears soft and mushy.
   b. Treatment.
      (1) Give protamine sulfate slowly, 1 mg/kg IV (may cause hypotension).
      (2) Repeat dose if coagulation tests continue to indicate heparin excess.
2. Dilution of coagulation factors.
   a. Laboratory tests.
      (1) PT and PTT moderately prolonged.
      (2) Clot forms slowly and is of poor quality.
      (3) TT moderately prolonged but corrected by 1:1 dilution with fresh plasma.
   b. Treatment.
      (1) Give fresh plasma, 10 ml/kg.
3. Thrombocytopenia or platelet dysfunction.
   a. Laboratory tests.
      (1) PT, PTT, and TT normal.
      (2) Clot forms promptly but does not retract over 15 to 20 minutes.
      (3) Platelet count low but may be low normal (approximately 100,000/mm³).
      (4) Oozing from surgical wounds.

   b. Treatment.
      (1) Give platelet concentrate, 1 unit/5 kg up to 10 units maximum.
4. Increased fibrinolysis.
   a. Laboratory tests.
      (1) PT, PTT, TT, and platelets normal.
      (2) Clot forms and may retract but then lyses within 1 hour.
      (3) Prolonged euglobulin lysis test (difficult to obtain).
   b. Treatment.
      (1) Give ϵ-aminocaproic acid, 200 mg/kg IV and then 150 mg/kg every 2 hours for a total of 12 hours.
5. DIC (see Chapters 14 and 20).

Surgical bleeding
1. Diagnosis.
   a. Continued chest tube drainage greater than 3 ml/kg/hr for 3 hours.
   b. Normal coagulation studies.
   c. Chest roentgenogram often shows widening of mediastinum or accumulation of blood in the pleural space, since clotting occurs normally. In coagulopathy, blood usually remains liquid and is drained more completely by the chest tubes.
2. Management.
   a. Reexploration.

Cardiac tamponade

Cardiac tamponade occurs when the pericardial pressure is sufficiently high to impair cardiac filling and thus reduce cardiac output. A free communication between the pleural space and the pericardium, an opening in the pericardium, or the presence of mediastinal chest tubes does not ensure the absence of cardiac tamponade. In the postoperative period, tamponade must be considered whenever there is evidence of low cardiac output, especially if there has been excessive chest tube drainage.

The diagnosis of tamponade can be difficult. Even though atrial filling is being impaired by an extrinsic clot and atrial blood pressures should increase, in the face of previous bleeding the atrial blood pressures may not be abnormally elevated as a result of concomitant hypovolemia.

Exact guidelines to the diagnosis of tamponade cannot be established since myocardial failure may produce all of the findings of tamponade, but certain findings make the diagnosis highly probable:

1. Excessive chest tube drainage (>3 ml/kg/hr) that ceases suddenly and is followed by systemic hypotension.
2. Rising left and right atrial blood pressures with systemic arterial hypotension.
3. Systemic hypotension in a patient not expected to have myocardial insufficiency.

Diagnosis. Once the suspicion has been established, the degree of systemic hypotension determines if time is available for further diagnostic maneuvers or if immediate mediastinal exploration is indicated. There is no single confirmatory noninvasive test to establish the presence of tamponade. The following maneuvers may be of considerable help:

1. Measurement of intrapericardial pressure through the chest tube.

a. Materials.
   (1) CVP manometer.
   (2) Three-way stopcock.
   (3) Sterile 20-gauge needle.
   (4) Sterile 0.9% sodium chloride solution.
b. Procedure (Fig. 54-1).
   (1) Clamp latex tubing between chest tubes and chest drainage system.
   (2) Fill manometer with 0.9% sodium chloride solution and insert needle into latex tubing proximal to clamp.
   (3) Measure pressure by observing height of fluid in the manometer, using midchest as zero level.
c. Interpretation.
   (1) If the pressure is equal to or less than atrial blood pressure, tamponade is highly unlikely.
   (2) If the pressure is higher than atrial blood pressure, there is tamponade or the chest tube is clotted. Either situation warrants exploration.
2. Chest roentgenogram.

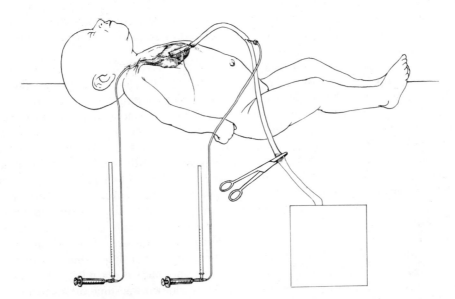

Fig. 54-1. Technique of measurement of intrapericardial pressure. A water manometer is attached to a clamped intrapericardial tube. Pressure is compared with LAP or CVP.

a. Widening of the mediastinum is highly suggestive of undrained and mediastinal hemorrhage, which may be the cause of tamponade.

Management

1. Volume replacement with blood is indicated to support cardiac filling until exploration can be performed.
2. Only in an extreme emergency situation should anyone other than a thoracic surgeon reopen the chest incision in the PICU.
3. Procedure: the lower one third of the incision is prepared with an iodine solution and reopened, and the fascial sutures are cut. The index finger is inserted under the sternum to elevate it, and a tonsil sucker connected to suction is used to evacuate blood from the substernal space and the space inferior to the heart. The hemodynamic response should be nearly instantaneous.
4. The patient is then transported to the operating room for complete reexploration and closure.

Residual cardiac disease

Palliative surgery. Residual cardiac disease is always present after palliative cardiac operations and may be a cause of low cardiac output in the postoperative period. A common example is congestive heart failure after a systemic-pulmonary arterial shunt operation for diminished pulmonary blood flow. The sudden increased pulmonary blood flow causes volume overload of the heart (usually the left ventricle). This is manifested clinically by tachycardia, gallop rhythm, hepatomegaly, and pulmonary congestion (active and passive) revealed by chest roentgenogram. Management should include digoxin, diuretics, fluid restriction, and assisted mechanical ventilation when indicated (see Chapter 13). If these measures are ineffective, reoperation to diminish the shunt size is indicated. In most patients, a period of medical management is successful in allowing the left ventricle to adjust to the increased volume load, and reoperation is not necessary. The opposite

problem exists after pulmonary artery banding in patients with an increased pulmonary blood flow. If the pulmonary artery band is too tight, there will be inadequate pulmonary flow, which can result in hypoxemia and low cardiac output. The chest roentgenogram will reveal oligemic lung fields. Prompt reoperation is indicated, since this state is not tolerated well. If cardiac arrest occurs, resuscitative efforts are usually unsuccessful.

Corrective surgery (usually open heart). Inadequate repair of congenital or acquired cardiac lesions should be detected intraoperatively and appropriate treatment undertaken before the patient is transferred to the PICU. When a patient has significant residual cardiac disease after open heart surgery (e.g., severe residual right ventricular outflow obstruction after repair of tetralogy of Fallot), it usually impairs cardiac performance and causes low cardiac output. These patients should be given as much support as possible, including assisted mechanical ventilation. The use of inotropic agents such as digoxin, dopamine, or isoproterenol may be indicated, and if cardiac output does not improve with their use, early repeat cardiac catheterization and reoperation must be considered to diagnose residual correctable lesions.

Myocardial damage

Myocardial injury can occur during open heart surgery, either inadvertently or as a result of the ventriculotomy needed for cardiac repair. Some degree of myocardial damage occurs in many patients as a result of cardiopulmonary bypass, regardless of the techniques employed. Myocardium that was preoperatively abnormal (e.g., severe left ventricular hypertrophy) is especially susceptible to ischemic damage during cardiopulmonary bypass. Injury to coronary arteries, such as may occur to an aberrant anterior descending coronary artery in some patients with tetralogy of Fallot, can severely impair postoperative cardiac performance and is associated with a high risk of intraoperative and/or postoperative mortality. All of these patients need some form of inotropic agent for cardiac support, and care should be taken to avoid, when possible, agents (such as epinephrine) that can produce tachycardias and other dysrhythmias that can further impair cardiac performance.

Pulmonary hypertension and arteriospasm

Patients with pulmonary arterial hypertension and pulmonary vascular disease represent high surgical risks and require special postoperative management. The PAP should be monitored by an indwelling pulmonary arterial catheter, and assisted mechanical ventilation should be used for at least the first 24 to 48

hours after surgery. Because of the marked degree of pulmonary arterial smooth-muscle hypertrophy present, there is the danger of pulmonary arteriospasm, with a sudden decrease in cardiac output leading to rapid cardiac arrest. A pulmonary vascular bed of this type is extremely sensitive to stimuli such as hypoxia, hypoxemia, and acidosis, and these must be carefully avoided postoperatively. The risks of arteriospasm are high during endotracheal-tube or orotracheal suctioning, which produces a rapid drop in Pa_{O_2}. Hyperoxygenation by manually hyperventilating the patient with 100% oxygen should always be done before suctioning. Sudden pulmonary arteriospasm manifested by a

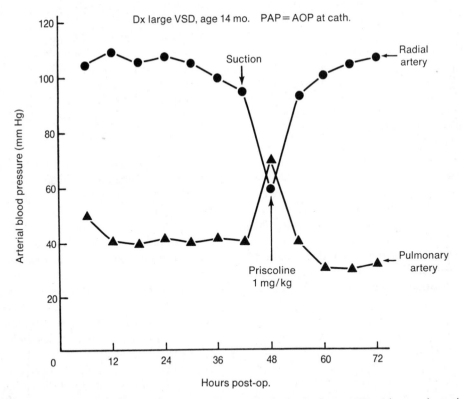

Fig. 54-2. Postoperative pulmonary arteriospasm after closure of a large VSD. After endotracheal suctioning 40 hours after surgery, (PAP) rose and P_{sa} fell. After infusion of tolazoline (Priscoline) directly into the pulmonary artery catheter PAP fell and P_{sa} returned to normal levels. *AOP*, aortic blood pressure; *cath*, cardiac catheterization; *Dx*, diagnosis; *PAP*, pulmonary arterial blood pressure; *VSD*, ventricular septal defect.

rise in PAP and a fall in P_{sa} and cardiac output should be promptly treated with hyperoxygenation and infusion of a pulmonary vasodilator into the pulmonary artery catheter. Tolazoline, 1 mg/kg, infused slowly over a period of several minutes, has been found effective in relieving pulmonary arteriospasm in some patients (Fig. 54-2).

Dysrhythmias

Dysrhythmias can occur after heart surgery, and although generally transient and well tolerated, they can impair cardiac performance. Their occurrence is more common in the presence of electrolyte imbalance (especially hypokalemia), metabolic acidosis, excess digitalis, preexisting or residual cardiac disease, and hypoxemia. These factors should be corrected when diagnosed.

Dysrhythmias that impair cardiac performance are bradycardias, tachycardias, and ventricular extrasystoles (see Chapter 5). Bradycardias with rates less than 80 beats/min should be increased by pacing to rates of 120 to 140 beats/min in young infants and to rates of 90 to 110 beats/min in older children, preferably by sequential atrial and ventricular stimulation, to provide the most efficient cardiac output. Tachycardias reduce cardiac output by decreasing ventricular filling time and thereby reducing stroke volume. Supraventricular tachycardias, such as paroxysmal atrial tachycardia or atrial flutter and fibrillation, should be treated with electrical cardioversion (see Chapter 5). Prompt termination of such tachydysrhythmias is indicated, because extremely rapid rates (250 to 350 beats/min) are poorly tolerated in the postoperative patient. Atrial pacing at faster rates can often capture the pacemaker control and interrupt the dysrhythmia. Ventricular tachycardia always reduces cardiac output significantly and should be promptly converted either by rapid pacing or more often by a combination of drugs, such as lidocaine (1 mg/kg dose IV, may be repeated up to 6 times at 10 minute intervals) or procainamide (5 to 8 mg/

kg/dose every 6 hours), and cardioversion (see Chapter 5). Ventricular extrasystoles can be treated with lidocaine or rapid pacing to interrupt the dysrhythmia. Complete atrioventricular dissociation is usually transient but should be treated with ventricular pacing to provide an adequate ventricular rate.

Transvenous pacemaker insertion

1. Equipment.
   a. Transvenous catheter (inserted like a CVP or pulmonary artery catheter).
   b. Cutdown tray (see venous cutdown procedure, p. 509).
   c. Battery pacemaker (check the date battery last replaced).
   d. ECG leads, electrodes, and monitoring unit.
2. Method.
   a. Usually the insertion of a transvenous catheter is done in emergency situations when drugs have been tried and are ineffective in increasing the heart rate and epicardial pacemaker wires have not been placed at the time of surgery.
   b. The pacemaker wire may be inserted percutaneously but usually will be inserted via a cutdown and the tip advanced to a length estimated to place it in the apex of the right ventricle.
   c. After insertion, attach the positive lead to the positive electrode and the negative lead to the negative electrode (Fig. 54-3).
   d. Set pacemaker rate, mode, sensitivity, and milliamperage (ma). The ma should be set at twice the level required to achieve capture.
   e. Note ECG pattern on the monitor, checking for pacing spikes before each QRS complex (Fig. 54-4). If spikes are difficult to see, get a paper copy of the rhythm strip. The tip of the catheter may have to be repositioned if complete capturing is not present.
   f. Secure the catheter and dress the insertion.
   g. Cover the pacemaker with a large surgical

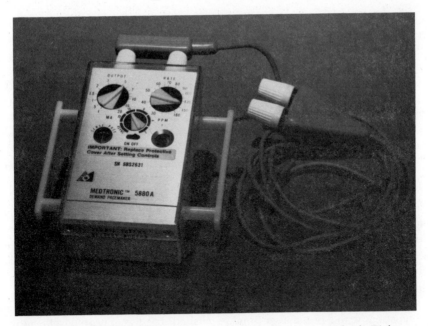

Fig. 54-3. Medtronic demand pacemaker battery, external, with wires attached. Dials: upper left, *MA* is the battery output in milliamps; upper right, the heart rate desired; lower left, pacing or sensing indicator; lower right, off-on safety catch; center, demand or fixed-rate setting; bottom center, off-on switch.

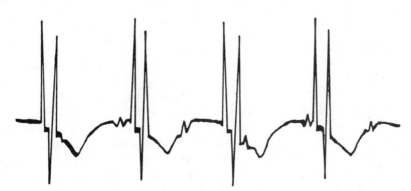

Fig. 54-4. Note pacemaker artifact just before each QRS complex in a patient with a functioning pacemaker.

glove to prevent water, blood, or other debris from coming in contact with the wires or connections and causing malfunction of the pacemaker.

h. Secure the pacemaker to the child's bed so that no tension will be applied to wires or connections.

i. Obtain a chest roentgenogram to check catheter tip position.

Internal pacemaker

1. Equipment. Since most patients who have undergone open heart surgery will return from surgery with pacing wires in place, the only equipment needed is ECG leads, elec-

trodes, and the monitoring unit. For internal pacing, one of two types of pacemakers will accompany the patient: demand or AV sequential.

  a. A demand pacemaker unit senses the rate of the patient's QRS complex, allowing the patient's heart to function and emitting pacing impulses only when the patient's spontaneous rates become less than a preset rate.

  b. The AV sequential unit will pace both the atria and the ventricles with an adjustable AV interval. An attempt to achieve atrial pacing alone should be made first, then, if there is an AV block, AV pacing should be established. An AV interval of 100 to 150 msec is usually optimal. The asynchronous mode is not likely to achieve a smooth response.

2. Receiving the patient with a pacemaker from surgery.

  a. The pacemaker is usually connected and pacing at the rate set in surgery. When the patient arrives, note the pacemaker rate, sensitivity, and ma and whether it is sensing or pacing.

  b. Connect the patient's leads to the monitor and note the presence of pacer spikes.

  c. Cover the pacemaker with a large surgical glove.

  d. Secure the pacemaker to the child's bed so that no tension will be applied to wires or connections.

CAUTION: With the pacemaker on, the heart rate monitor will sense the pacemaker spikes and display a heart rate (e.g., 120 beats/min), and thus the alarm will not sound even if the patient's heart has no intrinsic electrical activity. These patients may also be on a mechanical respirator and therefore may not have apnea. In any such patient, *always note the arterial pressure tracing* to document adequacy of cardiac output.

If a previously functioning pacemaker fails to capture and conduct a stimulus that initiates a QRS complex, the following steps should be taken, in order, until the problem is resolved:

1. Check that all connections are dry and secure.
2. Increase the milliamperage (ma).
3. Insert a fresh battery.
4. Check a chest roentgenogram to determine if the wires have become dislodged or broken.
5. Insert a transvenous pacemaker.

Infection

Prophylactic antibiotics. Prophylactic antibiotics are used routinely in patients having open heart surgery. The only clear evidence for the appropriateness of this practice is studies involving prosthetic heart valves in adults. Since intracardiac patches, pledgets, and suture lines are difficult to rid of infection once established, the use of prophylactic antibiotics seems justified. The most important factor in prophylaxis is adequate levels of antibiotic in blood and tissue at the time of incision. Gram-positive organisms are the most common offenders; therefore, an antibiotic with gram-positive activity is chosen.

Current practice is to give a cephalosporin IM 4 to 6 hours before surgery in a dose of 25 mg/kg. An IV bolus in the same dose is given in the operating room as soon as an IV route is established. Erythromycin lactobionate, 10 mg/kg IV given in the operating room, is used in patients with known or suspected sensitivity to cephalosporin. The IM route is not used in small infants who have inadequate muscle mass for deep injection. Antibiotics are continued only as long as central IVs and chest tubes remain, usually 2 to 3 days.

Prosthetic endocarditis. Infection of an intracardiac prosthesis is a serious complication; it is associated with high mortality. The majority of reported infections involve valve replacements; infection of intracardiac patches, baffles, and conduits is fortunately rare. Since eradication of established infection on foreign material is extremely difficult, prevention of infection is of major importance.

The role of prophylactic antibiotics in such patients is discussed above. Careful attention to asepsis in all phases of care is critical. IV catheters, CVP catheters, transthoracic monitoring catheters, temporary pacing wires, and chest tubes all provide entrance routes for bacteria. All IV tubing should be changed daily and the skin entry site cleansed with an iodine solution. The need for a urinary bladder catheter and for arterial, central venous, left atrial, and pulmonary artery catheters should be reviewed daily, and they should be removed as soon as possible. Protracted use of prophylactic antibiotics beyond the period of potential contamination may favor the appearance of endocarditis by opportunistic bacteria and fungi.

The specific management for established prosthetic infection cannot be reviewed here. Even with the best therapy, early onset (within 60 days) of prosthetic infection has a mortality greater than 50%. Early reoperation may improve the survival rate.

Wound and mediastinal infections. Wound and mediastinal infections are fortunately rare after open heart surgery. The reported incidence in adults is between 1% and 2%. Most infections can be related to certain predisposing factors, including prolonged perfusion time, excessive postoperative bleeding, depressed cardiac output in the postoperative period, and a history of reexploration for bleeding. Most infections are caused by gram-positive organisms.

Incisions must be carefully examined daily for erythema, drainage, or instability. If significant doubt exists, needle aspiration can be performed to establish the diagnosis.

Once mediastinal infection is diagnosed, surgical intervention is indicated. If the infection is detected early, the wound is reopened, debrided, and reclosed, with irrigation and drainage catheters in the anterior mediastinum. Continuous irrigation with antibiotic solution for 7 to 10 days may be adequate to allow pri-

mary healing. Initially, triple antibiotic solution is used (neomycin, bacitracin, polymyxin), and the solution is changed to a specific antibiotic when culture results and organism sensitivity are known.

If the infection is advanced and there is considerable soft-tissue involvement, extensive debridement of all involved bone and cartilage is essential. The wound is left open, all foreign material is removed, and antibiotic dressings are applied. Healing is by second intention. Patients can usually tolerate the open sternotomy if the wound is well packed and supported with a snug dressing.

Wound dehiscence. Wound separation in the absence of infection may occur in the early postoperative period and is usually the result of poor tissue strength, prolonged mechanical ventilator support, or overvigorous CPT. The skin may remain intact, with separation of the underlying muscles. The presence of swelling, serosanguineous drainage, or a palpable defect establishes the diagnosis. If the skin has separated, a sterile dressing should be applied. Definitive treatment is prompt resuturing in the OR.

Renal failure

Acute tubular necrosis occurring as a result of a transient period of low cardiac output is the most common cause of renal failure in the postoperative period and is more likely to occur in patients with preexisting renal disease. It is manifested by a decreasing urinary output and elevated levels of BUN and serum creatinine in the face of normal LAP and P_{sa} and other signs of adequate cardiac output. Management should include a trial of increased fluids and diuretics (furosemide, up to 4 to 8 mg/kg IV, and mannitol, 1 g/kg IV), and if urinary output does not increase, failure management should be instituted (see Chapter 17).

Diuresis is usual in the period immediately after termination of cardiopulmonary bypass. This is caused by the large fluid load imposed by transfusion of the extracorporeal circuit fluid prime at the end of the procedure. This diuresis will often occur in the face of depressed cardiac output and does not ensure against later renal insufficiency or low output state. Considerable amounts of potassium may be lost during this diuresis and should be replaced. A safe maximum dose of potassium chloride, 0.5 mEq/kg/hr, can be administered through a central venous catheter. Frequent monitoring (every 1 to 2 hours) of the serum potassium level is essential, especially if the possibility of diminished renal function exists.

Postcoarctation repair syndrome

After repair of coarctation of the aorta, patients can develop systemic hypertension to levels greater than preoperative measurements. This hypertension is usually transient, but if the blood pressure is greater than 160/100 mm Hg, it should be treated. Reserpine, 0.07 mg/kg IM every 12 hours, is usually effective in lowering P_{sa}. Occasionally a single dose results in permanent lowering of P_{sa}, but treatment is generally required for several days. Nitroprusside infusion is also effective if intra-arterial monitoring is being performed. Hypertension that occurs after coarctation of the aorta is occasionally associated with a syndrome of abdominal pain, paralytic ileus, and/or bloody diarrhea that is believed to be secondary to a mesenteric arteritis. Treatment should consist of lowering of P_{sa}, NG suction, and appropriate IV fluids until symptoms subside. Perforation of the bowel has been reported with this syndrome, but this is rare.

CNS dysfunction

Neurologic impairment in the postoperative period, which may be manifested by local or diffuse neurologic signs, is usually the result of either an intraoperative air embolism or a hypotensive episode with CNS injury occurring secondary to low cardiac output. Embolization of particulate matter, such as platelet or fibrin thrombi, fat, calcium, or other material, is a less common cause of CNS injury because of the use of special blood filters in the extracorporeal circuit. Regardless of the cause, most abnormalities will disappear in the postoperative period, so that adequate support will often result in complete neurologic recovery. Specific measures to reduce cerebral edema or treat seizures should be instituted (see Chapters 9 and 10). If hemiplegia or paraplegia develops, appropriate physiotherapy should be promptly instituted to prevent contractures.

Postpericardiotomy syndrome

A syndrome characterized by fever, pericardial friction rub, precordial pain, and occasionally signs of congestive heart failure (such as hepatomegaly and fluid retention) can occur in some patients after cardiac surgery. It typically appears 7 to 21 days after surgery but may appear within the first 48 hours, while the patient is still in the PICU. Studies have shown the syndrome to be an autoimmune phenomenon resulting from the production of heart antibodies in response to the surgical procedure. It is usually self-limited and can be managed with nonsteroidal agents such as indomethacin or by rapidly tapering doses of corticosteroids, but occasionally it can cause significant pericardial effusion and even cardiac tamponade, requiring prompt pericardiocentesis. This syndrome needs to be differentiated from other causes of fever in the postoperative period, particularly sepsis. Recovery usually occurs in a few days to a few weeks, and there do not appear to be any sequelae.

ADDITIONAL READING

Bove, E.L., and Behrendt, D.: Open heart surgery in the first week of life, Ann. Thorac. Surg. 29:130-134, 1980.

Buckberg, G.D., Towers, B., Paglia, D.E., and others: Subendocardial ischemia after cardiopulmonary bypass, J. Thorac. Cardiovasc. Surg. 64:669-684, 1972.

Casali, R., Simmons, R.L., Najarian, J.S., and others: Acute renal insufficiency complicating major cardiovascular surgery, Ann. Surg. 181:370-375, 1975.

Cordell, A.R., and Ellison, R.G.: Complications of intrathoracic surgery, Boston, 1979, Little, Brown & Co.

Fordham, M.E.: Cardiovascular surgical nursing, New York, 1962, Macmillan, Inc.

Harrison, D.C.: Action of drugs in patients early after cardiac surgery. I. Comparison of isoproterenol and dopamine, Am. J. Cardiol. **35:**656-659, 1975.

John, E.G., Levitsky, S., and Hastreiter, A.R.: Management of acute renal failure complicating cardiac surgery in infants and children, Crit. Care Med. **8:**562-569, 1980.

Kouchoukos, N.T., and Karp, R.B.: Management of the postoperative cardiovascular surgical patient, Am. Heart J. **92:**513-531, 1976.

Kouchoukos, N.T., Sheppard, L.C., and Kirklin, J.W.: Effect of alterations in arterial pressure on cardiac performance early after open intracardiac operations, J. Thoracic. Cardiovasc. Surg. **64:**563-572, 1972.

Midgley, F.M.: Recent advances in postoperative care of the pediatric patient, Crit. Care Med. **8:**559-561, 1980.

Parr, G.V.S., Blackstone, E.H., and Kirklin, J.W.: Cardiac performance and mortality early after intracardiac surgery in infants and young children, Circulation **51:**867-874, 1975.

Waldo, A.L., MacLean, W.A.H., Karp, R.B., and others: Sustained rapid atrial pacing to control supraventricular tachycardias following open heart surgery, Circulation **51** and **52**(Suppl. II):11-13, 1975.

55 Neurosurgery

Perioperative principles

FREDERICK H. SKLAR

GENERAL PRINCIPLES
Intracranial pressure

In the management of critically ill neurosurgical patients it is necessary to monitor and manipulate numerous interrelated physiologic variables, particularly ICP (see Chapter 10). To review briefly, the brain is enclosed in a rigid container, the skull, which limits the total volume of its contents. Under normal circumstances the intracranial compartment consists of brain tissue, CSF, and circulating blood. A slowly expanding mass lesion can displace CSF or blood from the intracranial compartment. Once compensatory mechanisms fail, normal ICP cannot be maintained, and a small volume increment (such as that from flush solutions) results in a large pressure response. The volume change responsible for intracranial decompensation may be due to the mass lesion itself or to a change in brain bulk related to another physiologic variable, such as vascular engorgement secondary to hypercarbia (see below). Traumatic subdural, epidural, or intraparenchymal hematomas as well as brain tumors, focal and diffuse areas of brain swelling, and perioperative blood clots are a few examples of space-occupying lesions. Obstruction of the CSF pathways can also result in intracranial decompensation. The cerebral circulation is very sensitive to changes in Pa_{CO_2}. Hypercarbia increases cerebral blood flow by vasodilation, resulting in an increase in brain bulk and ICP if compensatory mechanisms are inadequate. Conversely, hypocarbia causes vasoconstriction and brain relaxation. Hypoxia can also result in vasodilation and can increase brain edema.

Fever

Blood in the subarachnoid space frequently causes an aseptic meningitis, and fever after craniotomy or head trauma is common. Cerebral metabolic demands increase with fever, and this can aggravate existing neurologic deficits. Therefore, fever is treated aggressively with antipyretics and a cooling blanket. A possible infectious cause of the fever cannot be overlooked, and this suspicion increases if fever persists several days after surgery. However, aseptic meningitis can result in fever that lasts 10 days or more.

Diabetes insipidus and ISADH

Diabetes insipidus and ISADH occur not infrequently after craniotomy or head trauma (see Chapters 51 and 52).

Seizures

Seizures also occur frequently in these patients and may be associated with significant morbidity. Seizures may result in a Valsalva maneuver and apnea and may increase ICP to dangerous levels. Interference with respiration can result in hypoxemia and hypercarbia that cause the brain to become engorged with blood, increasing cerebral edema and ICP. Decerebrate posturing may also increase ICP.

Existing transtentorial herniations and foramen magnum pressure cones may be enhanced by these events.

Hydrocephalus

Because hydrocephalus is frequently associated with midline tumors and can develop acutely after posterior fossa surgery, intraventricular pressure is usually monitored in these patients. Sudden intracranial decompensation related to acute hydrocephalus can result in respiratory or cardiac arrest.

MONITORING

See also Chapter 4.
1. The patient's level of consciousness, equality and reactivity of the pupils, and the strength of the arms and legs are evaluated frequently. It is important to stimulate the child in order to assess accurately his neurologic status. Often a lethargic child will brighten up significantly when he is simply propped up in bed. Children with a depressed level of consciousness may require pinching of the trapezius muscle to arouse them or to observe their response to noxious stimuli. Rubbing the sternum should be avoided, since it leaves disfiguring bruises.
2. An indwelling peripheral arterial catheter provides continuous measurement of systemic arterial blood pressure and ready access to arterial blood samples.
3. A bladder catheter allows for hourly monitoring of urinary output and specific gravity.
4. Direct measurement of ICP with a ventricular or subdural catheter or a subarachnoid bolt is frequently done in critically ill neurosurgical patients (see Chapter 92). Palpation of the fontanelle is also an important part of the evaluation of ICP in infants. The risks of direct ICP measurement must be weighed against the benefits; ICP measurements are not routinely used in all neurosurgical patients.

MANAGEMENT
Intracranial pressure

See also Chapter 10.
Pupillary dilation may be a sign of brain herniation and requires immediate neurosurgical reassessment. Decerebrate and decorticate posturing may also indicate neurologic deterioration.

CSF drainage. CSF may be drained from a ventricular catheter when ICP exceeds 15 mm Hg. Since acute hydrocephalus may be of etiologic importance in cardiorespiratory arrest, always open the ventricular catheter to drain CSF if an arrest situation should occur. If a ventricular catheter is not in place, a ventricle is tapped through a twist drill hole or existing shunt (see Chapter 92).

Position. Patients should be positioned with the head elevated approximately 30 degrees to improve venous return from the brain. Do not flex the neck.

Fluids. IV fluids should be restricted (50% to 60% maintenance) but must be adjusted to maintain a minimum urinary output of 0.5 ml/kg/hr. IV fluids should be given cautiously by an infusion pump to prevent accidental fluid overload.

Other modes of treatment
1. Medical adjuncts to control increased ICP include dexamethasone, mannitol, furosemide, and hyperventilation (see Chapter 10).
2. The extremities should be restrained to prevent the child from dislodging the various tubes and monitoring devices. The unrestrained and confused child can fall from the bed and complicate his condition.
3. There should be no restrictive bands or tape around the neck, such as to secure an endotracheal tube.

Fever

Patients are treated with acetaminophen (1 gr/yr) for a temperature greater than 38.2° C and, in addition, with a cooling blanket for a temperature greater than 39.0° C.

Seizures

See also Chapter 9.

Most patients who undergo craniotomy or who have a serious head injury receive anticonvulsants prophylactically. When they occur, seizures are treated aggressively. With frequent seizures and status epilepticus it may be necessary to use pancuronium and mechanical ventilation to avoid ICP increases. In addition, patients who have generalized seizures while on a volume ventilator may develop a pneumothorax or pneumomediastinum. Forced ventilation against a rigidly fixed chest cage can be avoided by a protective respiratory pressure valve or by the use of pancuronium and controlled mechanical ventilation.

56 Burns

RONALD M. SATO

DEFINITION AND PHYSIOLOGY

The severity of a burn is determined by (1) the type of injury (flame, liquids, chemicals, electrical, radiation), (2) the duration of contact, (3) the area injured including percent of total body surface and location (vital anatomic areas), (4) associated injuries, and (5) preexisting illnesses or conditions.

Any child with a severe burn should be referred to a specialized burn facility as soon as his condition has been stabilized by securing the airway and IV infusions. A severe burn is defined as: (1) covering greater than 15% of body surface area, (2) involving the face or perineum, (3) second- or third-degree burns of the hands or feet, (4) circumferential burns of extremities, (5) deep second- and third-degree burns requiring early excision, (6) inhalation injury resulting in carbonaceous sputum, bronchospasm, and declining pulmonary function. Severe burns are often caused by bathing infants in hot water, and this may be associated with child abuse. The percentage of the body surface area burned may be estimated by the "rules of nines," which states that for adults each upper extremity is 9% of the body surface area, each lower extremity is 18%, the anterior trunk is 18%, the posterior trunk is 18%, the head is 9%, and the perineum is 1%. Second- and third-degree burns are combined in this estimation. In infants the head is 18% at birth, decreasing by 1% for the first nine years.

MONITORING

See also Chapter 4.
1. Temperature must be monitored closely, since body heat is easily lost through the burn wound, especially during dressing changes. A sudden rise in temperature between the fifth and seventh day postburn may herald the onset of burn wound infection.

MANAGEMENT
Integument

1. Give a tetanus booster if indicated. Give oral penicillin, 50,000 to 100,000 units/kg/day in three divided doses, for 5 days.
2. For analgesia use codeine, 0.5 to 1.0 mg/kg/dose PO every 4 hours, or meperidine (Demerol), 1 to 1.5 mg/kg/dose IM or IV every 4 hours, as necessary.
3. Initially cleanse the burned area with an iodine solution (Betadine) or a mild soap, and debride it, removing all loose skin and broken blisters. Small intact blisters may be left intact.
4. Apply 1% silver sulfadiazine cream (Silvadene) and a sterile dressing to protect the wound and prevent contamination. Change the dressing at least every 24 hours, reapplying the Silvadene cream. Observe for cellulitis and areas trapping pus. Obvious third-degree burns should be excised and grafted. Biologic dressings such as a porcine heterograft may be used over superficial second-degree burns to decrease pain and promote healing.

Systemic

1. Increased fluids, either oral or parenteral (Ringer's lactate) may be needed to maintain adequate urine output of at least 1 ml/kg/hr. The Parkland or Baxter formula (4 ml/kg/

345

percent burn) may be used as a guide for resuscitation of a major burn. There is approximately a 15% incidence of hypoglycemia during the first 48 hours in infants subjected to a major burn. Small amounts of glucose may be needed if signs of hypoglycemia are seen.

2. Because of the increased metabolic demands caused by the burn injury, nutrition is an important part of burn care. Daily calorie counts may be necessary. An estimation of the total caloric requirements is (60 calories × weight in kilograms) + (35 calories) × (percent burn).

ADDITIONAL READING

Gordon, M.D.: Nursing care of the burned child. In Artz, C.P., Moncrief, J.A., and Pruit, B.A., Jr., editors: Burns, a team approach, Philadelphia, 1979, W.B. Saunders Co., pp. 390-409.

57 Necrotizing enterocolitis

WILLIAM DAMMERT

DEFINITION AND PHYSIOLOGY

Necrotizing enterocolitis is an ischemic disorder of the gut that occurs in susceptible infants, especially stressed premature infants. The cause of the disease is unknown although several mechanisms have been suggested, including a vascular reflex that produces selective ischemia of the gut to protect the brain, heart, and kidneys during periods of asphyxia (the diving-seal reflex). Also suspected are infections, hyperosmolar feedings, polycythemia, lack of maternal milk, and umbilical artery and umbilical vein catheters. There is an association between the occurrence of necrotizing enterocolitis and PDA. This may be due to ischemia to the bowel secondary to the large diastolic run-off into the pulmonary vascular bed and/or due to splanchnic vascular constriction caused by digitalis, which in the past was frequently used in the management of preterm babies with large PDAs causing congestive heart failure. One study suggests that some affected infants have few of the usual risk factors and may have a history positive for placenta previa but not have respiratory disease. It is probably prudent to consider necrotizing enterocolitis as a syndrome with multiple causes.

The onset of signs is usually at 3 days of age. Patients have gastric retention, vomiting, abdominal distention, and bloody stools. Roentgenographically, distended loops of bowel with thickened walls and ascites are suggestive of the diagnosis, and intramural air (pneumatosis intestinalis), portal vein gas, and free intraperitoneal air are pathognomonic. With progression of the disease, bowel ischemia leads to necrosis, perforation, peritonitis, sepsis, shock, DIC, and death.

MONITORING

See also Chapter 4.

Gastrointestinal tract

1. Monitoring must be started as soon as any newborn patients are admitted. Detecting early signs is critically important for preventing a fatal progression of the disease.
2. Measure abdominal girth every 8 hours from the time of admission.
3. Note the character and frequency of vomiting.
4. Check for gastric residuals before feedings.
5. Note volume of NG drainage when the tube is in place.
6. Check any suspicious-appearing gastric residuals or stools for blood by Hematest. Once the patient is suspected of having necrotizing enterocolitis or is at exceptionally high risk (sick preterm infants, asphyxiated infants, infants with umbilical vessel catheters, infants with congenital heart disease causing low output, infants with PDA), test all gastric residuals and stools for blood. If the result is only slightly positive, test the specimen by the less sensitive (fewer false-positives) guaiac method.
7. Obtain abdominal roentgenograms, anteroposterior and cross-table lateral, if abdominal distention or bloody stools occur. If findings are suspicious, repeat roentgenograms every 6 hours until normal.
8. Inspect the anterior abdominal wall for signs

347

of cellulitis (edema and erythema), which is characteristic of perforation and peritonitis.

Renal-metabolic system

Once the diagnosis is established, increase the frequency of routine monitoring and include frequent blood pH determinations. These patients can be extremely unstable.

Hematologic system

1. WBC count with differential analysis initially and every 12 to 24 hours until stable.
2. Platelet count initially and every 12 to 24 hours until stable.
3. PT and PTT initially; repeat if abnormal.
4. Type and crossmatch.

MANAGEMENT
Gastrointestinal tract

1. Management is initially medical.
2. Give the patient nothing by mouth and establish continuous NG drainage on low suction.
3. Remove umbilical catheters.
4. Treat with systemic antibiotics (see Chapter 41).
5. Barium or Gastrografin enemas are contraindicated.
6. The duration of treatment is controversial. If soft signs (distention, slightly positive Hematest results on stools) are present, after 24 to 48 hours remove the NG tube, and if signs do not recur in 24 hours, introduce feedings cautiously. Use small volumes of dilute, low osmolality formula (e.g., one-fourth or one-half strength Special Care). If intramural air or signs of sepsis (glycosuria, thrombocytopenia, abnormal WBC count, temperature instability) are present, treat for 24 to 48 hours after these conditions revert to normal. If the blood culture is positive, treat for 7 to 10 days after a repeat blood culture shows no growth or until specific clinical signs have resolved.

7. If signs of bowel necrosis or perforation exist, surgery is indicated.
8. Late stricture formation will develop in 5% to 10% of patients, and clinical and radiologic signs of obstruction may be observed.
9. Hyperalimentation may need to be considered if multiple or prolonged episodes of necrotizing enterocolitis occur.

Renal-metabolic system

1. Maintain a neutral thermal environment.
2. Maintain urine output at a minimum of 1 ml/kg/hr. This may require 1½ to 2 times maintenance fluids.
3. Identify and correct hyponatremia, hyperkalemia, hypocalcemia, and metabolic acidosis.
4. Maintain Dextrostix between 45 and 90 mg/dl.
5. Check TSP or A/G ratio and correct any hypoproteinemia (FFP, 10 ml/kg). This may have to be done on a daily basis until hypoproteinemia resolves.

Cardiorespiratory system

1. Shock is frequently associated with bowel necrosis, perforation, and peritonitis. Hypovolemia and hypoproteinemia are the major problems (see "Hypovolemic shock," p. 74).
2. If volume replacement is achieved but hypotension and oliguria persist, use dopamine, 5 to 10 μg/kg/min IV, to increase systemic arterial blood pressure without diverting blood flow from the gut or kidneys. Do not use epinephrine or isoproterenol to support systemic arterial blood pressure.
3. Intubation and assisted mechanical ventilation may be necessary in patients who are stressed or in shock.

Hematologic system

1. Patients may become anemic from blood loss. Maintain Hct at 35% to 40%. Do not increase Hct to more than 55%, since hyper-

viscosity may cause or contribute to the pathophysiology of necrotizing enterocolitis (see Chapter 38).

2. Treat DIC as previously indicated (see Chapter 20).

ADDITIONAL READING

Bell, M.J., Fernberg, J.L., Askin, F.B., and others: Intestinal stricture in necrotizing enterocolitis, J. Pediatr. Surg. **11**:319-327, 1976.

Bell, M.J., Kosloske, A.M., Benton, C., and Martin, L.W.: Neonatal enterocolitis: prevention of perforation, J. Pediatr. Surg. **8**:601-605, 1973.

Cohn, R., Sunshine, P., and deVries, P.: Necrotizing enterocolitis in the newborn infant, Am. J. Surg. **124**:165-168, 1972.

Dudgeon, D.L., Coran, A.G., Lauppe, F.A., and others: Surgical management of acute necrotizing enterocolitis in infancy, J. Pediatr. Surg. **8**:607-614, 1973.

Harrison, M.W., Connell, R.S., Campbell, J.R., and Webb, M.D.: Fine structural changes in the gastrointestinal tract of the hypoxic puppy: a study of natural history, J. Pediatr. Surg. **12**:403-408, 1977.

Kirks, D.R., and O'Byrne, S.A.: The value of the lateral abdominal roentgenogram in the diagnosis of neonatal hepatic portal venous gas (HPVG), Am. J. Roentgenol. Radium Ther. Nucl. Med. **122**:153-158, 1974.

Kliegman, R.M., and Fanaroff, A.A.: Neonatal necrotizing enterocolitis: a nine-year experience. I. Epidemiology and uncommon observations, Am. J. Dis. Child. **135**:603-607, 1981.

Kliegman, R.M., and Fanaroff, A.A.: Neonatal necrotizing enterocolitis: a nine-year experience. II. Outcome assessment, Am. J. Dis. Child. **135**:608-611, 1981.

Santulli, T.V., Schullinger, J.T., Heird, W.C., and others: Acute necrotizing enterocolitis in infancy: a review of 64 cases, Pediatrics **55**:376-387, 1975.

Stevenson, J.K., Oliver, T.K., Jr., Graham, C.B., and others: Aggressive treatment of neonatal necrotizing enterocolitis: 38 patients with 25 survivors, J. Pediatr. Surg. **6**:28-35, 1971.

Touloukian, R.J., Poach, J.N., and Spencer, R.: The pathogenesis of ischemic gastro-enterocolitis of the neonate: selective gut mucosal ischemia in asphyxiated neonatal piglets, J. Pediatr. Surg. **7**:194-205, 1972.

Virnig, N.L., and Reynolds, J.W.: Epidemiological aspects of neonatal necrotizing enterocolitis, Am. J. Dis. Child. **128**:186-190, 1974.

Wilson, S.E., and Woolley, M.M.: Primary necrotizing enterocolitis in infants, Arch. Surg. **99**:563-566, 1969.

58 Esophageal atresia

THEODORE P. VOTTELER

DEFINITION AND PHYSIOLOGY

In esophageal atresia there is an abnormal separation of the esophagus from the trachea some time after the twenty-fourth day of gestation. There are four anatomic configurations (Fig. 58-1); proximal esophageal atresia with a fistula between the distal esophageal segment and the trachea, just superior to the carina, is the most common form (87%).

During fetal life the normal mechanism for swallowing amniotic fluid may be disrupted, and approximately 35% of these infants have a prenatal history of polyhydramnios. Shortly after birth they develop respiratory difficulties due to inability to swallow oral secretions, inhalation of these secretions into the lungs, and regurgitation of stomach contents through a distal fistula into the trachea. Infants may also have respiratory distress due to associated cardiac or pulmonary anomalies or to prematurity and hyaline membrane disease. If one attempts to feed these infants, they exhibit dysphagia and may inhale the feeding, exacerbating the respiratory distress. It may be difficult to provide adequate alveolar ventilation in patients with decreased lung compliance, since the gas can flow more easily through the fistula into the more compliant stomach.

Esophageal atresia occurs in approximately one out of 4,500 live births and is frequently associated with cardiac defects (25%), imperforate anus (12%), agenesis or hypoplasia of the lung (4%), and gastrointestinal anomalies (4%). In addition, patients with identifiable chromosomal abnormalities, such as trisomy 13, 18, and 21, polysplenia syndrome, and VATER syndrome (vertebral anomalies, anal atresia, tracheoesophageal fistula, radial dysplasia, and renal dysplasia) have a high incidence of esophageal atresia. These other anomalies may require evaluation before definitive surgery for the esophageal atresia. Patients who have cyanotic congenital heart disease, especially those who have lesions that may require immediate attention, such as D-transposition of the great vessels (balloon atrial septostomy) or pulmonary atresia (PGE_1 infusion followed by systemic-pulmonary shunt) and patients in whom a lesion incompatible with survival is suspected, such as aortic atresia, should be evaluated prior to correction of the esophageal atresia.

In addition to the clinical signs, the diagnosis is established by an inability to pass an NG tube and by roentgenographic identification of the blind esophageal pouch. Although the use of a radiopaque NG tube and air contrast may be adequate in establishing the diagnosis roentgenographically, it is important to identify an upper pouch fistula. An experienced radiologist should carefully instill 1 ml of contrast material (barium) into the proximal pouch, using fluoroscopic control. The contrast material should be aspirated from the pouch after adequate roentgenograms are made, so that barium is not accidentally introduced into the lungs. Air in the stomach and intestine revealed by roentgenogram indicates the presence of a tracheoesophageal fistula in addition to esophageal atresia.

Occasionally, a tracheoesophageal fistula may be present without the occurrence of esophageal atresia (H-type fistula). These patients have cough or apnea with liquid feedings,

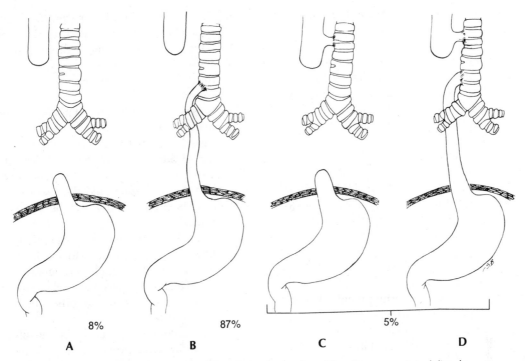

Fig. 58-1. Types of esophageal atresia. **A,** Esophageal atresia without an associated fistula; **B,** Esophageal atresia with distal tracheoesophageal fistula; **C,** Esophageal atresia with proximal fistula; and **D,** Esophageal atresia with proximal and distal fistulas.

abdominal distention with crying, and/or unexplained pneumonia. The diagnosis is established by an esophagram with cinefluoroscopy, since there is a possibility of multiple H-type fistulas. If the esophagram does not establish the diagnosis, endoscopy with bronchoscopy and esophagoscopy may be necessary. In some cases, the finding of an increased gastric oxygen concentration may be helpful. A posterior laryngeal cleft may be characterized by similar signs.

MONITORING

See also Chapter 4.

Gastrointestinal system

1. Preoperative: note quantity of oral secretions.
2. Postoperative:

a. Note quantity and character of oral secretions.
b. Aspirate the NG tube or gastrostomy tube for gastric residuals every 4 hours. Do not move the NG tube. Passing it over the anastomotic site may disrupt the suture line.
c. Observe for signs of breakdown of esophageal anastomosis, including mediastinitis (temperature instability, elevated WBC count), pneumothorax, and pneumomediastinum.

Cardiorespiratory system

1. Preoperative:
a. Obtain a chest roentgenogram and look for atelectasis, pneumonia, and cardiac or pulmonary anomalies.

b. Measure arterial blood-gas tensions and pH.

2. Postoperative:
   a. Obtain chest roentgenogram immediately after surgery and daily thereafter. Atelectasis and pneumonia are not uncommon. Chylothorax can occur. After feedings containing fat are introduced, send a specimen of tube drainage for fat stains and triglyceride level if chylothorax is suspected.
   b. Measure arterial blood-gas tensions and pH every 2 hours if respiratory distress is present and/or mechanical ventilation is needed.

Other systems

1. Preoperative:
   a. Measure serum creatinine and BUN if a renal anomaly is suspected.
   b. Consider chromosome analysis if indicated by physical examination.

MANAGEMENT
Gastrointestinal system

1. Preoperative:
   a. Place the patient in the head-up position to minimize inhalation of gastric contents through the tracheoesophageal fistula into the lungs.
   b. Insert a double-lumen tube with multiple vents at the tip (Replogle tube) into the esophagus to suction and empty the blind upper pouch. Place the tube on low continuous suction. This will minimize inhalation of oral secretions.
   c. Do not attempt to feed the patient. Give maintenance fluids, minerals, and glucose via an IV line.
2. Preliminary gastrostomy:
   a. In patients with severe respiratory distress that does not improve with initial management, a gastrostomy and fistula ligation may be done as initial steps, to avoid inhalation of stomach contents and to provide adequate alveolar ventilation.

b. Patients with multiple severe congenital anomalies may need gastrostomy only.
   c. Patients with associated distal gastrointestinal obstruction may need a gastrostomy for decompression.
3. Postoperative:
   a. Suction the pharynx with a catheter marked in such a manner that if it is inserted orally the tip will not be introduced into the esophagus and disrupt or stress the suture line. The anastomosis between the upper and the lower esophagus is often taut and can be easily disrupted.
   b. Perform a hypaque esophagram on the fifth postoperative day to establish the integrity of the esophageal anastomosis.
      (1) Minimal esophageal leaks may require no treatment other than delayed feedings.
      (2) Large esophageal leaks usually require reoperation.
   c. Feedings are begun 2 to 3 days after surgery, by slow continuous infusion into an NG tube placed at the time of surgery. The tube position should be checked roentgenographically before feedings are started. If the tip is not in the stomach, the tube should not be manipulated across the esophageal suture line. If the esophagram is normal, oral (nipple) feedings may begin on the fifth or sixth day.

Cardiorespiratory system

1. Preoperative: severe respiratory distress may require intubation, suctioning, and mechanical ventilation.
2. Postoperative:
   a. A nasotracheal tube should remain in place for one night after surgery, to provide an adequate means of suctioning. Avoid high CPAP unless indicated by severe respiratory distress. Should the endotracheal tube become dislodged and need to be replaced, reintubation must be done by skilled personnel to avoid

undue stretch on the esophagus and rupture of the suture line.

b. Patients with pulmonary parenchymal disease may require prolonged ventilatory support (see Chapters 34, 35, 96, and 97).

c. Vigorous suctioning and CPT may be required for 2 to 3 days after surgery.

d. If chylothorax occurs, continued drainage of the chest by thoracostomy tube is required. Small holes in the thoracic duct may seal spontaneously if flow through the defect is decreased by an enteral diet free of fat or by IV TPN. If this is unsuccessful, surgical closure may need to be attempted.

e. Surgical or medical management of congenital cardiac anomalies may be required.

ADDITIONAL READING

Abe, K., Shimada, Y., Takezawa, J., and others: Long-term administration of prostaglandin E$_1$: report of two cases with tetralogy of Fallot and esophageal atresia, Crit. Care Med. 10:155-158, 1982.

Barry, J.E., and Auldist, A.W.: The vater association, Am. J. Dis. Child. 128:769-771, 1974.

Bedard, P., Tirvan, D.P., and Shanding, B.: Congenital H-type tracheoesophageal fistula, J. Pediatr. Surg. 9: 663-668, 1974.

Cumming, W.A.: Esophageal atresia and tracheoesophageal fistula, Radiol. Clin. North Am. 13:277-295, 1975.

David, T.J., and O'Callaghan, S.E.: Cardiovascular malformations and oesophageal atresia, Br. Heart J. 36:559-565, 1974.

German, J.C., Mahour, G.H., and Woolley, M.M.: Esophageal atresia and associated anomalies, J. Pediatr. Surg. 11:299-306, 1976.

Greenwood, R.D., and Rosenthal, A.: The cardiovascular malformations associated with tracheoesophageal fistula and esophageal atresia, Pediatrics 57:87-90, 1976.

Kluth, D.: Atlas of esophageal atresia, J. Pediatr. Surg. 11:901-919, 1976.

Koop, C.E., Schnaufer, L., and Broennle, A.M.: Esophageal atresia and tracheoesophageal fistula: supportive measures that affect survival, Pediatrics 54:558-564, 1974.

Korones, S.D., and Evans, L.J.: Measurement of intragastric oxygen concentration for the diagnosis of H-type tracheoesophageal fistula, Pediatrics 60:450-452, 1977.

Meyers, N.A.: Oesophageal atresia: the epitome of modern surgery, Ann. R. Coll. Surg. Engl. 54:277-287, 1974.

59 Gastroschisis and omphalocele

WILLIAM DAMMERT

DEFINITION AND PHYSIOLOGY

Gastroschisis is an anterior abdominal wall defect 1 to 2 inches in diameter, usually to the right of an intact umbilical cord, and through which the intra-abdominal organs herniate. There is no covering sac, and the intestine is shortened, malrotated, leathery thick, and grossly edematous, with occasional areas of atresia (Fig. 59-1). The amount that the intra-abdominal organs herniate through the defect is variable. Embryologically, the defect results from failure of migrating muscles from dorsal myotomes to invade completely the embryonic abdominal wall. Because a large proportion of the intra-abdominal contents may be externalized in utero, the abdominal cavity may be small after birth. Concomitant anomalies are rare.

An omphalocele is a midline abdominal wall defect through which intra-abdominal organs herniate into the umbilical cord and are thus covered by fetal amniotic membrane (Fig. 59-2). Omphaloceles vary greatly in size; some are slightly larger than an umbilical hernia, whereas others can be huge, containing virtually all the bowel, liver, and spleen. The intestine will show some degree of malrotation. Associated anomalies are found in over 50% of patients, including anencephaly, congenital heart disease, spina bifida, diaphragmatic hernia, hydrocephalus, and chromosomal disorders.

The physiologic consequences of these two lesions before correction are similar. The large exposed surface area, particularly with gastroschisis, increases the infant's metabolic require-ments; heat, fluid, and protein are all lost from the gastrointestinal tract. Energy requirements and caloric expenditure may increase enough to cause hypoglycemia from depletion of hepatic glycogen, fluid loss may result in dehydration, and both of these may diminish cardiac output or cause respiratory distress. Circulation in the exposed bowel may be compromised secondary to fluid loss, poor perfusion, or strangulation, and bacterial invasion must be suspected. If a portion of the bowel has perforated, chemical meconium peritonitis may be present.

MONITORING

See also Chapter 4.

Gastrointestinal system

1. Preoperative: check for bowel viability. The defect may be small, and if the bowel fills with gas and/or becomes edematous, it may strangulate.
2. Postoperative:
   a. Measure abdominal girth every 8 hours.
   b. Check NG drainage.
   c. Check gastric residuals when feedings are started. Peristalsis may be impaired for a variable period.
   d. Examine the abdomen for signs of obstruction, perforation, and peritonitis (e.g., erythema or edema of bowel wall, abnormal bowel sounds, increasing girth, vomiting).
   e. Obtain a roentgenogram of the abdomen

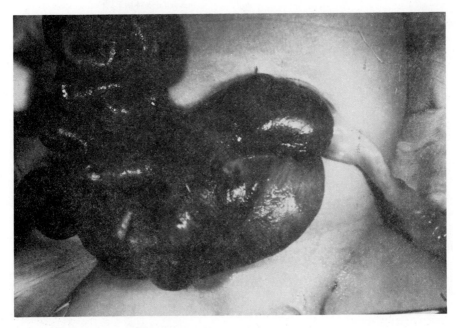

Fig. 59-1. Patient with gastroschisis.

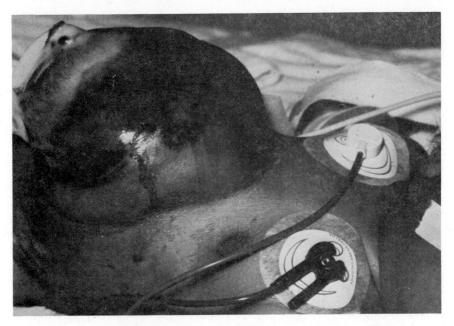

Fig. 59-2. Patient with a large omphalocele.

(anteroposterior and cross-table lateral) if signs of the above conditions appear.

Renal-metabolic system

1. Preoperative:
   a. Check temperature every hour until surgery; patients can lose an enormous amount of heat from exposed bowel surfaces. If the defect is large, placement of a skin probe for servocontrol of a radiant heat source may be impossible, and incubator temperature may have to be checked more frequently than usual.
   b. Check Dextrostix initially and every hour until surgery. Patients become hypoglycemic from stress and from caloric expenditure used in an attempt to maintain body temperature.

Cardiorespiratory system

1. Preoperative: measure arterial blood gas tensions and pH.
2. Postoperative:
   a. Closure may cause a significant elevation of diaphragms and seriously compromise ventilation by decreasing FRC and TLC. Obtain arterial blood-gas tensions and pH every 1 to 2 hours until stable or every 2 to 4 hours if mechanical ventilation is needed. An indwelling arterial catheter may be necessary.
   b. Observe for signs of inferior vena cava compression presenting as mottled, cyanotic, edematous lower extremities and systemic hypotension.

Hematologic system

1. Blood culture.
2. Hct every 8 hours.
3. WBC count with differential analysis initially and repeat if infection is suspected.
4. Platelet count initially and repeat if infection or DIC is suspected.

MANAGEMENT
Gastrointestinal system

1. Transport:
   a. Place an NG tube to keep gas out of bowel.
   b. Wrap bowel with sterile, warm, moist saline sponges and cover with Saran Wrap or an intestinal bag or enclose entire lower body including bowel in plastic bag.
   c. With gastroschisis, if bowel strangulation seems imminent, use sterile scissors to enlarge the constricting fascial and skin ring, being careful not to incise the bowel wall.
2. Surgery:
   a. Primary fascial skin closure is attempted but cannot always be accomplished.
   b. Skin closure without fascial closure may be accomplished. In this case the fascia can be repaired later.
   c. If neither of the above can be accomplished, a prosthetic (Silon) sac is sewn to the fascia and encompasses the herniated organs (Fig. 59-3, A). This is suspended over the patient (a silo) and, using surgically aseptic technique, is gradually squeezed down over a period of 5 to 10 days as the bowel wall edema regresses (Fig. 59-3, B). The skin and fascia are closed and the prosthetic sac removed when the majority of the intra-abdominal contents have been returned to the abdomen.
   d. Forcing the abdominal contents into the abdomen before edema has regressed and the abdominal cavity can accommodate them can cause inferior vena caval compression with hypotension as well as diaphragmatic elevation with respiratory failure. Either condition alone or a combination of the two may be fatal.
3. Postoperative:
   a. Record NG drainage.

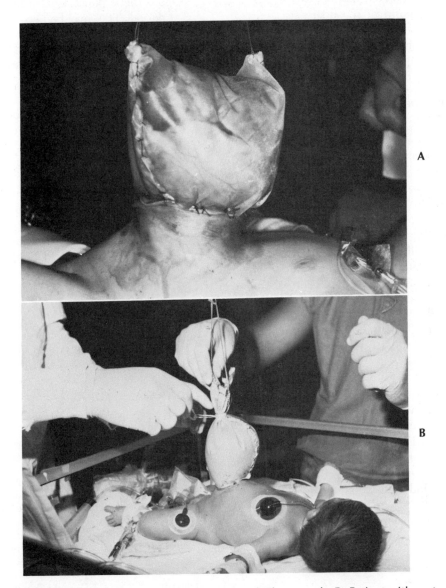

Fig. 59-3. A, Patient with gastroschisis after placement of Silon pouch. **B,** Patient with gastroschisis and Silon pouch 2 days after surgery. The abdominal contents have been returning to the abdominal cavity, and the pouch has been constricted twice.

b. Record number of stools. In the immediate postoperative period, stools may be guaiac positive secondary to surgical manipulation of the bowel.

c. Give ampicillin and gentamicin for 5 days (see Chapter 41).

d. Relieve bowel obstruction as indicated.

Renal-metabolic system

1. Transport:

a. Use an exogenous heat source to maintain normal body temperature.

b. Give $D_{10}W$ IV to maintain dextrose between 45 and 90 mg/dl.

c. Fluid losses from the bowel surface may be great, and the rate of IV infusions must be adjusted to maintain an adequate urine output (>1 ml/kg/hr) and normal heart rate and systemic arterial blood pressure. The rate of fluid administration should be at least 100 to 120 ml/kg/24 hr.

2. Postoperative:

a. Maintain body temperature.

b. Maintain Dextrostix between 45 and 90 mg/dl.

c. Maintain urine output at a minimum of 1 ml/kg/hr. This may require 1½ to 2 times maintenance fluids.

d. The patient may require multiple transfusions of FFP, 10 ml/kg, to maintain TSP at greater than 5.0 mg/dl. This is especially true for patients with a Silon pouch, who tend to have large external protein losses.

e. Patients may require multiple alterations of electrolytes in IV solutions to replace losses from the NG tube and moist dressings, especially if a prosthetic pouch is used.

f. Give maintenance calcium gluconate at 200 mg/kg/24 hr. More may be needed to keep the serum Ca at greater than 7.5 mg/dl.

g. If bowel function does not return or if a prosthetic pouch is used for a prolonged period, TPN may be necessary.

Cardiorespiratory system

1. Preoperative: cardiorespiratory failure is usually not a problem.

2. Postoperative:

a. Tachycardia and hypotension may be due to inferior vena caval compression, requiring surgical relief, or due to hypovolemia and hypoproteinemia, requiring volume replacement.

b. Tachypnea and poor color may be caused by inferior vena caval compression and/or respiratory failure due to diaphragmatic elevation; both require intubation and mechanical ventilation, and surgical intervention may be necessary to relieve the situation.

Hematologic system

1. Maintain Hct between 40% and 45%.

2. Diagnose and treat DIC (see Chapter 20).

ADDITIONAL READING

Firor, H.V.: Omphalocele: an appraisal of therapeutic approaches, Surgery 69:208-214, 1971.

Girvan, D.P., Webster, D.M., and Shandling, B.: The treatment of omphaloceles and gastroschisis, Surg. Gynecol. Obstet. 139:222-224, 1974.

Gray, S.W., and Skandalakis, J.E.: Embryology for surgeons, Philadelphia, 1972, W.B. Saunders Co.

Gross, R.E.: A new method for surgical treatment of large omphaloceles, Surgery 24:277-292, 1948.

Gutenberger, J.E., Miller, D.L., Dibbins, A.W., and Gitlin, D.: Hypogammaglobulinemia and hypoalbuminemia in neonates with ruptured omphaloceles and gastroschisis, J. Pediatr. Surg. 8:353-359, 1973.

Philippart, A.I., Canty, T.G., and Filler, R.M.: Acute fluid volume requirements in infants with anterior abdominal wall defects, J. Pediatr. Surg. 7:553-558, 1972.

Schuster, S.R.: A new method for the staged repair of large omphaloceles, Surg. Gynecol. Obstet. 125:837-850, 1967.

60 Intestinal atresia and imperforate anus

THEODORE P. VOTTELER

DEFINITION AND PHYSIOLOGY

Intestinal atresia is a lack of patency of a segment of bowel, which may be of any length and which is usually single but may be multiple. The atretic segment is thought to be secondary to an insufficient vascular supply to that area. Duodenal (1:3,500), jejunal (1:5,000), and ileal atresias (1:4,000) are not rare, but colonic atresia (1:20,000) is uncommon. The diagnosis of a high atresia is suspected in an infant who has lack of progression of air through the bowel as shown by roentgenogram and who has repeated vomiting that may be bile stained if the obstruction is distal to the ampulla of Vater. These infants may pass meconium. The diagnosis of a low atresia is suspected in an infant who has abdominal distention and lack of stools; vomiting may or may not be present. Abdominal roentgenograms show an obstructed pattern with dilated loops of bowel and air-fluid levels. Special positional views of the abdomen with air or radiopaque material may be needed to define the exact point of atresia. These should be done after consultation with a pediatric radiologist and a pediatric surgeon.

Imperforate anus includes a spectrum of findings, from a single membrane covering the anal orifice to anal or rectal agenesis or rectal atresia. These are related to whether the bowel terminates distal to, at, or proximal to the puborectalis sling of the levator ani musculature. The cause of these lesions is not known. They occur in approximately one out of 1,500 live births. The diagnosis is established by careful inspection of the perineum during the initial newborn examination. Approximately 70% of affected males have a fistulous connection, usually to the urethra, and 90% of the females have a fistula to the perineum or the vagina. Roentgenographic studies are necessary to establish the level of the atresia and the presence and location of a fistula.

MONITORING

See also Chapter 4.

Gastrointestinal system

1. Preoperative:
   a. Note vomitus for color and quantity.
   b. Note presence of meconium or stools.
   c. Measure abdominal girth.
2. Postoperative:
   a. Note color and quantity of NG aspirate.
   b. Note presence of stools.
   c. Measure abdominal girth every 8 hours.
   d. Auscultate for bowel sounds.
   e. If stools are loose or excessive, use TesTape to determine excess glucose loss.

Renal-metabolic system

1. Preoperative:
   a. Measure serum Na, K, Cl, Ca, and glucose. Infants, especially those with repeated vomiting, may become dehydrated, electrolyte depleted, and alkalotic.
   b. Measure arterial or venous blood gas ten-

359

sions and pH to document acid-base status.

c. Perform an IV pyelogram and a cystogram in patients with imperforate anus.

2. Postoperative: measure Na, K, and Cl concentrations in gastric secretions if electrolyte imbalance occurs or output is excessive.

MANAGEMENT
Gastrointestinal system

1. Preoperative:
   a. Place an NG tube for gastric decompression, using a double-lumen tube of adequate size. Attach the tube to continuous or intermittent low-pressure suction.
   b. Irrigate the tube every 2 hours with 2 to 3 ml of 0.9% sodium chloride solution to remove plugs.
   c. Do not attempt to feed the infant.
2. Postoperative:
   a. Leave the double-lumen NG tube in place and irrigate as above. Check the position of the tube by roentgenograms.
   b. If the patient vomits or becomes distended, check the patency of the tube and the adequacy of suction.
   c. Measure the NG drainage and record every 4 hours.
   d. The presence of green (biliverdin) gastric secretions is due to stasis and is a contraindication to removal of the NG tube. The exception to this is in patients with duodenal atresia and an incompetent pylorus.

e. When the patient passes stool or air (per rectum or ostomy site), the NG tube may be removed.

f. Gastric residuals of up to 6 to 8 ml every 4 hours are acceptable after the NG tube has been removed.

g. Feedings are begun after the patency and function of the gastrointestinal tract have been established as indicated above.

Renal-metabolic system

1. Give maintenance fluids, minerals, and glucose.
2. Additional fluids and minerals need to be given to correct deficits, to account for postoperative losses, and to replace NG drainage (see Chapter 16).
3. Excessive loss of protein or blood is not usually a problem with these defects.

ADDITIONAL READING

Adkins, J.C., and Kiesewetter, W.B.: Imperforate anus, Surg. Clin. North Am. **56:**379-394, 1976.

Santulli, T.V., Kiesewetter, W.B., and Bill, A.H.: Anorectal anomalies: a suggested international classification, J. Pediatr. Surg. **5:**281-287, 1970.

Santulli, T.V., Schullinger, J.N., Kiesewetter, W.B., and Bill, A.H.: Imperforate anus: a survey from the members of the surgical section of the American Academy of Pediatrics, J. Pediatr. Surg. **6:**484-487, 1971.

Stephens, F.D., and Smith, E.D.: Anorectal malformations in children, Chicago, 1971, Year Book Medical Publishers, Inc.

Wangensteen, D.H., and Rice, C.O.: Imperforate anus: a method of determining the surgical approach, Ann. Surg. **92:**77-81, 1930.

61 Diaphragmatic hernia

WILLIAM DAMMERT

DANIEL L. LEVIN

DEFINITION AND PHYSIOLOGY

In diaphragmatic hernia there is a displacement of abdominal contents through the diaphragm into the thoracic cavity. There are five types as depicted in Fig. 61-1.

Bochdalek hernia. This defect is posterolateral. It is the most common diaphragmatic defect and is on the left in 85% to 90% of patients. A sac covers the abdominal contents in only 10% to 15% of patients. The defect results from a failure of closure of the triangular pleuroperitoneal canal.

If abdominal organs migrate into the thoracic cavity early in gestation, the left lung fails to develop and is extremely hypoplastic. The heart is pushed into the right hemithorax, and the right lung is smaller than normal. Clinically, these patients are in severe respiratory distress from birth, have dextroposition of the heart, and have a scaphoid abdomen (Fig. 61-2). At first the left hemithorax is opaque on chest roentgenogram, but as the patient swallows air, bowel loops may be seen in the chest (Fig. 61-3). Patients with hypoplastic lungs have small pulmonary vascular beds, a decreased number of pulmonary resistance vessels per unit of lung tissue, and increased pulmonary vascular smooth muscle, all resulting in elevated pulmonary vascular resistance. Hypoxemia and hypercarbia further increase pulmonary vascular resistance, and all these factors cause significant R → L shunting via a PDA. These patients continue to shunt R → L even after the defect is repaired, and those with severe pulmonary hypoplasia have an extremely poor prognosis.

If the abdominal organs do not migrate upward through the diaphragmatic defect until later in gestation, lung development may proceed relatively normally. Although the defect may be large, these infants tend to have less distress than do those with hypoplastic lungs, and they also do better postoperatively.

Between these two extremes, some infants with moderate to severe hypoplasia and prolonged postoperative courses eventually survive. They exhibit some increase in lung volume with age but may still have an inadequate pulmonary vascular supply to the affected lung.

In 10% to 15% of patients with Bochdalek hernias the defect is on the right. In most of these patients the liver fills the defect and on roentgenogram appears to be a mass in the right lower lobe (Fig. 61-4). These patients usually have mild respiratory distress and present at several days or weeks of life or even later. Some patients with right-sided diaphragmatic hernia have large defects with bowel loops in the chest and pulmonary hypoplasia with the same problems as patients with left-sided defects (Fig. 61-5). Rarely, the defects are bilateral (Fig. 61-6).

Malrotation of the gut commonly occurs in association with diaphragmatic hernia. The differential diagnosis includes eventration of the diaphragm and adenomatoid cystic lung malformation.

Morgagni hernia. This type of defect is parasternal and is a rare lesion. There is a higher incidence of this lesion in patients with Down's syndrome. The defect is usually on the right, and there is usually a sac covering the abdomi-

361

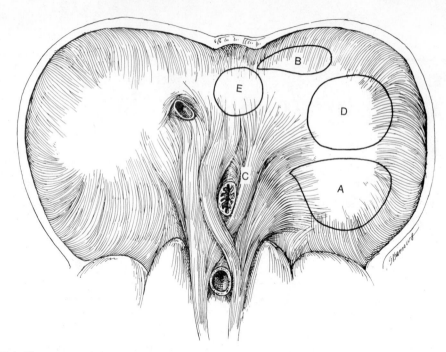

Fig. 61-1. Five types of diaphragmatic hernia: *A*, Bochdalek; *B*, Morgagni; *C*, esophageal hiatus; *D*, congenital absence of the diaphragm; and *E*, central tendon defect.

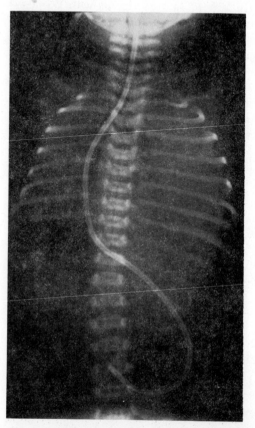

Fig. 61-2. Roentgenogram taken shortly after birth of an infant with a left-sided diaphragmatic hernia and hypoplastic lungs. The density in the left chest is not due to atelectasis alone, however, since the esophagus is shifted to the right (note NG tube) and the heart is dextropositioned. The mass effect is due to bowel in the left chest.

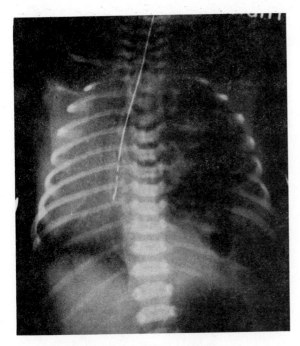

Fig. 61-3. Roentgenogram of the same infant as in Fig. 61-2 after bag and mask ventilation for respiratory distress. Now the bowel loops filled with air are visible in the left chest.

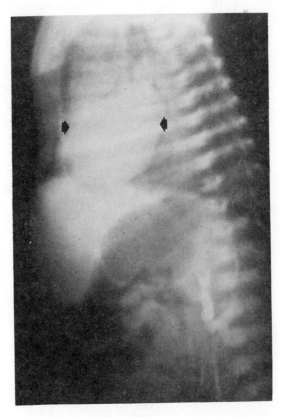

Fig. 61-4. Lateral chest roentgenogram of infant with right-sided diaphragmatic hernia. Note the apparent infiltrate (arrow). The infant was referred for persistent right lower lobe pneumonia.

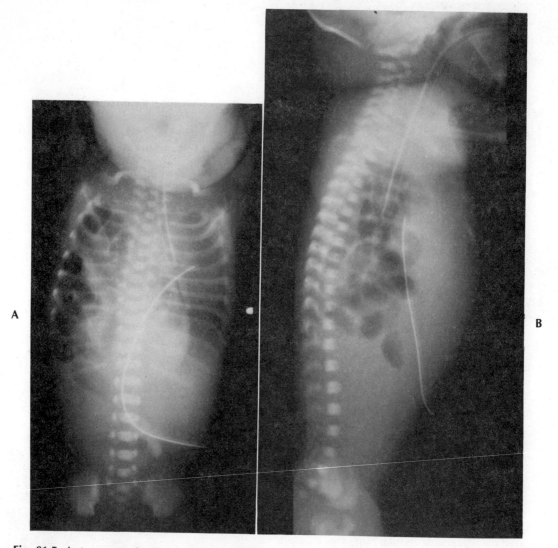

A

B

Fig. 61-5. Anteroposterior **(A)** and lateral **(B)** roentgenograms of premature infant with respiratory distress at birth. Note the right-sided diaphragmatic hernia with air-filled bowel loops in the right hemithorax.

nal organs. The lesion results from a failure of complete muscularization of the diaphragm. Signs of distress are usually mild or absent.

Esophageal hiatus hernia. This is a lesion in which the stomach can migrate upward through the esophageal opening in the diaphragm. It is a common lesion. Eighty percent of these lesions are sliding, so that the stomach may be partially

in the mediastinum or it may return completely to the normal position, and the other 20% are paraesophageal, or due to a short esophagus pulling the stomach up into the mediastinum. Signs include vomiting and a parasternal mass revealed by chest roentgenogram.

Congenital absence of the diaphragm. This lesion is usually unilateral and is most common-

Cardiorespiratory system

Measure arterial blood-gas tensions and pH every 1 to 2 hours. This usually requires an intra-arterial catheter. Since there may be massive R → L shunting via a PDA, obtain simultaneous arterial blood samples from preductus arteriosus and postductus arteriosus sites (see Chapter 39). $(P[A - a]O_2)$ greater than 500 mm Hg has been correlated significantly with a poor prognosis. These studies were done by obtaining blood samples from a postductus arteriosus (lower body) site.

Gastrointestinal system

If suspected, the diagnosis can be made antenatally by contrast fetography. Obtain an abdominal roentgenogram for signs of obstruction.

Hematologic system

1. Platelet count, PT, and PTT. DIC is commonly associated with shock (see Chapter 20).
2. Type and crossmatch.

MANAGEMENT
Gastrointestinal system

1. Surgical correction of the defect is of immediate concern. With Bochdalek hernias the patients are usually in respiratory distress, and surgery should be performed as an emergency procedure.
2. If signs of malrotation exist, surgical correction will be necessary before feeding is attempted.

Cardiorespiratory system

1. If the patient is in respiratory distress, intubate him and place an NG tube to prevent accumulation of air in the bowel, which would further impair pulmonary function.
2. Correct metabolic acidosis (pH <7.10 to 7.20) with sodium bicarbonate by giving one-half the calculated deficit (½ deficit = 0.3 × body weight in kg × base deficit) at a rate of 1 mEq/kg/min.

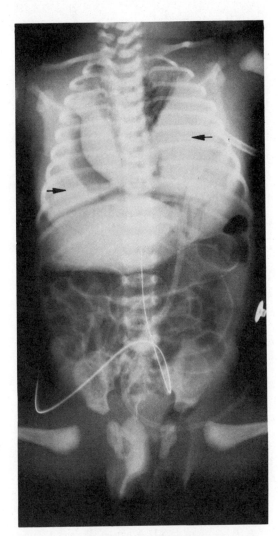

Fig. 61-6. Anteroposterior roentgenogram of infant with severe distress at birth. At autopsy there was no diaphragm and the liver was in both hemithoraces (arrows).

ly on the left. It is a rare lesion. Clinically it is similar to a Bochdalek hernia.

Central tendon defect. This is a defect in the tendinous (nonmuscular) portion of the diaphragm. It is a rare lesion.

MONITORING

See also Chapter 4.

3. Correct respiratory acidosis (Pa_{CO_2} >45 mm Hg) with mechanical ventilation. The lungs are hypoplastic, and the risk of pneumothorax is great, especially on the side of the more compliant lung. To decrease the risk of pneumothorax:

   a. Paralyze the patient with d-tubocurarine 0.5 mg/kg, or pancuronium (Pavulon), 0.1 mg/kg.

   b. Use low peak inspiratory and low end expiratory pressures (e.g., 20/2 cm H_2O).

   c. Use fast respiratory rates, as high as 100 breaths/min, to provide adequate alveolar ventilation.

4. If R → L shunting via a PDA is documented by simultaneous preductus and postductus arteriosus arterial blood oxygen samples (see Chapter 39), several regimens have been suggested that have had variable success. In most patients, the success of such regimens may be determined by the size of the pulmonary vascular bed more so than by the reversal of pulmonary arterial vasospasm.

   a. Use the alpha blocker tolazoline hydrochloride (2 mg/kg/hr continuous IV infusion) to dilate the pulmonary vascular bed.

   b. Ligate the ductus arteriosus and infuse tolazoline hydrochloride into the pulmonary artery. (We do not recommend this procedure.)

   c. Vasoactive agents that increase pulmonary vascular resistance should be avoided (see Chapter 14).

Renal-metabolic system

1. Patients are frequently hypotensive secondary to hypovolemia and hypoproteinemia. Postoperative fluid management may require 1.5 to 2 times maintenance to maintain urine output at a minimum of 1 ml/kg/hr. Give protein in the form of FFP, 10 ml/kg, or albumin, 1 g/kg, to maintain TSP levels at greater than 5 mg/dl.

2. When the patient starts to recover and mobilize fluid sequestered in tissues, furosemide, 1 mg/kg, may be necessary to reduce edema.

3. Shock may result in acute renal tubular damage (see Chapter 17).

4. Patients are frequently hypocalcemic and may require large doses (200 to 400 mg/kg/24 hr) of IV calcium gluconate to maintain serum calcium levels at greater than 8.0 mg/dl.

Hematologic system

1. Patients in cardiorespiratory distress should be provided with an optimal oxygen-carrying capacity (HCT >45%).

2. DIC should be promptly diagnosed and vigorously managed (see Chapter 20).

ADDITIONAL READING

Bell, M.J., and Ternberg, J.L.: Antenatal diagnosis of diaphragmatic hernia, Pediatrics 60:738-740, 1977.

Bloss, R.S., Turmen, T., Beardmore, H.E., and Arand, J.V.: Tolazoline therapy for persistent pulmonary hypertension after congenital diaphragmatic hernia repair, J. Pediatr. 97:984-988, 1980.

Levin, D.L.: Morphologic analysis of the pulmonary vascular bed in diaphragmatic hernia, J. Pediatr. 92:805-809, 1978.

Levy, R.J., Rosenthal, A., Freid, M.D., and others: Persistent pulmonary hypertension in the newborn with congenital diaphragmatic hernia: successful treatment with tolazoline, Pediatrics 60:740-752, 1977.

Naeye, R.L., Shochat, S.J., Whitman, V., and Maisels, M.J.: Unsuspected pulmonary vascular abnormalities associated with diaphragmatic hernia, Pediatrics 58:902-906, 1976.

Ohi, R., Susuki, H., Kato, T., and Kasai, M.: Development of the lung in fetal rabbits with experimental diaphragmatic hernia, J. Pediatr. Surg. 11:955-959, 1976.

Raphaely, R.C., and Downes, J.J.: Congenital diaphragmatic hernia: prediction of survival, J. Pediatr. Surg. 8:815-823, 1973.

Wohl, M.E.B., Griscom, N.T., Strieder, D.J., and others: The lung following repair of congenital diaphragmatic hernia, J. Pediatr. 90:405-414, 1977.

62 Gastrointestinal bleeding

ALAN D. STRICKLAND

DEFINITION AND PHYSIOLOGY

Gastrointestinal bleeding is usually divided into upper gastrointestinal bleeding (proximal to the ligament of Treitz) and lower gastrointestinal bleeding (distal to the ligament of Treitz). This division is based on the possibility of vomiting blood or finding blood in the stomach. These findings usually mean that the site of bleeding is proximal to the ligament of Treitz; bleeding distal to this point rarely produces blood in the stomach. Gastrointestinal bleeding is further classified based on the amount of blood. Thus, the vomiting of large amounts of clots or bright red blood is known as hematemesis, while coffee ground emesis usually indicates a smaller amount of blood loss from the upper gastrointestinal tract. Hematochezia, the defecation of bright red blood or clots, suggests a lower gastrointestinal bleeding point or a massive upper intestinal bleeding point such as a perforated duodenal ulcer. Melena, the defecation of tarry, black stools, suggests a high, slow bleeding point with some digestion of the blood. Occult rectal bleeding is the defecation of stools that appear normal but have abnormal amounts of blood in them, and it indicates a slow bleeding from a gastrointestinal site.

More than 10% of gastrointestinal bleeding results from causes outside the gastrointestinal tract. Included in these causes are bleeding from the nose, inherited coagulopathies, sepsis with DIC, and thrombocytopenia from idiopathic thrombocytopenia purpura (ITP) or leukemia. The gastrointestinal causes for bleeding are given in Tables 62-1 and 62-2, in their approximate order of incidence.

Physiologic changes depend on the amount of blood lost and the duration of the bleeding. Slow blood loss over a long period of time usually causes thirst. The patient responds by ingesting water or other hypotonic fluids, which worsen anemia and cause hypoproteinemia, hyponatremia, and occasionally orthostatic hypotension that is manifested by dizziness and syncope. Patients may also report weakness, loss of energy, apathy, and decreased activity. Massive, acute blood loss results in sudden loss of central venous blood volume, which leads to decreased blood pressure, peripheral vasoconstriction, increased heart rate, and orthostatic hypotension. Decreased blood supply to the brain may cause confusion or obtundation. Retinal artery spasm may follow decreased blood supply and result in permanent blindness. Myocardial ischemia may cause some chest pain and ECG changes. Oliguria results from the body's effort to retain fluid and support the blood volume.

Blood in the gastrointestinal tract serves as an irritant, causing vomiting when the blood is in the stomach or increased motility and diarrhea when the blood is in the bowel. Removal of blood from the stomach therefore decreases the mechanical trauma to the bleeding site and improves the chances for hemostasis. There is also some evidence that the presence of blood in the stomach interferes with the local clotting mechanism.

MONITORING

See also Chapter 4.

367

Table 62-1. Causes of upper gastrointestinal bleeding

Newborns	Infants	Children
Swallowed maternal blood	Superficial stress ulcers	Esophageal varices
Superficial stress ulcers	Gastritis	Superficial stress ulcers
Gastritis	Arteriovenous malformations	Peptic ulcers
Mallory-Weiss syndrome	Peptic ulcers	Gastritis
		Mallory-Weiss syndrome
		Esophagitis

Table 62-2. Causes of lower gastrointestinal bleeding

Newborns	Infants	Children
Anal fissures	Intussusception	Polyps
Necrotizing enterocolitis	Anal fissures	Anal fissures
Bacterial colitis	Bacterial colitis	Bacterial colitis
	Meckel's diverticulum	Intussusception
	Inflammatory bowel disease	Inflammatory bowel disease
	Intestinal duplications	Meckel's diverticulum
		Hemorrhoids
		Arteriovenous malformations

Cardiovascular system

1. Monitor heart rate and systemic arterial blood pressure. An ECG may be helpful if severe hypovolemia or chest pain is present.
2. Check Hb and Hct initially and every 2 hours until active bleeding has ceased.
3. Type and crossmatch for whole blood if hypovolemia is present or for packed RBCs if bleeding is less vigorous and anemia is predominant. If the patient is actively bleeding, keep at least 2 to 4 units of blood available in the blood bank.
4. Monitor urinary output. Bladder catheterization may be necessary.

Hematologic system

1. Carefully search for any history of the patient taking salicylates or steroids recently.
2. Measure PT, PTT, and platelet count. Diagnose any bleeding dyscrasias.
3. Measure WBC as an indication of the degree of stress on the bone marrow.

4. Monitor the platelet count if transfusions are needed.

Gastrointestinal system

1. Place an NG or orogastric tube to determine the presence of blood in the stomach.
2. Monitor the recurrence of blood in the stomach by placing an NG tube to gravity drainage for 4 to 12 hours after bleeding initially stops.
3. Check all stools for the presence of blood by the guaiac method.

MANAGEMENT
Cardiovascular system (see also Chapter 106)

1. Transfuse whole blood or packed RBCs to maintain the Hb >10 g/dl.
   a. Rapid bleeding indicates the patient is losing whole blood; so give whole blood or packed RBCs and FFP.
   b. Severe anemia with a decreased TSP due

to both chronic blood loss and hemodilution after rapid saline replacement would require packed RBCs and FFP or whole blood.

c. For severe subacute or chronic anemia without an emergency saline infusion, one may use packed RBCs and the patient will probably not require FFP.

2. Provide adequate IV fluids to establish and maintain a urinary output greater than 1 ml/kg/hr.

Hematologic system

1. Treat specific bleeding dyscrasias with the appropriate clotting factor or FFP.
2. If PT and PTT are prolonged, administer vitamin K (1 to 5 mg/24 hr, IV). Do not assume treatment is adequate: repeat PT and PTT.

Gastrointestinal system

Upper gastrointestinal bleeding

1. Remove blood from the stomach by lavage with water or saline at room temperature. After bleeding has stopped leave the NG tube in place for monitoring of rebleeding.
2. Vasoconstriction may be necessary if lavage does not stop the bleeding. This can be done in two ways. One method is effective but uncontrolled and uses norepinephrine. The other method is more precise but has more systemic effects; it uses vasopressin.
   a. Norepinephrine
      1. Mix 8 mg norepinephrine in 1 dl 0.9% sodium chloride solution.
      2. Dose is 60 to 75 ml/m^2 surface area.
      3. Place norepinephrine solution in stomach for 30 minutes, then remove gastric contents and repeat infusion.
      4. Several infusions may stop bleeding with few systemic effects.
   b. Vasopressin
      1. Mix 6 to 12 ml of Pitressin (20 units/ml) with D$_5$W to make 1 dl.
      2. Administer intravenously at rate to give 0.2 to 0.4 units/min.

3. This regimen avoids excess sodium load and is effective in stopping gastrointestinal bleeding.
4. Systemic side effects include hypertension and oliguria; infusions of D$_5$W continued for long periods of time may cause hyponatremia.
5. Once bleeding is stopped, the vasopressin dose is reduced decrementally and discontinued after 4 days.

3. Diagnose the source of the bleeding by endoscopy and/or barium-contrast roentgenography.
4. Give an antacid in a dose of 10 to 30 ml, orally or per NG tube, every 1 or 2 hours or cimetidine in a dose of 20 to 40 mg/kg/24 hr, IV or PO, in four divided doses to help prevent repeat bleeding from esophagitis, gastritis, Mallory-Weiss syndrome, superficial stress ulcers, or peptic ulcers. Sucralfate (1 tablet given orally every 6 hours) may be more effective than antacids or cimetidine for the short-term treatment of peptic ulcers.
5. Invasive procedures may be necessary if bleeding cannot be stopped or if frequent bleeding episodes occur. Repeated bleeding from esophageal varices may be handled by endoscopic or transhepatic sclerosis. Occasional patients may require portasystemic venous shunts to prevent repeated variceal bleeding. Use of the Blakemore tube has a 20% mortality rate, so it should be avoided if possible. Peptic ulcers require surgical intervention if bleeding is massive and cannot be stopped or if persistent bleeding recurs while optimal medical treatment is being given.

Lower gastrointestinal bleeding

1. Proctosigmoidoscopy should be performed, since many polyps are within reach of the proctoscope. The diagnosis of ulcerative colitis, bacterial colitis, amebic colitis, or rectal trauma may also be established by proctosigmoidoscopy.
2. Barium enema should be performed for bleeding from above the reach of the procto-

scope. Confirmation of a diagnosis with colonoscopy or angiography is occasionally useful.

3. Colitis and necrotizing enterocolitis require appropriate antimicrobial therapy.

4. Intussusception may be reduced during a barium enema or may require surgical reduction.

5. Colonic polyps usually may be removed by colonoscopy.

6. Surgery is required for correction of volvulus, Meckel's diverticulum, duplications of the bowel, or perforations of the bowel.

7. Inflammatory bowel disease is treated initially with corticosteroids and sulfasalazine (Azulfidine).

ADDITIONAL READING

Conn, H.O., and Simpson, J.A.: Excessive mortality associated with balloon tamponade of bleeding varices, J.A.M.A. **202**:135-139, 1967.

Johnson, W.C., Widrich, W.C., Ansell, J.E., and others: Control of bleeding varices by vasopressin: a prospective randomized study, Ann. Surg. **186**:369-374, 1977.

Lopez-Torres, A., and Wayne, J.D.: The safety of intubation in patients with esophageal varices, Am. J. Dig. Dis. **18**:1032-1034, 1973.

Ponsky, J.L., Hoffman, M., and Swaynagim, D.S.: Saline irrigation of gastric hemorrhage: the effect of temperature, J. Surg. Res. **28**:204-205, 1980.

Resnick, R.H., Iber, F.L., Ishihara, A.M., and others: A controlled study of the therapeutic portacaval shunt, Gastroenterology **67**:843-857, 1974.

Wilson, D.E., and Chalmers, T.C.: Management of emergencies. XII. Acute hemorrhage from the upper gastrointestinal tract, N. Engl. J. Med. **274**:1368, 1966.

63 Gastroesophageal reflux

ALAN D. STRICKLAND

DEFINITION AND PHYSIOLOGY

Gastroesophageal reflux (GER) denotes a condition of decreased pressure in the lower esophageal sphincter (LES) with frequent passage of gastric contents into the esophagus. This is distinct from vomiting or retching in that there is no alteration of peristalsis of the stomach or the small intestine and no feeling of nausea. Rather than nausea, older patients with GER report feelings of a burning sensation in the lower chest or of a bolus of food being lodged in the esophagus. Gastroesophageal reflux also differs from vomiting in frequency. Vomiting is usually episodic, while GER usually occurs several times per hour.

The lower esophageal sphincter is confined to the final 3 to 5 cm of the esophagus, usually encompassing the Z line where squamous esophageal mucosa meets columnar gastric mucosa (Fig. 63-1). The LES pressure does not depend on the diaphragm, the amount of esophagus in the abdomen, or the angle at which the esophagus enters the stomach. A muscular origin of the LES has, therefore, been postulated, though anatomic dissection does not reveal a well-developed muscle. The thin circumferential muscle found here is the presumed LES. (The opossum, because it hangs by its tail, has a thick, circumferential LES with a much higher LES tone than humans.) The LES tone increases from values less than 5 mm Hg in infants less than 1 month of age to values of 15 to 20 mm Hg, which remain stable from the second month of postnatal life through adult life. There is a good correlation between low LES pressure and GER, but use of the pressure as a diagnostic tool for GER has many false-positive and false-negative results.

In spite of this failure of LES pressure to precisely determine which patients will reflux, the muscular nature of the LES is still supported by several observations. For example, Chrispin and Friedland reported a child who had a colonic interposition of the mid-esophagus after lye ingestion. During one phase of the child's care, the upper esophagus was exteriorized on one side of the neck to drain swallowed saliva. The colonic interposition was exteriorized separately on the neck and connected to the intact lower portion of the esophagus. During fluoroscopy, a bolus of radiographic dye was introduced into the colonic interposition. It traveled to the lower esophagus and remained in the lower esophagus. The child then drank liquid, which passed out the upper exteriorization onto the neck. Shortly after the swallow, the LES relaxed, allowing the radiographic dye to pass into the stomach. Thus, the LES appears to be muscular and is under central neural control.

Numerous experiments have documented the effect of adrenergic and cholinergic drugs on the esophagus and the LES. Muscarinic parasympathomimetic agents such as bethanechol cause the LES to constrict. Nicotinic parasympathomimetic agents such as carbachol or nicotine relax the LES, though the effects vary with the dosage and large doses are frequently less effective than small doses. Thus, the amount of nicotine in two after-dinner cigarettes will relax the LES and cause eructation whereas larger numbers of cigarettes will not usually

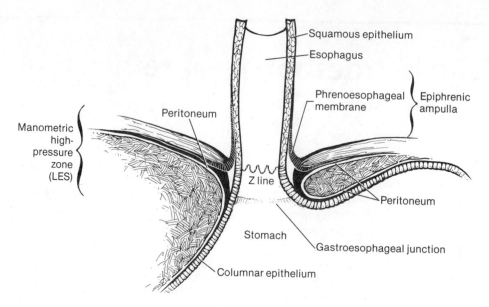

Fig. 63-1. Lower esophageal sphincter.

cause eructation. No effect on the LES has been found from alpha-adrenergic agents. Beta-adrenergic agents such as isoproterenol or CNS stimulants such as theophylline lower the LES pressure and increase the possibility of GER. Serotonin increases LES pressure. Histamine has not yet been studied in humans, but it increases LES pressure in animals.

LES pressure can also be altered by non-neuropharmacologic agents. Gastrin increases LES pressure, and since alkaline substances in the antrum stimulate gastrin release, they also increase LES pressure. However, alkaline substances introduced into the gastric fundus lower LES pressure. Prevention of gastric acid production by administration of cimetidine has no effect on LES pressure. The oils from anise, caraway, cinnamon, cloves, dill, fennel, garlic, ginger, peppermint, rosemary, spearmint, and turpentine relax the LES.

Infants with severe GER may have difficulty retaining enough food to allow weight gain. Vomiting is frequent and is worst immediately after feedings and during sleep. Thus,

much of the intake is lost. Occasional infants have recurrent inhalation pneumonia in association with GER. Older children with asthma that responds poorly to traditional therapy have been found to have GER, and resolution of their asthmatic condition occurs after correction of the reflux. Apnea occurs in many infants with GER, but both conditions are probably symptoms of neurologic immaturity rather than of GER causing apnea. Resolution of reflux has not had an effect on the incidence of apnea in these infants.

Gastroesophageal reflux affects 25% to 35% of all infants. Most of these infants have mild symptoms and do not require any diagnostic studies or therapeutic measures. The natural history of GER is that 85% of infants with GER will stop having reflux by 12 months of age and 95% by 24 months of age.

Diagnostic studies include barium swallow examination, Tc^{99m} swallow examination, esophageal manometry to determine LES pressure, esophagoscopy to document the presence of esophagitis, the Tuttle test (placing 173.4

ml/m² of 0.1M HCl into the stomach and monitoring esophageal pH for 15 to 60 minutes; two episodes of pH less than 4 in 15 minutes is a positive result), and prolonged esophageal pH monitoring. Esophageal pH monitoring in normal children has documented that reflux episodes occur in normal children, that the number of reflux episodes occurring normally is about 10 times higher within 2 hours of filling the stomach than when the patient is fasting, and that position (upright versus supine) and state of consciousness alter the number of reflux episodes. Thus, any test done solely within 2 hours after placing material in the stomach will have poor sensitivity and selectivity. For this reason, prolonged esophageal pH monitoring is currently thought to be the best diagnostic test for GER.

The majority of infants with GER have mild symptoms and require only outpatient therapy for poor growth. Those infants, regardless of gestational age or size, who have severe pulmonary symptoms require hospitalization. The procedures below are intended for these severely affected infants.

MONITORING

See also Chapter 4.

Respiratory system

1. Frequent or continuous monitoring for distress or apnea associated with inhalation of stomach contents.
2. Frequent auscultation of the chest to check for bronchospasm and pneumonia.
3. Chest roentgenograms as needed to define areas of hyperinflation and pneumonia and to follow the resolution or progression of abnormalities.

MANAGEMENT
Gastrointestinal system

1. Place the child in an upright posture (60 to 90 degrees from horizontal) the entire time. Since reflux may occur at any time of day, this position must be maintained 24 hours a day. A chalasia board is the preferable method of obtaining this position.
2. Thicken the feedings. An infant less than 6 months of age should have 2 to 4 tablespoons of rice cereal powder added to each 4 ounces of formula, resulting in a mixture thin enough to be sucked or gavaged but thick enough to lower the occurrence of reflux. Infants and children older than 6 months of age should always have solids whenever liquids are given in order to thicken gastric contents.
3. Esophagitis with burning pain is best treated with an antacid, 10 to 30 ml every 2 hours. Cimetidine, 20 to 40 mg/kg/24 hr PO, may also be used but does not raise LES pressure as antacids do.
4. Bethanechol (9 mg/m²/24 hr in 3 divided doses or 0.5 to 1.0 mg/kg/24 hr in 4 divided doses, PO) should be given to increase LES pressure.
5. If symptoms of reflux continue after adequate medical therapy has been tried for 2 weeks, a surgical antireflux procedure, such as the Nissen fundoplication, should be considered.

Respiratory system

1. Antibiotics with broad Gram-negative coverage should be used for inhalation pneumonia (see Chapter 41).
2. CPT should be used if infiltrates or atelectasis are present.
3. A trial of theophylline may be used for apparent bronchospasm. Since theophylline decreases LES pressure, it should be stopped if no improvement follows its institution (see Chapter 28).

ADDITIONAL READING

Berquist, W.E., Rachelefsky, G.S., Kadden, M., and others: Gastroesophageal reflux—associated recurrent pneumonia and chronic asthma in children, Pediatrics 68:29-35, 1981.

Crispin, A.R., and Friedland, G.W.: A radiological study of the neural control of oesophageal vestibular function, Thorax, 21:422-427, 1966.

Euler, A.R.: Use of bethanechol for the treatment of gastroesophageal reflux, J. Pediatr. 96:321-324, 1980.

Hill, J.L., Pelligrini, C.A., Burrington, J.D., and others: Technique and experience with 24-hour esophageal pH monitoring in children, J. Pediatr. Surg. 12:877-887, 1977.

Jolley, S.G., Johnson, D.G., Herbst, J.J., and others: An assessment of gastroesophageal reflux in children by extended pH monitoring of the distal esophagus, Surgery 84:16-24, 1978.

Walsh, J.K., Farrell, M.K., Keenan, W.H., and others: Gastroesophageal reflux in infants: relation to apnea, J. Pediatr. 99:197-201, 1981.

64 Hyperbilirubinemia

CHARLES E. MIZE

DEFINITION AND PHYSIOLOGY

Bilirubin is an end product of heme metabolism, derived from the breakdown of hemoglobin of erythrocytes or erythrocyte precursors in neonates and in small quantities from other tissue heme proteins. Hepatic bilirubin disposition is normally accomplished by converting free water-insoluble bilirubin to water-soluble bilirubin mono- and di-glucuronides and secreting these glucuronide derivatives through the biliary ductal outflow system. The van den Bergh diazotization reaction used in clinical laboratories for estimating direct- and indirect-reacting bilirubin generally, but not exactly, parallels an estimate of the bilirubin glucuronates (or conjugated bilirubin) and the free bilirubin (or unconjugated bilirubin). Transcutaneous measurement of bilirubin may be of additional aid. Based on this fractional bilirubin determination, clinical definitions of hyperbilirubinemic states differentiate between those states with (1) predominantly unconjugated bilirubin and those with (2) predominantly conjugated bilirubin. Hyperbilirubinemia results from (1) excessive bilirubin production beyond normal hepatic secretory capacity or (2) deficient hepatic bilirubin conjugation or secretion.

The predominantly unconjugated hyperbilirubinemic conditions most commonly encountered in the PICU are associated with bilirubin overproduction and impaired transport of bilirubin or hepatic clearance. Extravascular hemolysis (e.g., enclosed hematomas, petechial or organ hemorrhages, swallowed blood) and intravascular hemolysis (e.g., isoimmune hemolytic anemia, the polycythemia of maternal-fetal or feto-fetal transfusion or delayed umbilical cord clamping) reflect such bilirubin overproduction. Chemical or bacterial hemolysis (e.g., vitamin K analogues, coliform and staphylococcal products in septicemia) also lead to excessive bilirubin production, and red cell abnormalities (e.g., spherocytic and nonspherocytic anemias, hemoglobinopathies) lead to accentuated hemolysis and bilirubin overproduction. Moreover, free bilirubin increases in blood when an impaired transport of bilirubin on albumin occurs in hypoxemia and acidosis or as a consequence of hypoalbuminemia in premature infants. Significant displacement of bilirubin may potentially occur with drugs (e.g., sulfa) or free fatty acids generated from inadequately metabolized parenteral lipid. Less commonly, impaired hepatic uptake and consequent blood rise of bilirubin develops when hepatic venous sinusoidal perfusion is diminished after term due to congestive heart failure, extrahepatic portal vein thrombosis, or a functionally patent ductus venosus. Occasionally hepatic clearance is impaired as a result of hypothyroidism, intestinal obstruction (with delayed meconium or stool passage), antibiotics, and in infants of diabetic mothers. Unconjugated hyperbilirubinemia is seen in metabolic disorders when glucuronyl transferase is either inhibited (Lucey-Driscoll syndrome or in some infants fed lipase-rich breast milk) or genetically deficient (Gilbert syndrome, Crigler-Najjar syndromes I and II). Hyperbilirubinemia associated with delayed feeding in neonates seems related to a combination of decreased intestinal motility and delayed passage of meconium coupled with decreased bile flow and relative substrate deficiencies for bilirubin metabolism.

Physiologic jaundice of the newborn, clinically an important condition of predominantly unconjugated hyperbilirubinemia, reflects a complexity of physiologic events in the neonate:

1. There is increased bilirubin challenge to the liver. Persistence of the enterohepatic circulation of bilirubin may occur when intestinal β-glucuronidase hydrolyzes conjugated bilirubin to the readily reabsorbed unconjugated bilirubin. Red cell survival is diminished, red cell volume is relatively high, and there seems to be increased formation of heme from nonhemoglobin sources.

2. Bilirubin conjugation is diminished. Low glucuronyl transferase and uridine diphosphoglucose (UDPG) dehydrogenase activities in neonatal liver, competing enzymic pathways for UDP-glucuronic acid, and depleted glycogen stores or deficient glucose for UDPG may each retard conjugation.

3. Bilirubin hepatic clearance appears to be decreased. The hepatic cell bilirubin-binding protein, ligandin, may be low and such binding proteins may be preferentially bound initially by other anions. Moreover, short-term persistence of the fetal hormonal environment (especially estrogens) can suppress hepatic excretory mechanisms.

A recurring pattern of physiologic jaundice is recognized: In term infants, bilirubin peaks at approximately the third day of life (<10 mg/dl), followed by a fairly stable concentration between ages 5 and 8 days (<5 mg/dl), with a slow decline to normal levels by or before age 12 to 14 days. In preterm infants, the peak concentration may reach 12 to 15 mg/dl by age 4 to 6 days, and bilirubin levels remain elevated longer (3 to 4 weeks). Fasting can exaggerate unconjugated hyperbilirubinemia under normal conditions as well as during intercurrent infection.

The danger of excessive free or unconjugated bilirubin concentration in the newborn is the risk of irreversible brain damage, namely bilirubin encephalopathy or kernicterus, involving especially the basal ganglia, subthalamic nuclei, or inferior olives. The clinical signs of bilirubin neurotoxicity encompass a spectrum of deficits. In the neonate, they can range from minimal or nonspecific signs to a described sequence: lethargy, poor suck, and hypotonia in the first week, followed by relative hypertonia, possible fever, and opisthotonus, and then progressively decreasing muscle tone thereafter. Later clinical signs (after 1 year of age) include hypotonia, choreoathetosis, neurosensory deafness, cognitive function deficits, impairment of conjugate vertical gaze, and occasionally seizures. The essential factors in evaluating the risk of irreversible brain damage are (1) the serum bilirubin concentration, (2) the bilirubin transport or binding capacity of serum albumin, (3) associated conditions that increase cell and membrane susceptibility to bilirubin toxicity (e.g., acidosis, hypoxia), and possibly (4) prematurity, in which pathophysiologic mechanisms discussed above may be accentuated. The concentration of unbound bilirubin binding sites on plasma albumin relative to the free bilirubin concentration is particularly important, since this unbound, unconjugated bilirubin (possibly as a free fatty acid complex) is thought to enter the brain (and other tissues) more rapidly when the binding capacity of circulating albumin is exceeded. Associated hypoxia, acidosis, infection, and hypoglycemia may particularly predispose low-birth-weight infants to bilirubin-induced neurotoxicity, frequently with minimal clinical findings, and neural damage may occur at low bilirubin serum concentrations (<10 mg/dl) in low-birth-weight infants if such associated conditions are present. It is thus not possible to state an absolute minimum level of free bilirubin that will lead to tissue toxicity. A total bilirubin to plasma protein ratio less than or equal to 3.7 may suggest minimal risk unless hemolysis is occurring, while a serum bilirubin level of 10 mg/dl at age 24 hours, 15 mg/dl by 48 hours, or 20 mg/dl at any time must be considered high risk. A variety of saturation or binding indices have been described to estimate serum protein binding capacity for bilirubin. Their use is of potential importance in evaluating neonatal jaundice as it reflects subsequent long-term neurologic development.

Pharmacologic alteration of the unconjugated bilirubin concentration is possible under certain circumstances with selected drugs and/or with light irradiation:

1. A variety of drugs that stimulate proliferation of hepatic endoplasmic reticulum and mixed-function oxidase metabolism can stimulate hepatic glucuronidation of bilirubin. Phenobarbital is the most widely employed agent of this type, and it is most effective when liver tissue is relatively mature. Infants of gestational age less than 32 to 34 weeks generally do not respond with enhanced bilirubin conjugation and secretion. Hepatic immaturity in low-birth-weight infants thus effectively prevents this pharmacologic response. Charcoal, cholestyramine, or agar may bind bilirubin that reaches the intestinal lumen and prevent reabsorption.

2. Blue light (420 to 500 nm) appears to produce significant hydrogen-bond molecular alterations (photo-isomerization) and/or some degree of photo-oxidation of bilirubin in the fraction of the bilirubin pool primarily within the skin. The modified bilirubin products that are more water-soluble than bilirubin itself are excreted in urine or bile. Intermittent radiation appears to produce these overall changes as effectively as continuous radiation.

Side effects that can occur during or following cessation of such light or phototherapy include significantly increased insensible water loss, an evolving conjugated hyperbilirubinemia (the bronze-baby syndrome), and loose bowel movements. Other potential tissue injury (e.g., hemolysis, skin rashes, burns, or retinal damage due to uncovered eyes) must be recognized. In human cells in vitro, DNA strand breakage has been described as a result of radiation commonly used in neonatal phototherapy, and the presence of bilirubin (as a photosensitizer) enhances this effect. While repair of strand breakage is rapid at physiologic temperatures, the absence of long-term harmful effects has not been unequivocally established.

The most common causes of conditions with predominantly conjugated hyperbilirubinemia encountered in the PICU are infection and clinical injury to the liver, which result in deficient bilirubin secretion. Genetic and metabolic disorders are less frequent causes of conjugated hyperbilirubinemia, but they are important because several of these diseases if diagnosed early are treatable (e.g., galactosemia, fructose intolerance, tyrosinemia). Although anatomic disorders of the bile ducts are uncommon, a careful search should be made to diagnose them since they are potentially treatable lesions. Deficiency of α-l-antitrypsin presents as neonatal jaundice, and patients with cystic fibrosis develop obstructive jaundice, though rarely in the neonatal period. Although conjugated hyperbilirubinemia is considered nontoxic, it is a warning signal of the underlying hepatobiliary involvement. The pathophysiologic consequence of these pathologic conditions is cholestatic jaundice, in which conjugated hyperbilirubinemia is invariably coupled with a reduced bile flow and a reduced secretion of other anions (e.g., bile acids); also, bile pigment is frequently present in hepatic parenchymal cells.

Because clinical, pathologic, and general laboratory data frequently do not distinguish infectious liver disease from other causes of liver dysfunction and conjugated hyperbilirubinemia, it is imperative to seek specific infectious etiologies. Most agents that cause intrauterine or perinatal infection can produce hepatic inflammation. Frequently a mixed hyperbilirubinemia (conjugated and unconjugated) occurs in sepsis, since hemolysis and bilirubin overproduction accompany the process.

Finally, the conjugated hyperbilirubinemia

that may occur during treatment with certain drugs may relate to immaturity of metabolic pathways coupled with drug hypersensitivity or toxicity (e.g., herbal tea pyrrolizidine alkaloids). Hyperbilirubinemia during TPN may be the result of hepatocellular and canalicular cholestasis associated with a bile secretory defect, but it is frequently difficult to dissociate other potential pathophysiologic causes in the types of patients receiving IV alimentation.

MONITORING

See also Chapter 4.

Hepatic system

1. Unconjugated hyperbilirubinemia.
   a. Bilirubin (direct and indirect) initially, and daily thereafter (more frequently if bilirubin is rising by 5 mg/dl/24 hr or more).
   b. Serum albumin initially and daily.
   c. Serum bilirubin-binding sites (if available).
2. Conjugated hyperbilirubinemia.
   a. Bilirubin (direct and indirect) initially, and every 24 to 48 hours thereafter.
   b. Estimated size of liver by percussion.
   c. Laboratory tests initially and every 24 to 72 hours: SGOT, SGPT, alkaline phosphatase, serum albumin.
   d. PT and PTT initially and every 24 to 72 hours, depending on deficiency status.
   e. Viral hepatitis antigen and/or antibody identifications; toxoplasmosis, rubella, cytomegalic inclusion disease, herpesvirus hominis (TORCH) titers, and serologic test for syphilis (patient, mother).
   f. Toxicology screen, if appropriate; review herb tea history.
   g. Duodenal tube intubation for bilirubin identification.
   h. Portal tract sonography, nuclear medicine biliary duct excretion study, liver biopsy.

Cardiorespiratory system

1. Unconjugated hyperbilirubinemia: pH and base deficit every 24 to 72 hours.
2. Conjugated hyperbilirubinemia: pH and base deficit every 24 to 72 hours.

Metabolic system

1. Unconjugated hyperbilirubinemia.
   a. During phototherapy: careful body temperature monitoring to avoid hyperthermia; cover thermistor probes exposed to lamps.
   b. Plasma free-fatty-acid concentration initially and during bilirubin rising phase, if available; daily triglyceride during lipid infusion, if available.
   c. Maternal drug history (e.g., salicylates, sulfa).
   d. Review dietary intake and stooling pattern.
   e. T_4, T_3, and TSH.
   f. Consider determining intestinal transit time (by charcoal).
2. Conjugated hyperbilirubinemia.
   a. Urinary reducing substances for galactose while patient is receiving oral feedings of this sugar; specific identification of reducing substance, if present.
   b. Plasma and urinary amino acids initially.
   c. Sweat chloride test.
   d. Serum protein electrophoresis, BUN and amylase.
   e. Serum α-l-antitrypsin.
   f. Urinary and stool urobilinogen three times.

Hematologic system

1. Unconjugated hyperbilirubinemia.
   a. Blood type and Rh (patient, mother) and Coombs' test (direct, indirect); special antibody testing (RBC eluate) if unusual hemolysis is suspected.
   b. CBC, red cell morphology, reticulocyte count initially and every day.

c. Platelet count initially and per clinical indications.
d. Blood cultures.
e. Consider glucose-6-phosphate dehydrogenase screen, CT scan (extravascular blood loculation).
2. Conjugated hyperbilirubinemia.
   a. CBC and RBC morphology.
   b. Blood culture initially; TORCH titers and serologic test for syphilis (patient, mother).
   c. Platelet count initially and as indicated clinically.

Neurologic system

1. Unconjugated hyperbilirubinemia.
   a. Daily general neurologic evaluation.
   b. Specific attention to hypotonia, lethargy, rigidity, opisthotonus, high-pitched cry, seizures, poor suck, excessive yawning.
   c. Consider sonography or CT scan to diagnose CNS hemorrhage.
2. Conjugated hyperbilirubinemia: observe for cerebral edema or impending coma (see Chapter 19).

MANAGEMENT
Hematologic system

1. Unconjugated hyperbilirubinemia.
   a. Provision of satisfactory oxygen-carrying capacity (Hct ≥ 40% for neonates and ≥35% for children)
   b. Phototherapy and/or exchange transfusion according to guidelines (Fig. 64-1). The following precautions must be taken when phototherapy is used as a mode of therapy:
      (1) Routine maintenance checks of the lights should be made to ensure proper function and delivery of proper wavelength.
      (2) Infant precautions:
         (a) Both eyes must be patched to prevent retinal damage. Patches

should be removed and lights turned off for some time (several minutes) during parental visits.
         (b) Use an ultraviolet filter (plastic shield) between the light and the infant.
         (c) Variables that evaluate fluid loss must be rigorously monitored because of increased water loss with phototherapy.
         (d) Continuous temperature monitoring and control via a servomechanism are desirable because of increased potential for hyperthermia.
         (e) Efficiency is improved by undressing the infant and turning him from front to back every 2 hours.
      (3) Laboratory determinations that would be affected by light (e.g., bilirubin values) should be performed with the phototherapy unit off.
      (4) Since rebound hyperbilirubinemia may occur when phototherapy is discontinued, a bilirubin determination should be done within 4 hours of discontinuing phototherapy.
   c. Exchange transfusion (see Chapter 107).
   d. TSP should be kept at greater than 5.0 g/dl by giving protein as plasma, 10 ml/kg, or as 25% albumin, 1 g/kg.
2. Conjugated hyperbilirubinemia.
   a. Antibiotic coverage for sepsis or other infectious processes (see Chapter 41).
   b. Packed RBC transfusion for significant anemia.

Neurologic system

1. Unconjugated hyperbilirubinemia.
   a. Any time clinical signs of kernicterus appear, exchange transfusion is indicated regardless of the level of bilirubin.
   b. Diazepam is contraindicated for concomi-

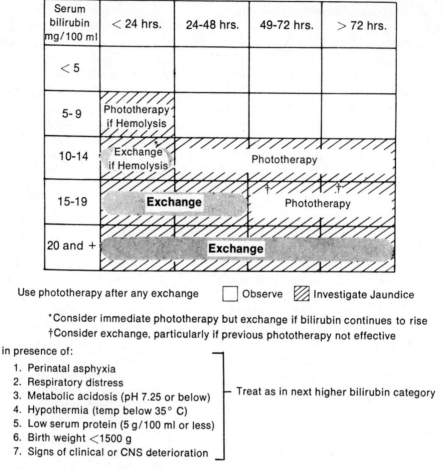

Serum bilirubin mg/100 ml	< 24 hrs.	24-48 hrs.	49-72 hrs.	> 72 hrs.
< 5				
5-9	Phototherapy if Hemolysis			
10-14	Exchange if Hemolysis	Phototherapy		
15-19	Exchange		Phototherapy	
20 and +	Exchange			

Use phototherapy after any exchange   ☐ Observe   ▨ Investigate Jaundice

*Consider immediate phototherapy but exchange if bilirubin continues to rise
†Consider exchange, particularly if previous phototherapy not effective

in presence of:
1. Perinatal asphyxia
2. Respiratory distress
3. Metabolic acidosis (pH 7.25 or below)   ⎤ Treat as in next higher bilirubin category
4. Hypothermia (temp below 35° C)
5. Low serum protein (5 g/100 ml or less)
6. Birth weight <1500 g
7. Signs of clinical or CNS deterioration ⎦

Fig. 64-1. General guidelines for the management of hyperbilirubinemia. (From Brown, A.K.: Jaundice. In Behrman, R.E., editor: Neonatology; diseases of the fetus and infant, St. Louis, 1973, The C.V. Mosby Co.)

tant seizure control. The benzoate preservative displaces bilirubin from albumin.
2. Conjugated hyperbilirubinemia: See Chapter 19.

Renal system

1. Unconjugated hyperbilirubinemia.
   a. Ensure adequate fluid intake to cover maintenance, losses, and insensible water loss (especially during phototherapy).
   b. Attempt to maintain urinary specific gravity ≤1.015.
2. Conjugated hyperbilirubinemia.
   a. Maintain fluid intake to prevent decreased excretion of conjugated bilirubin.
   b. With significant ascites, consider careful diuresis (see Chapter 19).

Metabolic system

1. Unconjugated hyperbilirubinemia.
   a. Consider phenobarbital (3 to 5 day lag),

3 to 5 mg/kg/24 hr initially, with relatively mature hepatic development or autosomal dominant glucuronyl transferase deficiency. CAUTION: Monitor for oversedation.

b. If infant is being breast-fed, consider temporary interruption and/or supplemental free water with sugar-electrolyte solution or formula.

c. Discontinue drugs that may inhibit conjugation (e.g., chloramphenicol).

d. Maintain blood glucose ≥90 mg/dl.

e. Avoid fasting.

f. Consider oral agar, 0.5 to 1.0 g/kg/24 hr, or cholestyramine, 0.5 g every 6 hr, for luminal binding.

2. Conjugated hyperbilirubinemia.

a. For prolonged PT give vitamin K 3 to 5 mg IV initially; 5 to 10 mg menadione daily PO thereafter to correct vitamin K deficiency. Reassess PT to determine response.

b. Discontinue potentially hepatotoxic drugs.

c. During parenteral alimentation, consider reduction or cessation of IV amino acid and/or lipid infusion; resume enteral feeds as early as possible.

d. With presumptive anatomic biliary obstruction, consider laparotomy and operative cholangiogram.

e. Use dietary medium-chain triglycerides as caloric source; give supplemental lipid-soluble vitamins enterally or parenterally as indicated.

f. To increase bile flow, consider phenobarbital, 5 to 10 mg/kg/24 hr, and/or cholestyramine, 1 to 2 g every 6 hr; these are not indicated with untreated extrahepatic biliary atresia.

ADDITIONAL READING

Barrett, P.V.D.: Effect of caloric and noncaloric materials in fasting hyperbilirubinemia, Gastroenterology 68:316-369, 1977.

Brodersen, R.: Bilirubin transport in the newborn infant, reviewed with relation to kernicterus, J. Pediatr. 96:349-356, 1980.

Brodersen, R.: Free bilirubin in blood plasma of the newborn—effects of albumin, fatty acids, pH, displacing drugs and phototherapy. In Stern, L., Oh, W., and Frus-Hansen, B. editors: Intensive care in the newborn, vol. 2, New York, 1978, Masson Publishing U.S.A., Inc., pp. 331.

Cashore, W.J., Gartner, L.M., Oh, W., and Stern, L.: Clinical application of neonatal bilirubin-binding determinations—current status, J. Pediatr. 93:827-832, 1978.

Committee on the Fetus and Newborn: Standards and recommendations for hospital care of the newborn infant, Evanston, Ill., 1977, American Academy of Pediatrics, p. 95.

Huxtable, R.J.: Herbal teas and toxins: novel aspects of pyrrolizidine poisoning in the United States, Perspect. Biol. Med. 24:1-14, 1980.

McDonagh, A.F.: Phototherapy: a new twist to bilirubin, J. Pediatr. 99:909-911, 1981.

Odell, B.B.: Neonatal hyperbilirubinemia, New York, 1980, Grune & Stratton.

Pearlman, M.A., Gartner, L.M., Lee, K.S., and others: Absence of kernicterus in low-birth-weight infants from 1971 through 1976: comparison with findings in 1966 and 1967, Pediatrics 62:460-464, 1978.

Rosenstein, B.S., and Ducore, J.: Enhancement by bilirubin of DNA damage induced in human cells exposed to phototherapy light, Pediatr. Res. 18:32-37, 1984.

Thaler, M.M.: Jaundice in the newborn: algorithmic diagnosis of conjugated and unconjugated hyperbilirubinemia, J.A.M.A. 237:58-62, 1977.

65 Starvation in the PICU

CHARLES E. MIZE

DEFINITION AND PHYSIOLOGY

Exigencies of PICU care may preclude normal modes of feeding or nutrition support, despite the recognition that increased metabolic demands are usually present. With patients who were previously well nourished and not chronically ill, endogenous body stores may be utilized effectively for a period of days without overt body wasting. Preexisting undernutrition from any cause shortens this period of endogenous supply, however, and the risk of significant body mass wasting even during initial PICU management is increased. Anthropometric parameters that help define in-hospital undernutrition indicate that the frequency of nutritional depletion in the PICU may be 50% greater than in the hospitalized but non-PICU population. Repetitive stress periods requiring prolonged PICU hospitalization without adequate substrate support can clearly contribute to this occurrence. The low-birth-weight infant possesses diminished reserves to handle acute substrate demands and may exhaust those reserves rapidly. Consequently, the risk of an evolving substrate deficit or unnoticed relative starvation built around protein-energy malnutrition may be high during acute and protracted PICU management. Specific risk factors that contribute to this potential in the PICU include:

1. Increased basic nutritional needs secondary to increased metabolic requirements of severe illness (e.g., respiratory insufficiency with increased work of breathing, fever, infection, trauma).
2. Protracted nutrient losses (e.g., short bowel syndromes, chronic diarrhea, Fanconi's syndrome).
3. Significant preexisting low body weight or recent weight loss of 10% or more (e.g., small-for-gestational-age infant, tumor, cachexia).
4. Protracted periods of zero enteral intake while a patient is receiving simple, extremely low–substrate density IV solutions (e.g., periods receiving only 5% glucose–electrolyte solutions).
5. Intake of drugs with catabolic or nutrient-antagonist properties (e.g., tetracyclines, antimetabolite agents).

The quantitative needs for nitrogen, energy (calories), and cofactors may be unexpectedly high in physiologic response to stress and disease, superimposed on basic endogenous rates of metabolism. Increased energy expenditures, ranging from 20% to 100% above basal, occur in essentially all PICU patients as a consequence of the hypermetabolic states associated with surgery and severe medical illness (Table 65-1).

Catabolism of body tissue can provide substrates to support this exaggerated metabolic response, which may in turn support initial tissue repair, wound healing, and key protein synthesis. This occurs because the turnover of body protein proceeds whether the patient is malnourished or not. In severe childhood protein-energy malnutrition, the rates of total body protein synthesis and degradation approximate 4 g/kg/24 hr; they rise to 9 to 10 g/kg/24 hr in a rapid rebuilding state, and stabilize at 6 to 7 g/kg/24 hr in a postrecovery state. An important feature of protein dynamics, nonetheless, is that

Table 65-1. Estimating energy requirements

Category	Clinical status	Percent of resting metabolic energy
Hypometabolism	Marasmus, cachexia	80%-100%
Well child	Normal population	100%
Low stress	Anemia, fever, mild infection	100%-120%
Medium stress	Skeletal trauma, debilitating chronic disease	120%-140%
High stress	Sepsis, severe musculoskeletal trauma	140%-170%
Severe stress	Burns	170%-200%

as exogenous protein input declines, the rate of body protein catabolism appears to increase, with an unchanged protein synthesis rate. Relative immobilization can induce net nitrogen loss. Thus, the body protein pool and the closely correlated muscle mass can be significantly depleted when inadequate precursors for new protein are provided. Moreover, in relatively acute hypermetabolic states, protein turnover is increased even though there are generally increased protein synthetic demands of stress. The flux leading to potential nitrogen depletion can thus be accelerated.

Other body constituents that are essential for tissue synthesis and breakdown (e.g., minerals) may reflect similar turnover kinetics. Vitamins and essential cofactors in this metabolic flux cannot be synthesized, and though prior storage of some of these is possible, relative starvation for these nutrients will rapidly deplete such stores. Clinical vitamin and mineral deficiencies subsequently develop.

The energy base for these reactions, ATP production, comes from the oxidation of glucose and fatty acid. Endogenous fatty acid derives indirectly from a quantitatively variable adipose triglyceride store, providing free fatty acids as a major transported fuel for peripheral tissue oxidation. Such lipid oxidation, associated with elevated blood catecholamines and cortisol, appears to continue even when glucose is available in critically ill patients. Endogenous glucose derives indirectly from a minimal glycogen store and directly via gluconeogenesis from renew-able gluconeogenic amino acid stores primarily derived from skeletal muscle. The latter source, when used for glucose production, can remove effectively gluconeogenic amino acids from the amino acid pool used for protein synthesis; and this removal results in a progressive quantitative loss of alpha-amino-nitrogen. If insufficient glucose is provided during relative starvation periods to maintain glucose requirements, this loss of nitrogen can account for continuing body-protein depletion and ultimately declining rates of endogenous protein synthesis. Lipid does not serve as a source of net carbohydrate production. Unless adequate nutritional intervention ultimately provides these several resources exogenously, the rates of other metabolic functions in the cell economy are altered, a net body mass depletion commences, and a variety of organ system deficits attendant to starvation or selective undernutrition develop. The general clinical consequences of such metabolic changes that evolve in association with suboptimal nutritional input may modify resistance to infection, specific protein synthesis, oxygen delivery to tissues, and individual organ functioning capacity (Table 65-2).

Changes that occur in general organ function during mild to moderate undernutrition may be minimal but can reflect significant and occasionally major dysfunction, depending on the severity and selectivity of the nutritional deficit. Marasmus and kwashiorkor, either alone or together, are rare, but a marginal protein-energy deficit, with or without selective nutrient, min-

Table 65-2. Organ system functions affected in starvation

Lymphoreticular function	Respiratory capacities
Intestinal transport	Hepatic substrate and drug metabolism
Endocrine adaptation	Hematopoietic synthesis
Cardiac hemodynamics	
Nervous system transmission	

eral, or cofactor deficits, may account for a variety of marginal or suboptimal organ system dysfunctions.

Intestinal dysfunction and/or deficient intestinal surface area, either of which may be a primary cause of inability to absorb sufficient substrates enterally, may become more severe as a consequence of an ongoing malnutrition that diminishes intestinal muscle mass and microvillus protein synthesis. Villus transport may be seriously diminished. Cellular immunity specifically, but also secretory as well as humoral immunity, may be depressed or aberrantly expressed; for example, antibody response to new antigens can be impaired. Bacterial or fungal overgrowth within the intestine may emerge, and the risk for sepsis, for specific localized infections, and for delayed healing of local infections and wounds is increased with even relative starvation. Respiratory capacity diminishes with diminished and weakened respiratory accessory and intercostal muscle mass; diminished gas flow rates and lessened ability to mobilize lung secretions may contribute to a heightened risk for pneumonitis. Hematopoietic stem cell maturation is retarded, anemia and diminished oxygen-carrying capacity occur, and diverse hematologic aberrations can appear, e.g., altered erythrocyte membrane transport and increased susceptibility to DIC associated with enhanced antithrombin activity. Peripheral nerve conduction may be slowed, and over even relatively short periods, head growth may be retarded. Hepatic albumin synthesis can ultimately be reduced. Functional hepatic metabolic adaptations such as

hepatic drug handling may be significantly altered when selective hepatic drug-metabolizing enzyme systems manifest reduced activity, yielding longer biologic drug half-lives or altered pharmacokinetic clearances, for diverse drugs ranging from cefoxitin and chloramphenicol to phenobarbital and thiopental. Blood volume increase occurring with severe protein deprivation will enhance the risk for heart failure. Cardiac hemodynamics may be further affected as myocardial mass is depleted with significant protein starvation. Pancreatic exocrine dysfunction, selective endocrine changes, (e.g., increased thyroxine-binding globulin), renal dysfunction with increased risk for bacteriuria, aberrant body temperature control, and psychomotor changes have all been variously reported in long term nonselective pediatric undernutrition. In some instances, these effects may only reflect different aspects of disordered separate nutrition factors, but in other instances severely suboptimal nutrition may allow many of these to be evident sequentially and/or concomitantly. Superimposed on these symptom complexes may be specific vitamin and/or mineral deficiency syndromes.

Substrate needs

Recommended daily nutritional and mineral needs based on parenteral estimates are discussed in Chapter 111. Enterally, allowance must be made for intestinal absorption efficiency.

The low-birth-weight (LBW) infant presents special nutritional problems, since the infant has not accrued the full complement of body minerals and stores of the full-term infant, and depletion of these body reserves occurs relatively rapidly compared to full-term infants and older infants and children. The maturing organ systems of low-birth-weight infants may metabolize minerals and substrates at varying rates, and absorption of nutrient materials is generally less efficient than in more mature infants and children. Recognition of these differences in net metabolizable energy from respective energy

Table 65-3. Basic calorimetric and energy data: infants (calories per gram)

	Gross energy*	Digested energy†	Metabolizable energy‡, oral	Metabolizable energy, IV
Glucose	3.74	3.7	3.7	3.4
Starch	4.18	4.1	4.1	
Long chain triglyceride avg.	9.45	8.0	8.0	9.4
Medium chain triglyceride	8.75	7.5	7.5	
Protein avg.	5.65	5.1	4.0	4.4
Glycine	3.12	3.0	2.1	(2.2)

*Bomb Calorimetric Data.
†Digested energy = Gross energy − Fecal energy loss.
‡Metabolizable energy = Digested energy − Urine energy loss.

resources will help define nutrition restitution needs more accurately (see Table 65-3).

The caloric equivalent of weight gain in the normal low-birth-weight infant has been estimated to be approximately 4.5 to 5.5 calories/g weight gain. Adult estimates average 3 to 4 calories/g during early weight loss, and 6 to 8 calories/g during progressive weight loss. The energy cost of depositing obesity tissue is estimated to be 7 to 8 calories/g. When patients are severely ill and manifest a hypermetabolic state, additional input of energy and nutrients must be supplied. Even without evident initial undernutrition, large numbers of calories are required to provide the energy for the hypermetabolism engendered by the illness. Direct measurements in severely ill pediatric patients are not generally available, but extrapolation from adult data yields estimates that can be applied to the PICU population. The calorie needs appear to vary depending on the particular pathophysiologic state (Table 65-1).

The energy needs have been reasonably well established clinically for recovery from classic childhood marasmus and are 200 or more calories/kg/24 hr. Increased oxygen consumption and increased metabolic flux or turnover of body components have furnished estimates of the energy needs during severe ill-

ness (see Table 65-1). The addition of appropriately balanced exogenous amino acid mixtures to resupply the pool for new synthesis and to reduce the net conversion of amino acids to catabolic end products will most efficiently bring about protein sparing and positive nitrogen balance. The needed levels of trace minerals have not been established, and the specific metal-substrate interactions or competitions that affect gut absorption of these minerals have not been defined. The importance of these trace minerals is illustrated by the role that one such mineral, zinc, plays in cellular immunity. Enzymic cofactor and structure roles exist for other trace minerals, and kinetic fluxes dictate the need for nutritional repletion and maintenance, although at requirement levels that are poorly defined at present. Essential fatty acid needs are similarly recognized for precursor and possibly structural membrane roles; the recommended daily requirement in the Nutrition Act of 1980 of 2.7% of the net daily enteral calorie intake (for normal metabolic processes) is based on normal intestinal absorption; more may be required during nutritional restitution.

Complications and risks of nutritional restitution

Although not preventing relative or absolute starvation in the hospitalized patient risks

Table 65-4. Nutritional restitution: complications and risks

1. Infection: primarily parenteral catheter–associated
2. Metabolic consequences: vitamin E/EFA imbalances, hypophosphatemia, hypercalciuria, osteopenia, rickets (with growth), hypercarbia (with increased glucose load), lactic acidosis, cardiac overload/failure, cholestasis residua, nitrogen imbalance
3. Technical difficulties: primarily catheter mechanical problems such as breakage, blockage, perforation/tissue migration

heightened morbidity, if not ultimate mortality, because of disassembly of the affected organ systems as noted above, certain risks have also been recognized with nutritional restitution and maintenance (Table 65-4). Infectious complications can occur with total parenteral nutrition (TPN), and a priority for TPN programs should be to minimize the risk of infection (see Chapter 111).

Metabolic risks of nutritional restitution often result from a need for a different balance of nutrients during repletion than during normal nutrition and this need is either not perceived or is not easily achieved. For example, during active anabolism the requirement for macrominerals, (e.g., potassium and phosphorus) may significantly increase. If exogenous supplies are not increased, plasma levels of these minerals may fall to low levels. A requirement for tocopherol and unsaturated essential fatty acid (EFA) in a ratio of tocopherol/EFA of 0.4 or greater has long been recognized. Insufficient provision of either may be associated with the development of mild to severe essential fatty acid deficiency. Occasional patients receiving high glucose input may develop lactic acidosis. Patients with severe pulmonary function abnormalities may be particularly sensitive to high glucose input either enterally or parenterally and have increased risk for hypercarbia be-

cause of the oxidation of glucose to carbon dioxide (Chapter 111, Table 111-2). Critically ill patients may have glucose intolerance due to an apparent insulin-resistance, with hyperinsulinemia and elevated catecholamine and/or cortisol blood levels; exogenously provided insulin may help overcome this resistance (see Chapter 111).

Moreover, while it may not be possible or desirable to initiate nutritional support with high–caloric density enteral or parenteral solutions, too great an input of nutrient solutions or a formula of low caloric or substrate density given in a legitimate attempt to provide sufficient net nutrients may increase the risk for fluid overload. Such risk is enhanced in a situation of increased intravascular volume, which develops in severe protein malnutrition. Cardiac muscle wasting, which can develop during malnutrition, may also predispose the patient to heart failure if too rapid refeeding is instituted.

Osteopenia, which may be evident in low-birth-weight infants, may evolve toward overt rickets which will develop in the absence of sufficient mineral deposition as growth occurs. Cholestasis can develop in the course of TPN, but rarely occurs with total enteral nutrition (TEN) support (see Chapter 111). Finally, technical problems of nutrient supply occasionally contribute to morbidity associated with nutritional support, but can generally be anticipated or readily recognized for corrective intervention (see Chapters 111 and 112).

MONITORING

See also Chapter 4.

Optimally, assessment of nutritional status is initiated when the patient is first seen, and this assessment should be repeated at regular intervals during a protracted hospitalization.

1. Thorough history, with an estimate of the duration of stress and nutritional deprivation and an estimate of actual nutrient intake over a defined period (monthly or more fre-

quently). Special arrangements may have to be made with the dietary department to achieve accurate calorie counts.

2. Physical clues to nutritional integrity (continuous observation).
   a. Energy and/or protein: estimate adipose mass and muscle mass (separately) by clinical examination and by objective anthropometric measures.
   b. Cofactors (vitamins, minerals, essential fatty acids): hair character, mucous membrane and skin changes, nailbed and ear cartilage changes.

3. Objective anthropometric measurements (weekly).
   a. Simple grid-charted percentiles for height, weight, head circumference, and length (and the age at which the measurement coincides with the 50th percentile).
   b. Percentage of expected weight adjusted for length and/or age. An estimate of expected weight (kg) for length (when length is between 50 and 95 cm) may be derived as follows:

   Male weight = (0.24 × Length) − 8.28
   Female weight = (0.24 × Length) − 8.13

   For example, a boy of length 81.9 cm would be expected to have a weight of 11.4 kg (50th percentile).
   c. Midarm circumference/head circumference ratio (each measured in cm). The normal from infancy to age 4 years is 0.33 or greater.
   d. Triceps skinfold thickness. Compare with normal graphs for age.
   e. Consider, if available, tomography and total body potassium, water, or electrical conductivity to estimate more accurately lean body mass.

4. Laboratory indices.
   a. General: Hb, albumin, glucose, and serum K and PO_4 should be assessed frequently.
   b. Specific: Measure serum proteins with shorter half-lives than albumin, to assess more rapid changes in hepatic protein synthesis (e.g., prealbumin, retinol-binding protein) and measure blood levels of trace minerals (e.g., zinc, copper, manganese, selenium, iodine, chromium), to assess unexpectedly large losses or unusual requirements.
   c. Timed urine collections (continuing at least 24 hours) for urine urea nitrogen (UUN) to estimate gross nitrogen balance, urine creatinine excretion to estimate sequential muscle mass restitution, and urine methylhistidine excretion (on exactly known intake) to estimate gross muscle catabolism.
   d. Obtain blood drug levels to estimate biologic serum decay or half-life (e.g., blood levels at two or more times following the drug injection in order to calculate logarithmic blood concentrations as a function of time).
   e. Periodic long-bone roentgenograms to assess the occurrence of osteopenia or rickets.
   f. Consider recall antigen skin tests of cellular immunity (when prior antigen exposure can be expected to have sensitized the patient adequately) to assess immune competence.

5. Continuing estimates of metabolic energy requirements (daily).
   a. Percentage increments for degree of expected hypermetabolic status, if present (Table 65-1).
   b. Amounts attributed to presence of fever (12% per degree C), muscular activity, and respiratory (muscle) efforts.
   c. Ongoing normal growth and development of organ systems.

MANAGEMENT

The clinical goals of nutritional intervention therapy include wound healing, nonfluid weight gain associated with positive nitrogen balance and protein accretion, and brain growth. The management decisions to achieve these ends should be based on a management plan that progresses through the following steps on a regular and recurring basis:

1. Nutritional evaluation (assessment of status).
2. Diagnosis of qualitative and quantitative nutritional deficits (energy, protein, minerals, vitamins).
3. Detailed plan (qualitative and quantitative) of substrate needs.
4. Nutritional therapy implementation by the enteral and/or parenteral route (see Chapters 111 and 112).

ADDITIONAL READING

Buchanan, N., Davis, M., Danhof, M., and Breimer, D.: Antipyrine metabolite formation in children in the acute phase of malnutrition and after recovery, Br. J. Pharmacol. **10:**363-368, 1980.

Chandra, R., Stiehm, E., Good, R., and Beisel, W.: Nutritional deficiency, immune responses, and infectious illnesses, Fed. Proc. **39:**3086-3108, 1980.

Cole, D., and Zlotkin, S.: Increased sulfate as an etiological factor in the hypercalciuria associated with total parenteral nutrition, Am. J. Clin. Nutr. **37:**108-113, 1983.

Hill, G.L.: Nutrition and the surgical patient, New York, 1981, Churchill Livingstone, Inc.

Kanawati, A., and McLaren, D.: Assessment of marginal malnutrition, Nature **228:**573-574, 1970.

Krieger, I.: Pediatric disorders of feeding, nutrition, and metabolism, New York, 1982, John Wiley & Sons, Inc.

Mehta, S., Nain, C., Sharma, B., and Mathur, V.: Steady state of chloramphenicol in malnourished children, Indian J. Med. Res. **73:**538-542, 1981.

Phillips, A., and Baetz, H.: Diet and resistance to disease, New York, 1981, Plenum Publishing Corp.

Pollack, M., Wiley, J., Kanter, R., and Holbrook, P.: Malnutrition in critically ill infants and children, J. Par. Ent. Nutr. **6:**20-24, 1982.

Viteri, F., and Alvarado, J.: The creatinine height index: its use in the estimation of the degree of protein depletion and repletion in protein-calorie malnourished children, Pediatrics **46:**696-706, 1970.

POISONINGS AND INGESTIONS

66 Poisoning
General principles

FRANCES C. MORRISS

Recent statistics from the National Clearinghouse for Poison Control Centers indicate that every year 86,500 children less than 5 years of age and 50,000 children greater than 5 years of age are victims of accidental poisonings. Though children less than 5 years old visit emergency rooms more frequently, only 12% show signs of toxicity while 52% of older children are symptomatic. Table 66-1 enumerates the most common toxins in this age group and relative mortality rates for hospitalized victims. Note that the majority of these agents were probably ingested orally.

For the toddler, any inviting substances, particularly those resembling food (e.g., ferrous sulfate tablets that look like M & M's) or those stored in familiar containers (e.g., Old English furniture polish in a pop bottle), are fair game. Not only are children this age naturally inquisitive, they also tend to explore, experiment, and imitate when they are bored, tired, or left unattended. Thus arises the familiar situation of the toddler, recuperating from a minor illness, who ingests a household product or a parent's prescribed medication.

Poisoning in older children, especially ado-

Table 66-1. Common poisons in children

Agent	Percent total poisonings		Percent mortality in hospitalized patients	
	<5 yrs	>5 yrs	<5 yrs	>5 yrs
Medicines				
Combinations	—	15*	—	0.5
External	11	5.5	0	0
Internal	41	35	0.5	0.6
Acetylsalicylic acid	4	2	0	0
Pesticides	5	5	0.9	3
Turpentine, paints	4	3	0	1.6
Cleaning and polishing agents	15	8	0.9	0
Petroleum products	3	4.7	0.8	0
Cosmetics	11	1.7	0	0
Gases and vapors	0.1	2	12.5†	4
Plants	12.6	3.6	0	0
Miscellaneous/unknown	8	19	0	1.7

Compiled from tabulations of 1979 poison control case reports, Nat. Clgh. Poison Control Cent. Bull. 25:1-10, 1981.
*This category may be indicative of suicide attempts or drug experimentation.
†Includes mortality from carbon monoxide and smoke inhalation.

lescents, must be viewed as suicide attempts or gestures or as the manifestation of a possible habituation. In either case, acute treatment must be supplemented by investigation of the psychosocial situation and by appropriate referral for continued emotional support and therapy.

Diagnosis of accidental ingestion must be entertained in any child who has bizarre symptoms or in whom the symptom complex is puzzling. Unexplained tachypnea, sudden cardiovascular collapse, or CNS symptoms such as convulsions, delirium, hallucinations, stupor, or coma should suggest an acute intoxication.

Since many toxins remain unidentified, a general approach to monitoring and therapy is given in this chapter. Toxins of specific interest are considered individually in subsequent chapters.

MONITORING

See also Chapter 4.

In most instances of accidental ingestion or exposure, anticipatory intensive monitoring will be unnecessary; however, when a highly toxic substance or a large volume of material has been introduced, close attention to all systems is mandatory. Multisystem involvement is common, and failure of several organs is not unlikely. Systems should be monitored as symptoms referable to specific organs appear. The frequency of monitoring suggested here can be decreased when stability of the organ system in question has been established.

Respiratory system

1. Arterial blood-gas tensions and pH initially and as indicated.
2. Blood oxygen saturation, P_{50}, and carbon monoxide and methemoglobin levels as indicated.

Central nervous system

1. EEG as indicated in the comatose patient.
2. Continuous monitoring of ICP if sustained

intracranial hypertension is suspected, documented, and being treated (see Chapters 10 and 92).
3. CSF analysis as indicated.
4. Frequent neurologic examinations.

Hepatic function

1. SGOT, SGPT, alkaline phosphatase, bilirubin, TSP with A/G, and NH_3 initially and twice weekly if abnormal or if a hepatotoxin has been identified.
2. Gastrointestinal function: abdominal roentgenograms initially if gastrointestinal symptoms are present or if the patient fails to respond to attempts to eliminate an ingested toxin. Massive ingestion of drugs or chemicals seen with suicide attempts may cause stomach concretions.

Skin and musculoskeletal systems

1. Careful and repeated inspection of burned or abraded areas or cutaneous sites of toxin involvement. Such inspection may need to include mucous membranes or fluorescein ophthalmologic examination.
2. Serum CPK if rhabdomyolysis is suspected.
3. If urinalysis is positive for occult blood, obtain urine and serum myoglobin.
4. Long-bone roentgenograms for heavy-metal ingestion.

Other systems

1. Serum amylase.
2. Serum lactate and pyruvate if persistent acidosis is present.
3. BUN, serum creatinine, Na, K, and Cl.
4. Serum glucose.

MANAGEMENT

The management of accidental poisoning is aimed at identifying the poison, decreasing its absorption, increasing its elimination from the body, and supporting all organ systems that may be affected. Few toxic agents have specific antidotes, and a much more favorable outcome is derived from close attention to and treatment of symptoms as they emerge. Since most toxins are capable of damage to multiple organs, repeated physical and chemical evaluation and alteration of therapy are necessary. Specific supportive measures are not detailed here (refer to Chapters 6, 9, 10, 11, 14, 16, and 17).

Poison identification

Although important, identification must not take precedence over treatment of the victim should there by any instability of vital signs. Symptomatic supportive treatment should be undertaken at once, and as soon as the patient's condition is stabilized, specific measures directed to the toxin can be instituted.

Interrogation. Conduct a thorough interrogation of the family, babysitter, etc. about the circumstances of the poisoning, with special attention to the amount ingested, the amount of time since ingestion or exposure, presenting symptoms, and initial treatment efforts and results. Acid substances will be rapidly absorbed from the stomach, but bases will not because of their degree of ionization in the acidic gastric environment. Absorption is impeded by the presence of food in the stomach; liquids are absorbed more rapidly than tablets unless they are enteric preparations or time-release capsules. Establish the time and conditions of the ingestion in order to determine whether induced emesis may be successful or not.

Sample and container. Obtain a sample of the agent and its container. A family member or a policeman may have to return to the home to search for a possible toxin. The label on a container may be the single most useful item in determining the potential toxicity of a product. The Federal Hazardous Substances Act of 1960 requires most dangerous household chemicals to bear a label that plainly lists ingredients. The Federal Insecticide, Fungicide, and Rodenticide Act of 1947 set up a signal word labeling requirement that aids in estimating potential toxicity (Table 66-2). The information

Table 66-2. Definitions of toxicity rating: toxicity rating chart

Signal word	Toxicity rating or class	Probable lethal dose (human) for 70-kg man (150 lb)
No label	1 Practically nontoxic	Above 15 gm/kg—more than 1 qt
No label	2 Slightly toxic	5 to 15 gm/kg—between 1 pt and 1 qt
Caution	3 Moderately toxic	0.5 to 5 gm/kg—between 1 oz and 1 pt (or 1 lb)
Warning	4 Very toxic	50 to 500 mg/kg—between 1 tsp and 1 oz
Danger Poison	5 Extremely toxic	5 to 50 mg/kg—between 7 drops and 1 tsp
Danger Poison	6 Supertoxic	Under 5 mg/kg—a taste (less than 7 drops)

From Mofenson, H.C., and Greensher, J.: The unknown poison, Pediatrics **54:**337, 1974. Copyright American Academy of Pediatrics 1974.

on labels concerning antidotes and initial therapy for overdosage is often inaccurate, and a more definitive source such as a Poison Control Center should be consulted; so-called chemical antidotes such as vinegar or baking soda may produce harmful chemical reactions with the toxin.

Standard references. The following standard references are particularly useful for determining the toxicity of an agent and selecting proper therapy:

1. Arena, J.M.: Poisoning: toxicology, symptoms, treatment, Springfield, Ill., 1974, Charles C Thomas, Publisher.
2. Gleason, M.N., Gasselin, R.E., and Hodge, H.C.: Clinical toxicology of commercial products, Baltimore, 1976, The Williams & Wilkins Co.
3. Goodman, L.S., and Gilman, A., editors: The pharmacologic basis of therapeutics, ed. 5, New York, 1975, Macmillan, Inc.

4. Grant, W.M.: Toxicology of the eye, ed. 2. Springfield, Ill., 1974, Charles C Thomas, Publisher.
5. Hardin, J., and Arena, J.: Human poisoning from native and cultivated plants, Durham, N.C., 1974, Duke University Press.
6. Lampe, K.: Common poisonous and injurious plants, U.S. Department of Health and Human Services Pub. No. (FDA) 15, 81-7006, Washington, D.C., 1980.
7. National Clearing House for Poison Control Centers Bulletin 23:2-14, 1979. (List of emergency phone numbers provided by manufacturers.)
8. Windholz, M., editor: The Merck index: an encyclopedia of chemicals and drugs, ed. 9, Rahway, N.J., 1976, Merck and Co., Inc.
9. American Association of Zoological Parks and Aquariums Antivenom Index Center, Oklahoma City, Okla., phone 405/271-5454. (Index of emergency information on antivenins; 24-hour, 7-day-a-week service.)
10. Telephone number of the nearest poison control center.
11. Poisindex, Microfiche System Micromed Ex., Inc., Denver, Colo.

Samples of blood, urine, and vomitus. Samples of blood, urine, and vomitus (or gastric lavage) should be sent for toxicology screens. Specific information about the suspected nature of the toxin (e.g., phenothiazine, petroleum distillate, antihistamine) needs to accompany the sample in order that as accurate a determination as possible can be made. In general, quantitative identification is not as useful as qualitative information in planning treatment because the time of ingestion is often unknown.

Decreasing toxin absorption

This mode of treatment applies only to ingested agents.

Emptying the stomach. This may be ineffective if the ingestion has occurred more than 4 hours earlier unless the ingested agent was taken with food or is known to delay gastric emptying. Emptying the stomach is contraindicated if the ingested toxin is a corrosive, a mineral acid, strychnine, or a high-viscosity petroleum distillate; hematemesis may also be a relative contraindication.

Induce emesis with syrup of ipecac (not fluid extract of ipecac), 10 to 15 ml in an infant, 20 to 30 ml in a child, followed by several hundred milliliters of fluid orally. Do not use carbonated beverages, which may cause gastric distention, or milk, which may retard the emetic effect of ipecac. Emesis is more successful if the stomach is full. Ipecac in a 30-ml dose may be obtained without a prescription and thus may be administered at home. It has been shown to be effective in 97% of children receiving it; complete evacuation of the stomach occurs within 20 minutes. If vomiting does not occur within ½ hour, the dose may be repeated. Retention of this amount of ipecac will not usually be a cause of further toxicity; ipecac contains a diotoxin (emetine) that in large doses is capable of producing conduction abnormalities, atrial fibrillation, and myocarditis. However, prolonged vomiting may occur, and the child should be observed for at least 45 minutes after the initial episode of emesis.

Produce emesis with apomorphine, 0.1 mg/kg IM (3 mg/m^2), preceded by several hundred milliliters of fluid orally. Emesis occurs within 5 minutes, and as with ipecac, gastric emptying is effective. Apomorphine may also promote reflux of contents from the upper intestine. After emesis has occurred, a narcotic antagonist (naloxone, 0.01 mg/kg IM) may be administered to counteract any respiratory depression secondary to apomorphine. Because it is administered parenterally, apomorphine cannot be given at home.

Gastric lavage is indicated if emesis cannot be induced or if the patient is convulsing or comatose and removal of stomach contents is deemed necessary (i.e., in cases of ingestion of a highly toxic agent or of a large volume of an agent). To minimize chances of inhalation, the patient should be placed on his left side with the head slightly lowered and the feet elevated.

Check the mouth for foreign objects. A sumped NG tube that is as large as possible should be gently passed through a nostril; this may be facilitated by use of a water-miscible jelly or by immersion of the tube in cold water. If the patient can cooperate, ask him to swallow frequently while the catheter is being advanced. It may be helpful to estimate the length of the catheter needed to reach the stomach by marking a length equal to the distance from the bridge of the nose to the xiphoid. When the NG tube is inserted to this length, aspirate and save the first (most concentrated) sample for analysis. Lavage fluid should be 0.9% or 0.45% sodium chloride solution, to prevent loss of electrolytes from the stomach. Small amounts of fluid should be used until the lavage fluid is clear; large amounts of fluid may promote passage of the toxin into the duodenum or distend the stomach. Care must be taken to retrieve all fluid instilled into the stomach; otherwise, gastric dilation may occur. Comatose patients, who lack protective airway reflexes (gag, cough, swallow) should be intubated with an endotracheal tube before institution of gastric lavage. It should be noted that this method of emptying the stomach is less effective than emesis. Under some circumstances, a fluid other than saline solution may be preferred for gastric lavage. The following is a list of such nonspecific antidotes and situations in which their use is appropriate.

1. Tannic acid, a mild acid, precipitates a large number of organic and inorganic compounds, including alkaloids (such as apomorphine, strychnine, and chinchona), glucosides, and the salts of heavy metals such as aluminum, lead, and silver. The precipitated toxin-tannate compound can redissolve and hydrolyze; therefore, the tannic acid solution must not be left in the stomach or the toxin may be absorbed. Use only a solution made from 30 to 50 g tannic acid in 1 L water.

2. Potassium permanganate is an oxidizing agent that neutralizes strychnine, nicotine, physostigmine, and quinine. It is a strong irritant, and a 1:10,000 solution with *no* undissolved particles should be used.

3. Dairy or evaporated milk may be used when a demulcent is needed to coat gastric mucosa and decrease pain from burns caused by ingestion of organic acids, copper sulfate, or croton oil.

4. Sodium bicarbonate (5%) can be used to combine with ingested ferrous sulfate to form the insoluble substance ferrous carbonate, which can then be mechanically removed. Otherwise, bicarbonate is not recommended to neutralize acids, since the production of carbon dioxide causes gastric distention and heat released by the reaction may be damaging to an irritated gastric mucosa.

5. A 10% solution of calcium lactate or gluconate may be used in fluoride and oxalate poisonings to precipitate the toxin.

6. Starch solution, 80 g in 1 L of water, neutralizes iodine; lavage should be continued until the return solution is not blue.

7. Ammonium acetate or ammonia water, 5 ml in 500 ml water, reacts with formaldehyde to form methenamine, which is nontoxic.

Use of activated charcoal, USP. Activated charcoal (Norit A, American Norit Company; Nuchar C, West Virginia Pulp and Paper Company; Charcoal, Merck) is the residue from destructive distillation of various organic materials treated to increase its absorptive capacity. If given within 3 hours of ingestion, and preferably within 30 minutes, it is a potent absorbant effective for most chemicals, except cyanide (Table 66-3). Absorbancy is unaffected by the wide range of pH found in the gastrointestinal tract; absorbed material is retained tenaciously. Activated charcoal should not be used concomitantly with syrup of ipecac, which is inactivated by charcoal. Use of activated charcoal after induced emesis has been shown to be more effective in decreasing absorption of toxins than use of charcoal or emesis alone. The most effective ratio of charcoal to poison is

Table 66-3. Some substances effectively absorbed by activated charcoal

Organic compounds		Inorganic compounds*
Aconite	Muscarine	Antimony
Alcohol	Nicotine	Arsenic
Antipyrine	Opium	Iodine
Atropine	Oxalates	Lead (to limited
Barbiturates	Parathion	extent)
Camphor	Penicillin	Mercuric chlo-
Cantharides	Phenol	ride
Cocaine	Phenolphtha-	Phosphorus
Delphinium	lein	Potassium
Digitalis	Quinine	Potassium per-
Elaterin	Salicylates	manganate
Hemlock	Stramonium	Silver
Ipecac	Strychnine	Tin
Methylene blue	Sulfonamides	Titanium
Morphine	Veratrum	

From Arena, J.: Treatment and specific antidotes, Mod. Treatment **8:**475, 1971.

*Cyanide is a known exception; it poisons the charcoal. Other compounds not absorbed are alcohols, boric acid, corrosives, and ferrous sulfates.

5 parts charcoal to 1 part toxin. If the toxin was ingested with a meal, a more appropriate ratio is 10:1 (1 g/kg in at least 250 ml water may also be a reasonable dose). The charcoal is given as a slurry mixed with water. Although it is an unpleasant looking concoction, most children will accept it when offered in a firm, pleasant manner. Repeated administration of charcoal exerts no greater benefit than a single dose. Burned toast or other forms of charcoal are ineffective; use only activated charcoal, USP.

Use of universal antidote. Universal antidote, which is a mixture of charcoal (burned toast), tannic acid (tea), and magnesium oxide (milk of magnesia), is ineffective and may be toxic in and of itself.

Use of olive oil. For ingested petroleum distillates or lipid-soluble products, olive oil (30 to 60 ml) may act as an absorbant. Mineral oil, alcohol, and milk should be avoided, since these agents may increase gastric absorption.

Increasing elimination of toxins

Cathartics. Cathartics may be useful in hastening elimination of a toxin from the gastrointestinal tract, particularly if the toxin is present in a bound form. Saline cathartics are usually recommended. Their mechanism of action depends on the fact that certain salts are poorly absorbed. Increased intraluminal osmolality thus causes retention of water and indirectly stimulates peristalsis and increases defecation. The most common saline cathartics are magnesium sulfate (Epsom salt), milk of magnesia, magnesium citrate, sodium sulfate, and potassium phosphate. A full dose should produce a semifluid bowel movement in 3 to 6 hours; repeated administration may lead to dehydration. Some absorption of salt may occur, especially with magnesium salts (up to 20% of the dose); however, if renal function is intact, excretion is rapid. Magnesium salts are contraindicated in patients with impaired renal function, as are sodium salts in patients with poor cardiovascular function. Dosage is as follows: milk of magnesia, 0.5 ml/kg/dose; magnesium sulfate (Epsom salt), 250 mg/kg/dose; sodium sulfate, 200 mg/kg/dose (or 30 to 50 g).

Lubricant cathartics of the mineral oil type promote defecation by softening feces and are not recommended. The mineral oil may at times act as a lipid solvent, and the effect on absorption of a lipid ingestant is unpredictable. Inhalation of mineral oil can cause a lipoid pneumonia. If stomach concretion is diagnosed by abdominal roentgenogram, castor oil may dissolve it and increase elimination.

Osmotic catharsis may be induced by giving 10% to 20% mannitol orally in a dose of 10 to 100 ml. Toxicity is low.

Forced diuresis or manipulation of urinary pH. Increased urinary elimination of a renally excreted toxin may be accomplished by forced diuresis or manipulation of urinary pH, usually alkalinization in the case of an acid toxin.

Forced diuresis decreases tubular reabsorption by decreasing the osmotic gradient between blood and urine and by shortening the exposure time of a drug to the resorptive site. This form of treatment succeeds only if renal excretion is the predominant route of drug elimination and renal function is intact. Clearance of alcohols, amphetamines, bromides, isoniazid, phencyclidine, phenobarbital, salicylates, and strychnine can be increased by forced diuresis.

Forced diuresis is accomplished by parenteral administration of large fluid volumes, 1.5 to 2 times maintenance requirements. Urine output should be 3 to 6 ml/kg/hr and specific gravity less than 1.010. Urine and serum electrolytes and osmolalities must be monitored frequently with particular attention to potassium. CVP monitoring may be helpful. An osmotic diuretic, mannitol (1 g/kg IV over 20 minutes as a single dose), may also be used to increase urinary output, particularly because fluid overload and water intoxication are complications of forced diuresis. The possible benefits of this mode of therapy should clearly be greater than the hazard of fluid overload before a decision to institute therapy is made. Pulmonary or cerebral edema and renal disease are contraindications to forced diuresis.

Only nonionized drugs can be reabsorbed in the distal renal tubule; the fraction of ionized drug present is determined by the urinary pH, which ranges normally from 6.5 to 7.8 in the tubular fluid. Acidic compounds (e.g., salicylates, phenobarbital) are eliminated more quickly in an alkaline urine (i.e., there is increased ionization of the drug and less tubular reabsorption), whereas bases such as amphetamine are cleared quickly in an acid urine. Acids with a pK_a value between 3.0 and 7.5 are sensitive to urinary pH changes; the corresponding pK_a values for bases are 7.5 to 10.5. Alkalinizing agents include sodium bicarbonate, sodium lactate, tromethamine (THAM) buffer, and carbonic-anhydrase inhibitors (acetazolamide), which block renal excretion of sodium bicarbonate.

The usual agent employed is sodium bicarbonate, 2 mEq/kg IV over 1 hour followed by 2 mEq/kg as a constant infusion over the next 6 to 10 hours. The urine pH should remain greater than 7.0; 3 to 4 mEq bicarbonate per kg may have to be given to achieve this goal. The hazards of this form of therapy are hypernatremia, hyperosmolality, and the development of systemic alkalosis, which can precipitate tetany. Alkalinization cannot be accomplished in the presence of hypokalemia; serum potassium must be monitored and kept within a normal range by addition of potassium chloride to IV fluids. Therefore, alkalinization should not be undertaken without the ability to monitor serum acid-base status (i.e., arterial blood-gas tensions and pH) and serum electrolytes. Acetazolamide, 5 mg/kg IV, may be given if a brisk diuresis has been established. However, it may increase a preexisting metabolic acidosis because tubular secretion of hydrogen ions is decreased. In addition to serum and urine pH monitoring, serum and urine potassium must be checked frequently, since large amounts of potassium will be excreted and must be replaced. Alkalinization of the urine should not be undertaken if systemic alkalosis or hypokalemia are present.

The agents most commonly used to acidify the urine in order to increase the excretion of bases such as strychnine, amphetamines, and phenothiazines are ascorbic acid and ammonium chloride. Ascorbic acid may be given orally or IV, usually 500 to 1000 mg every 4 to 6 hours for a total of 4 to 6 g/24 hr. Ammonium chloride, slowly or orally, is given 75 mg/kg/24 hr in 4 divided doses with maximum of 6 g/24 hr. Urine pH should be monitored frequently and should be maintained between 4.5 and 5.5. Ammonium chloride is contraindicated in patients with renal or hepatic dysfunction; hyperammonemia and systemic acidosis with hyperchloridemia can complicate its use as well.

Other methods. Less conservative methods of drug elimination are hemodialysis, lipid dialysis, hemoperfusion with lipid absorbents or charcoal, peritoneal dialysis, and exchange transfusion. The usual indications for any of these procedures are failure of more conservative treatment regimens, renal or hepatic failure, or such life-threatening toxicity (clinical signs of severe toxicity, ingestion of lethal dose, prolonged coma with deterioration) that more conventional therapy should be bypassed. For hemodialysis in particular, a clear indication should exist.

Hemodialysis. Hemodialysis is the most efficient method for removal of a dialyzable toxin, but the expertise required for successful completion of this technique often limits its use. Toxins circulating in the blood or reversibly bound to tissues or colloids can be effectively removed. Table 66-4 is a compilation of known dialyzable agents. Each year the Proceedings of the American Society for Artificial Internal Organs (ASAIO) publishes an updated summary of experience with toxic drugs and dialysis as a mode of treatment. Abnormalities of coagulation with bleeding are a major contraindication to hemodialysis.

Charcoal hemoperfusion. Toxins such as barbiturates, glutethimide, tricyclic antidepressants, digoxin, and theophylline can be removed from circulation by passing blood through a column of adsorbent material (charcoal or Amberlite [(XAD-4 resin]). The technique requires an arteriovenous shunt and anticoagulation but is simpler than hemodialysis. Although a controversial technique, hemoperfusion has been used successfully to decrease the duration of coma and cardiorespiratory support seen with lethal plasma concentrations of drugs. Problems with the technique include charcoal microemboli (prevented by adequate filtration), thrombocytopenia, bleeding, coagulopathies and hypocalcemia.

Lipid dialysis. Lipid dialysis is a technique devised for removal of lipid-soluble substances, such as glutethimide or camphor, that cannot be eliminated by other means. The technique is similar to that for aqueous dialysis, except that an oil such as soybean oil is circulated on the dialysate side of the membrane.

Peritoneal dialysis. Peritoneal dialysis, though not as efficient as hemodialysis, is more common because of its simplicity and easy availability. Contraindications include peritoneal infection and recent abdominal surgery. Since only unbound, ionized drugs are dialyzable, the efficiency of the procedure may be increased by adding albumin to the dialysate (if the drug is protein-bound) or by manipulating dialysate pH (see Chapter 110).

Exchange transfusion. Exchange transfusion is effective for agents that remain in the bloodstream rather than become fixed to tissues. Specifically, drugs that are bound to RBCs (e.g., carbon monoxide) or that produce methemoglobinemia (aniline dyes, nitrites, nitrates, bromates, chlorates, sulfanilamide, phenazopyridine, and nitrobenzene) are good indications for exchange transfusion. Besides removing the agent, exchange transfusion restores normal oxygen-carrying capacity. Availability of blood and the size of the child are obvious limiting factors to its use. In general, hemodialysis or peritoneal dialysis are preferable to exchange transfusion (see Chapter 107).

Nonorally absorbed toxins (exposed body surfaces)

See also Chapter 26.

Inhaled toxins. Inhaled toxins are usually absorbed directly through the lungs. The reaction of pulmonary parenchyma varies with the inhaled toxin but may include:
1. Acute chemical pneumonitis secondary to direct injury to tracheobronchial tube.
2. Hypersensitivity reaction to exposure to proteins or protein conjugates.
3. Restrictive disease secondary to chronic exposure. Asphyxiation occurs when 20% to 30% of gases inhaled are toxic fumes; death occurs when inspired oxygen is less than 10%.

The most effective measures to eliminate the toxin include removal of the patient to a toxin-free environment, removal of clothing carrying traces of toxin, administration of oxy-

Table 66-4. Known dialyzable poisons*

Barbiturates
Barbital
Phenobarbital
Amobarbital
Pentobarbital
Butabarbital
Secobarbital
Cyclobarbital

Glutethimide

Depressants, sedatives, and tranquilizers
Diphenylhydantoin
Primidone
Meprobamate
Ethchlorvynol
Ethinamate
Methyprylon
Diphenhydramine
Methaqualone
Heroin
Gallamine triethiodide
Paraldehyde
Chloral hydrate
Chlordiazopoxide

Antidepressants
Amphetamine
Methamphetamine
Tricyclic secondary amines
Tricyclic tertiary amines
Monomine oxidase inhibitors
Trancylopromine
Pargyline
Phenelzine
Isocarboxazid

Alcohols
Ethanol
Methanol
Isopropanol
Ethylene glycol

Analgesics
Acetysalicylic acid
Methylsalicylate
Acetophenetidin
Dextropropoxyphene
Paracetamol

Antibiotics
Streptomycin
Kanamycin
Neomycin
Vancomycin
Penicillin
Ampicillin
Sulfonamides
Cephalin
Cephaloridine
Chloramphenicol
Tetracycline
Nitrofurantoin
Polymyxin
Isoniazid
Cycloserine
Quinine

Metals
Arsenic
Copper
Calcium
Iron
Lead
Lithium
Magnesium
Mercury
Potassium
Sodium
Strontium

Halides
Bromide
Chloride
Iodide
Fluoride

Endogenous toxins
Ammonia
Uric acid
Tritium
Bilirubin
Lactic acid
Schizophrenia
Myasthenia gravis
Porphyria
Cystine
Endotoxin
Hyperosmolar state
Water intoxication

Miscellaneous substances
Thiocyanate
Aniline
Sodium chlorate
Potassium chlorate
Eucalyptus oil
Boric acid
Potassium dichromate
Chromic acid
Digoxin
Sodium citrate
Dinitro-ortho-cresol
Amanita phalloides
Carbon tetrachloride
Ergotamine
Cyclophosphamide
5-Fluorouracil
Methotrexate
Camphor
Trichlorethylene
Carbon monoxide
Chlorpropamide

From Arena, J.: Treatment and specific antidotes, Mod. Treatment **8**:478, 1971.
*This list is complete at press time. Undoubtedly many more compounds will be found to be dialyzable as time passes. Agents that are highly bound to plasma protein (and hence, poorly dialyzable, at least theoretically) may actually be removed in significant quantities because of a rapid equilibrium between the bound and unbound drug fractions. It is possible, therefore, that many compounds not listed as dialyzable may very well be removed by dialysis. Peritoneal dialysis, by rewarming the "core," has produced recovery from profound hypothermia.

gen to dilute any toxin remaining in the lung, and support of ventilation mechanically if the patient is asphyxiated. Inhaled particulate matter may require bronchoscopy for removal.

Arterial blood gas tensions and pH, a chest roentgenogram, and an ECG should be done to determine the extent of toxicity. If symptoms (chemical or physical) persist, a radioactive xenon scan will diagnose the degree of parenchymal damage.

Common inhaled toxins include smoke, steam, dust, carbon monoxide, mercury vapor, ammonia, butane, propane, hydrogen sulfide, and toxic fumes liberated by the inappropriate mixture of acid-type toilet bowl cleaners and sodium hypochloride bleaches (Chlorox). Such mixtures may liberate chlorine and chloramine gas ($NaOCl + H^+ \rightarrow Cl_2 + H_2O + NaCL + NH_2Cl + NaOH$). Both gases are highly irritating and capable of causing pulmonary edema, although they are so toxic that the victim is usually driven from the vicinity.

Cutaneous and transcutaneous absorption. Toxins applied to the skin should be removed with copious amounts of water after the victim has been stripped of all contaminated clothing. Specific treatment of any burns or dermatitis should then be instituted. Agents capable of producing systemic toxicity from transcutaneous absorption include chlorinated and organophosphate insecticides, halogenated hydrocarbons, caustics, and corrosives. Chemical antidotes should not be applied to the skin, since heat released secondary to the reaction between toxin and antidote may exacerbate the original injury.

Toxins introduced into the eyes should be washed out with large amounts of water.

1. Recommend irrigation with tap water or any innocuous watery solution at hand to patients phoning in.
2. After administration of a local anesthetic, flush the affected eye continuously with 0.9% sodium chloride solution for 1 to 2 minutes. Prolonged flushing will only irritate the eye and should be avoided unless the contaminant is chemically active or has an oily or viscous base.
3. Test the conjunctival sac with wide-range pH test paper. The normal pH is 7.0. An alkaline pH between 11 and 12 (from hair neutralizers, phosphate-free detergents, organic amines, lye, potash) causes the greatest eye injury (e.g., corneal erosions, scarring, and permanent opacity). Irrigation should continue until the effluent pH is between 8.0 and 8.5.
4. Use flourescein to discover epithelial damage. (Only sterile strips should be used, since fluorescein solution is a rich media for bacteria.)
5. If solid particle contamination is present, evert lids and make a careful search of the conjunctival sac. Continue irrigation if alkaline coagulation has occurred; a cotton-tipped applicator moistened with sterile antibiotic ointment may be used to remove particles adherent to tissue.
6. Consult an ophthalmologist for further diagnosis and treatment.

Toxins and specific antidotes

Specific antidotes are not numerous and can usually be identified by the Poison Control Center. The following is a partial list of toxins and their specific antidotes.

Narcotics. The antidote for narcotics (morphine sulfate, meperidine, methadone, diphenoxylate, alphaprodine, anileridine, hydromorphone, and pentazocine) is naloxone (Narcan); the usual dose is 0.01 mg/kg IV. This dose may need to be titrated to individual patients, since there is a broad dose-response curve. The suggested maximum is a total of 0.03 mg/kg in 3 divided doses. The peak effect occurs within 2 minutes after IV administration and lasts 30 to 45 minutes. Via the IM route, the peak effect occurs at 10 minutes and the duration is 2.5 to 3 hours. Naloxone has no respiratory or cardiac depressant activity and may be safely used as a diagnostic test for coma induced by an unknown drug. For longer-acting narcotics such as morphine, several reversal doses may be necessary and the patient should be hospitalized.

Warfarin and coumadin derivatives found in rodenticides. Give vitamin K (phytonadione), 25 to 150 mg IV, rate not exceed 10 mg/min.

Organophosphate insecticides. Give atropine sulfate and pralidoxime chloride (Protopam) (see Chapter 73).

Heavy metals. Give chelating agents (see Chapter 74).

Methyl alcohol (methanol). Alcohols and their derivatives are metabolized by the hepatic enzyme alcohol dehydrogenase; however, ethyl alcohol (ethanol) is the preferred substrate even in the presence of other alcohols. Ingested methanol or ethylene glycol such as may be found in solvents, paint thinners, antifreeze, dry cleaning fluid, and solid canned heat will be metabolized to glyoxalic acid, formic acid, oxalate, and other potent systemic toxins. As little as 2 teaspoons (orally) or 2 parts per million (inhaled) of these agents can be fatal. Patients appear to be inebriated without having the characteristic ethanol odor to the breath; many may have visual symptoms, and hypoglycemia may occur. A profound metabolic acidosis occurs, and a pH of less than 7.1 must be treated aggressively until definitive therapy can be effective.

The definitive therapy is administration of ethyl alcohol (ethanol) to bind hepatic enzyme sites and prevent the formation of toxic metabolites of ingested alcohols. Ethanol therapy should be begun immediately, though a blood sample for ethanol, methanol, and ethylene glycol should be drawn. If serum methanol levels exceed 25 mg/dl, hemodialysis should be considered. Ethanol therapy should be stopped if a significant ethanol level is documented (i.e., this episode may represent the more standard case of ethanol ingestion). Administer ethanol as follows:

1. Loading dose 0.8 g/kg (1 ml/kg) by one of the following routes:
   a. Oral or NG: 20% to 30% concentration.
   b. IV: 5% to 10% concentration (higher concentration causes thrombophlebitis).
2. Maintenance to begin immediately after loading dose: 130 mg/kg/hr (0.15 ml/kg/hr) orally or IV. If patient is placed on hemodialysis, maintenance should be 250 to 350 mg/kg/hr.
3. Check serum ethanol levels serially to ensure blood level of 100 to 150 mg/dl.
4. Check arterial blood-gas tensions and pH serially and treat acidosis.
5. Monitor closely for signs of fluid overload if the IV route is used.
6. Calcium oxalate crystals may be precipitated in urine; if present, check serum Ca.
7. Thiamine, 100 mg IM or IV, and pyridoxine, 50 mg IM or IV every 6 hours, may shunt the metabolism of ethylene glycol from the formation of oxalate and formate to the formation of less toxic metabolites.

Acute tubular necrosis secondary to precipitation of oxalate or to direct damage from toxic metabolites may occur, as well as hypocalcemia, tetany, and cardiopulmonary failure.

Cyanides. Free cyanide groups (CN^-) are handled by one of three pathways:

1. Reaction with methemoglobin to form cyanmethemoglobin. This is a very rapid reaction if significant amounts of methemoglobin are available, and methemoglobin competes with other binding sites for free cyanide.
2. Reaction with tissue cytochrome oxidase, the result of which is inactivation of the enzyme and inhibition of cellular respiration, resulting in tissue hypoxia.
3. Conversion by hepatic and renal rhodanase to thiocyanate, which is then excreted in the urine. This reaction is relatively slow unless an exogenous sulfur substrate (usually thiosulfate) is supplied. Vitamin B_{12} (cyanocobalamin) may be a coenzyme for this reaction.

The objective of treatment is to produce a high concentration of methemoglobin by the administration of sodium nitrate ($HbFe^{++} + NaNO_2 \rightleftharpoons HbFe^{+++}$). Methemoglobin then binds free cyanide ($HbFe^{+++} + Cn^- \rightleftharpoons HbFeCN$). Actual detoxification is then achieved by the action of rhodanase plus thiosulfate to form thiocyanate (SCN^-) ($Na_2S_2O_2 + HbFeCN \rightleftharpoons SCN^- + HbFe^{+++} + Na_2SO_3$). To form methemoglobin, administer sodium nitrite, 0.005 to 0.01 mg/kg IV by slow injection over 3 to 4 minutes. Then give sodium thiosulfate by slow IV injection, 150 to 200 mg/kg over 10 minutes. For recurrent symptoms, repeat the same procedure, halving the doses. The patient may be given amyl nitrite to inhale while the sodium nitrite and thiosulfate are being assembled; gastric lavage with potassium permanganate (1:10,000 solution) should be considered if cyanide was ingested orally. Some recommend, in addition, administration of vitamin B_{12}. Sources of cyanide include insecticides, rodenticides, silver polish, laetrile, photographic supplies, and seeds from apples, peaches, plums, cherries, and apricots. With liver dysfunction or depletion of thiosulfate, administration of sodium nitroprusside (Nipride) results in cyanide intoxication, initially manifested as unexplained systemic acidosis and failure to change blood pressure with increasing doses of the drug.

Belladonna alkaloids (scopolamine, hyoscine, atropine). Physostigmine is a tertiary amine capable of crossing the blood-brain barrier. It acts as an anticholinesterase, inhibiting the hydrolysis of acetylcholine at the junction of cholinergic fibers; its central effect is comparable to continuous cholinergic stimulation. Clinically, it reverses disorientation, delirium, hallucinations, and somnolence secondary to toxic doses of belladonna compounds as well as the peripheral anticholinergic signs (dilated pupils, tachycardia, bowel atonia). Because of its central cholinergic stimulation, physostigmine has been recommended in the treatment of overdoses of sedatives and CNS depressants, whose action may include cholinergic depression, and it is the drug of choice for toxicity from tricyclic antidepressants and phenothiazines, although all authors do not agree with this recommendation (see also Chapter 69). A partial list of drugs for which anecdotal evidence of reversal of CNS depression exists includes also diazepam, antihistamines, droperidol, and antiparkinsonian drugs. Physostigmine's central cholinergic-stimulating properties may or may not be useful. Reversal of respiratory depression or return of obtunded reflexes will not necessarily occur with its administration, and all usual supportive measures should be employed with sedative overdoses. Its use should probably be reserved for cases of severe intoxication manifested by CNS or cardiac symptoms. The usual dose is 0.5 mg (or 0.01 to 0.03 mg/kg) in increments of 0.1 mg IV over 2 to 3 minutes and may be repeated up to a total of 2 mg every 5 minutes with cardiac monitoring. Rapid IV administration (greater than 0.01 mg/kg/min) can cause bradycardia, seizures, and hypersalivation. A response within 5 minutes should be seen; since physostigmine has a short half-life, repeat doses may be needed at 30- to 60-minute intervals. In the presence of cholinergic toxic effects (bradycardia, miosis) physostigmine should be withheld.

Treatment of CNS depression. Nonspecific cortical or medullary stimulants such as caffeine, nikethamide, picrotoxin, bemegride, ethamivan, and doxapram are not recommended for CNS depression. The dose necessary to stimulate depressed respiration is only slightly less than the dose required to cause grand mal seizures. In addition, side effects such as hypertension, bradycardia with dysrhythmias, hyperthermia, toxic psychosis, nausea, and vomiting are common. The peak effect occurs at 30 minutes, and the duration of action is 1 to 4 hours, depending on the route of administration. Repeated doses must be given to sustain respiration. The role of analeptic agents in acute intoxication is practically non-existent. Securing the airway and support of ventilation are the preferred forms of treatment.

Prevention of poisonings

The environmental situation that promoted the overdose needs to be investigated, particularly for the older child or an adolescent who may be gesturing for help. There may be undesirable social forces (neglectful parents, financial inability to provide adequate supervision of infants) present in the home, or the poisoning episode may have been the result of ignorance. It has been shown that families experiencing a poisoning episode exhibit twice as many major stresses as families not experiencing such an episode. Social and emotional problems are also more common in families in which a child has ingested toxins more than once. Children who repeatedly ingest substances exhibit hyperactivity, temper tantrums, aggression, stubbornness, and negativism more often than noningestors, and the purposefulness of the behavior leading to ingestion has been proved. Appropriate parental education as to storage of harmful products, emergency treatment of future ingestions, or appropriate child supervision should be undertaken. In second or subsequent episodes of poisoning, a home visit by a public health nurse or referral to a social service or child welfare agency may be warranted to clarify the situation and remedy home problems.

ADDITIONAL READING

Abramowicz, M., editor: Cyanide intoxication from nitroprusside in anesthesia, Med. Lett. Drugs Ther. 18:68, 1976.

Arena, J.M.: Current status: the management and treatment of poisoning, Mod. Treatment 8:461-625, 1971.

Arena, J.M.: The treatment of poisoning, Clin. Symp. 30:1-47, 1978.

Bottenfield, G., and Cohen, S.E.: Therapeutics in the pediatric emergency room, Pediatr. Clin. North Am. 26:867-881, 1979.

Coleman, A.B., and Alpert, J.J., editors: Poisoning in children, Pediatr. Clin. North Am. 17:1, 1970.

Elenbaas, R.M., issue editor: Poisonings and overdoses, Crit. Care Q. 4:1-104, 1982.

Finge, E.: Cathartics. In Goodman, L.S., and Gilman, A., editors: The pharmacological basis of therapeutics, ed. 4, New York, 1971, Macmillan, Inc.

Goldfrank, L., and Bresmitz, E.: Toxic inhalants, Hosp. Physician 15:54-60, 1979.

Heisterkamp, D.V., and Cohen, P.J.: The use of naloxone to antagonize large doses of opiates administered during nitrous oxide anesthesia, Anesth. Analg. 53:12-18, 1974.

Holt, L.E., and Holz, P.H.: The black bottle, J. Pediatr. 63:306-312, 1963.

Holzgrafe, R.E., Vondrell, J.J., and Mintz, S.M.: Reversal of postoperative reactions to scopolamine with physostigmine, Anesth. Analg. 52:921-925, 1973.

Mofenson, H.C., and Greensher, J.: Controversies in the prevention and treatment of poisonings, Pediatr. Ann. 6:717-725, 1977.

Mofenson, H.C., and Greensher, J.: Physostigmine as an antidote: use with caution, J. Pediatr. 87:1010-1011, 1975.

Poison control statistics, Federal Drug Administration, 1974.

Post, K.M., Jaeger, R.W., and deCastro, F.J.: Eye contamination: a poison center protocol for management, Clin. Toxicol. 14:295-300, 1979.

Rogers, J.: Recurrent childhood poisoning as a family problem, J. Fam. Pract. 13:337-340, 1981.

Rosenbaum, J.L., Kramer, M.S., Raja, R.M., and others: Current status of hemoperfusion in toxicology, Clin. Toxicol. 17:493-500, 1980.

Shirkey, H.: Ipecac syrup: its use as an emetic in poison control, J. Pediatr. 46:139-140, 1966.

Swinyard, E.A.: Noxious gases and vapors. In Goodman, L.S., and Gilman, A., editors: The pharmacological basis of therapeutics, ed. 4, New York, 1971, Macmillan, Inc.

Tinker, J.H., and Michenfelder, J.D.: Sodium nitroprusside: pharmacology, toxicology and therapeutics, Anesthesiology 45:340-354, 1976.

67 Salicylism

FRANCES C. MORRISS

PHYSIOLOGY

Overdose of salicylates, which account for 3.8% of all poisonings in children, may be acute or chronic. The incidence has steadily decreased as a result of child-proof safety caps. Salicylates are rapidly absorbed from the gastrointestinal tract, hydrolyzed to free salicylic acid, and metabolized by the liver. Renal clearance of metabolites (salicyluric acid, salicylate glucuronide) is rapid. The concentration of free salicylate ion is the main determinant of toxicity. Distribution of salicylate, a weak acid, depends on serum pH; the nonionized lipid-soluble form penetrates biologic membranes easily. An alkaline environment favors dissociation (ionization) of salicylates and trapping of the drug in the alkaline milieu. Acidemia does not promote ionization and facilitates movement of salicylates from the vascular and extracellular fluid spaces into cells, the main site of toxic reactions.

The major toxic effects include (1) local gastrointestinal irritation, (2) direct stimulation of the respiratory center, (3) generalized increase in metabolic rate, (4) interference with intermediate carbohydrate metabolism, and (5) interference with mechanisms of coagulation. The usual signs of salicylism include marked hyperventilation, vomiting, fever, dehydration, CNS dysfunction, and polyuria followed by oliguria; with severe toxicity, there may be bleeding, pulmonary edema, respiratory depression, and coma with convulsions. There is a tendency for younger patients to have an acid serum pH; with increasing age, the number of patients who have acidosis decreases.

Salicylates have three separate actions on acid-base status. First, primary stimulation of the respiratory center increases minute ventilation and decreases serum carbon dioxide concentration. This action is independent of age. Second, there is a generalized stimulation of oxidative metabolism by means of uncoupling of mitochondrial oxidative phosphorylation, leading to increased oxygen consumption, increased carbon dioxide production, and heat production. It is this increased heat production that is responsible for fever in infants. These first two actions of salicylate are seen in older children and adults. The increase in minute ventilation usually precedes the increase in carbon dioxide production, so that Pa_{CO_2} is lowered, pH increased, and the bicarbonate buffer system depleted. If salicylism is chronic, renal compensation may produce a normal serum pH. Third, in the child less than 4 years of age, interference with intermediate metabolism (Krebs' cycle and carbohydrate production) causes increased production of organic acids, metabolic acidosis, ketonemia, and ketonuria. In addition, the younger child has a diminished capacity to buffer organic acids. The relative contribution of metabolic acidosis and respiratory alkalosis to the ultimate pH may thus be varied. The most severe acidosis is seen in the small child and in those with chronic overdoses; severe acidosis in the adult is a poor prognostic sign.

Dehydration is the consequence of increased insensible water loss secondary to the hypermetabolic state described above and to an obligatory water loss imposed by excretion of excess urinary solutes (organic acids, ketones). There are also urinary losses of sodium and potassium, the most common deficit being that of potassium compounded by increased cellular permeability to potassium and intracellular ion shifts. ISADH has been described in cases of severe toxicity. Interference with intermediate metabolism also leads to disorders of serum glucose; young children most often have hypoglycemia, although mild hyperglycemia (less than 200 mg/dl) can be seen. The CSF glucose concentration may be low in the absence of low serum glucose and may be one cause of coma and seizures.

Hemorrhagic problems result from local gastric irritation and from multifactorial coagulation defects, including increased capillary fragility, impaired platelet aggregation, decreased levels of factor VII, and inhibition of prothrombin production.

MONITORING

See also Chapter 4.

Serum salicylate level

Measurement of serum salicylate level is most useful in instances of acute ingestion. The salicylate level correlates poorly with the severity of intoxication, because toxic manifestations are determined by the peak level of salicylate and the rapidity with which it declines. Since the rate of metabolism is fairly predictable, a rough estimate of the peak level can be made for victims who have ingested a single dose. A nomogram has been developed for this purpose and can be used to predict the expected severity of the intoxication on the basis of a single blood salicylate level determination (Fig. 67-1). The classifications according to the nomogram are: asymptomatic (occasional subjective but no objective symptoms), mild (mild to moderate hyperpnea with lethargy), moderate (severe hyperpnea, prominent neurologic manifestations), and severe (severe hyperpnea, coma, and convulsions). For the best prediction the exact time of the ingestion must be known. Note that this nomogram may not apply to time-release capsules.

Respiratory system

Measure arterial blood gas tensions and pH initially and every 2 to 4 hours until normal.

Hematologic system

1. Perform coagulation studies, including Hct, PT, PTT, bleeding time, and platelet count; repeat as needed. Obtain type and crossmatch if there are overt signs of bleeding.
2. Check status of gastric bleeding with an NG tube.
3. Check stool (guaiac method).

Renal-metabolic system

Measure serum Na, K, Cl, and HCO_3 initially and serially if alkaline therapy is instituted.

MANAGEMENT

See also Chapter 66.

Specific measures

1. Decrease absorption (induce vomiting, give saline cathartic, use activated charcoal, or, if the patient is comatose, use gastric lavage). Since toxic doses delay gastric emptying, these measures can be effective up to 6 hours after ingestion. Lavage with bicarbonate will delay the absorption of aspirin time-release capsules retained in the stomach.
2. Increase excretion of salicylate (establish adequate alkaline urine output).
   a. The respiratory center will still be influenced by salicylate, and Pa_{CO_2} will continue to be depressed despite a high serum pH. Alkalinization of the urine may require large amounts of sodium bicarbonate and may quickly lead to systemic alkalosis for which the respiratory system cannot compensate. This form of therapy should only be used for patients with signs of severe toxicity (bleeding, coma, respiratory depression) or for those in whom the serum level indicates severe toxicity. Serum pH, BUN, electrolytes, and osmolality must be known before ini-

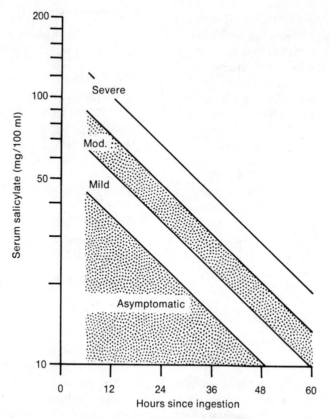

Fig. 67-1. Nomogram relating serum salicylate concentration and expected severity of intoxication at various intervals after the ingestion of a single dose of salicylate. (From Done, A.K.: Pediatrics **26:**800, 1960.)

tiation of bicarbonate therapy and must be reevaluated frequently thereafter. Alkalinization with bicarbonate is contraindicated in patients with systemic alkalosis. In addition, in the young patient there is almost always hypokalemia, which must be corrected if excretion of an acid moiety in the urine is to be successful (the ion exchanged for H^+ in the distal tubule is K^+). Continuous ECG monitoring is necessary if large amounts of potassium must be given rapidly. Acetazolamide is not recommended for alkalinization of urine in children with salicylism.

3. Artificial removal of salicylate (hemodialysis,

peritoneal dialysis, or exchange transfusion in newborns) should be considered when salicylate levels are greater than 100 mg/dl or when coma, renal failure, or failure to respond to conservative therapy occurs.

Supportive measures

Institute supportive measures as outlined in previous chapters on organ failure, with special reference to the following:

1. Administration of parenteral fluids will depend on the degree of dehydration and the extent of electrolyte abnormalities. Sudden death secondary to profound hypoglycemia has been reported in younger children, and

therefore glucose-free IV solutions should never be used. If systemic acidosis exists, a solution containing sodium lactate has better buffering capacity than a saline-based solution (lactate is metabolized via Krebs' cycle to carbon dioxide, which is then converted to bicarbonate ion).

2. Vitamin K may partially reverse the bleeding disorder (1 to 5 mg IV).
3. Iced saline lavage may be useful in controlling bleeding secondary to gastric irritation (see Chapter 62).
4. Treat hyperpyrexia with sponging or an ice mattress rather than with antipyretics.
5. Acute administration of anticonvulsants may be necessary to control seizure activity; however, chronic anticonvulsant therapy is unnecessary.

ADDITIONAL READING

Done, A.K.: Salicylate intoxication: significance of measurements of salicylate in blood in cases of acute ingestion, Pediatrics 26:800-807, 1960.

Done, A.K., and Temple, A.R.: Treatment of salicylate poisoning, Mod. Treatment 8:528-551, 1971.

Feuerstein, R.C., Finberg, L., and Fleishman, E.: The use of acetazolamide in the therapy of salicylate poisoning, Pediatrics 25:215-227, 1960.

Oliver, T.K., and Dyer, M.E.: The prompt treatment of salicylism with sodium bicarbonate, Am. J. Dis. Child. 99:553-565, 1960.

Pierce, A.W.: Salicylate poisoning, Pediatrics 54:342-347, 1974.

Reimold, E.W., Worthen, H.G., and Reilly, T.P.: Salicylate poisoning, Am. J. Dis. Child. 125:668-674, 1973.

Winters, R.W.: Salicylate intoxication. In Winters, R.W., editor: The body fluids in pediatrics, Boston, 1973, Little, Brown & Co.

68 Acetaminophen overdose

FRANCES C. MORRISS
ALAN H. HALL
BARRY H. RUMACK

PHYSIOLOGY

Acetaminophen (Tylenol, Tempra) has been recommended as the antipyretic of choice for children because of its relative lack of serious side effects as compared with aspirin. Acetaminophen given in an appropriate therapeutic dose produces minimal adverse or hypersensitivity reactions; when it is ingested in excessive amounts, severe hepatotoxicity may result. Acetaminophen overdoses are becoming increasingly common. In 1983, there were 11,179 cases reported to the American Association of Poison Control Centers, National Data Collection System, with over 50% of these overdoses occurring in children 6 years of age or younger. Acetaminophen is rapidly absorbed from the stomach, with peak serum concentrations being reached in 1 to 2 hours, but with overdose, peak serum concentrations sometimes are not reached for as long as 4 hours. Rate of absorption is influenced by rate of gastric emptying and type of preparation (liquid versus tablet). Elimination half-life varies from 1 to 3 hours; metabolism occurs rapidly by biotransformation in hepatic microsomal systems. Eighty percent of the dose is conjugated with glucuronic acid and to a lesser extent with sulfates. These conjugated metabolites lack biologic activity. Minor metabolites are formed by hydroxylation and deacetylation in the cytochrome P-450 mixed-function oxidase chain. This hydroxylated metabolite is a highly reactive arylating agent that is detoxified by conjugation with hepatic glutathione and is subsequently excreted in the urine as a conjugate of cysteine and mercapturic acid. The rate of formation of these minor metabolites is increased when inducers of drug metabolism are ingested and when the usual conjugating pathway is overloaded (i.e., with overdose).

Ingestion of large quantities of acetaminophen causes excessive formation of intermediate metabolites in the liver. If hepatic glutathione is depleted to less than 70% of normal by conjugation of these intermediate products, the reactive arylating metabolite will bind to cellular macromolecules, causing hepatic necrosis, particularly in the centrilobular areas. Induction of hepatic enzymatic systems by such agents as barbiturates, hydantoins, and narcotics will increase the likelihood of formation of intermediate reactive compounds. In a national study, potentially hepatotoxic plasma levels of acetaminophen were observed to have fewer hepatotoxic effects on young children than on adults. This observation and animal studies suggest that young children may possess a degree of protection against acetaminophen hepatic toxicity. The mechanisms may include a higher rate of glutathione turnover, which determines the capacity to increase hepatic glutathione after depletion, and a shift from predominance of sulfate conjugation to glucuronide conjugation in children between 9 and 12 years of age. Additional evidence suggests that the concomitant acute ingestion of alcohol (a frequent excipient in oral acetaminophen preparations) may confer a degree of hepatoprotection.

Hepatic injury may be seen within 36 to 48 hours after ingestion of a single large dose; a toxic dose may be 150 mg/kg or greater. There may be no signs or symptoms in the first 24 hours after ingestion, or the patient may manifest anorexia, nausea, vomiting, and diaphoresis. Symptoms may abate. After 24 hours there are increases in transaminases and bilirubin and prolongation of clotting time. Abdominal pain secondary to hepatic enlargement follows after 48 hours. Hypoglycemia, jaundice, metabolic acidosis, and clotting abnormalities characterize severe hepatic damage. If hepatotoxicity develops, the maximal changes in liver function indicating necrosis usually occur 2 to 4 days after ingestion; therefore, early clinical improvement or lack of symptoms *does not* indicate absence of severe hepatic damage. If liver function tests are entirely normal after 48 hours, significant hepatic damage is unlikely. Fulminant hepatic failure with encephalopathy may occur in 4 to 6 days. (See Chapter 19.) In the immediate postingestion period the plasma concentration of acetaminophen in relation to the time of the ingestion has a prognostic value for potential hepatotoxicity and hence is used to determine the need for treatment. A nomogram of plasma acetaminophen levels (single acute dose) versus time has been developed for prediction of toxicity (Appendix C, Fig. C-1).

Involvement of other organ systems includes renal tubular necrosis with oliguria. This rare complication may be exaggerated by the antidiuretic effect of acetaminophen and by excessive fluid loss from vomiting. Myocardial necrosis and subendocardial hemorrhage may cause decreased cardiac output and ECG changes (ST abnormalities, T-wave flattening); dysrhythmias also may be associated with hepatic failure. Hyperosmolar coma secondary to hyperglycemia is an uncommon complication but must be carefully delineated from coma secondary to hepatic encephalopathy because of difference in treatment. Note that signs and symptoms of acetaminophen toxicity resemble those of Reye's syndrome.

The ingestion of alcohol and other drugs such as antihistamines, codeine, or anticholinergics is associated with an alteration of mental status that is not seen with the ingestion of acetaminophen alone.

MONITORING

See also Chapter 4.
1. Plasma acetaminophen level.
2. Toxicology screen, if other ingestants are suspected.
3. Hepatic, renal, and cardiac function.
   a. Daily SGOT, SGPT, bilirubin, PT, and PTT for at least 2 days. If abnormalities are documented, continued and more extensive evaluation of hepatic function should occur.
   b. Blood sugar initially, in 48 hours, and as needed.
   c. BUN, serum creatinine, and electrolytes initially and in 48 hours or when renal problems are manifest.
   d. Twelve-lead ECGs as baseline and with symptoms of cardiac dysfunction.

MANAGEMENT

See also Chapter 66.

Specific measures

1. Decrease absorption. Emesis after ingestion is common in young children but should be induced or gastric aspiration and lavage performed. Activated charcoal and cathartics should be avoided if oral acetylcysteine is to be used, because they may decrease the effectiveness of the antidote. If charcoal has been given, relavage until the stomach contents are clear.
2. Increase elimination.
   a. Forced diuresis is of no benefit and may lead to fluid overload in view of the antidiuretic effect of acetaminophen.
   b. Hemodialysis and peritoneal dialysis are effective in removing acetaminophen but have no effect on severity of hepatic damage (an intracellular process) or mortality.
   c. Sorbent hemoperfusion does not affect

the course of acetaminophen toxicity.
3. Specific antidote *N*-acetylcysteine (20% solution) is the treatment of choice.
   a. Dose:
      (1) Loading dose of 140 mg/kg orally *followed by*
      (2) 70 mg/kg orally every 4 hours for 17 additional doses (for a total dosing time of 72 hours).
      (3) If a dose is vomited within an hour of administration, repeat the dose.
      (4) Dilute the 20% solution to a 5% solution with a palatable juice or soda pop. If the dose is to be given by nasogastric tube, dilute to 5% solution with water.
   b. Indications (Appendix C, Fig. C-1):
      (1) Plasma acetaminophen level indicates hepatotoxicity by nomogram 4 to 24 hours after ingestion.
      (2) Inability to determine plasma acetaminophen level within 16 hours of ingestion and more than 150 mg/kg has been ingested.
   c. Mechanism of action: *N*-acetylcysteine is a glutathione precursor that increases availability of intracellular glutathione. In addition, *N*-acetylcysteine directly conjugates through a sulfhydryl bond with reactive metabolites of acetaminophen. In animal models it has been shown to supply a source of sulfate, thereby maintaining a nontoxic pathway (sulfate conjugation) for clearance. Glutathione is ineffective as an antidote because the exogenously administered form fails to penetrate hepatocytes.
   d. Safety:
      (1) The most common side effect of oral treatment is vomiting.
      (2) Oral *N*-acetylcysteine has proved to be safe and effective treatment in several large series.
      (3) Intravenous *N*-acetylcysteine has been associated with anaphylaxis, including fatal reactions.
      e. Intravenous *N*-acetylcysteine is undergoing a multicenter clinical trial in the United States. A 48-hour protocol with doses similar to those of the oral protocol are being used. The oral preparation of *N*-acetylcysteine is *not* to be used intravenously. Information about the nearest center able to administer intravenous *N*-acetylcysteine may be obtained by calling the Rocky Mountain Poison and Drug Center, Denver, Colo., 1/800/525-6115.

Supportive measures

Supportive measures are directed at treatment of effects of other ingested drugs and of any renal and hepatic problems that occur. For aid in interpreting plasma levels and determining the course of treatment, consultation with a regional poison center is recommended. (See Chapters 17 and 19.) Note the following:
1. Antihistamines, barbiturates, steroids, and ethacrynic acid enhance acetaminophen toxicity and should be avoided.
2. Give careful attention to fluid administration to maintain adequate hydration and avoid fluid overload.
3. IV fluids may be necessary for persistent vomiting.
4. See Chapter 19 for differential diagnosis.

ADDITIONAL READING

American Academy of Pediatric Committee on Drugs: Commentary on acetaminophen, Pediatrics 61:108-112, 1978.

Greene, J.W., Craft, L., and Ghishan, F.: Acetaminophen poisoning in infancy, Am. J. Dis. Child. 137:386-387, 1983.

Mant, T., Tempowski, J.H., Volans, G.N., et al.: Adverse reactions to acetylcysteine and effects of overdose, Br. Med. J. 289:217-219, 1984.

Miller, L.F., and Rumack, B.H.: Clinical safety of high oral doses of acetylcysteine, Semin. Oncol. 10(suppl. 1):76-85, 1983.

Rumack, B.H.: Acetaminophen overdose in young children: treatment and effects of alcohol in 417 cases, Am. J. Dis. Child. 138:428-433, 1984.

Veltri, J.C., and Litovitz, T.L.: 1983 Annual Report of the American Association of Poison Control Centers National Data Collection System, Am. J. Emerg. Med. 2:420-443, 1984.

69 Tricyclic antidepressant overdose

FRANCES C. MORRISS

DEFINITION AND PHYSIOLOGY

Tricyclic antidepressants (imipramine, desipramine, amitriptyline, nortriptyline, doxepin, amoxapine) are rapidly and completely absorbed from the gastrointestinal tract. After absorption, 73% to 98% of the dose is bound by serum protein, then metabolized by the liver, and excreted into the biliary system. Complete demethylation or interruption of the tricyclic ring causes loss of pharmacologic activity. Monodismethyl metabolites, however, are active and can contribute to toxicity. With overdose, hepatic enzyme systems may become saturated and cause prolonged serum half-life; in addition, metabolites excreted into the gastrointestinal tract may be reabsorbed and redistributed. Because of high lipid solubility and tissue protein binding, the potential volume of distribution for the drug is huge. The variability in rate of metabolism, protein binding, redistribution, and potential toxicity of metabolites makes a fatal dose level difficult to establish, but ingestions in adults of greater than 1,000 mg (approximately 15 mg/kg) cause severe toxicity.

Pharmacologic actions are myriad and include:

1. Anticholinergic effects (tachycardia, mild hypertension, mydriasis, fever, urinary retention, dry mucous membranes, hallucination, agitation, seizures, coma, and myoclonic muscle twitching are secondary to competitive blockade of acetylcholine at cholinergic receptors.

2. Adrenergic stimulation (tachycardia and hypertension) is followed by adrenergic depletion (severe bradycardia and hypotension). Tricyclics block the re-uptake of released norepinephrine at adrenergic nerve endings, resulting in norepinephrine excess initially and then, as it is metabolized, in a depleted state.

3. Direct quinidine-like effect on the myocardium results in decreased conduction velocity, increased refractory period, decreased automaticity, and decreased contractility. Correlating ECG changes are prolonged QRS and QT intervals, ST elevation, T-wave changes, right bundle-branch block, and various degrees of atrioventricular block, including asystole. The mechanism of these changes involves inhibition of adenosine triphosphate phosphohydralase and thus interruption of the sodium-potassium balance of myocardial contractile membrane.

Symptoms may be seen as soon as 4 hours postingestion but may occur as rapidly as 30 minutes postingestion in very young children. A brief period of CNS excitation may precede the ensuing CNS and cardiac depression. Anticholinergic effects are prominent; respiratory depression is seen. Hypotension is more common than hypertension, and a variety of cardiac dysrhythmias, often life threatening, are common. Late (3 to 7 days) cardiac complications, including sudden death, have been described in patients with severe symptomatology and incomplete resolution of dysrhythmias (i.e., persistent tachycardia and/or atrio-ventricular conduction defects).

MONITORING

See also Chapter 4.

Cardiorespiratory system

1. Initial and serial ECGs in addition to continuous monitoring until 48 hours after all abnormalities have resolved.
2. Frequent systemic arterial blood pressure determinations: an intra-arterial catheter may be necessary for good monitoring.

Other systems

1. Sequential neurologic evaluation.
2. Serum tricyclic antidepressant levels do not correlate well with symptoms, ECG changes, or outcome; a high degree of serum and tissue protein binding and variables in metabolism lead to large amounts of drug in the liver and myocardium in spite of low serum concentrations.

MANAGEMENT

See also Chapter 66.

1. Induce vomiting in the awake patient or institute gastric lavage in comatose patient; these procedures are much less effective 2 to 3 hours postingestion because of rapid absorption.
2. Administer activated charcoal. One gram of charcoal will absorb 250 mg of amitriptyline. Repeated doses (every 4 to 6 hours) may prevent reabsorption of metabolites that have been excreted into the bowel via the enterohepatic route.
3. It is unknown whether cathartics are effective in increasing elimination of the charcoal-drug complex. Peritoneal dialysis and hemodialysis are not useful because of the high rate of tissue and protein binding; the role of adsorbent hemoperfusion is unknown.
4. Meticulous attention to support of affected organ systems cannot be overemphasized; even though physostigmine is a fairly specific antidote, not all signs and symptoms may be reversed with its use.
   a. Cardiac support. Because myocardial contractility is depressed, attempts to increase preload as a method of supporting the blood pressure may result in volume overload. Hypotension may be secondary to norepinephrine depletion or primary myocardial depression and it may be treated with vasopressors (see Chapter 14). Reasonable choices would be dopamine (increases contractility and may cause release of peripheral norepinephrine) or, with severe hypotension, norepinephrine.
   b. Dysrhythmias.
      (1) Sinus tachycardias do not need treatment unless they contribute to hypotension. Propranolol, because of negative inotropic effects, is contraindicated; physostigmine (a quaternary amine anticholinesterase) is equally as effective for control.
      (2) Ventricular dysrhythmias and atrioventricular nodal abnormalities may be treated with alkalinization of blood to pH 7.5, accomplished by hyperventilation and administration of sodium bicarbonate (1 to 3 mEq/kg). The mechanism of action is unknown, but alkalinization may increase the binding of tricyclic antidepressants, thus decreasing the concentration of free active drug.

      Physostigmine is also effective clinically, though no explanation exists, since cholinesterase inhibitors have no effect on ventricular conduction. If dysrhythmias result from imbalances of cholinergic and adrenergic myocardial stimulation, cholinergic stimulation may restore the balance; acetylcholine may also be involved in the release of norepinephrine.

      Dose: adult, 2 mg IV over 2 to 3

minutes and repeated every 10 to 15 minutes until therapeutic result is achieved or cholinergic symptoms ensue. Effective dose as established above may be repeated frequently for recurrent dysrhythmias. Pediatric, 0.5 mg IV over 2 to 3 minutes. Repeat every 10 to 15 minutes as above. The use of physostigmine is controversial; some authors recommend the use of phenytoin (Dilantin), 5 mg/kg IV.

Quinidine, lidocaine, and procainamid may all contribute to myocardial depression and enhance tricyclic toxicity.

(3) Bradycardias (late sign of toxicity). Physostigmine as above. Electrical pacing, which depends on endogenous norepinephrine release to transmit impulses, is usually ineffective.

c. Respiratory support may be needed.

d. CNS support. Physostigmine is the treatment of choice for prolonged coma, seizures, hallucinations, and delirium. Coma with tricyclic antidepressant intoxication usually lasts 24 to 36 hours and generally requires no therapy other than support. Physostigmine administered to diagnose tricyclic-induced coma is nonspecific, since patients with coma of multiple etiologies will show arousal.

5. Patients should be hospitalized for observation and ECG monitoring until absence of symptoms is unequivocally proved (minimum of 6 hours for the patient who presents with no initial symptoms; 24 to 48 hours after ECG returns to normal for patients who show signs of cardiotoxicity).

ADDITIONAL READING

Bailey, D.N., and Shaw, R.F.: Tricyclic antidepressants: interpretation of tissue and blood levels in fatal overdoses, J. Anal. Toxicol. 3:43-46, 1979.

Brown, T.: Sodium bicarbonate treatment for tricyclic antidepressant arrhythmias in children, Med. J. Aust. 2:380-382, 1972.

Burks, J.S., Walker, J.E., Rumak, B.H., and others: Tricyclic antidepressant poisoning: reversal of coma, choreoathetosis and myoclonus by physostigmine, J.A.M.A. 230:1405-1407, 1974.

Callahan, M.: Tricyclic antidepressant overdose, J.A.C.E.P. 8:413-425, 1979.

Crammer, J., and Davis, B.: Activated charcoal in tricyclic drug overdose, Br. Med. J. 4:527, 1972.

Hollister, L.E.: Tricyclic antidepressants, N. Engl. J. Med. 299:1106-1109, 1978.

Manoguerra, A.S.: Tricyclic antidepressants, Crit. Care Q. 4:43-52, 1982.

Thompson, W.L.: Poisoning: the twentieth-century black death. In Shoemaker, W.C., and Thompson, W.L., editors: Critical care: state of the art, vol. 1, 1980, Society of Critical Care Medicine, Fullerton, Cal., pp. N36-N39.

Tobis, J., and Das, B.N.: Cardiac complications in amitriptyline poisoning: successful treatment with physostigmine, J.A.M.A. 235:1474, 1976.

70 Plant poisoning

FRANCES C. MORRISS

PHYSIOLOGY

The 1981 Bulletin of the National Clearinghouse for Poison Control Centers indicates that plants, excluding mushrooms and toadstools, are the most commonly ingested agent by children less than 5 years of age and represent 12% of all reported ingestions in this age group. Although plant ingestions are common, mortality is low, hospitalization is infrequent, and side effects are minimal. Accurate statistics are difficult to obtain because of incomplete reporting and difficulty in identifying the plant ingested. Most physicians are unfamiliar with principles of plant identification, specimens presented are often insufficient for proper identification (e.g., seed, flower, or leaf rather than the entire plant), and frequently only a vague description or common name of a plant is known. In addition, the available literature on phytotoxicity is confusing; many myths and pieces of inaccurate information have been perpetuated. The best resource individuals for critical plant poisonings may be found in local college departments of botany, biology, or agriculture, or on the staff of a botanical garden, park department, or arboretum. Nurserymen or florists are good resources in a small community. An individual thoroughly familiar with botanical keys for identifying plants and preferably one who can accurately identify a plant from fragments should be sought. The most difficult plants to identify are mushrooms because distinguishing morphologic features are subtle; a distant expert may be needed if there is no readily available mycologist. Sources of information include:

1. Hardin, J.W., and Arena, J.A.: Human poisoning from native and cultivated plants, ed. 2, Durham, N.C., 1974, Duke University Press.
2. Kingsbury, J.M.: Poisonous plants of the United States and Canada, Englewood Cliffs, N.J., 1964, Prentice-Hall, Inc.
3. Lampe, K.E., and Fogerstrom, R.: Plant toxicity and dermatitis; a manual for physicians, Baltimore, 1968, The Williams & Wilkins Co.
4. Smith, A.: The Mushroom Hunter's Field Guide, Ann Arbor, Mich., 1974, The University of Michigan Press.
5. Tampion, J.: Dangerous plants, New York, 1977, Universe Books.
6. Two poison control centers specialize in plant toxicology:
   a. Texas State Poison Center, University of Texas Medical Branch, Galveston, Tex., (713) 765-1420
   b. Pittsburgh Poison Center, Pittsburgh, Pa., (412) 681-6669

A few types of toxins and symptom complexes commonly encountered in plant poisonings are presented below.

1. Alkaloids are crystalline organic compounds containing nitrogen and having an alkaline pH (generally not caustic). Atropine, nicotine, and colchicine are examples.
2. Cyanogenic glycosides react with enzymes to yield free cyanide.
3. Cardiac glycosides (digitalis) affect smooth muscle, particularly cardiac muscle.
4. Phytotoxins, large protein molecules related to bacterial toxins and snake venom, are highly toxic.

5. Toxalbumins are proteins similar to phytotoxins.
6. Irritant glycosides can burn and ulcerate mucous membranes.
7. Saponins are compounds that form soap when mixed with water and produce severe gastrointestinal symptoms.
8. Oxalates may exist in plants in crystalline form as insoluble calcium oxalate crystals or as soluble oxalic acid. The sharp crystals, usually not absorbed, cause mechanical irritation and pain rather than systemic oxalic poisoning.
9. Resinoids, semisolid substances produced by plants, produce a variety of symptoms including CNS effects such as hallucinations.
10. Hematologic glycosides affect the coagulation system.

Many plants contain more than one toxic compound; therefore common symptom complexes have been grouped below.

Gastrointestinal irritants. Gastrointestinal irritation is the most common symptom seen after plant ingestion and may range from local mucous membrane manifestations, such as intense burning, to a severe enteritis with vomiting, cramping, and profuse diarrhea. The extent and onset of symptoms depend on the chemical nature of the toxin, whether biologic activation occurs after ingestion, the amount of toxin ingested (this in turn may depend on what part of the plant was eaten, since toxins may be concentrated in seeds or roots), and often the age of the victim. Agents considered nontoxic in adults may produce severe symptoms in children. Fatalities caused by this group of toxins are usually secondary to fluid depletion and cardiovascular collapse (hypovolemia, electrolyte-related dysrhythmias). Plants associated with prominent gastrointestinal problems are included in Table 70-1.

Plants containing cardiac glycosides. Many plants (*Convallaria majalis* [lily-of-the-valley], *Neruim oleander* [oleander], *Digitalis purpurea* [foxglove], *Actaea* [baneberry]) contain digitalis or related glycosides in such amounts that ingestion of berries, leaves, flowers, or water from vases containing oleander flowers can be fatal. Intoxication is similar to an overdose of digitalis, with cardiac conduction effects predominating over increased automaticity.

Treatment is based on the specific dysrhythmia encountered. Gastrointestinal and CNS symptoms may accompany the cardiac effects, with the first of these probably being due to saponins rather than glycosides.

Plants containing atropine. Atropine and related alkaloids are produced by a number of plants. Signs of toxicity secondary to parasympathetic antagonism are easy to identify and include mydriasis, loss of accommodation, dryness of mouth, dysphagia, flushed, dry skin, and tachycardia. Patients with severe intoxication exhibit hyperpyrexia, delirium, hallucinations, convulsions, and coma. Fatalities are uncommon, and symptoms may be reversed with physostigmine (see Chapter 66). Plants containing atropine or related substances are:

1. *Datura stramonium* (jimsonweed, thorn apple), in the seeds, flowers, and leaves.
2. *Atropa belladonna* (deadly nightshade).
3. *Hyoscyamus niger* (henbane).
4. *Lantana camara* (wild sage). The unripe berries contain lantanin, acute ingestion of which resembles atropine intoxication. In addition, there is acute photosensitization of skin. Four to five berries may be lethal; symptoms may be delayed up to 24 hours.
5. Myristicin, the active agent found in nutmeg, causes atropine-like symptoms, hallucinations, and delirium and can be fatal. Morning glory seeds produce the same symptom complex.
6. Colchicine is found in bulbs and seeds of *Colchicum autumnale* (autumn crocus). Symptoms may be delayed in onset, and anticipatory hospitalization is advised.

Plants containing nicotine and related alkaloids. The alkaloids such as nicotine, cytisine,

Table 70-1. Plant poisoning: plants causing gastrointestinal symptoms

Plant	Toxic part	Toxin	Comment
Abrus species (rosary bean)	Seeds	Abrin	Also causes hemolysis; seeds found in jewelry made in tropics
Aesculus (horse chestnut)	Nuts		
Arnica species	Flowers and roots		Houseplant
Arum family (calla lily, *Caladium, Dieffenbachia, Philodendron,* elephant's ear)	All parts	Calcium oxalate crystals, toxic resinoids	Common houseplants; systemic oxalate poisoning does not occur; rather, mechanical irritation; swelling of mucus membranes sometimes a problem
Buxus Sempervirins (box)	Leaves	Daphnin, coumarin-like compounds	Lethal
Caltha palustris (cowslip)	Leaves, stems		Contains a vesicant causing mucous membrane blisters
Daphne species (spurge laurel)	All parts, especially berries		
Euphorbia (poinsettia)	Leaves, stems, flowers	Sap is a skin irritant	
Hedera (English ivy)	Leaves	Saponin	
Hyacinth (hydrangea)	Bulb	Cyanide-releasing compound	Severe symptoms
Ilex (holly)	Berry		Mild symptoms
Iris	Bulb		
Lathyrus (sweet pea)	Peas, pods	Toxic amine	Paralytic syndrome with large ingestion
Ligustrum (privet)	Berries		
Menispermum canadense (Virginia creeper)	Leaves	Oxalic acid	
Mistletoe	Berries	Toxic amines	
Narcissus	Bulb		
Phytolacca species (pokeweed)	All parts; toxin concentrated in roots	Saponin, glycoprotein	Severe, often fatal
Podophyllum (May apple)	Unripe fruit	Resinoid	Ripe fruit edible
Poinciana (bird of paradise)	Pods		
Prunus species (cherries, apricots, peaches, plums, nectarines)	Twigs, foliage, seeds, fruit pits	Cyanide-releasing compound	Fruit edible
Ranunculus species (buttercup)	All parts	Vesicant	Severe symptoms
Rheum rhaponticum (rhubarb)	Leaf blades	Oxalate	Stalks are edible

Table 70-1. Plant poisoning: plants causing gastrointestinal symptoms—cont'd

Plant	Toxic part	Toxin	Comment
Ricinus species (castor bean)	Seeds	Ricin	Severe symptoms including gastrointestinal hemorrhage; can be fatal; often symptoms may be delayed
Robinia species (black locust)	Bark, foliage, seeds	Phytotoxin	
Sambucus species (elderberry)	Leaves, shoots, bark	Sambunigrin (cyanide-releasing compound)	
Solanum species (woody night shade, European bitter-sweet, Jerusalem cherry, eggplant, sweet potato, bull nettle)	Leaves	Solanine	Large dose lethal
Symplocarpus foetidus (swamp cabbage)	All parts		
Veratrum species (false hellebore, bear grass)	All parts		
Wisteria	Pods	Resinoids, wisterin	

taxine, and coniine cause symptoms similar to the atropine group of toxins. However, the symptoms arise from stimulation of autonomic ganglia. Fatalities secondary to respiratory failure are not uncommon. Patients usually experience emesis shortly after ingestion, followed by profuse salivation, headache, confusion, incoordination, muscle weakness, hyperpyrexia, tachycardia, mydriasis, and occasionally convulsions. This type of alkaloid is found in the following plants:

1. *Nicotiana* species (weed tobacco), in the leaves.
2. *Laburnum anagyroides* (golden chain tree), in the seeds.
3. *Conium maculatum* (poison hemlock), in the leaves and seeds.
4. *Taxus* species (English yew, Japanese yew), in all parts; concentrated in seeds.
5. *Dicentra* species (bleeding heart), in all parts

(contains isoquinoline alkaloids, apomorphine, protopine).
6. Heath family (azaleas, laurels, rhododendron), in all parts.
7. *Gelsemium sempervirens* (jessamine), in all parts; nectar toxic as well.
8. *Aconitum* (monkshood) and *Delphinium* species (larkspur) in leaves, seeds, and roots.

Atropine may be needed for treatment of reflex bradycardia.

Treatment is usually symptomatic and supportive.

Convulsants. The naturally occurring convulsant (cicutoxin) is found in *Cicuta* species (water hemlocks), a group of plants that resemble wild parsnips and grow in wet, swampy areas. Within a half hour of ingestion, nausea, vomiting, salivation, and tremors appear. Grand mal convulsions follow shortly afterward, and fatalities are secondary to prolonged periods of anoxia accompanying the tonic contractions. Treatment consists of effective seizure control.

Mushrooms. Mushrooms are the traditionally fatal plant; if identification is in doubt, the ingestion of a wild mushroom should be treated as potentially serious until its nontoxic nature is established. Mushroom intoxications have been divided into two subgroups based on the appearance of symptoms in relation to the time of ingestion. Symptoms (usually gastroenteritis) that appear within 6 hours are rarely serious. Treatment is directed toward management of fluid and electrolyte disturbances. Many mushrooms contain muscarine, the effects of which (sweating, salivation, colic, and rales) can be reversed by atropine; if untreated, circulatory failure, convulsions, and coma may supervene (see Chapter 73). Other mushrooms, notably *Amanita muscaria*, contain a potent hallucinogen whose effects, including central agitation, last 3 to 4 hours; the victim may require sedation and provision of a nonstimulating environment. Increased severity may be seen with concomitant ingestion of alcohol.

In fatal poisonings (from mushrooms of the *Amanita phalloides* group), the symptoms usually appear after a 12-hour latent period; two classes of thermostabile cyclic polypeptides, amatoxins and phallotoxins, cause the symptom complex seen. Initially, phallotoxins induce nausea, emesis, abdominal cramping, and profuse watery diarrhea, all of which are easily controlled with routine supportive care. After the onset of symptoms, removal of mushrooms from the gastrointestinal tract is not helpful. Three to five days after ingestion a dose-dependent response to amatoxins occurs; this consists of renal tubular necrosis (minimal exposure) or a hepatorenal syndrome (massive exposure) with liver and renal failure that is commonly fatal. Treatment is difficult but should include initial gastric lavage with a solution of tannic acid (1:400) or potassium permanganate (1:5000) to precipitate alkaloid toxins as well as administration of atropine for para-sympathetic overactivity. Hemodialysis has been used successfully to support renal function, and a high protein diet, IV nutritional supplementation with protein hydrolysate, and corticosteroids may decrease the severity of hepatic damage. Thioctic acid, an investigational drug that seems promising, may be obtained from the National Institutes of Health (NIH).

MANAGEMENT

See also Chapter 66.

1. Plant identification, though frustrating, should be attempted; a complete specimen of the plant is most useful to the person attempting a precise botanical classification. Otherwise, the victim may receive unnecessary treatment for ingestion of a harmless substance.

2. Establish the time of ingestion, the specific portion of the plant ingested, and the quantity, if possible.

3. Procedures to eliminate the toxic substance should be instituted (emesis, activated charcoal, and saline catharsis). Often the ingestant will have produced emesis already, and ipecac may be withheld. If irritation and burning are prominent, administer a demulcent such as milk to coat mucous membranes. See Chapter 66 for treatment of cyanide poisoning if plant ingested contained a cyanide-releasing compound.

4. Symptomatic treatment should be aimed at correction of fluid and electrolyte abnormalities, with close monitoring of cardiovascular variables and should include a long enough period of observation to rule out other common sequelae, including convulsions, cardiac dysrhythmias or conduction abnormalities, autonomic stimulation, respiratory failure, and hallucinations. If the patient is symptomatic or the side effects of the toxic substance are known to have delayed onset, a minimum of 24 hours of observation is warranted.

ADDITIONAL READING

Arena, J.M.: The treatment of poisoning, Clin. Symp. **30**:1-47, 1978.

Ellis, M., Robertson, W.O., and Rumack, B.: Plant-ingestion poisoning from A to Z, Patient Care **11**:86-140, 1979.

Kingsbury, J.M.: Phytotoxicity. I. Major problems with poisonous plants, Clin. Pharmacol. Ther. **10**:163-169, 1969.

Kingsbury, J.M.: Phytotoxicity. II. Poisonous plants and plant-caused emergencies, Clin. Toxicol. **2**:143-148, 1969.

Lampe, K.F.: Mushroom poisonings in children, Paediatrician **2**:83-86, 1973.

Lampe, K.F.: Systemic plant poisoning in children, Pediatrics **54**:347-351, 1974.

National Clearinghous for Poison Control Centers: Bulletin **25**:1-4, 1981.

71 Petroleum distillate ingestion

FRANCES C. MORRISS

PHYSIOLOGY

In children less than 5 years of age, 4% to 10% of ingestions involve petroleum distillates, and the mortality in these patients is high. A rational approach to treatment requires knowledge of the type of hydrocarbon ingested, the amount ingested, and whether any additives are present. Table 71-1 lists common hydrocarbons and their approximate toxicity.

Toxicity takes the following forms.

Respiratory system

Pneumonitis is the most common symptom, occurring in 25% to 40% of patients. The initial sensation is a burning in the mouth and throat followed by gagging, choking, and coughing. Continued nonproductive cough is indicative of severe involvement and is usually followed within 30 minutes by tachypnea, cyanosis, retractions, and grunting. Respiratory failure may supervene. Pulmonary involvement usually progresses over 24 hours, plateaus, and begins to subside within 2 to 5 days. (If no roentgenographic evidence of pulmonary involvement occurs by 6 hours postingestion, the likelihood of severe pneumonitis is small.) A chest roentgenogram reveals either bilateral basilar infiltrates or fine perihilar infiltrates that may extend laterally and progress to a picture of pulmonary edema. Consolidation of infiltrates is common. Air trapping, pleural effusion, and pneumatoceles may also be seen. Roentgenographic abnormalities commonly persist after clinical symptoms cease. In general, there is poor correlation between the severity of clinical symptoms and the roentgenographic findings. Arterial blood-gas analysis reveals an early hypoxemia usually accompanied by hypocarbia, suggesting ventilation/perfusion abnormalities. Autopsy studies reveal hyperemia, hemorrhagic pulmonary edema, interstitial inflammation, and necrotizing bronchopneumonia. Survivors may have residual small airways obstruction.

Pulmonary lesions are most likely caused by inhalation of the hydrocarbon and not by gastrointestinal absorption. Animal studies have shown no pulmonary damage from gastric instillation of sublethal doses of hydrocarbon when vomiting and inhalation were prevented by esophageal ligation. The lethal-dose ratio of oral to intratracheal hydrocarbon is large, suggesting that only huge oral doses of hydrocarbon could cause enough absorption to lead to pulmonary lesions. The roentgenographic manifestations of hydrocarbon pneumonitis resemble inhalation pneumonia rather than the uniform distribution expected of an absorption pneumonitis. The rapid onset of symptoms and immediate pulmonary changes (15 to 20 minutes) strongly suggest inhalation. Absorption with excretion into the lungs cannot be ruled out but is probably less frequent than inhalation.

The physical and chemical characteristics of the hydrocarbon influence the extent of the pulmonary injury; the risk of lung damage from inhalation increases with decreased surface tension, decreased viscosity, and increased volatility. Low surface tension promotes rapid movement of the hydrocarbon over the surface contacted, and low viscosity increases penetration of the fluid into the distal airways. Increased

Table 71-1. Common hydrocarbons

Product	Synonym	Main use	CNS depression	Pulmonary pathology
Benzene	Benzol	Paint thinner	4+	1+
Toluene		Paint remover		
Xylene (aromatic hydrocarbons)		Solvent		
		Plastic, rubber cement		
Turpentine (volatile oil)	Oil of turpentine	Paint thinner	3+	1+
Petroleum ether	Benzine (not benzene)	Rubber solvent	4+	0
Gasoline	Petroleum spirits	Fuel	3+	2+
Petroleum naphtha	Ligroin	Cigarette lighter fluid	3+	3+
VMP naphtha	Varnish naphtha	Paint or varnish thinner	3+	3+
	Painter's naphtha			
Mineral spirit	Stoddard solvent	Dry cleaner	3+	3+
	White spirits	Solvent		
	Varsol	Paint thinner		
	Mineral turpentine			
	Petroleum spirits			
Kerosene	Coal oil	Charcoal lighter fluid	1+	2+
		Solvent		
		Fuel for stoves, lamps		
Fuel oil	Home heating oil	Fuel	1+	1+
Diesel oil	Gas oil			
Mineral seal oil	Signal oil	Furniture polish	1+	4+
Mineral oil (nontoxic)	Liquid petrolatum	Laxative	0	1+
		Suntan oil		
Lubricating oils (nontoxic)	Motor oil	Lubricants		1+
	Household oil			
	Cutting oil			
	Transmission fluid			
Triorthocresyl phosphate	Machine oil	Machine oil	Paralysis	
Shellac (5% methanol, 1% gasoline in ethanol)	Solox		3+	0
Asphalt	Asphalt		0	0
	Tar			

Modified from Done, A.K.: The toxic emergency, Emergency Med., April, 1974, p. 291; in Mofenson, H.C., and Greensher, J.: Controversies in the prevention and treatment of poisonings, Pediatr. Ann. **6:**719, 1977.

volatility causes direct introduction of the hydrocarbon into the lungs. The initial effect of intrapulmonary hydrocarbons is probably a change in alveolar surface tension (decrease in surfactant), leading to alveolar and distal airway instability, which produces the ventilation/perfusion inequalities. Later, absorption of lipid-soluble hydrocarbon contributes to parenchymal destruction. A secondary effect contributing to morbidity is a high incidence of bacterial infection. Hydrocarbons may significantly diminish the lung's ability to clear bacteria.

The presence of additives such as camphor, naphthalene, heavy metals, nitrobenzene, or trichloroethane markedly increase the toxicity of any given hydrocarbon.

Central nervous system

CNS toxicity is manifested by weakness, tremors, confusion, convulsions, and coma and is more likely to occur with highly volatile distillates or ingestion of more than 1 ounce of fluid. Animal studies have indicated that the most probable cause of CNS symptoms is hypoxia rather than direct damage.

Viscera

With large ingested volumes, visceral involvement occurs. The most common problems include gastrointestinal irritability with bloody diarrhea, myocardial irritability (dilation, atrial flutter, ventricular fibrillation), and hepatic and renal parenchymal destruction with organ failure. Occasionally bone marrow suppression is seen.

Skin

Hydrocarbons are primary skin irritants and defatting agents causing comedones, folliculitis, and photosensitivity. Although absorption through the skin may occur, organ damage via this route is rare.

MONITORING

See also Chapter 4.

Respiratory system

See Chapter 12.

MANAGEMENT

See also Chapter 66.

Specific measures

There is considerable controversy over the need to empty the stomach after a hydrocarbon ingestion, since vomiting predisposes the patient to inhalation of stomach contents. Frequently (in 35% of patients) vomiting occurs at the time of ingestion.

1. Emesis is contraindicated if the patient is comatose or convulsing, has absent gag reflex, dysrhythmias, or respiratory failure, or

Table 71-2. High-viscosity petroleum distillates

Asphalt
Cutting oil
Diesel oil
Home fuel oil
Glues
Greases
Lubricating oil
Mineral oil
Mineral seal oil (furniture polish)
Motor oil
Petroleum jelly
Rubber cement
Tar
Transmission fluid
Paraffin wax

From Mofenson, H.C., and Greensher, J.: Controversies in the prevention and treatment of poisonings, Pediatr. Ann. **6:**722, 1977.

has ingested a mineral seal oil or a hydrocarbon with a corrosive additive.
2. Emesis is unnecessary for high-viscosity petroleum distillates (Table 71-2).
3. Emesis is indicated if the hydrocarbon contains a dangerous additive (such as a heavy metal) or if the volume of an aromatic or turpentine type of hydrocarbon ingested exceeds 1 to 2 ml/kg (increased chance of systemic toxicity).
4. If emptying the stomach is judged necessary, syrup of ipecac should be used in the awake child. This should only be done under closely supervised conditions; do not advise the parent to induce vomiting at home. This method of induced emesis has been shown to be safe in such patients. If the patient is comatose or exhibits instability of other organ systems, the airway should be secured first with an endotracheal tube, preferably cuffed. Then a cautious gastric lavage with a large amount of 0.9% sodium chloride solution via an NG tube may be undertaken. Lavage with a lipid substance is not recom-

mended, because of the possibility of lipoid inhalation pneumonia.

If lavage has been done, 30 to 60 ml of olive oil may be placed in the stomach to decrease further absorption of remaining hydrocarbon. Mineral oil or alcohol should not be used, because both may increase absorption of the hydrocarbon. Charcoal is ineffective for hydrocarbons but may absorb additives.

Exposed skin should be cleaned with soap and water and covered with sterile mineral oil to decrease absorption from skin surface. Eyes should be flushed for 10 to 15 minutes to prevent burning.

Supportive measures

Supportive measures primarily involve the treatment of respiratory failure (see Chapter 12). The use of steroids in the treatment of hydrocarbon pneumonia has not been shown to be efficacious. The role of antibiotics remains controversial because of the frequency of secondary bacterial infection; many prefer to wait and treat such a complication when it occurs. If prophylactic antibiotics are preferred, give penicillin (50,000 to 100,000 units/kg/day in parenteral form) for 3 to 5 days.

ADDITIONAL READING

Anas, N., Namasonthi, V., and Ginsberg, C.: Criteria for hospitalizing children who have ingested hydrocarbons, J.A.M.A. **246**:840-843, 1981.

Bratton, L., and Haddon, J.E.: Ingestion of charcoal lighter fluid, J. Pediatr. **87**:633-638, 1975.

Eade, N.R., Taussig, L.M., and Marks, M.I.: Hydrocarbon pneumonia, Pediatrics **54**:351-356, 1974.

Gerarde, H.W.: Toxicological studies on hydrocarbons. V. Kerosene, Appl. Pharmacol. **1**:462-470, 1959.

Giammona, S.T.: Effects of furniture polish on pulmonary surfactant, Am. J. Dis. Child. **113**:658-663, 1967.

Marks, M.I., Chicoine, L., Legere, G., and others: Adrenocorticosteroid treatment of hydrocarbon pneumonia in children—a cooperative study, J. Pediatr. **81**:366-369, 1972.

Mofenson, H.C., and Greensher, J.: The correct new answer to an old question on kerosene ingestion, Pediatrics **59**:788, 1977.

Ng, R.C., Darwish, H., and Stewart, D.A.: Emergency treatment of petroleum distillate and turpentine ingestion, Can. Med. Assoc. J. **111**:537-538, 1974.

Shirkey, H.: Treatment of petroleum distillate ingestion, Mod. Treatment **8**:580-591, 1971.

Walsdorf, J.: Kerosene intoxication: an experimental approach to the etiology of the CNS manifestations in primates, J. Pediatr. **88**:1037-1040, 1976.

Wasserman, G.B.: Hydrocarbon poisoning, Crit. Care Q. **4**:33-42, 1982.

72 Exposure to household cleaning agents

FRANCES C. MORRISS

PHYSIOLOGY

Corrosive agents are common constituents of household cleaners; the most common ingestants are caustic alkalis rather than acids. Soaps, washing powders, bleaches, disinfectants, and toilet bowl cleansers commonly contain sodium hydroxide (lye, caustic soda), potassium hydroxide (potash), sodium and potassium carbonates, peroxides, and oxides. These agents are also found in glycosuria-testing tablets (Clinitest tablets). Many soaps and cleaning agents do not contain corrosives, and these are discussed briefly below.

Noncorrosive agents

Nonionic detergents. Toilet soaps and light-duty laundry products are nonionic detergents composed of polyether sulfates, alcohols, sulfonates, and monosterates. This type of preparation is nontoxic because in solution no reactive ions are released, and ingestion requires no treatment. Gastric irritation after ingestion of large volumes may be decreased by dilution with a demulcent such as milk. (A demulcent is an agent that counteracts irritative symptoms secondary to surface inflammation of mucous membranes or skin.) Statistically, the largest number of ingestions occur with this group of agents and these ingestions usually involve children less than 5 years of age in a home setting (see Tables 72-1 and 72-2).

Anionic detergents. Anionic detergents contain sodium, potassium, or ammonium salts of fatty acids, sulfonated hydrocarbons, or phosphorylated hydrocarbons. When placed in water, they release a cation (Na^+ or K^+). This type of detergent is common in laundry soaps, low-sudsing soaps for automatic washers, liquid hand soaps, and biodegradable soaps. Addition of surface-active agents, perfumes, and coloring agents does not increase systemic toxicity. This type of product usually contains insufficient amounts of bleach to cause mucous membrane damage. The primary symptoms after ingestion include local mucous membrane irritation (without burns), nausea, and vomiting that may be severe enough to cause dehydration. Treatment should include dilution of the ingestant with large quantities of water followed by oral administration of a demulcent such as milk or olive oil. The addition of a hydrocarbon (most commonly pine oil) to detergent increases toxicity, and then ingestion should be handled as a hydrocarbon ingestion (see Chapter 71). Esophageal burns with stricture formation have been reported secondary to ingestion of granular electric-dishwasher soaps as well as detergents containing tripolyphosphate. Although these are anionic detergents, the inorganic content is higher, the pH is higher, and caustic side effects are significant (see below for treatment).

Cationic detergents. (See Table 72-2.) Cationic detergents release an anion (Cl^- or Br^-) in solution. The highly reactive anion accounts for the increased toxicity of these agents. Most are quaternary ammonium compounds found as the salts of ammonium chlorides, bromides, iodides, and nitrates; and they are the active

Table 72-1. Soaps, detergents, cleaners, and bleaches

Toxicity	Product	Toxic ingredient or effect	Treatment*
High	Electric dishwasher granules†	Caustic (may be severe)	Treat as caustic burn†
	Ammonia†	Caustic; coma and convulsions	As caustic†; supportive
	Bleach, commercial	Boric acid or oxalate poisoning	Milk; calcium; supportive
	Bleach, oxygen	Boric acid poisoning	Supportive
Medium	Bleach, chlorine	Gastrointestinal irritation, some causticity	Demulcents ± treat as caustic burn
	Borax	Boric acid poisoning	Supportive
	Water softeners† (soluble)	Some caustic; hypocalcemia and acidosis possible	Milk; as for caustic†; supportive
	Liquid general cleaners:		
	Kerosene	Pneumonia, systemic toxicity	As for petroleum distillates‡
	Pine oil	Gastrointestinal and genitourinary irritation; depression and weakness	Supportive; demulcents
	Detergent granules† for laundry, dishes, and general use	Gastrointestinal irritation to causticity (some frankly caustic and have higher toxicity)	Demulcents; treat as caustic burn†
Low	Detergent powders†	Gastrointestinal irritation (causticity possible, but unlikely)	Demulcents ± treat as caustic burn†
	Liquid detergents	Gastrointestinal irritation	Demulcents
	Toilet soap	Gastrointestinal irritation	Demulcents
	Fabric softeners	None	None
	Window cleaners (liquid)	Alcohol	
Inhalation hazard	*Chlorine bleach mixed with:*		
	Strong acid (bowl cleaner)	Chlorine gas (intense respiratory irritation)	Oxygen
	Ammonia	Chloramine fumes (respiratory irritation, nausea)	Terminate exposure; supportive

From Done, A.K.: Poisoning from household products, Pediatr. Clin. North Am. **17**:577, 1970.
*In addition to evacuation of stomach (except with caustic burn) or removal from skin, when indicated.
†Products threatening caustic effects will be identified with a *caution* label. Details of treatment can be found elsewhere.
‡Details of treatment can be found elsewhere.

ingredients of antiseptics, disinfectants, bactericides, sanitizers, and deodorants. Toxicity is increased by the addition of phenols, hydrocarbon derivatives, and corrosive acids. In the concentrated form, such agents are rapidly absorbed, and 20 to 30 ml of a 10% solution can be fatal. Toxicity is secondary to inhibition of cellular metabolic processes and is compounded by whatever toxicity occurs because of the additives. Phenols (carbolic acid, creosote, Lysol, resorcinol) denature and precipitate cellular proteins; oxalic acid binds ionized calcium, causing development of tetany. Symptoms of cationic detergent ingestion may include vomiting (often bloody), epigastric pain, hepatic and renal failure, coma, convulsions, cardiovascular collapse, and death. Treatment is the same as outlined in Chapter 66: the stomach

Table 72-2. Disinfectants and deodorizers

Toxicity	Product	Toxic ingredient or effect	Treatment*
High	Naphthalene deodorizer (bathroom, toilet, garbage can)	Irritation, coma, convulsions, hemolysis, kidney damage	Supportive; alkalinize urine; transfuse as needed
	Acid disinfectant (boric, chloroacetic, formic, salicylic, etc.)	Corrosive, plus systemic effects of anion	Supportive and as caustic burn†
	Phenolic disinfectant	Phenols; hexachlorophene (gastrointestinal irritation, shock, coma; corrosion or kidney damage possible)	Treat as caustic burn† or anticipate renal failure
Medium to high‡	Alkali disinfectant (sodium or ammonium hydroxides)	Potentially caustic	Demulcents ± treat as caustic burn†
	Benzalkonium and other QAC§ disinfectants	Gastrointestinal irritation, convulsions, coma, respiratory distress, collapse	Supportive; demulcents; or milk
	Pine oil disinfectant	Gastrointestinal and genitourinary irritation; depression and weakness	Supportive; demulcents
	Halogen disinfectants	Hypochlorites or chlorinated hydrocarbons (irritation; excitation)	Demulcents ± treat as caustic burn†; sedation as needed
Medium	Wick deodorizers	Formaldehyde and hydrocarbons (gastrointestinal irritation, abdominal pain, shock, hematuria, coma, convulsions)	Supportive; demulcents; sodium bicarbonate
	Deodorizing cleansers	Pine oil or QAC§	(See above)
	p-Dichlorobenzene or sodium bisulfate deodorizer (bathroom, toilet, garbage can)	Irritation, abdominal pain, narcosis; liver, kidney damage possible	Supportive; demulcents
Low	Iodophor disinfectant	Detergent-iodine complex (gastrointestinal irritation)	Demulcents
Nil	Spray deodorizers	(Variable)	Symptomatic
	Refrigerator deodorizer	Charcoal (inert)	None

From Done, A.K.: Poisoning from household products, Pediatr. Clin. North Am. **17**:579, 1970.
*In addition to evacuation of stomach (except with caustic burn) or removal from skin, when indicated.
†Details of treatment can be found elsewhere.
‡Depending upon constitution and concentration.
§Quaternary ammonium compounds.

should be emptied if a corrosive agent has not been ingested; absorption should be decreased if possible; and multisystem support should be instituted (Tables 72-1 and 72-2). Giving a weak alkali (as has been recommended in the past) to counteract a weak acid may compound the gastric or mucous membrane injury because of the heat released by the neutralizing reaction. A demulcent should be given instead; milk will form a coagulum that insulates against thermal and further caustic injury; water may be given to dilute the ingestant. Both agents are readily available and have high patient acceptance. The use of mild soap solutions to precipitate quarternary ammonium compounds is no longer recommended because of the unavailability of pure soap in most households. Castor oil or olive oil retards absorption of phenols. Oxalic acid may be precipitated as calcium oxalate by gastric introduction of calcium in the form of milk, calcium gluconate, or calcium lactate. (See below for treatment of caustic acid ingestion.)

Solvents. Solvents such as those that are found in cleaning and polishing preparations contain mixtures of petroleum hydrocarbons and nonpetroleum solvents (carbon tetrachloride, acetone amyl acetate, ethylene dichloride, methyl alcohol, and trichloroethylene). In addition to the problem of hydrocarbon pneumonitis, the following symptom complexes may be seen after ingestion:

1. Carbon tetrachloride: hepatic and renal failure.
2. Ethylene dichloride: pulmonary edema.
3. Trichloroethylene: coma, acute ventricular dysrhythmias.
4. Methyl alcohol: respiratory depression, severe acidosis, coma, blindness.
5. Phenols: respiratory depression, cardiovascular collapse.

Treatment is aimed at preservation of organ function (see Chapter 66) and correction of hydrocarbon pneumonitis. Fats, oils, and alcohol given orally may increase absorption of these agents. Vomiting should not be induced, though careful gastric lavage may be indicated for highly toxic hydrocarbons.

Corrosive agents (see Table 72-3)

Acids. Although less common, ingestion of a corrosive acid (hydrochloric, sulfuric, boric, chloracetic, formic, salicylic acids) poses a serious problem. Acids produce coagulation necrosis, which develops an overlying protective eschar. Since most acids are taken in liquid form and in larger volumes than alkalies and do not cause an initial intense mucosal injury, the site of injury is the stomach rather than the esophagus. The exact location and extent of injury depend on the amount and concentration of the acid ingested, the position of the patient, the length of time the acid is in contact with gastric mucosa, and the presence or absence of food in stomach. Damage is usually most severe in the antrum, the most dependent portion, where pooling occurs; circumferential involvement may lead to pyloric obstruction, necessitating gastric resection. Esophagitis is very uncommon.

There are surprisingly few symptoms noted with acid ingestion though hematemesis and severe epigastric pain are reported. Lack of symptoms may mask the severity of damage. In one series 8% of patients required emergency surgery for development of perforation and/or peritonitis; 60% of patients had subsequent gastric surgery for pyloric obstruction. 15% of ingestions were fatal. Physical findings will be absent on examination of the pharynx and initial roentgenographic examination may be negative, though bubbles and streaks of gas may be seen in gastric fundus in severe cases. All cases should have fiberoptic endoscopic evaluation to assess the degree and extent of damage; the visual findings are black linear streaks of necrosis along the greater curvature extending into the antrum circumferentially and ulceration of the greater curvature with sparing of the lesser curvature.

Table 72-3. Common household corrosives

Type	Brand name	Corrosive chemical
Acids	Mister Plumer® (K-Lan Co.) (liquid)	Concentrated sulfuric acid
	Quaker House® Steam Iron Cleaner	Hydrochloric acid
	Sno Bol® Liquid Toilet Bowl Cleaner	Hydrochloric acid 15%
	Lysol® Liquid Toilet Bowl Cleaner	Hydrochloric acid 8.5%
		Ammonium chloride 1%
	ZUD® Rust and Stain Remover (granular)	Oxalic acid
	Sani-Flush® Toilet Bowl Cleaner (granular)	Sodium bisulfate 75%
	Vanish® Toilet Bowl Cleaner (granular)	Sodium acid sulfate 62%
	Rooto®	Sulfuric acid
Alkalies	Liquid Drano®	Sodium hydroxide
		Ammonium hydroxide
	Drano® (granular)	Sodium hydroxide
	Easy-Off® Liquid Oven Cleaner (liquid)	Sodium hydroxide
	Mr. Muscle® Overnight Oven Cleaner (liquid)	Sodium hydroxide
	Liquid Plumr®	Sodium hypochlorite, potassium and sodium hydroxide
	Minute® Mildew Remover	Calcium hypochlorite 48%
	Comet® Liquid Disinfectant Bathroom Cleaner	Tripotassium phosphate 1.8%
		Sodium hypochlorite 0.5%

From Graham, D.Y.: Corrosive injury to the stomach: the natural history and role of fiberoptic endoscopy, Am. J. Surg. **137:**803-806, 1979.

Alkalis. The major morbidity caused by ingestion of cleaning products occurs with ingestion of corrosive alkalis such as lye or bleaching compounds. Caustic alkalis combine with cellular proteins to form proteinates and combine with fats to form soaps, producing deep penetrating burns and liquefaction necrosis. The depth of the injury is directly related to the concentration of alkali and the duration of exposure. There is, in addition, an intense inflammatory response that can extend to the muscle layer of the tissue involved; in the esophagus, perforation and stricture formation are the end stage of these destructive processes. The height of the inflammatory process occurs within 48 hours. Ten days after ingestion, granulation tissue has replaced necrotic tissue; by 3 weeks there may be early contracture formation with replacement of the muscularis layer by fibrous tissue overlaid by squamous epithelium. Although they contain corrosive alkalis, chlorinated bleaches (Clorox, sodium hypochlorite) do not produce as severe a reaction. Esophageal injury is limited to edema, and stricture formation is uncommon.

Immediately after ingestion, the victim experiences an intense burning pain from the mouth to the stomach. This pain is so intense that only small amounts of liquid preparations can be tolerated before the patient spits them out or vomits. Concentrated granular preparations (e.g., Drano) must first dissolve on mucous membranes, and therefore large amounts can be ingested. Swallowing soon becomes impossible, partly because of spasm at the site of injury and partly because of esophageal obstruction from intense edema.

Physical examination reveals soapy white mucous membranes that eventually become brown and ulcerated. Vomitus may be bloody, containing shreds of mucous membranes. Shock, upper airway obstruction due to glottic edema, and esophageal perforation may all occur. The sequela of lye ingestion is esophageal stricture, which may be severe enough to necessitate colon interposition to replace the destroyed esophagus or the use of a stent placed shortly after ingestion to keep the esophagus open.

MONITORING

See also Chapter 4.

With esophageal perforation or pneumonitis, measure arterial blood-gas tensions and pH every 4 to 6 hours.

MANAGEMENT

See also Chapter 66.

Specific measures

1. Identify the corrosive agent; patients who ingest agents not associated with esophageal burns (e.g., Clorox) or stomach injury require only examination for local mucous membrane injury, demulcent therapy for membrane irritation, and symptomatic support. Administration of a weak acid to neutralize a weak alkali is no longer recommended by the National Clearinghouse for Poison Control Centers. Hospitalization will probably not be necessary unless the product contained a toxic additive.
2. Decrease absorption.
   a. Induction of vomiting and lavage are contraindicated, since protective airway reflexes may be absent secondary to second- and third-degree burns. Friable tissue may be perforated with passage of an NG tube. Any alkali reaching the stomach will be neutralized by gastric acid.
   b. Give a palatable liquid such as water or milk to dilute any alkali or acid remaining in the esophagus and stomach.
   c. Skin that has come in contact with the corrosive agent should be bathed with large volumes of water until the soapiness disappears. Any burns should be treated.

Eyes should be thoroughly irrigated until the pH of irrigant returning from eye is less than 8, and an ophthalmologist should be consulted immediately, since the damage may extend to penetration of the globe.
3. Local mucous membrane pain may be eased with a demulcent such as milk.
4. Treat esophageal injury from caustic alkali (protocol developed by Department of Surgery, Johns Hopkins Hospital).
   a. Esophagoscopy should be performed within 48 hours of ingestion (the sooner the better) to confirm the presence of an esophageal burn. The esophagus at this point is extremely friable, and perforation is highly likely after 48 hours. Therefore, the esophagoscope should be introduced only to the level of the burn; attempts to pass it beyond a circumferential burn may cause perforation. Laryngoscopy with the patient under anesthesia should be done at the same time to identify damage to the glottic and supraglottic structures. The patient must be hospitalized and fluids withheld. The presence or absence of burns in the mouth does not correlate well with the presence of esophageal burns, so examination of the esophagus is mandatory for planning therapy. If no esophageal burn is identified, the patient may be discharged as soon as oral intake is satisfactory. Follow-up in a month is necessary to make certain that there are no symptoms of esophageal dysfunction. Identification of a burn is followed by therapy for the inflammatory response.
   b. Treat the inflammation with steroids. Animal studies have shown that steroids given within 48 hours of the caustic burn will decrease granulation-tissue formation but will not prevent stricture formation. The efficacy of steroids in humans has not been conclusively proved; however, in view of the intense inflammatory

reaction associated with this injury, their use is not unreasonable. Prednisone, 2 mg/kg/day, or its equivalent is given for 3 to 10 weeks, depending on the extent of the burn and the results of repeat esophagoscopy.

c. Prophylactic antibiotics are recommended by many authors. The most common infective agent early in the course is a gram-positive coccus. Ampicillin (100 mg/kg/24 hr) or penicillin (50,000 to 100,000 units/kg/24 hr) may be given parenterally for the first 5 to 10 days. Infection is much more common in the event of esophageal perforation.

d. Follow-up esophagoscopy and careful cinefluoroscopy are used to assess the degree of inflammatory response 3 weeks after a burn. Early stricture formation may be diagnosed as well. Some authors advocate a cinefluorogram in the first 24 hours after a burn.

e. The use of silastic stent placed in the esophagus at the time of the initial esophagoscopy shows promise in managing the development of stricture. It is left in place for 3 weeks; esophagoscopy is done prior to stent removal.

f. Serial esophageal dilation is begun as soon as stricture formation is documented. Eighty percent of strictures occur within 10 weeks. Steroids are usually discontinued at this time.

5. Treat stomach injury (caustic acid).

a. Fiberoptic endoscopy should be performed as soon as possible. Endoscope should be passed only to the margin of the burn, where friable tissue makes perforation likely.

b. Induction of vomiting and gastric lavage are contraindicated. If large volumes of highly concentrated acid were ingested, it may not be buffered by the stomach and an antacid should be given for neutralization.

c. The roles of anti-inflammatory agents and antibiotics are unknown.

d. Oral fluids should be withheld and the patient hydrated intravenously until oral fluids can be safely taken.

e. Follow-up radiographic and/or endoscopic examination may be necessary.

f. The role of early gastric surgery is unknown.

Supportive measures

Once an esophageal or gastric burn has been documented, hospitalization is mandatory. The patient should be observed in an area where airway support is readily available. Burns and edema in the supraglottic area may cause total respiratory obstruction, necessitating a tracheostomy. Parenteral hyperalimentation and/or gastrostomy may be needed to supply adequate calories in the event of total esophageal destruction; emergency surgery for gastric perforation may be necessary.

ADDITIONAL READING

Arena, J.M.: Treatment of caustic alkali poisoning, Mod. Treatment 8:613-618, 1971.

Ashcraft, K.W., and Simon, J.L.: Accidental caustic ingestion in childhood, a review: pathogenesis and current concepts of treatment, Tex. Med. 68:86-88, 1972.

Chodak, G., and Passaro, E., Acid ingestion, J.A.M.A. 239:225-226, 1978.

Done, A.K.: Poisoning from household products, Pediatr. Clin. North Am. 17:569-581, 1970.

Haller, J.A., Andrews, H.G., White, J.J., and others: Pathophysiology and management of acute corrosive burns of the esophagus: results of treatment in 285 children, J. Pediatr. Surg. 6:578-584, 1971.

Lawrence, R.A., and Haggerty, R.J.: Household agents and their potential toxicity, Mod. Treatment 8:511-527, 1971.

Lowe, J.E., Graham, D.Y., Boisaubin, E.V., and others: Corrosive injury to the stomach: the natural history and role of fiberoptic endoscopy, Am. J. Surg. 137:803-806, 1979.

National Clearinghouse for Poison Control Centers: Bulletin 23:1-2, 1979.

73 Organophosphate insecticide poisoning

FRANCES C. MORRISS

PHYSIOLOGY

Organophosphate compounds are systemic inhibitors of the enzyme cholinesterase, which hydrolyzes the neurotransmitter acetylcholine into acetate and choline, thus inactivating it. The insecticide preferentially and tightly binds to the enzyme's active site, preventing access to acetylcholine. Initially the organophosphate reversibly phosphorylates the enzyme, but after several hours it forms a stable permanent monoalkylphosphoryl bond. After this sequence of reactions, the enzyme's activity is inhibited for several weeks until new serum cholinesterase can be synthesized by the liver; cholinesterase located in the CNS and at the neuromuscular junction is resynthesized more slowly (after several months).

Acetylcholine is the neurotransmitter that relays nerve impulses at the following cholinergic sites: (1) preganglionic to postganglionic neurons of the sympathetic and parasympathetic nervous systems, (2) postganglionic parasympathetic fibers to effector organs, (3) postganglionic sympathetic fibers to sweat glands, (4) motor nerves to muscle fibers, and (5) some poorly defined CNS synapses. The effect of acetylcholine accumulation is one of initial stimulation followed by loss of function. Symptoms referable to dysfunction of the parasympathetic nervous system include pupillary constriction, salivation, sweating, abdominal cramps, bronchorrhea, bronchospasm, bradycardia that may progress to heart block, hypertension, and loss of bowel and bladder control (sphincter dysfunction). CNS manifestations may include anxiety, restlessness, headache, emotional lability, drowsiness, difficulty in recall and concentration, coma, and convulsions terminally. The consequences of cholinergic stimulation at the neuromuscular junction can be fatal. Initially, fasciculations occur in striated muscle, first in extraocular muscles and progressing to larger muscle groups. Profound muscle weakness then follows, with development of ataxia, incoordination, and respiratory muscle paralysis in the most severe cases. Death is usually secondary to respiratory arrest and anoxia caused by a combination of bronchospasm, bronchorrhea, and paralysis of respiratory musculature.

The organophosphates as a group are among the most potent toxins known, and doses fatal within several hours may be introduced through the skin, lungs, and eyes as well as the gastrointestinal tract. The mean lethal dose can be as small as several hundred milligrams. The more common insecticides accounting for a majority of poisonings are parathion, malathion, tetraethyl pyrophosphate (TEPP), hexaethyltetraphosphate, and octamethyl pyrophosphoramide (OMPA), listed in order of increasing toxicity.

MONITORING

See also Chapter 4.

Respiratory system

Respiratory monitoring should be designed to detect early signs of respiratory failure.

429

1. Monitor respiratory rate continuously with audible apnea alarm.
2. Note any signs of compromised breathing (retractions, cyanosis, change in secretions, decrease in TV). Auscultate the chest hourly for signs of bronchospasm.
3. Measure arterial blood-gas tensions and pH as indicated.
4. If profound muscle weakness is present, VC and inspiratory force measurements may be helpful.

Renal-metabolic system

1. Check temperature every hour until stable; institute continuous monitoring if temperature is rising hourly.
2. Serial plasma and RBC cholinesterase levels at weekly intervals may be useful in determining the length of time full support may be needed.

Central and autonomic nervous systems

Central and autonomic nervous system symptoms may be vague, but nursing personnel should note any of the following signs, which may precede respiratory paralysis or indicate that therapy is becoming ineffective.
1. Changing state of consciousness.
2. Pupillary changes, especially if the patient is receiving atropine; miosis is an indication that atropine effect is diminishing.
3. Agitation, anxiety, restlessness.
4. Convulsions.
5. Excessive sweating and salivation.

Neuromuscular system

1. Observe patient for muscle fasciculations.
2. Check for muscle weakness with the following tests:
   a. Hand grip sustained for more than 30 seconds.
   b. Ability to hold head off of bed for more than 30 seconds.

MANAGEMENT

See also Chapter 66.

Speed is essential in treating organophosphate poisoning because of the rapid onset of action and extreme toxicity of the agent. Treatment is aimed at removal of the agent as rapidly as possible, administration of physiologic and chemical antidotes, and supportive therapy. The patient must be cared for in an area capable of immediate respiratory support, since provision of an artificial airway and mechanical ventilation are often necessary and lifesaving. Any signs of respiratory compromise should be an indication for this type of support. Treatment of the intoxication may not successfully reverse the effects at the neuromuscular junction.

Removal of intoxicant

Removal of the agent should be as thorough as possible. The patient should be stripped of all his clothing and bathed and shampooed with large amounts of soap and water (bar soap is more effective than liquid detergent in removing insecticide). Eyes and exposed mucous membranes should be lavaged liberally (see Chapter 66). Exposed body surfaces should then be wiped with alcohol to further remove traces of insecticides; all towels, clothes, etc. should be discarded (not reused). The usual methods of emptying the stomach should be employed if the agent was ingested orally, and catharsis should be instituted.

Antidotes

Atropine sulfate. The physiologic antidote for organophosphate compounds is atropine sulfate, a parasympatholytic agent that blocks the action of acetylcholine at parasympathetic receptors. Atropine counteracts only the peripheral parasympathetic effects of acetylcholine; symptoms caused by excessive stimulation in the CNS cholinergic sites may be partially alleviated while stimulation of the neuromuscular junction is unaffected (i.e., respiratory muscle paralysis, coma, and convulsions can occur despite atropine therapy). Atropine will alleviate bronchospasm, decrease the volume of secretions, reverse miosis and bradycardia, and diminish bowel symptoms. Patients with organophosphate poisoning are relatively tolerant to the effects of atropine, so that large doses are necessary and the patient needs to be titrated with atropine until signs of toxicity such as dilated pupils, tachycardia, flushing, and inhibition of sweating appear. Recommendations are variable based on age or weight of the patient.

1. The initial dose is 0.02 to 0.05 mg/kg repeated every 10 minutes until atropinization is accomplished. Atropine can be given IV, IM, or SC.
2. The following regimen may be used instead of the above: less than 2 years of age, 0.2 mg; 2 to 10 years of age, 0.5 mg; more than 10 years of age, 1 to 2 mg. Dose to be repeated every 10 minutes to desired effect.
3. Full atropinization should continue for 24 to 48 hours, depending on the severity of symptoms. Atropine effect may last 1½ to 4 hours, depending on the route of administration.
4. Caution should be used if atropine is given concomitantly with pralidoxime (see below).

Pralidoxime chloride. Pralidoxime chloride (2-pyridine aldoxime methyl chloride, 2-PAM chloride, Protopam) is the specific chemical antidote for organophosphate compounds. The molecule was specifically designed to occupy the active site of the phosphorylated esterase and thus reactivate the enzyme. It has no effect on the accumulated, unhydrolyzed acetylcholine. Since pralidoxime does not cross the blood-brain barrier, CNS cholinesterase is not reactivated, and *therefore respiratory compromise due to central depression of the respiratory centers will not be altered.* The specific antidotal activity lies in the oxime moiety and is independent of the salt; the chloride is preferred to the

iodide salt. Pralidoxime is non–plasma protein bound, partly metabolized by the liver, and partly excreted unchanged in the urine; its half-life is short. Toxicity is minor, consisting of headache, nausea, vomiting, blurred vision, dizziness, and hyperventilation. As an antidote, pralidoxime becomes much less effective when given 48 hours after exposure (because of the formation of the highly stable organophosphate-esterase compound) or when given to patients who have been chronically exposed (e.g., agricultural workers). In such instances, enzyme reactivation will be incomplete, and supportive therapy, particularly mechanical ventilation, may have to be continued on a long-term basis. Serum and RBC cholinesterase activity can be assayed on a weekly basis to determine the degree of activity. The activity of both enzymes is usually reduced by 50% or more after intoxication. Serum levels may be determined before therapy is started if the diagnosis is in doubt; treatment should not be delayed until these values come back.

1. The dose is 25 to 50 mg/kg IV as an infusion over 15 to 30 minutes, rate not to exceed 7 to 10 mg/kg/min; this dose may be repeated in 3 to 8 hours as needed. An effect (e.g., increase in muscle strength) should be seen within minutes.
2. Repeat doses may be given orally every 5 hours if gastrointestinal symptoms are minimal.
3. Therapy should be continued as long as signs of cholinesterase inhibition recur.
4. As the enzyme is reactivated, the patient may become more sensitive to atropine, since acetylcholine will begin to be hydrolyzed, and therefore less atropine will be needed to counteract its effects.
5. Renal insufficiency is a relative contraindication to use of pralidoxime.
6. High doses can cause neuromuscular blockade.
7. Tranquilizers, phenothiazines, narcotics,

and xanthine derivatives should not be given with pralidoxime.

Supportive therapy

Supportive therapy may be required in the following situations (see appropriate chapters).
1. Respiratory paralysis and failure, which require mechanical ventilation. Intubation equipment and skilled personnel *must* be immediately available.
2. Coma.
3. Dysrhythmias, particularly bradycardia severe enough to depress cardiac output.
4. Convulsions.

ADDITIONAL READING

Hayes, W.J.: Epidemiology and general management of poisoning by pesticides, Pediatr. Clin. North Am. **17:** 629-643, 1970.

Koelle, G.B.: Cholinesterase inhibitors. In Goodman, L.S., and Gilman, A., editors: The pharmacological basis of therapeutics, ed. 4, New York, 1971, Macmillan, Inc.

Zavon, M.R.: Poisoning from pesticides: diagnosis and treatment, Pediatrics **54:**332-336, 1974.

74 Intoxication from heavy metals

FRANCES C. MORRISS

PHYSIOLOGY

Intoxication due to heavy metals involves multiple organ system abnormalities because metals bind to tissue sites known as ligands to form soluble, dissociable complexes. A ligand is a molecule capable of functioning as a donor partner in one or more bonds. The most common preferential binding sites are those containing oxygen, nitrogen, sulfur, and phosphorus (i.e., OH^-, COO^-, $PO_4H_2^-$, SH, NH_2, and imidazole); the most stable complexes are formed with sulfur and nitrogen. Many of the toxic side effects of a ligand–heavy metal complex derive from inactivation of sulfhydryl groups, which are essential to the activity of many enzymes.

Table 74-1 is a summary of the more common features associated with toxic levels of heavy metals. Heavy metals are common constituents of many pesticides and fungicides, and they are capable of producing symptoms and death immediately if ingested in large quantities or even after weeks to months when taken in minute amounts. In general, the inorganic salts of metals are more toxic on an mg/kg basis; toxicity of organic metal complexes is often a combination of the toxicity inherent in the metal and in its organic carrier.

MANAGEMENT

See also Chapter 66.

In addition to the usual forms of symptomatic support, management of patients with heavy-metal toxicity involves the use of chelating agents that bind relatively tightly to the metal and prevent or reverse binding to tissue ligands. A chelate is a complex formed between the metal and a compound containing two or more preferential binding sites that have a stronger affinity for the metal than the comparable tissue binding sites. The end product of such a reaction is usually a stable heterocyclic ring that is excreted unchanged in the urine. Both free and soft tissue–bound metal can be removed. Chelating agents are more effective when given as close to the time of ingestion as possible. Irreversible damage to enzyme systems may occur if the heavy metal is bound to tissues for long periods of time; storage in tissues inaccessible to chelating agents (e.g., bone, hair) may occur. Inadequate doses of chelators may cause redistribution of the metal in the body and increase toxic effects. Therefore, therapy is aimed at providing an excess of chelating agent in order that all heavy metal is bound and excreted; timing of repetitive doses is based on rapidity of excretion. Patients who have ingested large amounts or highly toxic metals (e.g., arsenic, inorganic mercury) should receive the maximal dose of the appropriate agent. The common chelating agents include the following.

BAL

BAL (Dimercaprol, 2,3-dimercaptopropanol) forms a tightly bound nontoxic chelate with antimony, arsenic, mercury, and gold and probably with bismuth, copper, chromium, and nickel. Whether it effectively binds lead is controversial. All such BAL-metal complexes are dissociable to some degree, and BAL may be oxidized with release of the metal in its active form. BAL must be administered in such a fashion that there is always an excess available

Table 74-1. Characteristics of heavy metal intoxication

Metal	Source	Ingested dose*	Toxic levels Whole blood or serum	Urine
Antimony (Sb)	Herbicide, pesticide, tartar emetic (trivalent compounds more toxic than pentavalent ones), antiprotozoal medication	1 g or 15 mg/kg		
Arsenic (As)	Insecticides, paint, herbicides, rodenticides	>1.5 mg/kg orally (inorganic As)	Serum >3 mg/dl	>10 μg/24 hr
Bismuth (Bi)	Fungicide	15 g or 0.1 mg/m^2		
Cadmium (Cd)	Metal polish, alloys, rust-proof plate, alkali batteries, contaminated shellfish	1 g or 15 mg/kg		>100 μg/24 hr or >0.1 μg/ml
Copper (Cu)	Paint (with As), insecticides, fungicides	15 g or 200 mg/kg		
Gold (Au)	Therapeutic preparation			
Iron (Fe)	Therapeutic preparation (ferrous sulfate)		>175 μg/ml	>150 μg/24 hr
Lead (Pb)	Paint, putty, lead-glazed ceramics, batteries	10 g or 100 mg (in tetraethyl form)	Whole blood >10-40 μg/100 g	>80 μg/24 hr

*Minimal lethal dose of ingested organic salt—based on adult data.

Clinical features	Onset	Therapy
Local: papular, vesicular eruptions	Hours	BAL
Oral—systemic: emesis, pneumonia, arthritis, myocardial depression, abdominal cramps, hypotension	Hours	
Chronic exposure: bradycardia, hepatitis, anaphylaxis, arthritis	Weeks	
Vapor: bronchopneumonia + systemic effects	Immediate	BAL or D-penicillamine
Oral—acute: acute hemorrhagic gastroenteritis, shock, uremia, muscle cramps, convulsions	6-12 hr	
Oral—chronic: desquamation, erythema of extremities, eczematoid eruption, loss of hair and nails, hyperpigmentation, hyperirritability, apathy, anorexia, hypotonia, photophobia, abdominal pain, peripheral neuritis, hypertension, diarrhea, renal tubular damage, cirrhosis; subnitrite—methemoglobinemia	Weeks to months	
Chronic: ulcerative stomatitis, anorexia, headache, rashes, nephrosis, jaundice, hyperpigmentation, gastroenteritis, diarrhea, colic	Weeks	BAL
Vapor: pulmonary edema, bronchitis	Immediate	EDTA (BAL contraindicated)
Oral: emesis, renal failure, severe myalgia, diarrhea, abdominal cramps	Immediate	
Oral—chronic: osteomalacia, liver damage, anemia	Months	
Oral: emesis, capillary damage leading to hepatic and renal damage, mucous membrane necrosis	Immediate to hours	D-Penicillamine or EDTA
Parenteral: exfoliative dermatitis, bone marrow suppression, stomatitis, tracheitis, gastritis, colitis, vaginitis, eosinophilia, encephalitis, neuritis, hepatitis	1-3 mo	BAL or D-penicillamine
Oral:		Desferrioxamine preferred; DTPA, EDTA (BAL contraindicated)
Emesis, hemorrhagic gastroenteritis with profuse diarrhea	30-60 min	
Sudden cardiovascular collapse	12 hr	
Duodenal stenosis	Weeks	With CNS symptoms: BAL + EDTA
Oral—chronic: emesis, anorexia, incoordination, ataxia, iron deficiency anemia, apathy, increased ICP with encephalopathy and seizures, permanent brain damage, renal insufficiency, severe paroxysmal abdominal pain	Weeks to months	Without CNS symptoms: EDTA
		Subacute: D-penicillamine
		N.B.: EDTA most effective; BAL used only for immediate mobilization and to initially treat encephalopathy

Continued.

Table 74-1. Characteristics of heavy metal intoxication—cont'd

Metal	Source	Toxic levels		
		Ingested dose*	Whole blood or serum	Urine
Mercury (Hg)	Dyes, antiseptics, fungicides, contaminated fish (pike, perch, mackerel, bass, walleye)	15 mg/kg (inorganic Hg)	>0 μg/ml	>10 μg/24 hr
Nickel (Ni)	Petroleum refining, ? cigarettes	Inhaled: 1 part per million Oral: varies widely		
Radioactive metals (radium, strontium, uranium)	Fallout, medicinal			
Selenium (Se)	Insecticide, dermatologic preparation			
Thallium (Th)	Rodenticide	300 mg or 4 mg/kg		>0
Vanadium (V)	Industrial exposure, color picture tubes	>110 mg/kg (?)		
Zinc (Zn)	Galvanized containers, deodorants, disinfectants, pigments, talcum powder	15 g or 200 mg/kg		

to bind metal and compete with tissue ligands (particularly SH groups). The degree of effectiveness in reactivating enzyme systems is proportional to the length of time the system has been inactivated; BAL is ineffective in the presence of huge quantities of unbound metal. BAL-metal complexes dissociate in acid environments; thus, alkalinization of urine will protect the kidneys from damage secondary to free metal. Toxic reactions to BAL occur in 50% of patients receiving 5 mg/kg and may consist of headache, nausea, vomiting, conjunctivitis, salivation, lacrimation, perioral burning, sweating, abdominal and perineal pain, tachycardia, and

Clinical features	Onset	Therapy
Vapor: bronchopneumonia with hemoptysis and pneumonia	Immediate	BAL or D-penicillamine
Oral —acute: acute hemorrhagic gastroenteritis, shock, uremia (inorganic Hg)	Immediate	
Oral —chronic: desquamation, erythema of extremities, eczematoid eruption, loss of hair and nails, hyperirritability, apathy, anorexia, insomnia, hypotonia, photophobia, abdominal pain, tachycardia, hypertension, hemoconcentration, renal dysfunction, peripheral neuritis	Weeks to months	D-Penicillamine
Organic methyl Hg: potent teratogen, irreversible CNS damage	Months to years	D-penicillamine
Inhaled: frontal headache, dizziness, nausea and vomiting, cyanosis, chest pain, cough, weakness, diarrhea, distention, convulsions	Immediate to hours	Dithiocarb or BAL
Oral: capillary damage to brain and adrenals, myocardiopathy, renal dysfunction	Hours to days	(Conflicting evidence)
Chronic: vomiting, diarrhea, bone deformities, renal tubular dysfunction, eczematoid eruption	Weeks	DTPA preferred to EDTA
Oral: jaundice, cirrhosis, gastroenteritis, renal tubular dysfunction, myocardial necrosis	Hours to days	EDTA (?) (BAL contraindicated)
Oral:		Dithiocarb or Dithizion (organic reagent); BAL (?)
Nausea, vomiting, albuminuria	24 hr	
Renal tubular necrosis, convulsions, polyneuritis, ataxia, dementia, peripheral neuropathy, psychosis	3-14 days	
Hair loss, ataxia, nail changes, dry skin	Weeks	
Dust inhalation: cough, hemoptysis, bronchospasm	Immediate	EDTA + ascorbic acid; DTPA
Oral: anorexia, anemia, nausea, headache, tumor, tremor, blindness, psychic disturbances, renal dysfunction	Days	
Inhaled: pulmonary edema, bronchopneumonia	Immediate	EDTA
Oral:		
Gastroenteritis, shock, nephritis	Hours	
Esophageal or pyloric stricture	Weeks	

hypertension. If successful chelation occurs, enzyme systems containing heavy metals as prosthetic groups (catalase, carbonic anhydrase, carboxypeptidase, peroxidase, cytochrome *c*) can be inhibited.

1. Route: deep IM only.
2. Preparation: 10% solution in peanut oil.

3. There are several recommended dose schedules:
   a. For severe intoxication, 3 mg/kg IM every 4 hours for 2 days, then 2.5 to 3 mg/kg IM every 6 hours for 1 day, then 2.5 to 3 mg/kg IM every 12 hours for 4 to 12 days.

b. For mild intoxication, 2.5 mg/kg IM every 4 hours for 2 days, then 2.5 mg/kg IM every 12 hours for 1 day, then 2.5 mg/kg IM daily for 4 to 12 days.

c. The above schedules can be modified on the basis of severity of symptoms and the amount ingested. The effectiveness of therapy should be monitored by urine levels of the metal, and once urine is metal-free, therapy may be stopped. In cases of chronic intoxication, several courses of therapy may be necessary to effect excretion of metal that is mobilized from inaccessible body stores (e.g., bone) after concentration of metal in soft tissues has become low.

4. BAL may be given in the presence of renal failure but not in the presence of hepatic dysfunction.

5. Iron should not be given concomitantly, since it will form a toxic chelate with BAL.

Ca EDTA

Ca EDTA (ethylenediaminetetraacetic acid, calcium disodium edetate) forms a poorly dissociable ringlike complex with polyvalent metals that displace calcium from the original molecule. Because of rapid induction of profound hypocalcemia, this agent should always be given as the calcium disodium form, which will release calcium when the heavy metal is chelated. The half-life of the chelate is approximately 1 hour, with 50% urinary excretion in that time; at the end of 24 hours, 1% to 2% of the initial dose remains in the body. The principal toxic effect can be a dose-related massive renal tubular necrosis manifested as albuminuria, glucosuria, hematuria, casts, and oliguria. Minor effects include histamine reaction, with an erythematous rash, lacrimation, sneezing, ECG abnormalities, and local reactions at the injection site. Ca EDTA most effectively chelates lead, zinc, cadmium, cobalt, copper, vanadium, and manganese; there is no increased excretion of mercury.

1. Route: IV or IM (only when fluid restriction is a concern, as in the presence of cerebral edema such as seen with lead encephalopathy); oral absorption is poor

2. Preparation:

a. IV, 20% solution, 200 mg/ml; dilute with D_5W or 0.9% sodium chloride to a 0.2% to 0.4% solution (2 to 4 mg/ml).

b. IM, 20% solution mixed with procaine to make a 0.5% to 1.5% concentration of procaine.

3. Dose: the maximum safe dose is 75 mg/kg/ 24 hr, but since renal damage is possible, this dose is usually given only when very high levels of metals are present. The lower dose is 50 mg/kg/24 hr IV in two to three divided doses for 5 to 7 days. If the dose schedule is to be repeated, allow 2 to 3 days between courses of therapy.

4. Renal failure or failure to establish good urine output is a contraindication to the use of Ca EDTA.

5. Increased renal excretion of potassium occurs.

Desferrioxamine

Desferrioxamine (Desferal, deferoxamine mesylate) is a chelating agent specific for iron; its affinity for iron is so great that iron may be removed from ferritin, hemosiderin, and transferrin. Toxic effects include hypotension with rapid IV administration; ocular injury can be seen after long-term oral therapy. An occasional hypersensitivity reaction consisting of erythema and urticaria can be seen. Excretion is via the kidneys.

1. Route: IM is preferred; the IV route may be used as long as cardiovascular signs are monitored closely and rate of administration does not exceed 15 mg/kg/hr. The oral route is contraindicated because the iron chelate is readily absorbed from damaged intestinal mucosa and may increase serum iron levels. Recent evidence suggests that the subcutaneous route may be effective for long-term treatment of chronic iron overload states (e.g., thalassemia).

2. Preparation: 250- to 500-mg ampules of lyophilized agent to be reconstituted with sterile water.
3. Dose schedule:
   a. 20 mg/kg IM every 6 to 12 hours for 2 to 3 days, the maximum daily dose not to exceed 3.5 mg/m²; subsequent doses of 10 mg/kg IM every 4 to 12 hours should be given as needed. Injection should be done by a "Z" technique.
   b. For the patient in shock, 40 mg/kg IV over 4 hours, rate not to exceed 15 mg/kg/hr. Repeat this dose in 4 to 6 hours; then give 20 mg/kg as a continuous infusion over 8 to 12 hours.
4. Continue administration until the orange-pink discoloration of urine caused by the desferrioxamine-iron complex has cleared. Low urine levels of iron may not be detected with usual analytical methods.
5. In the presence of renal failure, chelated iron (but not free iron) may be removed by dialysis.

D-Penicillamine

D-Penicillamine (Cuprimine, β,β-dimethylcysteine) is a sulfhydryl amino acid that complexes with copper, lead, arsenic, mercury, zinc, magnesium, and calcium. Recent evidence indicates that it is effective in acute arsenic and mercury poisoning (i.e., the chelate-metal complex is stable). Its use for subacute plumbism is well established. Toxicity is low, but the occurrence of fever, erythematous or urticarial rashes, thrombocytopenia, or nephrosis, all manifestations of acute sensitivity to the drug, requires prompt discontinuance of the drug. Urinary excretion is rapid.
1. Route: oral, excellent absorption.
2. Preparation: 250-mg capsules (contents may be mixed with small amounts of fruit juice if the child is too small to take capsules).
3. Dose:
   a. Free base, 40 mg/kg/24 hr orally on an empty stomach at least 1½ hours before a meal, *or*

b. Hydrochloride salt, 50 mg/kg/24 hr, *or*
   c. 25 mg/kg/dose in 4 doses has been used for severe intoxication, with a maximum of 1 g/kg/24 hr for 5 days.
   d. A 3- to 4-day observation period should precede reinstitution of therapy.
   e. If the patient is in shock, chelation therapy should be begun with an alternate agent administered parenterally and D-penicillamine started later.
4. Oral dose is potentiated by simultaneous oral administration of alkali (sodium bicarbonate, 1% solution).
5. Renal insufficiency is a contraindication to its use.

DTPA

DTPA (diethylenetriaminepentaacetic acid) is a polyamino acid similar to EDTA and may be useful in cases of intoxication from heavy metals not chelated by EDTA. It has been found useful with some radioactive metals. DTPA binds calcium rapidly, and tetany may be seen after rapid IV administration. For this reason, the calcium disodium form is preferred. Chelate-metal complexes are rapidly excreted in the urine; as much as 40% of the dose is excreted in 2 hours and 50% to 70% in 4 hours.
1. Dose: 0.5 to 1.0 g as a 25% solution IV.
2. This dose may be repeated every 2 weeks.

Diethyldithiocarbamate

Diethyldithiocarbamate is an investigational drug manufactured by Rohm & Haas Co., Philadelphia; limited experience suggests that it eventually may be the agent of choice for chelation of thallium and nickel.

Dithizion

Dithizion is an organic solvent that may be obtained from a chemical supply company and may be efficacious in treating thallium intoxication. The dose is 10 mg/kg twice a day orally with 10 ml of 10% glucose solution for 5 days. The agent may be diabetogenic.

ADDITIONAL READING

Arena, J.M.: Poisoning: toxicology, symptoms and treatment, ed. 3, Springfield, Ill., 1974, Charles C Thomas, Publisher.

Center for Disease Control: Increased lead absorption and lead poisoning in young children, J. Pediatr. **87:**284-830, 1975.

Chisolm, J.J.: Poisoning due to heavy metals, Pediatr. Clin. North Am. **17:**591-615, 1970.

Chisolm, J.J.: Treatment of lead poisoning, Mod. Treatment **8:**593-611, 1971.

Done, A.K.: Specific antidotes for poisons. In Shirkey, H.C., editor: Pediatric therapy, ed. 6, St. Louis, 1980, The C.V. Mosby Co.

Gleason, M.N., Gosselin, R.E., Hodge, H.C., and others: Clinical toxicology of commercial products—acute poisoning, ed. 4, Baltimore, 1975, The Williams & Wilkins Co.

Levin, W.G.: Heavy metal antagonists. In Goodman, L.S., and Gilman, A., editors: The pharmacological basis of therapeutics, ed. 5, New York, 1975, Macmillan, Inc.

Peterson, R.G., and Rumack, B.H.: d-Penicillamine therapy of acute arsenic poisoning, J. Pediatr. **91:**661-666, 1977.

Robertson, W.O.: Treatment of acute iron poisoning, Mod. Treatment **8:**552-560, 1971.

75 Psychosocial aspects of pediatric intensive care

The parent

KATHERINE LIPSKY

DEFINITION OF THE PROBLEM

Families experience the circumstances surrounding the admission of a critically ill child to a PICU as a crisis situation. Psychologic crisis is defined as a sudden and urgent disturbance in a state of relative equilibrium. Individuals strive to maintain a state of psychic balance that is usually achieved through a constant series of adaptive maneuvers and characteristic problem-solving activities. The causative elements of a crisis are usually external and often catastrophic. The individual in crisis must respond to forces that originated outside of himself and his control while the demands of the situation tax his habitual patterns of coping. The result may be a temporary inability to manage, cognitive confusion, affective lability, disorganized behavior, and a dramatic rise in tension or anxiety. In response, tension-reducing adaptations develop: some are useful, others maladaptive; some lead toward personal growth, others toward increased vulnerability.

Comprehensive patient care requires the PICU staff to understand and cope with families' responses to a crisis situation. Although this discussion focuses on the identification and management of parental needs and stresses, similar principles apply to other members of the immediate family, such as older siblings, to members of the extended family, such as grandparents, and to other adults emotionally involved with the PICU patient.

Admission to a PICU is usually an unplanned emergency event allowing parents little time for emotional preparation. Moreover, the outcome for the patient may be unknown, and this uncertainty adds to the anxiety experienced by the family. Few parents possess a level of medical sophistication and emotional detachment sufficient for a thorough and undistorted understanding of their child's health problems and treatment plan. This lack of understanding can serve to increase parental confusion and concern. Parents are often aware that they cannot control what happens, or when it happens, to their gravely ill child. This adds a feeling of helplessness and hopelessness to the already high level of anxiety. Parents may be called on to prepare for the impending loss of a valued child in an unfamiliar and machine-dominated setting not conducive to the expression of grief. The need for hospitalization may add significant financial and environmental burdens to the already emotionally stressed family unit. Because PICUs are often located in regional centers, parents may be far from home and separated from familiar family and social support systems.

The above factors all combine to greatly increase the waiting parents' experience of anxiety. Often, however, it is the overwhelming intensity of this anxiety that allows parents to accept more readily timely interventions that reduce stress and strengthen coping skills.

Since defenses tend to be fluid and individuals tend to be particularly vulnerable during a crisis situation, PICU medical, nursing, and social work staff, acting as a team, have the opportunity to provide effective supportive intervention. Research indicates that a little help, rationally directed and purposely focused at such a strategic time, can be more effective than more extensive help given at a period of less emotional accessibility. Such intervention can help parents strengthen the personal resources and coping abilities necessary for successful crisis resolution.

MONITORING

Three general indices require monitoring to assess parents' adjustment to the PICU experience.

Cognitive understanding of the patient's physical condition, prognosis, and treatment plan. Although it is true that parents' understanding of their child's condition is affected by their intellectual capacities, sociologic background, personality type, and psychologic processes such as denial or anger, too often the cause of misunderstanding results from the hospital staff's failure to communicate. Members of the PICU staff need to be aware that it is their responsibility to convey pertinent medical and nursing information on a cognitive level appropriate for the parents. This requires patience and compassion. The best way to avoid both esoteric overkill and condescending oversimplification is to listen to the kinds of questions each parent is asking.

Affective adjustment to the patient's need for PICU care. Parents experience considerable emotional distress during a child's PICU hospitalization. Absence of signs of such emotional stress can signal that something is wrong in the parent-child relationship. Indeed, follow-up studies of discharged patients and their families indicate that in the case of neonates, the early and often prolonged separation caused by hospitalization can interrupt the natural parent-

infant bonding process and thus interfere with future parenting motivation and capacity. Because a considerable amount of parental emotional stress is ordinarily experienced and expected during a child's stay in the PICU, the aspect of affective adjustment that needs to be monitored is the appropriateness of the parents' emotional reaction in relation to the patient's physical condition and prognosis. Parents who underreact or overreact to the actual situation are the ones who usually need additional social work intervention and support. Certain families appear to be especially vulnerable to emotional difficulties during crisis. High-risk factors include single parent families, parents who have a previous history of psychiatric dysfunction, and parents experiencing residual grief from previous unresolved losses.

Many parents of critically ill children experience anticipatory grieving. This anticipatory grief can occur whether the child eventually recovers completely, recovers but with residual damage, or dies. The stages of anticipatory grief are similar to those experienced during grief following actual object loss as described by Kübler-Ross: (1) initial shock and denial characterized by refusal or inability to accept the real situation as it currently exists; (2) feelings of anger, rage, and envy when the question "Why me, why my child?" may be asked repeatedly; (3) bargaining, or an attempt to postpone the inevitable; (4) depression, in which previous anger is replaced by a feeling of sadness and a sense of great loss; and (5) eventual acceptance involving a decrease in previous agitation and the ascension of a degree of quiet expectation. These behaviors can be identified in parents' attempts to deal with an anticipated or actual death of a child. Stages need not, but tend to, unfold in sequence. More than one stage can be experienced simultaneously. Each stage may last for different amounts of time and may be experienced with varying intensity by each parent. Obviously, not all parents are able to work through conflicting feelings and reach an acceptance of their child's death during the course of a PICU hospitalization. These stages of grieving should be recognized by PICU staff and accepted as a normal part of parental affective adjustment.

Support systems available to parents. Support can come from (1) extended family members, (2) social, religious, and work affiliations, (3) hospital staff and other waiting PICU families, and (4) community mental health and social welfare agencies. It is important to assess sources of support available to parents during and following their child's hospitalization. It is also important to recognize that the presence of family and friends does not always mean that appropriate support is being offered. Well-meaning relatives and associates can be detrimental to parental adjustment by making additional emotional demands or by adding to parental confusion. It is helpful, therefore, to monitor the quality of support available to waiting parents and to try to mobilize the most positive, meaningful, and appropriate support available.

MANAGEMENT

PICU medical, nursing, and social work staff can take specific steps to support parents in their cognitive and affective attempts to master the crisis of a PICU hospitalization. Such supportive measures include the following.

Orientation. Parents should be oriented to the unit and its waiting area. Clarification of visiting procedures and hospital expectations helps reduce parental uncertainty and anxiety.

Access to patient. Access to a comfortable waiting area, liberal visiting hours, and unlimited telephone calls to the PICU provide needed physical comfort and psychologic reassurance and help to decrease feelings of alienation and increase a sense of trust.

Communication with personnel. Adequate communication during parents' visits to the PICU should be ensured. Introducing the unit personnel responsible for the patient's care

during each shift, explaining the various equipment and monitoring devices in use, candidly describing the patient's overall condition, and discussing treatment alternatives all serve to reduce parental anxiety and cognitive distortions.

Parent-child interaction. Opportunities for parent-child interaction should be facilitated. Parents should be encouraged to interact both verbally and physically with their child. Many parents can be given responsibility for the more routine health care tasks in their child's therapeutic regimen. When parents are able to spend time with their child and to participate even minimally in his care, their feelings of helplessness and hopelessness tend to be diminished.

Ventilation of feelings. Ventilation of parental feelings and concerns should be encouraged. Waiting periods between visits offer time for the expression of parental concerns. Many parents are reluctant to verbalize feelings of anger or frustration to staff members who directly care for their child because of the fear of retaliation through inadequate patient care. The PICU social worker, who is free from direct patient care responsibility, is in an excellent position to listen empathetically, reassure parents of the normalcy of their reactions, and give appropriate supportive counseling. When information given to the social worker is selectively shared with the PICU staff, accommodations can often be made that improve the quality of time parents spend with their child, thus reducing parental discontent and anxiety.

Referral. Families may benefit from referral to appropriate community agencies. The hospitalization of a child can aggravate a family's financial, environmental, and psychologic difficulties. Provision of appropriate community resources can often help to relieve parents of these additional burdens.

Guidance for siblings. Anticipatory guidance for siblings should be provided. Parents may be concerned about preparing siblings for the patient's possible death or survival with residual damage. Parents may also be experiencing difficulties due to siblings' behavioral reactions to parents' increased time and attention to the hospitalized child. Worry about their other children can add considerably to waiting parents' stress.

Expressions of grief. Expressions of grief should be facilitated. When the death of a pediatric patient seems inevitable, it is helpful to allow parents to express their feelings of anger, pain, and loss. Increased opportunity to spend time with the dying child may also be helpful. After a death, parents should be afforded the opportunity to be with their child's body if they so desire.

Follow-up. An opportunity for follow-up contact should be offered to the parents. This is especially important for parents who have lost a child in the PICU, because such continuing communication helps prevent feelings of abandonment. In those instances where permission for an autopsy has been granted, a conference between the parents, the attending physician, and the PICU social worker held 6 to 8 weeks after the patient's death to discuss results of the autopsy report offers the parents a chance to ask questions, clarify concerns, and air residual issues of self-blame and anger. Furthermore, such a conference provides the attending physician and PICU social worker with an opportunity to evaluate the family's recuperative coping abilities. When appropriate, further therapeutic interventions, such as follow-up community referrals, may be made if it is determined that the parents need professional help in managing their grief.

Parents of children who survived their illness but with residual damage also benefit from follow-up contact with the PICU staff. Parents of children with a chronic handicap have been described as suffering from "chronic sorrow," and follow-up studies indicate an increase in the incidence of family dysfunction that correlates with the severity and type of the child's disability. Continuing contact with the PICU social worker can ensure that ongoing community services arranged before the patient's discharge have been properly mobilized to meet the family's needs.

Ongoing contact with parents of healthy survivors can also be therapeutic. Many parents appreciate renewed opportunity to express their gratitude to PICU staff members. Others feel the need to bring their child back for a visit to demonstrate how well the child is doing and to show that they, as parents, are carrying on the fine care that was initiated during the patient's stay in the PICU.

ADDITIONAL READING

Barnett, C.R., Leiderman, P.H., Grobstein, P., and others: Neonatal separation: the maternal side of interactional deprivation, Pediatrics **45:**197-205, 1970.

Benfield, D.G., Lieb, S.A., and Reuter, J.: Grief response of parents after referral of the critically ill newborn to a regional center, N. Engl. J. Med. **294:**975-978, 1976.

Engle, G.L.: Is grief a disease? Psychosom. Med. **23:**18-22, 1961.

Goldberg, S.B.: Family tasks and reactions in the crisis of death, Soc. Casework **54:**398-405, 1973.

Hancock, E.: Crisis intervention in a newborn nursery intensive care unit, Soc. Work Health Care **1:**421-432, 1976.

Harper, R.G., Concepcion, S., Sokal, S., and Sokal, M.: Observations on unrestricted parental contact with infants in the neonatal intensive care unit, J. Pediatr. **89:**441-445, 1976.

Hill, R.: Generic features of families under stress. In Parad, H., editor: Crisis intervention: selected readings, New York, 1965, Family Service Association of America.

Kaplan, D., and Mason, E.: Maternal reactions to premature birth viewed as an acute emotional disorder. In Parad, H., editor: Crisis intervention: selected readings, New York, 1965, Family Service Association of America.

Kennell, J.H., Slyter, H., and Klaus, M.H.: The mourning response of parents to death of a newborn infant, N. Engl. J. Med. **283:**344-349, 1970.

Klaus, M.H., Jerauld, R., Kroger, N.C., and others: Maternal attachment—importance of the first postpartum days, N. Engl. J. Med. **286:**460-563, 1972.

Kliman, A.S.: Crisis: psychological first aid for recovery and growth, New York, 1978, Holt, Rinehart & Winston.

Kübler-Ross, E.: On death and dying, New York, 1969, Macmillan, Inc.

Kübler-Ross, E.: Living with death and dying, New York, 1981, Macmillan, Inc.

Lindemann, E.: Beyond grief: studies in crisis intervention, New York, 1979, Jason Aronson, Inc.

Lindemann, E.: Symptomatology and management of acute grief, Am. J. Psychiatry 101:141-148, 1944.

Nadelson, T.: Psychiatric aspects of the intensive care of critically ill patients. In Skillman, J.J., editor: Intensive care, Boston, 1975, Little, Brown & Co.

Olshansky, S.: Chronic sorrow: a response to having a mentally defective child, Soc. Casework 43:190-193, 1962.

Rappaport, L.: Crisis intervention as a mode of brief treatment. In Roberts, R.W., and Nee, R.H., editors: Theories of social casework, Chicago, 1970, University of Chicago Press.

Rappaport, L.: The state of crisis: some theoretical considerations. In Parad, H., editor: Crisis intervention: selected readings, New York, 1965, Family Service Association of America.

Rappaport, L.: Working with families in crisis: an exploration in preventative intervention. In Parad, H., editor: Crisis intervention: selected readings, New York, 1965, Family Service Association of America.

Schiff, H.S.: The bereaved parent, New York, 1977, Crown Publishers, Inc.

Solnit, A.J., and Green, M.: Psychologic considerations in the management of deaths on pediatric hospital services, Pediatrics 24:106-112, 1959.

Solnit, A.J., and Stark, M.H.: Mourning and the birth of a defective child, Psychoanal. Study Child 16:523-537, 1961.

Voland, R.L., editor: Counseling parents of the ill and the handicapped, Springfield, Ill., 1971, Charles C Thomas, Publisher.

76 Psychosocial aspects of pediatric intensive care

The patient

KATHERINE LIPSKY

DEFINITION OF THE PROBLEM

Admission to a PICU is a crisis situation for the pediatric patient as well as for his parents. Child patients can undergo some of the same psychological stresses and concerns that affect their parents. These conflicts were described in Chapter 75. However, unlike the waiting parents, the child himself is the actual target of unfamiliar, invasive, often painful procedures that are inflicted on him by unknown staff members in a frightening, noisy, and strange environment. The personal meaning and potential trauma of a PICU admission for each child depends on several variables. These include the severity of the illness, level of consciousness, chronologic age, and developmental level.

In evaluating and attempting to minimize the trauma of a PICU admission for a child, the staff needs to be aware of specific problems.

Phase vulnerability. This refers to particular vulnerabilities associated with specific ages and developmental stages. Those physical and psychologic functions and capabilities that are currently emerging or that have recently been established are most vulnerable to damage. Therefore, experiences as a patient in a PICU can have highly personalized, idiosyncratic meaning arising from underlying age-related fantasies and concerns.

Separation. Separation from parents may have profound effects on the hospitalized child. The devastating emotional and physical effects of early prolonged maternal separation on young children have been documented in studies on anaclitic depression and on separation anxiety. Patient care must include a careful evaluation of the child's response to separation from parents and its concomitant traumatic potential. Adequate time for visiting with parents must be provided because of the child's primary dependence on parents for emotional support and replenishment.

Cognitive development. Children's thinking tends to be characterized by the predominance of fantasy. This richness of fantasy contributes to the often significant disparity between the nature of diagnostic and therapeutic procedures and the child's perception of what is done to him and why it is being done. Such idiosyncratic distortion is complicated further by the child's poorly developed time sense and limited ability to delay, predict, or sense sequence.

Regression. Nearly every illness and hospitalization encourages regressive behavior in the patient. Such regression is often more frightening to the pediatric patient than to the adult patient because it involves the loss of newly acquired, and therefore precious, achievements. Regression is often compounded by impairment of motility, with consequent loss of motor discharge of aggression, curiosity, and general tension.

MONITORING

An assessment of the patient's adjustment to a PICU hospitalization requires the monitoring of three general indices.

Chronologic age, developmental level, and associated phase-related vulnerabilities. For example, the 18- to 30-month-old child, occupied with the separation-individuation struggle and experiencing conflicting needs for autonomy and dependence, may be especially vulnerable to prolonged periods of parental separation. Another example is the oedipal-age child. With an already heightened sensitivity to bodily harm, the oedipal-aged child may be particularly traumatized by the painful, invasive medical procedures that are often a part of a PICU admission.

Severity of illness and level of conscious awareness. Some children are so critically ill or neurologically damaged that they are unresponsive even to deep pain. It is important to remember, however, that many children who are unable to respond to the environment may, in fact, be taking in everything that happens to and around them.

Behavioral reaction to hospitalization. Pathologic behavioral reactions (both during and following the PICU experience) to organic problems and hospital experiences can have an adverse effect on the recovery process itself, make nursing and medical management more difficult, and prolong hospitalization.

MANAGEMENT

PICU medical, nursing, and social work staff can take specific steps to assist the patients in their attempts to master the experience of a PICU admission and to prevent or reduce associated psychologic trauma. Such measures include the following.

Orientation. Whenever possible, patients should be oriented to the PICU and the staff before admission. Because so many admissions are on an emergency basis, prior orientation is often not possible. However, preadmission tours through the PICU can be arranged for elective surgery candidates.

Positive environmental stimulation. Positive environmental stimulation should be provided to counteract much of the necessary negative stimulation in a PICU setting. Visual, aural, and tactile stimulation can all be utilized at age-appropriate levels. Even neonates can benefit from positive environmental input, such as a colorful mobile or soft radio music. Children of all ages respond to positive tactile stimulation (stroking, hugging, holding, etc.) designed to counteract the painful invasive tactile stimulation that they are subjected to during various procedures.

Information. Factual orienting information should be given. The nursing staff can do much to decrease a patient's fear and confusion by providing orientation to time and place, by explaining procedures step by step as they occur, by repeating routine procedures in an ordered way so that the patient can become familiar with them, and by honestly telling a child when a procedure may hurt and when it will not.

Parent-child interaction. Opportunities for parent-child interaction should be facilitated. Pediatric patients of all ages derive their chief emotional support from their families and need visiting time to be reassured that parents have not abandoned them.

Acknowledgment of frustrations. The patient's frustration due to lack of control over the situation should be acknowledged. Patients should be encouraged to make decisions whenever possible. Such action helps to compensate for their lack of control over their overall situation. Opportunities for decision-making must be appropriate to the patient's age and health care needs. Obviously, there is little room for patient input in many areas of care. Providing opportunities for decision-making is particularly therapeutic for the adolescent patient.

Ventilation of fears and concerns. An opportunity to ventilate fears and concerns should be offered to the patient. The nursing staff can encourage patients to express, either verbally or through behavior, their anger at being assaulted, hurt, and restrained. Clarifying what each specific experience means to each child can facilitate adjustment to the PICU. Some hospitals have a child life staff with specialists in child growth and development who can help patients master their traumatic experiences through therapeutic play. The duration and vigor of therapeutic play opportunities can increase as the patient's health improves and can continue after he has moved out of the PICU. If a child manifests severe or prolonged behavioral adjustment problems as a result of the hospitalization, a psychiatric consultation may be appropriate.

Tutoring. Provision of hospital-bound tutoring prevents the school-age pediatric patient from falling behind academically. Minimizing the differences between the ill child and other children decreases the risk of further social isolation after discharge from the hospital.

Follow-up. Follow-up contact with former PICU patients is encouraged. Such contact offers former patients the therapeutic opportunity to view the staff under relaxed, nonthreatening circumstances and can help the child place his hospital experiences in better perspective.

ADDITIONAL READING

Aradine, C.R.: Books for children about death, Pediatrics 57:372-378, 1976.

Bowlby, J.: Separation anxiety, Int. J. Psychoanal. 41:89-113, 1960.

Hoffmann, A., Becker, R.R., and Galriel, H.P.: The hospitalized adolescent, New York, 1976, The Free Press.

Mahler, M.: Thoughts about development and individuation, Psychoanal. Study Child 18:307-323, 1963.

Oremland, E.K., and Oremland, J.D., editors: The effects of hospitalization on children, Springfield, Ill., 1973, Charles C Thomas, Publisher.

Spitz, P.A.: Anaclitic depression, Psychoanal. Study Child 2:313-341, 1946.

77 Psychosocial aspects of pediatric intensive care

The staff

KATHERINE LIPSKY

DEFINITION OF THE PROBLEM

The crisis orientation of the PICU means that the staff must function is a physically and psychologically stressful environment. Since patient survival often depends on rapid and accurate responses to emergency situations, the staff must maintain almost constant vigilance. Although medical or surgical attending physicians bear the burden of ultimate responsibility for patient management decisions and although rotating house officers must respond to emergencies with quick and correct judgment in an unfamiliar setting, nursing personnel form the core of the patient care team and have to function effectively in the hectic PICU environment week after week. Physically, the nurse is the staff member who spends the most time within the PICU, and psychologically, it is the nurse who must interact effectively with the numerous medical and technical personnel who make transient appearances related to patients' specific health care needs. For these reasons, this chapter deals primarily with problems encountered by the nursing staff. However, several of the management suggestions have general applicability to all members of the PICU health care delivery team.

The PICU environment imposes extraordinary physical and emotional burdens on its nursing staff. Some of the specific pressures include the following.

External isolating factors. PICUs are often physically separated from other nursing units. PICU nurses may be required to wear distinctive uniforms, such as scrub suits, that further set them apart from their nursing colleagues. Not infrequently, floor nurses tend to regard the highly specialized PICU nurses with considerable ambivalence, which adds psychologic separation to geographic distance. This combination of factors tends to reduce opportunities for interaction with and support from the majority of hospital nursing colleagues and tends to place PICU nurses in the wearying position of defensive isolation.

Excessive sensory stimulation. The frenetic PICU environment exposes nurses to a massive array of sensory stimuli, some emotionally neutral and others highly charged. Because they work near blood, excreta, exposed genitalia, and wasted and unconscious bodies, nurses are bombarded with stimuli that are potentially able to mobilize every possible conflictual area at every psychologic developmental level.

Complex technical equipment. Nurses are required to operate intricate monitoring devices and to perform precise and complicated procedures. The possibility for error is always present, and the results of such error may be catastrophic.

Chronic latent anxiety. In an environment where every procedure is potentially lifesaving, any error in technique or judgment may be life-threatening. This knowledge places the PICU

449

nurse under the strain of chronic anxiety and self-doubt. Although this anxiety can increase alertness and sharpen nursing skills, it can also reduce efficiency and decision-making capacity if it exceeds optimal levels.

Incessant repetitive routine. Paradoxically, despite the emergency-oriented atmosphere of a PICU, nurses also are required to carry out repetitive routines such as monitoring and charting. PICU nurses are expected to make observations about patients' conditions, but they are often so involved in collecting and charting data that they have little time to interpret the information obtained, thus adding to their frustration and anxiety.

Presence of distraught relatives. Families of patients can take up nursing time and dissipate the nurse's emotional energy by making excessive demands for information and reassurance.

Repetitive contact with death. Imminent death is an ever present possibility in the PICU and an ongoing threat to nurses' feelings of potency. It is a constant reminder of the nurse's vulnerability and provides repeated episodes of object loss. The intensity of reaction to each loss parallels the degree to which the nurse becomes emotionally involved with the patient. Because of the tragic sense of unrealized potential, pediatric deaths are frequently difficult to assimilate. Many nurses protect themselves from painful object loss by denial, by relating more to machinery than to patients, and by excessive, even macabre, laughter and humor.

MONITORING

Ongoing attention to the following three indices is useful in assessing overall staff functioning in a PICU setting:

1. General emotional tone and morale level as expressed in verbal responses to job-related demands.
2. Frequency of incident reports. Fluctuations in the occurrence of incident reports can reflect both individual and group behavioral responses to job-related pressures.
3. Rate and flow of staff absences and resignations.

MANAGEMENT

Specific steps can be taken to increase job-related rewards and decrease job-related stresses. The following supportive measures can help develop more staff efficiency and satisfaction.

Provide orientation and ongoing education. A thorough initial period of training and orientation is essential. It should focus on the job characteristics specific to a PICU and must include both technical and psychologic aspects of patient care. Regularly scheduled ongoing educational opportunities serve to increase both feelings of confidence and actual competence.

Build in special benefits. Such benefits can enhance an appropriate sense of pride in performing a difficult job. Special privileges, e.g., a small pay differential or periodic brief extra vacations, can help bolster individual and group esteem.

Ensure delivery of appropriate positive feedback. Mechanisms to provide encouragement and positive reinforcement can have a significant impact on improving staff morale. Too often mistakes are pointed out while good work fails to be rewarded. The PICU social worker is often in an ideal position to pass on words of praise and gratitude from waiting families and fellow staff members that otherwise would have been unknown.

Facilitate group cohesiveness. Encouraging a feeling of group belonging and commitment offers the best basis for cooperative resolution of the multiple practical and emotional problems associated with working in a PICU. Management suggestions to promote group cohesion include the following.

Health team staffings. Weekly meetings can be held that are attended by PICU medical, nursing, and social work personnel. A patient is presented, problems are identified, and a treatment plan, including individual responsibilities, is discussed. Medical, nursing, and psychosocial aspects of the case are covered. The nursing plan is shared with all shifts. Those nurses who are unable to participate in the conference are thus recognized as contributors to the patient's overall health care planning.

Regular group meetings. These meetings can be designed to explore both the positive and negative aspects of the work experience. Communication must be focused on the PICU situation rather than expanding into more general self-exploration. Moreover, the interchange cannot be allowed to transcend limits that interfere with comfortable working together between sessions. Such group meetings can provide:

1. An avenue for ventilating intragroup hostilities and complaints.
2. Recognition that uncertainty and anxiety are shared, acceptable feelings.
3. Realization that minor mistakes are inevitable and need not be a source of paralyzing guilt or shame.
4. A sharing of techniques that individuals have found useful in dealing with problems arising on the job.
5. A forum for developing constructive solutions for problem areas and effective suggestions for improved communication.
6. An arena for positive feedback.

Planned social activities. Spontaneous informal socializing often occurs among staff members and can enhance PICU morale and cohesion. In addition, one or two large, planned annual social events can also increase solidarity and esprit de corps. For example, an annual Christmas alumni party held for patients who graduated from the PICU can serve as a tangible and rewarding testament to the staff's hard work and skill.

ADDITIONAL READING

Caldwell, T., and Weiner, M.F.: Stresses and coping in ICU nursing. I. A review, Gen. Hosp. Psychiatry 3:119-127, 1981.

Gardam, J.F.: Nursing stresses in the intensive care unit, letter, J.A.M.A. 208:2337-2338, 1969.

Hay, D., and Oken, D.: The psychologic stresses of intensive care unit nursing, Psychosom. Med. 34:109-118, 1972.

Kilgour, D.Y.: Nursing in intensive therapy units—personnel problems. In Walker, W.F., and Taylor, D.E.M., editors: Intensive care, London, 1975, Churchill Livingstone.

Kornfield, D.S.: Psychiatric view of the intensive care unit, Br. Med. J. 1:108-110, 1969.

Koumans, A.J.: Psychiatric consultation in an intensive care unit, J.A.M.A. 194:133-137, 1965.

Vreeland, R., and Ellis, G.: Stresses on the nurse in an intensive care unit, J.A.M.A. 208:332-334, 1969.

Weiner, M.F., and Caldwell, T.: Stresses and coping in ICU nursing. II. Nurse support groups on intensive care units, Gen. Hosp. Psychiatry 3:129-134, 1981.

78 Suicide

KENNETH M. WIGGINS

DEFINITION AND PHYSIOLOGY

Children and adolescents admitted to a PICU with injuries, poisoning, or metabolic imbalance may be suffering the results of suicide attempts. Children as young as 5 years of age frequently threaten suicide and make attempts, but the attempts infrequently result in death in children prior to 11 or 12 years of age. The suicidal behavior of adolescents is much more likely to result in death, and even though suicide is almost certainly underreported, it is the second leading cause of death among adolescents in the United States.

Suicidal behavior is often obvious, but it is quite possible for situations appearing to result from accidents or fate to be the result of suicidal behavior. The initial suicide attempt of any individual child or adolescent more often comes as a surprise to the patient's family and physician. Whether suicidal behavior is overt and obvious, disguised, or apparently accidental, any suicidal aspect of life-threatening conditions needs to be recognized, managed, and treated by PICU personnel. Conditions leading to a first or subsequent suicide attempt are likely to continue unless there is active intervention, and the fact that a child or adolescent attempts suicide usually complicates his life and makes subsequent attempts even more likely. A patient admitted to a PICU for conditions not resulting from a suicide attempt may become suicidal in the PICU because of his illness, his treatment, or his experiences in the PICU.

The choice of suicidal behavior as a method for solving problems is determined by many factors. Preadolescents are much more likely to threaten or attempt suicide because they want to strike back or get even with someone; they are often angry and see themselves as mistreated or rejected. The preadolescent is likely to view death as temporary. Because the desire for death for whatever reason is so common in preadolescents, it is fortunate that they are not usually very good at planning and executing lethal activities. Adolescents, however, become increasingly capable of inducing their own deaths. Some adolescents desire death because of their perception that they have fallen short of their own expectations or the expectations of other people important in their lives. Any combination of large numbers of problems seems to increase the risk for suicidal behavior in adolescence, whether these problems be frequent moves, multiple losses (especially of parents by divorce or death), school failure, alcoholism in the family, or parents or friends who have attempted suicide. Adolescents are probably more likely than preadolescents to be overtly depressed at the time that they make suicide attempts.

Suicidal behavior may arouse discomfort, disapproval, or rejection on the part of health care providers and family members. This fact, along with the frequent desire of the patient and/or family to minimize the significance of the episode, decreases the likelihood of successful intervention. However, an attempt to end one's life presents a crisis that also produces an opportunity for change in both the individual and his environment. The treatment of children and adolescents who have attempted to end their lives should always combine work with the individual and the family and/or other people important in the patient's environment. The younger the patient, the more necessary it will be to mobilize the family and others in the patient's environment.

MANAGEMENT

1. Provide medical and surgical treatment for the results of the suicide attempt as indicated to maintain the patient's life and return him to a state of health, if possible.
2. Provide appropriate treatment for any medical problems contributing to the suicide (diabetes mellitus, seizure disorder, organic brain syndrome, depression, schizophrenia, etc.).
3. Observe and control the patient while in the PICU to prevent further suicide efforts.
4. Be alert to the possibility of suicidal ideation and behavior, and acknowledge the reality of suicidal behavior.
5. If the presence of suicidal behavior has been determined, tactfully present this information to both the patient and his family. Do not be afraid to mention suicide, depression, anger, hostility, hopelessness, or death wishes to the patient or to his family.
6. Transfer the patient from the close supervision of the PICU only after it has been determined that the patient is no longer suicidal or that adequate suicidal precautions can be effected.
7. Either perform or obtain an assessment of the patient, his family, and his environment in order to determine suicidal potential and factors needing correction so that plans can be formulated and executed to correct contributing factors and to protect the life of the patient.

ADDITIONAL READING

Crumley, F.E.: Adolescent suicide attempts and melancholia, Dallas Med. J. 67:306-309, 1981.

Mattsson, A., Sesse, L.R., and Hawkins, J.W.: Suicidal behavior as a child psychiatric emergency, Arch. Gen. Psychiatry 20:100-109, 1969.

Orbach, I., and Glaubman, H.: The concept of death and suicidal behavior in young children, J. Am. Acad. Child Psychiatry 18:668-678, 1979.

Pfeffer, C.R.: Psychiatric hospital treatment of suicidal children, Suicide Life Threat. Behav. 8:150-160, 1977.

Pfeffer, C.R., Conte, H.R., Plutchik, R., and Jarrett, I.: Suicidal behavior in latency-age children, J. Am. Acad. Child Psychiatry 18:679-692, 1979.

Shaffer, D.: Suicide in childhood and early adolescence, J. Child Psychol. Psychiatry 15:275-291, 1974.

Teicher, J.D.: Suicide and suicide attempts. In Noshpitz, J.D., editor: Basic handbook of child psychiatry, vol. 2, New York, 1979, Basic Books, Inc., Publishers, pp. 685-696.

79 Child abuse and neglect

PAUL R. PRESCOTT

DEFINITION AND ETIOLOGY

Child abuse and neglect have existed throughout the centuries in all societies. The definition of what constitutes abuse and neglect depends to a great extent on individual cultural customs and the laws written to enforce them. In the United States during the first half of this century, efforts to control abuse were directed towards enforcing the then existing laws against child labor and assault. Many obviously abusive injuries were blamed on accidental trauma or spontaneous events. In 1946 Dr. John Caffey, a radiologist, pointed out the occurrence of subdural hematomas associated with multiple fractures of the ribs and long bones; however, the full implications of child abuse and neglect were not realized until 1962, when the term "the battered-child syndrome" was coined in an article by Dr. C. Henry Kempe and associates. Following this new exposure of a medical syndrome, the long-term denial of the existence of child abuse ceased, leading to the passage of laws now in effect in all fifty states, requiring the reporting of abuse and neglect.

The scope of the battered-child syndrome has grown enormously as more and better research has been accomplished. We now recognize that the problem is not limited to the physically abused and battered child but also includes nutritional deprivation, medical care neglect, physical neglect, sexual abuse, intentional drugging, emotional abuse, lack of supervision, abandonment, and educational deprivation. All but the last of these may result in intensive care admission.

Between 2% and 6% of the children in the United States experience some form of abuse each year, with an estimated annual incidence of 1 million cases. Approximately 4,000 children die each year as a result. Child abuse accounts for 10% of all trauma seen in pediatric emergency rooms in children less than 3 years of age and for 25% of all fractures in children less than 2 years of age. The long-term morbidity is staggering, resulting in learning and language deficiencies; developmental, mental, and growth retardation; blindness and deafness; psychosis; depression; suicide; juvenile and adult crime; prostitution; and drug abuse. As many as 30% of abused children may be functionally mentally retarded, with more than half experiencing neurologic damage. Even more critical is the finding that destructive behavior traits may be passed on from previously abused parents to their own children, resulting in a self-perpetuating cycle of abuse and neglect.

The causes of the battered-child syndrome are many and varied. Cultural factors invariably have an effect. Society has always recognized the right of family privacy and has been reluctant to intervene in domestic affairs. This is still evident in the relative ease with which appropriate steps can be taken to protect a child from physical abuse as opposed to the difficulties faced in getting society to recognize emotional battering or medical care neglect. Abuse is often rationalized by the "spare the rod" philosophy, which fails to distinguish between discipline and abuse, and the "man's home is his castle" attitude towards privacy. Given these attitudes it is not surprising that more than 90% of physical abuse is inflicted by parents, many of whom are less than 30 years of age. Although initial reactions may suggest that an abusive parent is

454

far from normal, only 10% are found to be psychotic or sociopathic. Abuse occurs in all income groups, with the poor being most highly represented, probably due to reporting factors. There is no racial difference in incidence.

In many cases the abusive parent has been abused in the past, feels isolated and distrustful, and has low self-esteem and poor impulse control. The parent may suffer from frustrated dependency needs, leading to distorted expectations and role reversal, with the child being viewed as existing to fulfill the parent's need for love and nurturance. Many abusive families are isolated from the community and supportive family or friends and are subjected to increased stress such as low income level, unemployment, or illness. The child may be viewed as being special or different if he is physically disabled, slow in development, or if he has a temperament different from his parents. The pregnancy may have been unwanted or unplanned. The infant may have been premature or may have required prolonged hospitalization following birth, resulting in poor bonding. Many families may be able to manage in spite of these factors until an additional crisis precipitates the abusive episode.

The above brief outline of a typical abusive family is not meant to imply that all abusive families fit this description. Despite these known characteristics of abusive families, we must recognize that, given the right circumstances and conditions, we are all capable of striking out in anger or fear. The potential for abuse may vary, but this fact must be recognized if all such cases are to be diagnosed.

The physician has three main responsibilities: detection, reporting, and acting as the child's advocate to ensure his protection, survival, and well-being.

Legal aspects

Because laws on child abuse vary somewhat from state to state, it is essential that physicians become familiar with the law in their particular states. Most states specifically require medical personnel to report cases, while others mandate that all citizens report. Despite various wordings of the individual laws, reporting is required in all cases in which child abuse or neglect is suspected; the diagnosis need not be absolute. The state agency that is required to receive and investigate reports also varies, but it is usually a division of the state welfare agency.

All state laws provide immunity from civil and criminal prosecution provided that the report is given in good faith. In addition, a penalty is usually provided for failure to report. Physicians may also be liable under malpractice laws because of failure to report suspected abuse or neglect. Under tort doctrines, failure to comply with a mandatory statute can constitute negligence in and of itself. That this malpractice liability is real was confirmed in a suit upheld by the California Supreme Court (*Landeros vs Flood*, 1976).

Unfortunately, physicians do not like to be involved in child abuse cases. They often fail to realize that abuse and neglect determinations fall under civil, not criminal, proceedings. Intent does not have to be proved. The primary purpose of the laws is to protect the child and prevent future injury, not to punish the abuser. The aim of child protective service personnel is to provide counseling and assistance to involved families so that the family can be reunited. A child should be permanently removed from the home only when counseling fails and obvious danger exists.

That reporting and investigation are necessary becomes clear when it is realized that a seemingly believable history offered to explain a child's injuries is often disproved when investigated. For example, a motor vehicle accident can cause a skull fracture and facial bruises only if it actually occurred; a fall to a tile floor may fracture an infant's skull only if the floor is actually tile. These are two examples of disproved histories obtained at our institution in a few months' time. A doctor has neither the time nor the legal right to check the validity of such histories. In all cases of significant trauma involving a child, the history should be independently verified. An abused child sent home without intervention has a greater than 50% chance of being reinjured, a 35% chance of suffering severe permanent damage, and a 5% chance of being killed.

Clinical and laboratory evaluation

History. Since most parents do not initially admit to child abuse, the physician must suspect it in any case of severe trauma. Certain types of histories that may be offered should be considered diagnostic of child abuse. These include:

1. Eyewitness history. If offered by the child or if one parent accuses the other and no custody dispute is involved, the history is usually true.
2. Allegedly self-inflicted injury. This is always suspect in children less than 2 years of age and diagnostic in a child who is not yet crawling.
3. Sibling-inflicted injury. Although this can occur, if the history is of repetitive injuries the family needs help in dealing with the sibling, and a report should be made to ensure that the family receives assistance.
4. History completely incompatible with the nature of the injuries.
5. Delay in seeking medical care. In 30% of abuse cases, care is delayed until the following morning. In an additional 30% the delay may be as long as 1 to 4 days. In severe accidental trauma no delay generally occurs.
6. No history. Abusive parents often deny any knowledge of how the trauma occurred or offer vague explanations such as "He might have fallen."
7. Partial confession. A parent may admit to striking a child but deny that the blow was hard enough to cause the injury in question.

Obtaining the history in child abuse cases is never an easy task. The following guidelines should be kept in mind:

1. Remain professional, be objective, and control any hostility that possible child abuse may provoke. The parents may be feeling angry or depressed, and ambiguity can be viewed as a threat.
2. Be supportive and understanding, never judgmental. At no time should the physician directly accuse a parent or another party of child abuse. The physician's input should be limited to medical facts, presented in an open, honest, and authoritative manner.
3. All discussions must be completely documented in the chart.
4. Histories should be obtained from all relevant caretakers and separately from each parent if at all possible. Record the name of the informant, the date, time, place, people present, and sequence of events surrounding the injury, and the parents' affect toward the child and the child's injuries. Note any changes in the history made by the parents or discrepancies between different histories, and any time lag before seeking medical care.
5. Obtain a detailed developmental history. Injuries are often claimed to be self-inflicted even though the stage of development obviously disproves this.
6. If nutritional neglect is suspected, the history should include past weights and heights, a 24-hour dietary recall, appetite, stool pattern, vomiting or regurgitation, and the parents' explanation for the failure to thrive.
7. If the injury involves water burns, note specific environmental details such as depth and estimated temperature of the water and length of exposure.
8. If medically possible, a separate, nondirective history should be obtained from all children greater than 3 years.
9. Inform the parents that, based on the nature of the injuries, a report will be made to the appropriate authorities. Explain that such a report is mandated by state law for the protection of all children and that other

people will be involved, including social workers and the police if required under the applicable statutes. If it appears that the parents may attempt to remove the child from treatment, they should be informed only after the child's admission, but before the protective services caseworker arrives.

10. Outline the investigative procedure as well as the nature of the injuries and the treatment plan.

Physical examination. The medical record needs to be complete and precise, especially in documenting the types of injuries present. A complete examination must be performed, paying special attention to the following:

1. Detailed plotting of height, weight, and head circumference.
2. Careful retinal examination. Retinal hemorrhage may indicate significant intracranial hemorrhage from violent shaking, even though there are no external marks. Any CNS trauma in infants and toddlers must be considered abusive until proved otherwise.
3. Describe all bruises, abrasions, and lacerations. Measure the size and note the location, shape, position, color, age, and special characteristics of each injury. If possible, state what the injury looks like or was caused by, for example, grab or pinch marks, blunt trauma, looped cord marks. Pathognomonic sites of injury include the buttocks and lower back, genitalia and inner thighs, cheeks, earlobes, and neck.
4. Bite marks. Note the location and age. Measure the distance between the midpoints of the canines. Adult bite marks measure greater than 3 cm.
5. Burns. Note the exact nature of the burn, including degree and area, clear or blurred margins, dry or weeping, and the presence or absence of splash marks in cases of liquid burns. If the burn is clearly of the dunking or stocking or glove type, this should be stated.
6. Diagram of the injuries listed in 3, 4, and 5.

Label the diagram with the information outlined.

7. Oral cavity. Note any injuries to the frenulum, lips, and teeth. Injuries in this area are generally pathognomonic of abuse.
8. Musculoskeletal system. Palpate all bones, including the ribs, for tenderness or swelling. Check range of motion of all joints.
9. Abdomen. This is easily overlooked when there is other, more obvious trauma. Examination must be complete and thorough with an assessment of bowel sounds, distention, tenderness, or masses. Injuries can include intestinal intramural hematoma, perforation, liver or spleen lacerations, and renal trauma without external bruising.
10. Genitalia. Note any bruises, abrasions, lacerations, swelling, erythema, or discharge. Trauma in this area is virtually pathognomonic of child abuse. In a female child sexual abuse should always be suspected and looked for.
11. Nutritional status. Not all abused children are neglected, but if neglect is suspected, then nutritional assessment should include measurements of subcutaneous fat.

MONITORING
Laboratory examination

1. Urinalysis to diagnose renal injury even in the absence of external abdominal trauma.
2. Serum amylase and lipase if external abdominal trauma, left upper quadrant mass or tenderness, hematuria, or left lower rib fractures are present.
3. CBC and differential.
4. Coagulation profile: platelet count, bleeding time, PT, PTT, fibrinogen level, thrombin time, and peripheral blood smear. Coagulation studies are rarely needed in practice, since ongoing bleeding from an organic cause is usually obvious and does not cause bruising limited to the buttocks, back, face, or genitalia as is generally seen in abuse cases. However, if the parents strongly claim that the child always bruises easily or if the

legal climate is known to lean heavily on such statements, then a full coagulation profile must be done.

Roentgenographic examination

1. Skeletal survey on all children less than age 5 years. After age 5 this can be limited to those children with bone tenderness, swelling, limited range of motion, or significant old external trauma. Injuries should be dated as accurately as possible. Ideally, all roentgenograms should be reviewed by a pediatric radiologist experienced in child abuse. Highly suspicious findings include any fracture in an infant; metaphyseal or epiphyseal injuries and rib fractures in infants and toddlers; exaggerated periosteal reaction, which may indicate repeated trauma; costochondral separations; multiple injuries, especially with different stages of healing; and common fractures associated with any of these.
2. Full facial series if significant facial trauma is present.
3. Other studies as indicated by the nature of the injury, laboratory results, or peripheral findings on a skeletal survey, such as free intraperitoneal air, blurred liver or psoas margins, or abnormal gas patterns.

Other measures

1. Height and weight. Monitor daily as accurately as possible in cases in which nutritional neglect is evident or suspected.
2. Skin. Check daily for the first few days for development of bruises that may not have been apparent on the initial examination. Previously noted bruises may assume a pattern that suggests a specific cause.
3. Abdomen. Examine initially and every few hours for signs of distention, decreased or absent bowel sounds, or masses, any of which may suggest previously unsuspected trauma.
4. Musculoskeletal system. Areas of tenderness or swelling that were discovered on the ini-

tial examination but which appeared normal on the initial skeletal survey should be reexamined in 2 weeks, when signs of healing make injuries obvious.
5. Vision and hearing assessment. In cases involving ocular or CNS trauma, permanent deficits often occur. Perform assessments prior to discharge so that future therapy and treatment needs are known and devices can be obtained if indicated.
6. Changes in affect and reactions of the parents and the child should be documented.
7. A record should be kept of hospital visits by parents, grandparents, and other relatives to aid in possible placement decisions.
8. More specific monitoring will depend on the types of injuries sustained, and the appropriate chapters should be consulted.

MANAGEMENT
Hospitalization

1. If the hospital has a child abuse and neglect team, notify it as indicated in its procedures.
2. Telephone a report to the state agency responsible for investigating child abuse. This should be done by the physician or a member of the abuse team so that pertinent medical findings can be provided.
3. In serious injuries temporary custody may be taken from the parents and placed with the child protective agency. In these cases, permission for any medical procedures must be obtained from the agency, not from the parents. The agency will usually ask for the parents' consent, but the parents may no longer have this right.
4. The hospital chart may be subpoenaed in subsequent legal proceedings during which it is possible that sequelae of the abusive episode may be blamed on the medical care received. Only careful, complete documentation can show this to be untrue.
5. Provide a written report or affidavit to the appropriate agency within 24 hours. Include your name and status; a detailed summary of

the pertinent history and physical, laboratory, and radiologic findings; the method of abuse or the object used if this can be determined from the medical evidence; and, most importantly, a firm statement of your opinion regarding the probability that the injuries were inflicted.
6. Color photographs are required by law in some states, and should be obtained in all cases to document physical findings.
7. There is a 20% risk that the siblings of an abused child have also been abused. All siblings should be examined within 12 hours.
8. Developmental and behavioral screening of the child should be performed as soon as medically possible to delineate the extent of permanent injury and to obtain a baseline for follow-up evaluations.
9. Cooperate with the agency investigating the incident, provide an opinion as to the medical and psychological follow-up the child will need, and aid in determining appropriate placement based on this assessment.

Court testimony

1. Advance preparation is a must. The entire case, including roentgenograms and special studies, should be completely reviewed. Be certain of specific dates.
2. A pretrial meeting with the prosecutor is helpful. For the physician testifying for the first time, a review of evidence and questions to be asked helps to organize his or her thoughts. This also presents an opportunity for the physician to educate the prosecutor on the medical facts and point out those that are the most significant.
3. Appear in court appropriately dressed. Leave scrub suits and laboratory coats behind.
4. Questions may be asked by the prosecutor and several others. If the parents are separated, each may have an attorney. Relatives requesting custody may be represented. In addition, an attorney is generally appointed guardian *ad litem* to protect the child's best interests. All of these attorneys have the right to examine and to cross-examine.
5. The physician should be a neutral expert witness and never appear antagonistic. Your duty is to present and to explain the medical facts, not to act as the prosecutor. You must remain objective and stay within your area of expertise.
6. As a witness, you have the right to understand all questions asked. If a question is not understood, it should not be answered. Ask that the question be rephrased; however, never do this in an attempt to avoid giving an answer.
7. Never guess at an answer. Admit what you do not know. However, if you are certain, say so, and do not waiver.
8. Never volunteer information. Listen to the question and answer what is asked.
9. It is always a good idea to hesitate a moment before answering a question in order to allow the prosecutor to raise an objection if he or she so desires.
10. If a yes-no question requires a more complex answer, explain this to the judge. You will usually be allowed to proceed with a more detailed reply.
11. Remain calm and collected, projecting an image of confidence and knowledge. Displays of anger only serve to lower your credibility and objectivity.

ADDITIONAL READING

Caffey, J.: Multiple fractures in long bones of infants suffering from subdural hematoma, Am. J. Radiol. **56:**163-173, 1946.
Caffey, J.: On the theory and practice of shaking infants, Am. J. Dis. Child. **124:**161-169, 1972.
Caffey, J.: The whiplash shaken infant syndrome: manual shaking by the extremities with whiplash-induced intracranial and intraocular bleedings, linked with residual permanent brain damage and mental retardation, Pediatrics **54:**396-403, 1974.

Ellerstein, N., editor: Child abuse and neglect: a medical reference, New York, 1981, John Wiley & Sons, Inc.

Ford, R.J., Smistek, B.S., and Glass, J.T.: Photography of suspected child abuse and maltreatment, Biomed. Commun. 3:12-17, 1975.

Giovannoni, J., and Becerra, R.: Defining child abuse, New York, 1979, The Free Press.

Helfer, R.E., Slovis, T.L., and Black, M.: Injuries resulting when small children fall out of bed, Pediatrics 60: 533-535, 1977.

Kempe, H., and Helfer, R., editors: The battered child, ed. 3, Chicago, 1980, University of Chicago Press.

Lenoski, E.F., and Hunter, K.A.: Specific patterns of inflicted burn injuries, J. Trauma 17:842-846, 1977.

Williams, G., and Money, J., editors: Traumatic abuse and neglect of children at home, Baltimore, 1980, The Johns Hopkins University Press.

Wilson, E.F.: Estimation of the age of cutaneous contusions in child abuse, Pediatrics 60:750-752, 1977.

80 Legal aspects of pediatric intensive care

BARTON E. BERNSTEIN

In an era when children's personal and constitutional rights are being formulated and formalized, numerous ethical and legal dilemmas face the pediatrician, especially when medical treatment is imperative and the legal overtones loom only hazily on the horizon. Today individuals live in an epoch of divorcing parents, custodial and noncustodial; mature and emancipated minors; and specific laws which vary from state to state relating to abortion, drug treatment, venereal disease, birth control, and battered and abused children. There is also increasing public interest in and awareness of malpractice, proper record keeping and confidentiality, and increasing media coverage of accepted and refused emergency medical treatment and the boundaries of informed consent. In each of these areas, law affects medicine, and therefore the relationship of law and medicine is a legitimate concern to medical personnel of all disciplines. A fundamental knowledge of legal issues is essential. Both law and medicine should focus more attention on how power and responsibility for children are allocated and should be allocated. Who decides now? Who should decide? These are the critical issues facing pediatric medicine.

PARENTAL CONTROL

Most state statutes provide for parental rights, privileges, duties, and powers, and these specifically include the duty to provide a child with medical care. Implicit in this duty is the power to consent to all reasonable and necessary medical care needed by the child and collaterally, in the absence of a court order, the right to refuse medical treatment whether, in the opinion of the physician, the denial of care is appropriate or not.

When parents are divorced, parental powers are divided, and the custodial parent (managing conservator) and the noncustodial parent (possessory conservator) each have a segment of parental power. The custodial parent retains the duty to provide the child with medical care while the noncustodial parent, during periods of possession or visitation, only has "the power to consent to medical and surgical treatment during an emergency involving an immediate danger to the health and safety of the child." [*Texas Family Code* 14.04 (3)] This power has been extended (5/20/83) to include "the right of access to medical, dental, and educational records of the child" to the same extent as the custodial parent. There are lingering questions concerning whether a medical or psychiatric evaluation is the same as treatment. The primary awareness needed is one of status. Where the parents are divorced, the relationship of the child to the presenting parent, relative, or friend must be determined so that legal consent for treatment can be obtained. Any of the persons listed below may consent to medical treatment of a minor when the person having the power to consent as otherwise provided by law cannot be contacted and actual notice to the contrary has not been given by that person:

1. a grandparent;
2. an adult brother or sister;
3. an adult aunt or uncle;

461

4. an educational institution in which the minor is enrolled that has received written authorization to consent from the person having the power to consent as otherwise provided by law;
5. any adult who has care and control of the minor and has written authorization to consent from the person having the power to consent as otherwise provided by law; or
6. any court having jurisdiction of the child. (*Texas Family Code* 35.01, 35.02)

For a minor child to be admitted to a mental hospital, the parent's consent or that of a legally appointed guardian or person *in loco parentis* is usually sufficient. However, the age of the child may determine if the child's consent is also needed, and this varies from state to state, the youngest age being 12. The same is true when considering release from a mental hospital. Consent forms must be signed by both parent and child if the child is over the statutory age, which varies from 12 years to majority. When considering the voluntary admission to mental hospitals, state laws vary concerning request for admission, release request, concurrence of the hospital superintendent, admission hearing, retention of the child after minority, age distinctions, and parental notice. (See Table 4G, p. 102, in *The Legal Status of Adolescents,* for a state-by-state summary of consent requirements.)

A recent modern innovation in custody litigation involves establishing joint custody over children. In joint custody arrangements the critical issue is that both divorced parents have an equal responsibility for making decisions that affect the child. However, the powers and duties are numerous, and the joint custody title may or may not include joint decision-making over medical care. The divorce decree must be perused to determine the actual powers and duties of each joint custodial parent. As a minimum the parent requesting treatment for a child must show that he or she has the legal authority to receive the medical treatment

requested and has the legal obligation to pay for it. The medical professional would be wise to inquire as to the legal status of the child and ask for some written evidence.

The biologic parent has the power to consent to medical treatment in the absence of a court hearing that specifically grants to another the right and/or duty to provide medical care. "Recently in the United States a child who had been raised from birth in a foster home was denied, by his biologic parents, an operation to correct his ventricular septal defect; he was, in effect, condemned to an early death." (*Canadian Medical Association Journal,* 1980) The biologic parents had the right. Should the medical community feel strongly enough that an operation is needed, it would have to have a guardian appointed with court-ordered power to provide medical care and treatment.

THE MINOR'S CONSENT

As a general rule, the minor's consent need not be obtained before providing medical treatment, since the consent of the parents or other lawfully authorized person satisfies the requirements of law. There are circumstances, however, when consent must be obtained from the minor, and consent of the parent alone is not sufficient. State statutes expressly stipulate that certain minors be treated differently. These include minors in the military and those who are emancipated or pregnant. Such statutes developed out of an awareness that in these circumstances, maturity and independence could be expected. In addition, the privacy right and the states' interest in the health and safety of others gave rise to specific laws and case precedents which deal with abortion, contagious reportable diseases, and the treatment of drug dependency, use, or addiction. These laws vary and their verbiage is often confusing. C. Dean Davis has assembled a chart which clearly outlines the various fact situations as well as the consent requirements and the party responsible for payment (Table 80-1). A similar chart to this should

Table 80-1. Consent requirements and payment responsibility in the state of Texas

If patient is	Is parental consent required?	Are parents responsible for cost?	Is minor's consent required?	May physician inform parents of treatment?
Under 18, unmarried, no special circumstances:	Yes	Yes	No	Yes
Under 18, married or previously married:	No	No	Yes	No
Under 18, emergency, and parents not available:	No	Yes	No	Yes
Emancipated (over 16), not living at home, manages own financial affairs:	No	No	Yes	Yes
Unmarried, pregnant, under 18 (care related to pregnancy):	No	No	Yes	Yes
Unmarried, pregnant, under 18 (care not related to pregnancy, and no other special circumstances):	Yes	Yes	No	Yes
Unmarried, under 18, determination if pregnant, no other special circumstances:	Probably not	Probably not	Probably yes	Probably yes
Under 18, on active duty with armed services:	No	No	Yes	Yes
Under 18, therapeutic abortion:				
Married or previously married:	No	No	Yes	Yes
Emancipated:	No	No	Yes	Yes
Not married or previously married, not emancipated:	No	No	Yes	Yes
Under 18, care for contagious reportable disease:	No	No	Yes	Yes
Birth control, under 18:				
Married or previously married:	No	No	Yes	No
Emancipated:	No	No	Yes	Yes
Care related to treatment of pregnancy:	No	No	Yes	Yes
Not married or previously married, not emancipated, care not related to treatment of pregnancy:	Yes	Yes	No	Yes
Under 18, examination and treatment for drug addiction, dependency or use (a recent Texas law states "if 13 or older"):	No	No	Yes	Yes

be assembled in each jurisdiction; the same information for other states is readily available in chart form. *The Legal Status of Adolescents, 1980,* published by the U.S. Department of Health and Human Services, contains easy-to-read summaries of all state laws assembled in tables under the title "Child's Abilities to Consent to Medical Treatment":

Table 4A, "Minor's Consent to General Medical, Surgical, Psychiatric and Health Services"

Table 4B, "Minor's Consent to Emergency Treatment"

Table 4C, "Minor's Consent to Treatment for Venereal Disease"

Table 4D, "Minor's Consent to Drug and Alcohol Abuse Treatment"

Table 4E, "Minor's Ability to Obtain Birth Control Services and to Consent to Treatment for Pregnancy"

Table 4F, "Minor's Consent to Abortion"

Table 4G, "Voluntary Admission of Minors to Mental Hospitals"

Recent public interest in "squeal laws" (the right or duty to inform and obtain consent from parents) has inspired litigation in this area.

Numerous cases are in court and on appeal. The law is therefore in a state of flux, and an attorney must be consulted for the current status of the law should a problem arise. These topic headings alert the professional that a problem area exists in a developing branch of the law.

Seeking the consent of minors, especially in areas where their consent is required for a particular treatment, raises problems not faced when seeking the consent of an adult. In accordance with the general principle of the right to self-determination, the law and therefore physicians are beginning to take seriously the idea that minors are entitled to some form of consent or dissent regarding the things that happen to them in the name of treatment, assessment, or other professional activities that have generally been determined unilaterally by adults in the minor's interest. When the consent of a minor is involved, the medical record and practitioner's notes should contain references to the conversations that preceded the consent and indicate that such consent was given knowingly, intelligently, and voluntarily. The mere signing of a form without a discussion of its contents is meaningless.

Knowing means that the minor understands the consensual meanings of the words and phrases of the discussion. In the discussion the physician should consider the minor's general intellectual capacity, familiarity with the content area, and linguistic background. The medical record should contain language indicating that the minor's developmental stage or maturity was adequate so as to enable him to consent to the treatment offered. Some such language may appear to be self-serving, but should a problem arise at a later date the medical record will be an excellent source of documented evidence.

There is little evidence that minors of age 15 and above, as a group, are any less competent to provide consent than are adults. In the age range of 11 to 14 years, existing research suggests caution regarding any assumptions about these minors' abilities to consider intelligently the complexities of legal alterna-

tives, risks and benefits, or to provide consent that is voluntary. Most research suggests that minors below age 11 generally do not have the intellectual abilities or are too prone to deferent response to satisfy a psychological interpretation of the legal standard for competent consent." *(Vierling, 1978).*

Thus the consent must be obtained if required, coordinated with the medical care involved, and reduced to writing in the medical history.

A few specific problems deserve mention. In a recent case, the United States Supreme Court held that a Missouri statute was unconstitutional because it provided for parental veto of an abortion decision made by a minor who was pregnant. *(Planned Parenthood v. Danforth,* 428 U.S. 52, 96 S.CT. 2831, 1976.) Also, there is some discussion concerning contraception advice for the child less than 16 years of age. Should the physician notify the parent or guardian that "the pill" has been prescribed? There would seem to be little danger that the physician would be prosecuted for his silence. Also, a physician could probably perform an abortion on a minor without the consent of the parents, the minor's husband, or the biological father. This is an evolving branch of law and the latest cases should be reviewed before making a decision.

INFORMED CONSENT—ELEMENTS

Consent is clearly needed prior to the medical treatment of any person in a nonemergency situation. When a malpractice claim is based on the failure of the patient to give informed consent, it is not sufficient for the defendant to offer expert opinion showing an adequate standard of care. The mere touching of a patient, if unauthorized, is a sufficient cause for a malpractice suit in and of itself. Furthermore, the phrase "informed consent" is a redundancy. Consent, if uninformed, is not consent at all in the legal sense of the word, and touching as a result of an uninformed consent can give rise to the civil tort of assault and/or battery under the theory that every person has a right to determine what should be done with his or her body.

The consent process should ideally include the following items:

1. A description of the proposed treatment in language that can be understood by the patient, his guardian, and/or his parents.
2. Alternatives to the proposed treatment.
3. Risks of death or serious bodily injury in the proposed treatment.
4. Problems of discomfort and recuperation that are anticipated.
5. Any additional information that other physicians would ordinarily disclose in similar circumstances.

The physician must disclose all information pertinent and relevant to the decision-making process, i.e., risks which would lead a reasonable person, in the patient's circumstances, to decline the treatment or to accept it. The physician concerned with protecting himself or herself legally should err on the side of overinforming.

The consent of the parent or child is presumed in an emergency and is implied when the parent does not object to procedures which are simple and whose risks are either common knowledge or extremely remote and commonly appreciated as remote. Also, a parent who, for personal reasons, wishes to place the responsibility for treatment solely in the hands of a physician can waive consent and ask not to be informed. For therapeutic reasons the physician can determine that it is in the patient's best interest not to be informed, in which case the medical record should substantiate the facts that support the physician's judgment. Should a patient not be competent to consent, an appropriate guardian must be judicially appointed to provide consent.

As previously noted, the obvious incompetence of most children requires that someone speak for them in consenting to medical care. This authority has generally been assigned to parents, but there are several circumstances in which this might be questioned. Parental consent is questioned in matters involving sexuality when the child is either emancipated or a ma-

ture minor with sufficient intelligence to understand the nature and consequences of the treatment to which he is consenting. Parental consent may not be legitimate when the parent appears not to be acting in the best interest of the child, as when the physician observes gross abuse or neglect. Where abuse, neglect, or child battering is observed, the law imposes additional legal restraints and affirmative duties on any person who has cause to believe that a child's physical or mental health has been or may be adversely affected. Failure to report abuse or neglect is a criminal offense and may also give rise to civil liability.

EMANCIPATION

An individual under the age of majority is a minor. Majority varies from state to state, generally from 18 to 21 years of age. The disabilities of minority may be removed by operation of law in several ways, so that the minor may consent to medical care as if he had reached the age of majority.

Emancipation describes the situation in which a child moves from dependence on his parents to economic self-sufficiency. This may also include medical independence. Emancipation occurs when the child enters into a valid marriage, reaches the age of majority, enlists for active duty with the military, or meets the criteria of a statute that the legislature has enacted to confer certain of the rights of majority on those below the general age of majority. If the child meets any of these requirements, conferral of the rights of majority is automatic; no further parental or state action is necessary. Again, the question is one of status. The status of the child must first be determined; then the appropriate consent can be obtained.

THE BATTERED OR ABUSED CHILD

The PICU must constantly be on the alert to recognize, diagnose, and report child abuse, often referred to as the "battered-child syndrome" (see Chapter 79). The battered-child syndrome describes the plight of young children who have suffered intentional, repetitive, and severe physical injuries inflicted by their parents or parent substitutes. All fifty states have enacted child abuse reporting laws which require physicians to report suspected incidents of child abuse to local protective departments or to the police. To stimulate disclosure, these statutes typically make the reporting physician immune from slander, libel, breach-of-confidentiality, or right-of-privacy lawsuits instituted by outraged parents. Moreover, in the majority of states, failure to report could result in criminal sanctions.

Some state laws also impose tort liability if a physician negligently fails to diagnose and report child abuse, based on the theory of the dual goals of tort liability: financial deterrence for careless behavior and compensation for injuries caused by such negligence. This civil liability arose in part because of the dearth of cases that imposed criminal liability on physician-defendants for failure to report. Civil liability thus afforded a greater possibility of relief to the child-plaintiffs, acting through their parents or court-appointed guardians *ad litem*. The civil cause of action and trial would, of course, be for money damages.

In tort cases the plaintiff must prove the presence of traumatic symptoms, the failure to diagnose, and the lack of treatment, including the failure to report, causing further injury to the child. General principles of tort law involve the issue of proximate cause and forseeability, i.e., that failure of the physician to act caused additional harm to the child and that the harm caused was forseeable.

There are specific circumstances that should alert all PICU staff to the possibility of child abuse, i.e., when the battered-child syndrome is appropriate as a formal diagnosis. Physical injuries resulting from abuse usually include cuts, burns, bruises, abrasions, contusions, shock, lacerations or ruptures of internal organs, scratches, multiple scars, hemorrhage, subdural hematoma, and fractures. The signs of

child abuse may also include malnutrition, anemia, poor skin hygiene, soft tissue swelling, and hematomas for which there is no plausable explanation. Child abuse victims are usually too young to defend themselves, and a majority are less than 3 years of age. The offenders are from all strata of society and, as a rule, have been apparently normal persons. The PICU intake person must relate the observable medical facts to the history given. Careful interviewing and recording are essential. All evidence must be documented, including photographs, if possible. Implausable explanations for injuries cannot be accepted at face value. The determination of whether a reasonably prudent physician, confronted with the infant or child's symptoms, would have suspected the battered-child syndrome, confirmed that diagnosis, and promptly reported the findings to authorities is to be made based on expert testimony and not as a matter of law. PICU staff persons must be trained to become familiar with the battered-child syndrome, since immediate state action can often protect the child from further harm by fostering medical treatment, removing the child from the home, and rehabilitating the offender. Medical personnel must be willing to make the personal time commitment involved in the litigation that results from the reporting. The ramifications of abuse are both legal, medical, and time consuming. A table listing child abuse prevention and treatment programs in each state appears in *The Legal Status of Adolescents, 1980* (Table 10C, p. 299).

MALPRACTICE

Malpractice has become an ogre on the medical horizon. Legal theory might indicate that medical practice would improve so long as each physician practiced with an awareness that negligence could lead to litigation and financial damages. There is some question as to the validity of this theory, since insurance provides pecuniary insulation and the litigation is more of a harassment or an annoyance. Nevertheless, no hospital, nurse, physician, professional corporation, or allied health professional can ignore the realities. Citizens are becoming more litigious and malpractice actions will continue to be filed against medical practitioners with increasing frequency.

Malpractice is to be distinguished from breach of contract or breach of warranty. These causes of action arise when a physician promises a result or makes a statement in contract form and the other person relies on the statement. Doctors can only offer reasonable care. They cannot warrant or guarantee results and should not offer unrealistic assurances. In addition, they should be aware that physicians have been liable for assault and battery, false imprisonment, defamation of character, fraud, invasion of privacy, and the infliction of mental distress. These are not common to the PICU practitioner but are still areas of potential liability that deserve mention.

Medical malpractice or negligence occurs when a health care provider fails to follow an accepted standard of care and fails to exercise that degree of care, skill, and learning expected of a reasonable, prudent health care provider in the same profession or class and acting in the same or similar circumstances, and such failure was the proximate cause of the injury. In the PICU context the standard encompasses not only medical care, but also failure to report child abuse, whether or not sufficient medical care was offered.

The standard of care or level of medical competence is based on a nationwide standard. Unless otherwise provided by statute, general practitioners are held to the standard of general practitioners and specialists are held to the standards of specialists with their particular medical expertise. Evidence of the level of competence which the practitioner should possess is offered on a case-by-case basis by an expert who by learning, training, and experience is qualified by the judge to offer opinion testimony. Until the judge accepts the witness as an expert, the witness may not offer opinion evidence or answer hypothetical questions. Thus, when a procedure or practice is called into question or reviewed, experts called by either or both adversarial parties testify concerning the state of the art and the application of the art to the particular patient.

The following four elements must be present in order for a plaintiff to recover damages due to negligence:

1. Duty to use due care: that a nurse/patient or physician/patient relationship exists; not a social or informal conversation or relationship.
2. Breach of that duty: failure to conform to or departure from a specific duty owed to the patient; negligently treating the patient.
3. Injury, including mental anguish.
4. Proximate cause: a causal relationship between the defendant's (e.g., nurse's, physician's) conduct and the damage suffered (i.e., the conduct caused the damage).

Physicians are liable for their own actions and are further liable for the actions of their employees when the employees are acting in the course and scope of their employment. In addition to possible liability for the acts of their employees, physicians might also be held liable when they refer cases to other physicians not in their employ. In general, physicians are not liable when substitute physicians or specialists take over their cases; but if they are careless in selecting the substitutes or specialists, they will be liable for their own negligence. If physicians continue to participate in the treatment of their patients, their legal status will be that of joint venturer, and they will be liable for the negligence of the other physicians. When there is a legitimate difference of opinion concerning medical treatment, the options available must be presented to the consenting party so that he or she can weigh the information, the risk and benefits, and make a decision. The risk of decision making rests with the party offering informed consent. The physician is responsible for seeing that the treatment is performed properly.

The major legal risks of hospitals include the duty to supervise and manage all employees, to select competent physicians, to avoid self-dealing and conflict of interest, to provide adequate facilities and equipment, to provide adequate insurance, to provide satisfactory patient care, to select a competent administrator, and to provide a safe working environment. Hospitals are liable for negligent acts of their employees that are committed within the scope of the employees' duties and obligations.

The major risks for physicians include lack of documentation, failure to properly diagnose, inadequate workup, treatment outside the field of competence, mistaken identity, misdiagnoses, abandonment (failure to follow up on acute patient care after the acute stage of the illness has subsided, or neglecting to give a patient or parents warnings or necessary instructions, premature termination of treatment, failure to ensure a patient's understanding that further treatment of a complaint is necessary), failure to obtain informed consent, failure to seek consultation or refer to a medical specialist, failure to choose alternative procedures, failure to order roentgenograms, failure to guard against infections, aggravation of an existing condition, misrepresentation and/or unnecessary surgery, and premature dismissal of a case.

The major legal risks of nurses include improper administration of drugs; failure to follow a physician's orders; failure to report significant changes in the patient's condition; failure to take correct telephone orders; sponge or instrument miscounts; burns by improper use of hot water bottles, sitz baths, heating pads, etc.; patient falls; failure to report defective equipment; failure to follow established procedures; and even the loss of patient valuables.

The above lists can be used by PICU personnel when reflecting on hospital, physician, or nurse liability. These lists are by no means inclusive, but they are designed to highlight areas that deserve medical concern. There are case precedents in all these areas.

EMERGENCIES

In most emergency situations the hospital or treating physician should make a reasonably diligent attempt to obtain the authorization of a relative and, failing to do so, may wish to seek a court order if it could be procured without delay that would threaten the life or seriously worsen the patient's condition.

But when treatment is required immediately to preserve the life of the patient or to prevent the impairment of the patient's health and it is impossible to obtain the consent of the patient or someone legally authorized to consent, the required procedure may be undertaken without any liability for failure to procure consent. Such a situation is an emergency, and the law furnishes the authorization to proceed with emergency medical treatment.

Since the existence of an emergency is a matter of fact, the hospital and the physician must make every effort to document the medical need for proceeding with treatment without consent. A consultation with a colleague or specialist should be ordered and the consultation documented if the physician has any question as to whether or not an emergency exists. The chart should indicate that a delay would result in greater injury. When an emergency exists and the parents refuse consent, this refusal should likewise be noted. Medical treatment may not be imposed on the children of nonconsenting parents. A court order is needed.

When a PICU is available in a community and holds itself out as offering emergency facilities, medical care cannot be refused to patients in an emergency situation, regardless of the patient-hospital history including the ability to pay or prior unpaid bills. Patients must be examined, diagnosed, and treated. Any PICU that establishes arbitrary standards for admission based on discrimination of any type would be extremely vulnerable should admission be refused and a patient's condition worsen. The hospital may establish standards based on its ability to treat patients and considering the facilities available.

PICU MEDICAL RECORDS

A medical record and chart should be established for every child presented to the PICU for examination, diagnosis, and treatment. Generally this includes data identifying the patient, a medical history, a provisional diagnosis, treatment notes, laboratory and tissue reports, formal diagnosis, and autopsy findings. The written record, like medical treatment in general, should meet current standards of professional practice. These standards will in most instances exceed specific legal requirements. The legal maxim "Absence of evidence indicates evidence of absence" applies especially to medical records. If a portion of the examination, diagnosis, or treatment is omitted from the record, that omission can be used as evidence that it did not take place.

Records should be confidential, secure, dated, current, authenticated, legible, and complete; the record department should be adequately directed, staffed, and equipped, and it should maintain a system of identification and filing to facilitate prompt location of each record.

The role of medical records personnel in patient care evaluation programs should be defined. Records should be signed, and spoken orders should later be reduced to writing and signed. The record should be completed shortly after discharge, and if a parent refuses to sign a discharge form or removes a child against medical advice, the circumstances of such removal should be clearly noted, together with accurate quotations from the parent that relate to the removal. Corrections must be lined out and initialed. Erasures or total obliterations should never be permitted. When a medical emergency is involved, the record should state all relevant data that lead to the conclusion that an emergency situation exists, and if the examination indicates battering or abuse, this too should be recorded together with a notation that the authorities have been alerted. In the PICU, as in other medical situations, the treating physician is expected to know what the record contains, especially immunities, allergies, or previous treatment.

Although hospital records are owned by the hospital, parents and court appointed guardians have a right to read, examine, and copy medical records at reasonable cost. The patient or his authorized representative has a legal right to the information in his medical record. Medical records are confidential. They should not be released without proper authorization or divulged to a third party without the consent of the subject of the information, his parent, or guardian. When used as a teaching tool, the medical record should be reviewed to ensure that the patient cannot be personally identified. Records are to aid the patient who has a right to be secure in the knowledge that his or her medical history is known only by the physician and those third parties with a legitimate concern or interest.

The accuracy and completeness of medical records cannot be overemphasized. They are the prime foundation of malpractice litigation. In most states they may be introduced into evidence by the affidavit and/or testimony of the medical records custodian or librarian as long as they are maintained in the regular course of business, each entry is made at or near the time of the act or event, and the records are maintained for the purpose they are intended to serve. Under these circumstances medical records are admissible as long as their authenticity is properly established. Microfilms would normally be admitted as evidence as would computer printouts.

Confidentiality

The discussions of minor's consent and record keeping touch on the issue of confidentiality of PICU medical records. The basic principle is that medical records and medical treatment are confidential. The contents or even the existence are to be revealed only to those parties who need to know and even then only with proper authorization for their release. Medical records may be released when the law requires them, such as in cases of child abuse, gunshot wounds, or reportable contagious diseases. Medical records, especially when established for children, form the beginning of a data bank that can follow a child for life, and for that reason extreme care must be taken in their creation, maintenance, and retention.

Invasion of privacy and wrongful disclosure of confidential information are wrongs that invade the right of a patient to personal privacy (e.g., when the patient is subjected to unwanted publicity). Hospitals, physicians, and nurses may become liable for invasion of privacy if they divulge information from a patient's medical record to improper sources or if they commit unwarranted intrusions into the patient's private affairs. A hospital could be sued for allowing pictures to be taken of a malformed or dead child. Comments concerning a patient's physical condition, as diagnosed by symptoms and reactions, should come from a physician and, since such matters involve protected information, all material to be disclosed should be with the specific permission of the parent, the mature minor when appropriate, a person *in loco parentis,* or a court-appointed guardian.

CONCLUSION

The PICU presents unique legal problems since the patient and the patient's rights in infancy are invested in third parties, parents, or guardians. As the infant matures, these rights change and more responsibility and authority shift to the child, who then has more input into his or her medical care. Finally, the child may become an adult by marriage, emancipation, or reaching the age of majority. The status of the child and the status of the law at the time of treatment should govern the actions of the PICU staff, and both vary from state to state and evolve constantly. This chapter has discussed general legal principles that affect the PICU. However, a lawyer familiar with medical law should be consulted whenever a specific problem arises.

ADDITIONAL READING

Brown, R.H.: The battered child, Medical Trial Tech. Q. 27:272-279, Fall 1980.

Clymer, J.N.: Torts: the battered child—a doctor's civil liability for failure to diagnose and report, Washburn Law Journal 16:542-551, Winter 1977.

Contraception and the under 16s, Br. Med. J. 281:318, July 1980.

Fast, N.: Informed consent. In Gelles, S.S., and Kagan, B.M., editors: Current pediatric therapy, Philadelphia, 1978, W.B. Saunders Co., p. 832.

Hoffman, A.D.: Is confidentiality in health care records a pediatric concern? Pediatrics 57:170-172, 1976.

The legal status of adolescents 1980, U.S. Department of Health and Human Services, Office of the Assistant Secretary for Planning and Evaluation, Washington, D.C., 1981.

Legal and Consent Manual, Austin, Tex., rev. 1971, Texas Hospital Association.

Leonard, J.J., Jr.: Medical negligence: perspective on the coming decade, The Forum 16:403-415, Winter 1981.

Life and death decisions about children—who has the right? Can. Med. Assoc. J. 123(1):54, 1980.

Mazura, A.D.: Negligence, malpractice—physicians' liability for failure to report child abuse, Wayne Law Review 23:1187-1201, March 1977.

Mnookin, R.H.: Children's rights: legal and ethical dilemmas, The Pharos 41(2):2, 1978.

Nehls, N., and Morgenbesser, M.: Joint custody: an exploration of the issues, Family Process 19(2):117-125, 1980.

Pozgar, G.D.: Legal aspects of health care administration, Germantown, Md., 1979, Aspen Systems Corp.

Southwick, A.F.: The law of hospital and health care administration, Ann Arbor, 1978, Health Administration Press, University of Michigan.

Texas family code, available from Business Management Division, Mail Code 413-X, Texas Department of Human Resources, P.O. Box 2960, Austin, Tex. 78769.

Vierling, L.: Minor's consent to treatment: developmental perspective, Professional Psychology 9(3):412, August 1978.

Warren, D.G.: Problems in hospital law, ed. 4, Germantown, Md., 1983, Aspen Systems Corp.

PART THREE
Equipment and techniques

81 The physical setting

DANIEL L. LEVIN

Each maximum intensive care bed should have a minimum of 75 square feet of floor space; 100 to 125 square feet per bed site is ideal. Mechanical ventilation and electrical monitoring with oscilloscopic display for heart rate, respiratory rate, and one, two, or three separate modes for pressure should be available at each bed site (Fig. 81-1). Each monitor should have the capacity for writeout either at the bedside or at a central station, and there should also be bedside and central station alarms. Each bed should be supplied with three oxygen, two air, and two vacuum outlets in addition to twelve regular electrical outlets and six grounding

sockets. In addition, there should be two monitor platforms with separate electrical outlets, a high-voltage x-ray outlet, two 220-amperage outlets for heating and cooling blankets, an intercom, a remote alarm system (residents' sleeping quarters, central station, recovery room), and individual light switches at each bed site. Electrical outlets should be identified numerically so that the corresponding circuit breaker can be found and switched by PICU personnel. Electrical outlets should be monitored for excessive current leakage, with an alarm to indicate when an electrically unsafe piece of equipment is in use. Each group of electrical outlets at one bed site should be connected to separate transformers so that the potential for losing all power at one site at one time is extremely low. All electrical outlets in the PICU should be on a backup emergency generator. The outlets at every patient module should be identical throughout the unit so that personnel can find the proper equipment, plug, or button almost instantly.

Adequate work space should be provided for clerks, aides, nurses, and physicians. Adequate space for offices, sleeping quarters, study, and storage should be provided. Provision of this type of space helps keep patient areas clean and uncluttered.

ADDITIONAL READING

Tooley, W.H., and Sutherland, J.M.: Hospital care of newborn infants, ed. 6, Evanston, Ill., 1977, American Academy of Pediatrics.

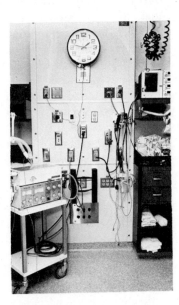

Fig. 81-1. Patient module.

82 Electrocardiographic and respiratory monitors

FRANCES C. MORRISS
CATHERINE P. MAST

INDICATIONS

All patients who are admitted to a PICU are unstable or potentially unstable. Rapid detection of abnormalities in vital signs is the key to preserving adequate organ function and eventual survival. Abnormalities in heart rate, ECG patterns, and respiratory rate are the most universally available signs for early recognition of major instability in the patient. These variables should be monitored continuously in all PICU patients.

TECHNIQUE
ECG monitoring system

The electrocardiograph is a device used to detect electrical activity of cardiac muscle and consists of a sensor system (electrodes), an amplifier, and a recorder. Since physiologic electrical activity is being measured directly, no transducer is needed.

Conduction of current through tissue occurs by migration of positive and negative ions from point to point. To measure the current in tissue, there must be a transfer of electrical energy from tissue ionic movements to electron conduction occurring in the measuring circuit. This transfer is accomplished by means of electrodes placed on or in the tissue whose electrical energy is to be measured.

The most common electrode used for continuous monitoring is the silver–silver chloride electrode, which consists of either a solid silver surface coated with a layer of silver chloride or a pellet of silver powder and silver chloride powder compressed together. The presence of the silver chloride prevents the formation of a large charge gradient between the electrode and the electrolyte solution (i.e., body surface) and increases the stability of the electrode by diminishing reaction between electrode and electrolyte. (Silver chloride dissociates into silver and chloride ions that migrate between the silver electrode and the electrolyte solution without significant transfer of charge or change in electrode potential.) Silver electrodes are preferred for use on the skin because they do not form toxic soluble metal salts with prolonged contact; tissue damage is minimal. Electrical stability of the electrode is maximized by mechanical stabilization of the electrode-tissue interface with the use of an electrolyte paste between the electrode surface and the skin.

Cardiac muscle contraction is accompanied by characteristic electrical events consisting of depolarization and repolarization (changes in electrical potential) of individual cells in response to impulses originating in the conducting system. Since these events occur almost simultaneously in the cells of the various chambers and produce a fairly uniform signal, the heart can be viewed as a generator of electrical impulses. This impulse formation can be recorded from the body surface because the body, which consists primarily of electrolyte solution, acts as a volume conductor. Thus, electrodes placed on the surface will detect changes in electrical potential generated elsewhere (e.g., in the heart); since the potentials so detected are of low amplitude, amplification is necessary to make the signal visible. In addition, a filtering system is incorporated in the amplifier to reduce "noise" (unwanted electrical signals). The American Heart Association standards provide for amplifier frequency response between 0.05 and 100 Hz, with low-frequency filtering between 0.05 and 0.14 Hz to eliminate patient motion and respiratory artifact, no filtering between 0.14 and 50 Hz, and high-frequency filtering above 50 Hz to eliminate 60-cycle alternating current and muscle artifact.

The amplified and filtered electrical activity in the form of a moving wave can then be displayed in a number of ways, the most usual being (1) continuous oscilloscopic display, (2) digital readout of heart rate computed from the QRS or T-wave deflection, and (3) continuous writeout of the waveform on paper to provide a permanent record. The recording equipment for this last method is usually remote from the patient's bedside. Standard ECG graph paper has vertical lines at 1-mm intervals with a recording speed of 25 mm/sec (thus, 1 mm equals 0.04 second) and a sensitivity of 10 mm vertical deflection per mV current produced. Physiologic bedside monitors usually are standardized to a sensitivity of 20 mm deflection per mV current produced, with a sweep speed of 50 mm/sec; however, sweep speed and degree of waveform deflection can usually be adjusted for individual needs. The configuration of the waveform so displayed depends on the placement of the electrodes (potential is measured as electrical activity between two electrodes on either side of the heart with reference to a zero electrode located remote from the heart). Standard placement includes electrodes on the right arm, right leg, left arm, and left leg, and a lead selector is incorporated into the system so that electrical potentials from different aspects of the heart (i.e., between different electrodes) can be analyzed according to the clinical situation. Most systems used in a PICU setting employ only three electrodes with no lead selection possible; in this case, electrode placement should be such to record maximal potential changes originating in the heart and consists of leads located at the base and apex of the heart (right upper lateral chest wall below the clavicle and left lower chest wall in the anterior axillary line below the point of maximal impulse formation), with the reference electrode being placed on the upper left chest wall. Such lead placement may need to be modified if simultaneous respiratory and ECG waveforms are being recorded from the same electrodes (see Fig. 21-1).

Proper technique for placement of the ECG electrodes includes (1) cleansing the appropriate areas on the chest with alcohol, (2) placing a small amount of conductive gel at each area of contact if pregelled disposable electrodes are not used, and (3) applying the electrode and lead wire firmly to completely dry skin.

Common problems seen are artifact, absence of ECG tracing, electrical interference, blurring of tracing, and nonadherence of electrodes to the skin. These may be eliminated by (1) recleaning the patient's skin with alcohol, (2) reapplying new electrodes, since the electrode gel may have become dried, (3) wiping off excess electrode gel, and (4) checking the electrode cable for breaks in insulation and proper attachment to the monitor. After correct placement of the leads and electrodes, the leads should be plugged into the lead cable, which contains three insertion points labeled RA (right arm), LA (left arm), and RL (right leg). Note that the ECG and respiratory tracings should appear clear and well defined. If the ECG or respiratory wave tracing is positioned too high or too low on the oscilloscope, no waveform will be seen. Absence of respiratory waveform may indicate that the electrodes measuring impedance are not on opposite sides of the thorax. If the monitor sensitivity control is set too low, the heart and respiratory rates may not appear. If a very small tracing is noted on the oscilloscope and no digital readout is seen, sensitivity may be set too low. If the respiratory module sensitivity is increased to a high level, the module may also sense the heart rate and override the apnea alarm. Sensitivity should be set as high as possible to detect most of the patient's breaths and avoid detection of weaker signals not generated by breaths. The monitor alarms should always be in the "on" position, and "high" and "low" alarm limits should be set appropriately for each child's age and condition so that tachypnea, apnea, bradycardia, and tachycardia can be readily detected.

Sources of error

Errors in measurement of electrical activity may be minimized by good design to decrease random error in circuitry and to increase stability of the baseline reference and the calibration system. Baseline stability is also increased by the methods of electrode stabilization referred to above. The response of the system in simulating the event being measured may be altered by the presence of noise (unwanted electrical signals that arise from sources other than the event being measured). Sources of noise may be (1) mechanical (vibration, physical impact), (2) electrical, arising from the monitoring system (thermal activity of components, failure to reject a common mode interference such as 60-cycle alternating current) or from the organism (action potentials from muscle, modulation of electrode output by the output of a second sensor), or (3) biologic, arising from events other than the one being measured that mechanically or electrically modify the desired signal.

Reduction of noise can be accomplished by stabilization of the device (permanent mounting, secure electrode application) to reduce mechanical noise, by filtration to reduce electrical noise, and by accurate electrode placement to maximize waveform, but biologic error and variations in physiologic variables cannot be eliminated. At the present time, the most common types of interference seen in a PICU are (1) 60-cycle/sec artifact, (2) artifact secondary to muscle contraction (shivering) or excessive patient movement, and (3) in the operating room, interference from the electrocautery.

Respiratory monitors

Methods of monitoring respiratory function that require patient cooperation and application of a breathing device (spirometry) or placement of a device in the airway are generally not useful in infants and children. Impedance pneumography provides continuous noninvasive surveillance of respiratory rate and pattern; although there is some correlation with depth of respiration, TV is not routinely measured by this method. Respiration can also be monitored by directly sensing the body motions that accompany breathing.

The impedance technique is based on the observation that variations of volume that occur within an electrical field during breathing are accompanied by changes in electrical resistance. When an alternating current source is used to create the electrical field, the measured resistance changes are called impedances and are measured as the changes appearing between a pair of electrodes placed on either side of the chest. With proper electrode placement, the impedance at 50 kc alters about 0.5% during quiet breathing. Thus, a small current passing through the chest is modulated by air entering and leaving the thorax.

By the use of suitable filtering circuits, ECG may be recorded from the same electrodes used to record transthoracic impedance, providing that electrode placement is appropriate. The measuring electrodes are placed on either side of the chest (anterior axillary line in the fourth or fifth intercostal space), with the reference electrode for the ECG placed on the manubrium or other suitable distant point. Oscilloscopic display of respiratory waveform often has a superimposed cardiac component that is easily identified if ECG and respiratory patterns are

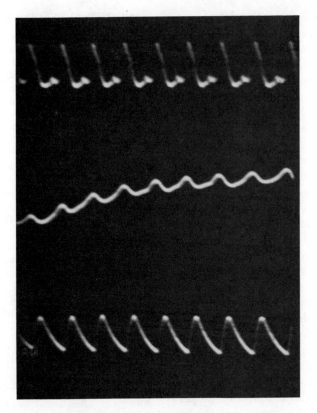

Fig. 82-1. Cardiac artifact in respiratory waveform *(top to bottom):* ECG, respiratory waveform with artifactual elevations corresponding to each heart beat, and systemic arterial blood pressure waveform.

displayed on the same screen (Fig. 82-1). The size of the respiratory waveform correlates grossly with the depth of respiration; thus, a patient receiving intermittent mandatory ventilation will have two respiratory waveforms: one arising from the ventilator and one from his own spontaneous activity. The inclusion of an alarm system that will signal if there is an absence of respiratory activity within a preset period (usually 6 to 10 seconds) allows this system to be used as an apnea monitor. Studies have shown an incidence of 2% false-positive alarms for apnea and 0% false-negatives with this system, so the sensitivity of the instrument is acceptable. It must be remembered that even with an obstructed airway, chest wall activity

due to respiratory efforts will register as respiratory activity in the absence of effective ventilation and will not trigger the alarm.

Electrode design (with the addition of a current source to create a known electrical field), amplification, and display characteristics are the same as described for ECG above. Sources of error in measurement are the same.

Breathing motions may be detected by (1) placing the patient on a pad or mattress that senses motion by displacement of air with weight shifts and converts it to an electrical signal, (2) monitoring changes in vertical pressure associated with respiration, (3) measuring capacitance change in wire mesh layers incorporated into a mattress, and (4) monitoring voltage alterations induced in a coiled wire secondary to movement of a magnet taped to the patient's abdomen or back. All these devices require that the patient lie on a sensing device usually incorporated into a mattress or pad. In general, these devices are less susceptible to cardiovascular artifact but may record physical impact, vibration, and body movements as breaths.

RISKS AND COMPLICATIONS

The main hazard in using an apnea alarm is too great a reliance on the device to detect respiratory problems; only absence of breathing will be detected. Obstructed or disorganized breathing must be detected by observation of the patient's efforts and by auscultation of breath sounds. Concomitant use of ECG to detect bradycardia may aid in detecting those apneic episodes that are accompanied by hypoxia and are therefore potentially life-threatening.

Any device that employs electrodes on the body surface can serve as a conductor of electrical energy to the patient from an outside source. All monitoring devices must be properly grounded and preferably should employ isolated circuitry so that such a situation does not arise. Should there be any doubt about grounding, the device should be disconnected during defibrillation or use of electrocautery. In addition, electrode placement may interfere with diagnostic roentgenograms, and patients with chest dressings may not be adequately monitored because of inappropriate electrode placement.

Patients with sensitive skin (e.g., premature infants) may display evidence of maceration, petechiae, or rashes beneath electrodes, especially if frequent changes are required.

ADDITIONAL READING

Daily, W.J.R., Klaus, M., and Meyer, H.B.P.: Apnea in premature infants; monitoring, incidence, heart rate changes and an effect of environmental temperature, Pediatrics **43**:510-518, 1969.

Emergency Care Research Institute: Evaluation: infant apnea monitors, Health Devices **4**:3-24, 1974.

Farman, J.V., and Juett, D.A.: Impedance spirometry in clinical monitoring, Br. Med. J. **4**:27-29, 1967.

Geddes, L.A.: The acquisition of physiological data in electronics in anesthesiology, Int. Anesthesiol. Clin. **3**:379-405, 1965.

Geddes, L.A., Hoff, H.E., Heckman, D.M., and others: The impedence pneumograph, Aerosp. Med. **33**:28-33, 1962.

Geddes, L.A., Hoff, H.E., Heckman, D.M., and others: Recording respiration and the electrocardiogram with common electrodes, Aerosp. Med. **34**:791-793, 1962.

Instrumentation Study Group: Electronic equipment in critical care areas. III. Selection and maintenance program, Circulation **44**:A247-A261, 1971.

Kramer, L.I.: Rapid accurate electrocardiogram and apnea monitoring, J. Pediatr. **87**:107-109, 1975.

Rudin, S.G., Foldvari, T.L., and Levy, C.K.: Bioinstrumentation—experiments in physiology, Millis, Mass., 1971, Harvard Apparatus Foundation, Inc., pp. 60-71.

Stein, I.M., and Shannon, D.C.: The pediatric pneumogram: a new method for detecting and quantitating apnea in infants, Pediatrics **55**:599-603, 1975.

Strong, P.: Biophysical measurements, Beaverton, Ore., 1970, Tektronix, Inc., pp. 1-26, 49-65, 219-247.

Uhl, R.R.: Monitoring: present concepts and future directions, Curr. Probl. Anesth. Crit. Care. **1**:1-47, 1977.

Vallbona, C.: Physiologic monitoring in children. In Ray, C.D., editor: Medical engineering, Chicago, 1974, Year Book Medical Publishers, Inc.

Wilber, S.A.: Errors in physiological measurement in electronics in anesthesiology, Int. Anesthesiol. Clin. **3**:407-416, 1965.

83 Pressure transducers

DANIEL L. LEVIN
CATHERINE P. MAST

INDICATIONS

In the PICU, pressure transducers are used to directly measure systemic and pulmonary arterial, left and right atrial, venous, esophageal, and intracranial pressures. Pressures should be measured directly when constant, accurate information is necessary because of the instability of the patient and the severity of his illness and when indirect or noninvasive measurements are impossible (e.g., LAP) or misleading (e.g., during peripheral vasoconstriction, funduscopic assessment of ICP).

TECHNIQUE
Transducers and strain gauges

1. By means of a linear relationship with a strain gauge, transducers convert mechanical or physical energy into electrical energy.
2. Physical input into a standard fluid-filled dome (or a miniature crystal) distorts a diaphragm (or the crystal) and stretches a small wire (strain gauge). The wire is charged with electrical current, and the stretch of the wire changes its resistance and therefore changes the amount of electrical current flowing through the device (Fig. 83-1, A). The diaphragm is sensitive and should not be touched with anything but fluid.
3. Redundantly isolated transducers have less chance of damage due to high electrical exposure during electrical cardioversion.

Amplification and recording

1. The electrical output produced by the change in resistance in the wire is small and noisy (full of irregularities).

2. Therefore, the signal is passed through a preamplifier to be filtered.
3. The signal then passes through an amplifier to be enlarged.
4. Then the signal passes to a recording or display device (digital or metered readout, oscilloscope, paper).

Zero

1. Attach the transducer to the input catheter and the pressure module.
2. By convention, zero for cardiovascular measurements is at the middle of the left atrium or midchest level.
3. Zero for ICP is at the level of the external auditory canal, which corresponds to the level of the third ventricle.
4. Turn the stopcock nearest the patient off to the patient and open transducer to room air.
5. Turn the zero dial so that the recorder reads zero.

Calibration

1. Most clinical recording devices have an electrical calibration that is done with the equipment in the zero position. This is the most convenient means of calibration.
2. Calibration is most accurately done by use of a mercury manometer. With the stopcock closest to the patient still turned off, insert the tubing from a mercury manometer into the system so that the pressure will be transmitted to the transducer. Pump up the mercury to 200, 100, 50, and 0 mm Hg and check the display or recorder for 200, 100, 50, and 0 mm Hg, respectively.

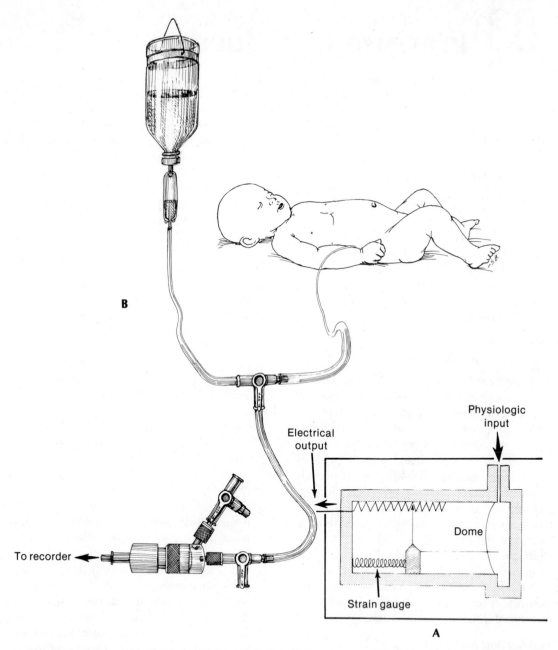

Fig. 83-1. A, Principle of the strain gauge. **B,** Intermittent arterial blood pressure readings with pressure transducer, fluid source, and three-way stopcock.

Oscilloscopic display

Catheter

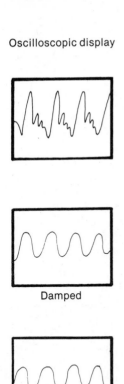

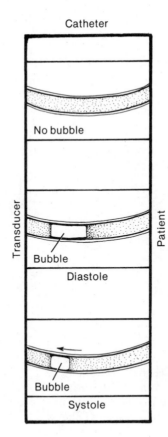

Damped

Damped

Transducer

Patient

No bubble

Bubble

Diastole

Bubble

Systole

Fig. 83-2. *Top,* With a fluid-filled catheter there is a normal systemic arterial blood pressure tracing with a dicrotic notch. *Middle,* With a bubble in the catheter, the tracing is damped. Note the size of the bubble during diastole. *Bottom,* During systole the bubble is compressed rather than transmitting the pressure wave along the fluid column. This accounts for the damped tracing.

3. Turn the stopcocks to close the transducer to air and to open it to the patient; the mercury manometer may be disconnected from the system.
4. Check the screen for a characteristic pressure wave (venous, arterial, intracranial).
5. Check the connections to be certain they are tight.
6. Check for gas bubbles or blood in the system. The presence of air or blood damps the pressure wave and therefore gives inaccurate readings (Fig. 83-2).

Fluid infusion

1. Recordings of pressure may be intermittent when a three-way stopcock is used (Fig. 83-1, *B*).

2. Readings may be continuous with the use of an Intraflow device. This plastic, disposable device has one portal to the input (patient) line, one to the fluid source (infusion pump or pressure bag), and one to the transducer. A resistance is interposed between the fluid source and the pressure transducer to allow continuous inflow of fluid from the fluid source to the patient and continuous display of the pressure (see Chapter 87). Always use a 3-ml/hr Intraflow when using a pressure bag. With a regulated infusion pump, a 3-ml/hr or a 30-ml/hr Intraflow may be used.
3. If the patient has more than one physiologic variable being measured, a manifold may be used to decrease the number of transducers needed. Label the catheters and tubing ap-

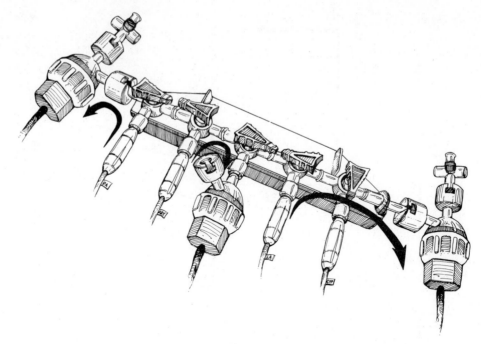

Fig. 83-3. This Cobe 5 stopcock manifold is connected to three transducers to give continuous readings of three pressure tracings simultaneously. High-pressure lines are connected on the left of the manifold, low-pressure lines on the right. In this illustration the PA (pulmonary arterial blood pressure) is displayed via the transducer on the left, and the ART (systemic arterial blood pressure) is displayed via the center transducer. On the right side either the LA (left atrial pressure) or the CVP (central venous blood pressure) can be displayed alternately by turning the stopcocks in the normal manner. Arrows indicate direction of flow from pressure source toward its transducer.

propriately so that medication or inappropriate infusions will not be given inadvertently (Fig. 83-3).

RISKS AND COMPLICATIONS

Indwelling catheters are always a possible source of infection, emboli, bleeding, and electrocution. Be especially careful to prevent introduction of air into catheters on the left side of the heart (e.g., left atrial catheters). Air emboli to the coronary arteries or brain may cause severe morbidity or mortality. The miniature crystal transducers and pressure bag reduce this risk. All electrical systems must be grounded and constantly monitored for excessive current leakage (>10 μamp). Catheters and pressure readings should be discontinued as soon as the patient is stable. If readings do not appear appropriate or are damped: (1) check the patient for stability, (2) check the level of the transducer, (3) check the connections to make certain they are secure, (4) check for blood in the catheter or transducer, (5) check for air in the catheter or transducer, (6) check for arterial spasm, and (7) gently aspirate and flush the catheter but do not forcibly dislodge a clot.

ADDITIONAL READING

Strong, P.: Biophysical measurements, Beaverton, Ore., 1971, Tektronix, pp. 93-100.

84 Infusion pumps

FRANCES C. MORRISS
DONNA S. BURNS

INDICATIONS

Infusion pumps may be useful for (1) ensuring constancy of the rate of infusion, as may be necessary with the administration of medication with a short half-life (e.g., catecholamines, insulin, lidocaine, thiopental), (2) ensuring constancy of volume administered per unit of time (e.g., TPN fluid, prevention of volume overload in the neonate), and (3) ensuring patency of the vessel, usually an artery.

TECHNIQUE

See also Chapter 111.

There are three types of constant infusion devices: one employing peristaltic propulsion of liquid through tubing sequentially compressed by rollers, one employing constant pressure on the plunger of a syringe, and one employing sequential low-volume filling from a volumetrically regulated cassette (i.e., slow constant-pressure infusion). In general, the cassette pumps provide greater constancy and accuracy of rate and volume to be administered. All types may be battery powered and all allow the rate of infusion to be changed. Battery operation provides for accurate delivery of fluids to the child during transportation between hospital departments. Pumps are available that will work on battery power for up to 8 hours and recharge within 20 to 30 minutes. Pumps are now available that can be set at a minimal rate of 0.1 ml/hr up to a rate of 999 ml/hr. Recent tests have shown that pump performance in terms of rate delivered is quite reliable, particularly when the infusion is given through a catheter as opposed to a butterfly needle of comparable diameter. A Metriset can be placed between the fluid source and the pump so that only 1 or 2 hours of fluid will be available for infusion. This protects the child from fluid overload should the pump malfunction. Some pumps are available with two sets of digital dials. One dial indicates the volume to be infused. This number corresponds to the amount of fluid contained in the Metriset to be infused over a 1- to 2-hour period. A second dial displays the rate at which the solution is to be infused. Most pumps incorporate specific alarm systems so that obstruction of the line, presence of air, low battery states, and completion of the infusion can be quickly identified. There is no reliable alarm as yet to detect the presence of infiltration.

RISKS AND COMPLICATIONS

Since most constant infusion devices do not employ a standard drip chamber, the patency of the catheter being used must be assessed at the site of insertion. The pump will continue to deliver fluid and medication despite an infiltration, and extravasation of medication or hypertonic solution into the skin can be severe. In addition, the consequences of interruption of a constant infusion of medication if occlusion of the line occurs or if the pump is turned off must be recognized. Alternative routes for glucose, vasoactive or inotropic agents, etc., must be reestablished quickly to maintain normal vital signs in such instances.

Careful observation of a piggyback solution

is necessary when the solution is dripping in by gravity and the primary IV solution is being infused through the pump. When the piggyback solution is completely infused, air will be carried by the primary IV solution to the patient from the piggyback bottle unless there is a diaphragm to close over the outlet and thus prevent air from entering the tubing.

ADDITIONAL READING

Abernathy, C.M., and Dickinson, T.C.: Massive air emboli from intravenous infusion pump: etiology and prevention, Am. J. Surg. **137**:274-275, 1979.

Chow, A.E.: Syringe pump malfunction, Anaesthesia **36**: 523-525, 1981.

85 Radiant warming devices

FRANCES C. MORRISS
MARY E. GRANDY
LARRY T. JOHNSON

INDICATIONS

Standard closed incubators control infant temperature by recirculation of warmed and humidified air. Disadvantages of this type of device include loss of heated environment when the incubator is opened, potentially wide swings in incubator and infant temperature during on-off cycles of the heating element, noisy patient environment, and relative inaccessibility of the infant. Though temperature and humidity can be kept constant, heat loss by radiation through incubator walls still occurs. Warming by radiant energy in the infrared spectrum is at least as effective as a standard incubator in maintaining infant temperature within a range that minimizes oxygen consumption and calorie expenditure.

All objects warmer than absolute zero emit radiant energy, the quantity and quality of which depend on that body's temperature. Heat loss by radiation occurs by emission of heat to a colder object, and heat gain occurs by absorption of the radiant energy emitted from a warmer object. Radiant energy in the far infrared spectrum (3 to 13 μ) is an effective source of heat for the human body because it is almost completely absorbed by dry skin to a depth of less than 1 mm. Radiant energy with wavelengths of less than 3 μ is ineffective because a portion of the energy is reflected by the skin. Heating of the skin causes vasodilation with increased blood flow to the skin; heat is transferred from the surface to the blood and thus to deeper structures. Any impairment of peripheral circulation may result in an inability to dissipate heat from the skin surface.

A radiant warmer consists of an electrically heated element that emits radiation in the infrared region of the electromagnetic spectrum from a location above the patient. The element may be a quartz heating tube, coil, or light and may be incorporated into a free-standing unit or a fixed open incubator. The quartz heating source is preferred for the following reasons: (1) rapid heating time, (2) resistance to thermal shock, (3) insensitivity to drafts, and (4) no emission of visible light, which decreases heating efficiency and interferes with assessment of patient skin color.

Radiant warmer incubators have certain advantages, including (1) easy access to the patient, (2) ease of cleaning and lack of water source in the unit, (3) a more efficient servo-control mechanism than most closed incubators whose heater output operates on an on-off principle rather than an output proportional to a preset patient temperature, (4) absence of emission in the visible spectrum, and (5) maintenance of an even surface temperature and minimal energy loss due to scattering of radiation (achieved by use of a parabolic reflector to reflect divergent energy toward the patient surface). Essential features that should be included in radiantly warmed incubators are: (1) uniform distribution of heat to the infant, (2) inability to heat the skin to temperatures greater than 45° C, the temperature at which direct tissue damage occurs, (3) emission of infrared energy be-

485

tween 3 and 13 μ, (4) adequate high and low patient-temperature alarms that cannot be silenced as well as an alarm for probe or heater-element malfunction, (5) constant display of infant skin temperature, (6) variable heater control mechanism (manual and automatic), (7) safe electrical conditions, including leakage current from the probe to the ground or from the chassis to the ground of less than 100 and 50 μamp respectively, inability of radiofrequency sources to interfere with the control unit, and inability of line voltage variation to interfere with heater output, and (8) convenient design features such as resistance to tipping, protection of the patient and personnel from hot surfaces, a tilting mattress, adequate work and storage space, space for roentgenographic plates, and phototherapy lights.

TECHNIQUE

1. If time allows, the incubator unit should be preheated. White linens will increase the efficiency of the unit (automatic control mode).
2. The infant should have a skin probe positioned appropriately as soon as he is placed in the incubator so that skin temperature monitoring (which controls the heater output) can be measured (manual servocontrol). The set point for the heater output is usually a skin temperature of 36.5° C for a term infant and 37° to 37.5° C for a preterm infant. The skin probe should never be placed between the infant and the mattress, because the probe will sense both the infant and mattress temperature and thus affect heater output. An adhesive strip covered with a heat-reflecting substance (foil) is preferred for attaching the probe to the skin; the skin thermistor is thus protected from sensing environmental heat. Only probes designed for a specific unit should be used with that unit; interchanging probes may alter heater output.
3. The manufacturer's recommendations for

maintaining proper space between the infant and the heating element should always be rigorously observed, especially with free-standing units.
4. The infant should never be left unattended in an open incubator and should never be left in an incubator without a probe attached.
5. Initially, the infant's axillary temperature should be checked frequently (every 30 to 60 minutes) to determine the particular temperature needed to keep the infant warm and to adjust the rate of heating if the infant was chilled. Once a stable thermal state has been achieved, temperature may be checked less frequently (every 2 to 4 hours). Probe position should be checked during every shift.
6. Sudden infant temperature changes, once rechecked, should be investigated.

Risks and complications

Overheating is the most serious complication of radiant warmers; undetected hyperthermia can result in permanent neurologic damage or death. To avoid this complication, radiant warmers must have adequate alarm systems, nursing personnel must be thoroughly familiar with the use of the manual and automatic control modes determining heater output as well as with thermistor placement, and a regular maintenance program to check heater output must be followed. In addition, conditions such as hypermetabolic states and inadequate peripheral circulation may predispose to overheating; alternate sources of temperature control should be utilized for such patients whenever possible. Portable units (warming lights) should always be placed at a proper distance from the patient's skin surface to avoid overheating and skin burns.

Increased insensible water losses, increased resting heat production, and increased oxygen consumption have all been documented in infants nursed in open radiant warmers. Fluid requirements may increase from 20% to 50%, particularly with the concomitant use of phototherapy lights. Consequently, fluid and electrolyte balance must be closely monitored.

The main adverse biologic effects attributed to infrared radiation are cataracts, flash burns of the skin from intense sources, and heat stress. The warm sensation occurring on the skin when radiant energy is absorbed normally provides adequate warning of overheating; however, an infant in a radiant warmer cannot respond to such an endogenous signal. In the near infrared spectrum (wavelengths greater than 1.4 μ), the cornea and aqueous humor absorb increasing amounts of radiation; at wavelengths greater than 1.9 μ, the cornea is the sole absorber. This energy is conducted to the interior of the eye, where heating of the iris and adjacent tissue is thought to induce opacities in the crystalline lens. Retinal lesions may be produced when energy of 0.7 to 1.5 μ in parallel rays is concentrated (by a factor of 100,000) by the cornea and focused on small areas of the retina. Sensory nerve endings in the cornea, iris, and internal ocular structures are very sensitive to temperature changes, which elicit pain and subsequently a protective blink reflex. However, with use of a continuous source of radiation, blinking may not provide adequate ocular protection. Because radiant warmers provide a drying environment, corneal scarring secondary to drying may also result, particularly if lid closure is impaired. To date, cataracts and retinal damage have not been reported in infants cared for in radiant warmers, but specific studies designed to investigate this point have not been done. Specific careful observation of the eyes for adequate blinking and closure should be included in routine nursing care of an infant in a radiantly warmed incubator.

Skin damage, specifically burns, has been documented in infants with poor peripheral circulation and in patients placed too close to the heat source. In addition, excessive drying of the skin may occur, particularly in very small preterm infants with delicate skin; such drying may predispose the patient to tissue breakdown over pressure points (buttocks, elbows, heels).

ADDITIONAL READING

Agate, F.J., and Silverman, W.A.: The control of body temperature in the small newborn infant by low-energy infrared radiation, Pediatrics **31**:725-736, 1961.

Bell, E.F., Gray, J., Weinstein, M.R., and Oh, M.H.: The effects of thermal environment on heat balance and insensible water loss in low-birth-weight infants, J. Pediatr. **96**:452-459, 1980.

Bell, E.F., Weinstein, M.R., and Oh, W.: Heat balance in premature infants: comparative effects of convectively heated incubator and radiant warmer, with and without plastic heat shield, J. Pediatr. **96**:460-465, 1980.

Committee on Environmental Hazards: Infant radiant warmers, Pediatrics **61**:113-114, 1978.

Infant radiant warmers, evaluation, Health Devices **3**:4-23, 1973.

Levison, H., Linsao, L., and Swyer, P.: A comparison of infrared and convective heating for newborn infants, Lancet **2**:1346-1348, 1966.

Marks, K.H., Gunther, R.C., Rossi, J.A., and Maisels, M.J.: Oxygen consumption and insensible water loss in premature infants under radiant heaters, Pediatrics **66**:228-232, 1980.

Ortiz, A., Knudson, R.P., Alden, R.E., and others: Oxygen consumption of infants under infrared radiant energy warmers, Pediatr. Res. **11**:539, 1977.

Porth, C., and Kaylor, L.: Temperature regulation in the newborn, Am. J. Nurs. **78**:169-193, 1978.

Sliney, D.H., and Freasier, B.C.: Evaluation of optical radiation hazard, Appl. Optics **12**:1-24, 1973.

Whiteside, D.: Proper use of radiant warmers, Am. J. Nurs. **78**:1694-1696, 1978.

86 Temperature-sensing devices

FRANCES C. MORRISS

INDICATIONS

Temperature is a measure of the intensity of heat, a physical property generated by the movement of the molecules (kinetic energy) composing any substance. A change in temperature of a substance may produce a change in one or more physical characteristics of that substance. All temperature-sensing devices, known as thermometers, are based on such changes.

Temperature is measured in terms of degrees, with the temperatures at which water boils (boiling point) and freezes (freezing point) being used as the fixed points from which the rest of the scale is determined. The two most commonly used scales are the Fahrenheit (°F), on which the freezing point is 32° and the boiling point is 212°, and the Celsius (°C), on which the freezing point is 0° and the boiling point is 100°. These two scales may be interconverted by the following equations:

$$°F = (°C \times {}^9/_5) + 32$$
$$°C = (°F - 32) \times {}^5/_9$$

Several physiologic temperatures may be of interest: (1) core (a reflection of basal metabolic energy production), usually measured in the rectum, mouth, or esophagus, (2) skin, and (3) CNS, measured in the nasopharynx or at the tympanic membrane. The mode of monitoring may be continuous or intermittent, depending on the degree of temperature aberration or the use of a servocontrol mechanism (see Chapter 18). In complex situations such as internal organ cooling or regulation of thermal environment, multiple temperature sensors (skin, esophageal, rectal) may give a truer picture of temperature and temperature gradients in patient.

TECHNIQUE AND SPECIFIC DEVICES

The most commonly used temperature sensors utilize the thermoexpansive and thermoresistive principles in transducing temperature.

Thermoexpansive thermometer

The prototype of all thermometers is the mercury thermometer, based on the volume expansion of a liquid that occurs with an increase in temperature. Mercury is used in thermometers that measure mammalian temperature because of its physical characteristics: (1) rapid heat conduction, (2) low freezing point (−40° C) and high boiling point (+357° C), so that mercury remains in a liquid state over a wide range of human, environmental, and physiologic conditions, (3) uniform and relatively large expansion per unit rise in temperature, (4) opacity, which increases visibility, and (5) cohesiveness when in contact with glass. The device consists of three portions: (1) a large thin-walled bulb containing mercury (or other liquid), (2) a stem containing a small-volume capillary tube attached to the bulb for expansion or contraction of the mercury as it heats or cools, and (3) a scale, usually etched in the glass stem. When the bulb of the thermometer is placed in contact with the medium to be measured, heat transfer occurs quickly through the thin wall of the bulb, and the fluid in the reservoir reaches equilibrium with the surrounding medium. Liquid in the reservoir then expands or contracts, forcing liquid into or out of the capillary tube. Most such thermometers have scales between 94° and 106° F and are inappropriate for measurement of extremes of temperature. In addition, they are easily broken, have relatively slow response, and cannot be used for continuous or remote temperature recording. Mercury thermometers are most useful for calibration purposes and in the care of patients with contagious diseases.

Thermistors (thermoresistive thermometers)

Certain conductors of electricity will exhibit an alteration in conductance with a concurrent change in temperature. Such a conductor can be used to transduce temperature, which is sensed by measuring the conductor's electrical resistance, the reciprocal of conductance. Most thermistors are oxides of heavy metals formed by fusing the powered oxide into rods, beads, or plates at high temperatures; the usual oxides are of nickel and manganese (NiO, Mn_2O_3), which have a sensing range of $-60°$ to $+100°$ C. They are extremely sensitive to small changes in temperature. When the flexible temperature probe tip, which contains heavy metal oxide attached to an insulated wire and leads to the monitor, is inserted into the medium to be measured, a change in electrical resistance occurs in the probe, and this change is measured by a Wheatstone bridge. Current flowing through the meter (directly calibrated for temperature) is proportional to the resistance in the measuring limb of the bridge, which in turn is proportional to the temperature of the transducer probe. To be accurate, the probe must be in direct contact with the medium being measured. Thermistors have a rapid response and are small, lightweight, inexpensive, and very sensitive to small temperature changes. Disadvantages include (1) instability (resistance in the probe gradually increases with time), (2) fragility because of its small size, and (3) nonisolated circuitry despite battery operation, which makes some types unsuitable for use with electrosurgical or defibrillating devices. This type of device is commonly employed in the continuous measurement probes used in servocontrolled incubators and heating blankets and in standard intermittent measurement sensors.

Adhesive strips containing liquid crystals sensitive to changes in skin temperature are available for monitoring trends. Changes in the crystals induce changes in numbered color indicators on the strip ranging from 86° to 102° F. Use of this device must be correlated with a more accurate thermistor or thermometer.

RISKS AND COMPLICATIONS

The main complication encountered in measuring temperature is inaccuracy due to inappropriate measurement technique. False elevations occur when the sensor is placed close to large blood vessels or other high-flow organs (e.g., over the liver, in the stomach). False depressions occur when (1) good thermal contact is prevented by feces or placement over a bony structure, (2) the temperature measured is iatrogenically altered (e.g., an esophageal probe may measure the temperature of cool gases in the trachea of a patient on mechanical ventilation or the temperature of cold gastric lavage fluid or cold blood being transfused into the right atrium; an improperly insulated skin probe may measure environmental temperature), or (3) a skin probe is used in the presence of vasoconstriction. In case of uncertain measurements, core temperature measured orally, rectally, or in the axilla should be obtained for verification.

Probes placed for the purpose of continuous measurement may cause mechanical irritation (skin breakdown, tympanic membrane rupture, nasal or anal ulceration) and, if they contain nonisolated circuitry, may provide a path for electrical current through the body.

ADDITIONAL READING

Dornette, W.L.: Thermometry in clinical practice, Int. Anesthesiol. Clin. 3:473-488, 1965.

Kuzucu, E.Y.: Measurement of temperature, Int. Anesthesiol. Clin. 3:435-449, 1965.

Levine, D.S.: Thermometry in anesthesia, Clin. Anesth. 2:108-118, 1964.

Schneider, A.J.L., Apple, H.P., and Braun, R.T.: Electrosurgical burns at skin temperature probes, Anesthesiology 47:72-74, 1977.

87 Arterial catheters

DANIEL L. LEVIN

CATHERINE P. MAST

INDICATIONS

Indwelling systemic arterial catheters are used in acute situations in patients who are unstable or potentially unstable for (1) frequent sampling of blood to determine oxygen and carbon dioxide tensions and pH, (2) continuous display of systemic arterial blood pressure, both numerically and by waveform, (3) exchange transfusion (at the withdrawal site), (4) rapid atraumatic accurate blood sampling for frequently obtained tests (e.g., serum electrolytes, Ca, Hb, Hct, serum acetone, and blood clot for type and crossmatch). The last is a relative indication and is usually not the sole indication for an indwelling arterial catheter.

TECHNIQUE
Site

1. In newborns, the umbilical arteries may be used and a polyvinyl chloride or Silastic catheter is introduced into the abdominal aorta. This route is preferred in emergency circumstances, in the delivery room, and in the PICU because the vessels are easily exposed and the catheter usually is easily introduced, even by the least experienced individuals. Because of a high complication rate with these catheters (13.5%), some authors no longer recommend their use in an elective situation when there is sufficient time to introduce a catheter into a small peripheral artery (complication rate of less than 1%) (Table 87-1).
2. For administration of medications (antibiotics, sodium bicarbonate, calcium) or glucose solutions in a concentration greater than 10%, the umbilical artery is not the route of choice because these compounds may cause damage directly to the aorta. A peripheral IV may be inserted for medications or a venous catheter with the tip in the superior or inferior vena cava or in the right atrium should be used for glucose in high concentrations.
3. Peripheral arteries such as the radial, posterior tibial, dorsal pedal, and temporal are the preferred sites (in that order). The brachial arteries and rarely the axillary arteries may also be used; however, because they are end arteries with larger areas of distribution, they are used infrequently.

Equipment (Fig. 87-1)

Umbilical artery catheterization

1. Single end-hole polyvinyl chloride (Argyle) catheters, either #3.5 French (for less than 1,500 g body weight) or #5.0 French (for more than 1,500 g body weight) in diameter. Smooth, soft Silastic catheters are also being produced.
2. An 18-gauge blunt needle.
3. Luer-Lok disposable stopcock (Pharmaseal K-69).
4. A 4-foot Luer-Lok Cobe tubing.
5. A 30-ml/hr disposable Intraflow (Sorenson Laboratories) or Bentley disposable monitoring system at the end of the Cobe tubing.
6. A constant infusion fluid source (I-Med pumps).

Table 87-1. Complications of arterial catheters

Umbilical artery
1. Bleeding from loose connections
2. Infection, local and systemic
3. Emboli to kidneys, bowel, spinal cord, and extremities
4. Spasm of iliac arteries
5. Thrombus formation with partial or complete occlusion of the aorta and its branches
6. Perforation of vessels with hemorrhage
7. Arterial intimal damage from trauma
8. Infusion of hypertonic and irritating solutions into misplaced catheters with necrosis of kidney, hip joint, buttock; hyperinsulinemia
9. Electrocution

Peripheral artery
1. Bleeding from loose connections
2. Infection, local or systemic
3. Local ischemia to small skin area
4. Arterial intimal damage with eventual occlusion of the lumen
5. Necrosis of distal parts due to infusion of hypertonic and irritating solutions
6. Electrocution
7. Possible cerebral embolism with temporal arterial catheters

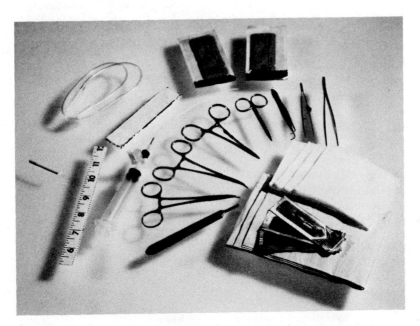

Fig. 87-1. Equipment necessary for umbilical artery catheterization (gauze sponges, suture, Dermick tape, and sterile measuring tape not shown).

7. A pressure transducer (see Chapter 83) and a pressure monitor.

8. Whatever fluid the infant will require, mixed with 1 unit of sodium heparin per 1 ml of fluid.

9. For introducing the catheter the following sterile instruments are needed on a sterile tray:
   a. Draping towels.
   b. Gauze sponges.
   c. A #11 surgical blade.
   d. Scalpel handle.
   e. A 4-0 silk suture on needle.
   f. Needle holder.
   g. Two 5-inch mosquito hemostats (very delicately curved).
   h. Toothed forceps.
   i. A 4-inch eye-dressing curved forceps.
   j. A 4-inch eye-dressing straight forceps.
   k. Small scissors.
   l. Dermick tape, 8 to 10 cm.
   m. A 5- to 6-ml syringe for flush solution.
   n. A 6- to 8-cm length of umbilical tape.
   o. Sterile measuring tape.

10. Good lighting.

11. Sterile gloves and surgical gown.

12. Surgical cap and mask.

Peripheral artery catheterization

1. A 22- or 24-gauge Deseret Teflon-coated Angiocatheter is adequate for all sizes of babies and has been introduced into the radial arteries of babies as small as 500 g. Larger catheters may be used in older children. It is rarely necessary to use a catheter larger than 20-gauge.

2. A 4-inch sterile Cobe tubing should be attached to the hub of the catheter so that the sampling port is not introduced directly onto the catheter. Sampling these few inches away will decrease movement of the catheter and prolong its life.

3. A 3-ml/hr intraflow or Bentley disposable monitoring system should be used on all peripheral arterial catheters.

4. All other equipment is identical to that used with the umbilical arterial catheters.

Catheter insertion

Umbilical artery (Fig. 87-2)

1. Monitoring of ECG, heart rate, and respiratory rate must be continued throughout all procedures.

2. Restrain the infant's legs and arms.

3. Clean the umbilical clamp, stump, and a wide area of the surrounding abdominal skin with an iodine solution for at least 2 minutes and allow to dry.

4. Drape the area so that only the umbilical cord is exposed.

5. Loosely place umbilical tape around the base of the cord. Do not include the skin. Do not tie the tape tightly. Tighten the tape only if there is bleeding.

6. Calculate 65% of the shoulder-umbilical length (add the length of the umbilical stump) and place the Dermick tape on the catheter at this distance from the tip. This should place the tip of the catheter at the third or fourth lumbar vertebra.

7. Cut the flared end of the catheter, insert the blunt needle, and attach the Luer-Lok stopcock.

8. Flush the stopcock and catheter with heparinized 0.9% sodium chloride solution (see above).

9. Use a scissors or surgical blade to cut the umbilical cord 1.5 to 2.0 cm above the skin, removing the cord clamp.

10. Hold the cord up with your fingers, the hemostats, or a toothed forceps.

11. Identify the umbilical arteries, which are small, thick walled, usually two in number, and caudally located on the cut cord surface.

12. Gently insert the closed tips of the curved eye-dressing forceps into the lumen of one artery until the bend in the forceps reaches the cut end of the artery. Allow the forceps

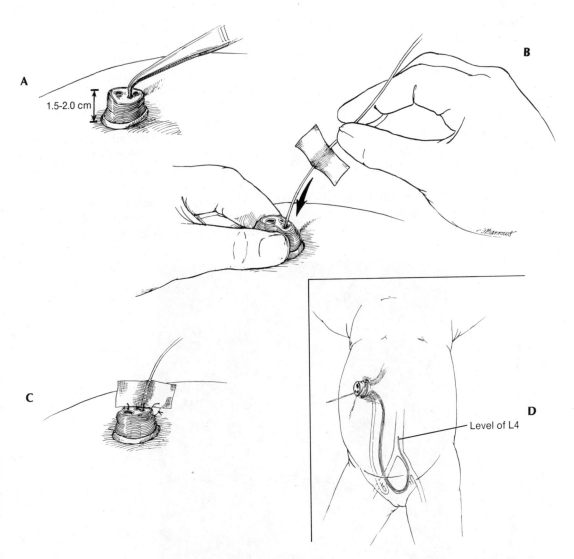

Fig. 87-2. Technique of umbilical artery catheterization: **A,** insert curved forceps into artery; **B,** introduce catheter to premeasured distance; and **C,** suture catheter into place. **D,** Course and proper position of tip of catheter.

to open and dilate the artery; repeat this several times.
13. Hold the catheter between the thumb and index finger or with the straight forceps about 1 cm from the tip and insert into the lumen of the artery.

14. Advance the catheter until the tape marker is at the cut surface of the cord. Use gentle, steady pressure if an obstruction is met, but do not force the catheter. Arteries can be perforated by the use of force. Normally the catheter will meet minimal or mild resis-

tance as it passes from the hypogastric artery into the femoral artery.

15. If the catheter cannot be advanced, try the other artery. If this is unsuccessful, consider an alternative route.

16. Once the catheter is in place, aspirate blood and any air and flush clear. Never introduce air into the catheter.

17. Flush the Cobe tubing with fluid and clear it of bubbles before connecting it to the catheter.

18. Attach the catheter to the 4-foot Cobe tubing and turn on the stopcock. Check the pressure waveform on the oscilloscope.

19. Observe the legs and buttocks for blanching, cyanosis, or mottling. Check the strength of the femoral pulses.

20. Suture the tape to the skin at the juncture of the abdominal wall and the umbilical cord. Use one suture on either side of the catheter (Fig. 87-2).

21. It is better to leave the cord exposed with a covering of iodine ointment so that it can be observed rather than to cover it with an occlusive dressing.

22. Obtain an anteroposterior roentgenogram of the abdomen to check the level of the catheter tip. It should be between the third

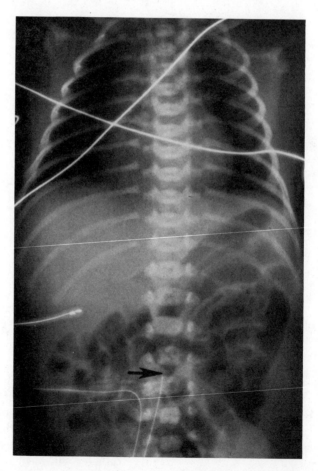

Fig. 87-3. Roentgenogram showing tip of umbilical arterial catheter at top of L-4.

and fifth lumbar vertebral bodies (Fig. 87-3. Higher catheters have an increased risk of thrombi and emboli to the kidneys, bowel, and spinal cord. Lower catheters or those turned posteriorly or inferiorly may cause vasospasm and ischemic necrosis of the hip or leg.

Peripheral artery

1. Fig. 87-4 shows the location of the various arteries.
2. Position the extremity on a small board, pad pressure points, and gently extend the wrist or ankle. If the temporal artery is used, shave the area.

3. Clean the skin for at least 2 minutes, using an iodine solution.
4. Drape the area with sterile towels.
5. Unless the patient cannot feel pain, use a 25-gauge needle and syringe to infiltrate the area with 1% lidocaine without epinephrine.

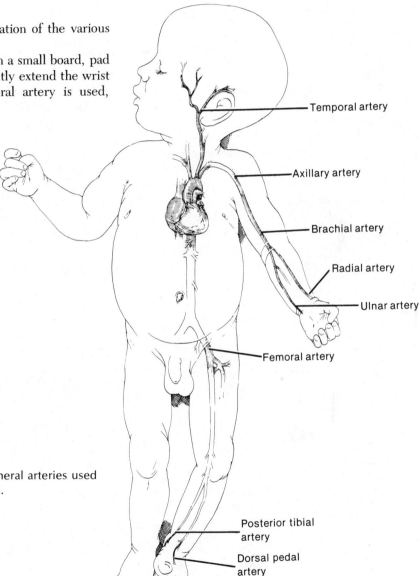

Fig. 87-4. Locations of peripheral arteries used for introduction of catheters.

Percutaneous catheterization

1. Palpate the artery, make a small skin incision using the tip of a 20-gauge needle, and thrust the catheter through the artery at a 30- to 45-degree angle (Fig. 87-5).
2. Slowly withdraw the catheter.
3. When blood is observed in the lumen of the catheter, hold the stylet and advance the catheter into the lumen of the artery. Withdraw the stylet.
4. Attach the 4-inch Cobe tubing.
5. Aspirate blood and flush the catheter and tubing with heparinized 0.9% sodium chloride solution.
6. Attach the 4-inch Cobe tubing to another 4-inch or a 4-foot Cobe tubing for easy placement of the equipment near the patient.
7. Attach the Intraflow or Bentley disposable monitoring system, fluid source, and pressure transducer.
8. Securely tape the catheter in place. Do not use an occlusive dressing. Leave the skin over the course of the catheter exposed to enable observation of blanching or inflammation.
9. Check the pressure waveform on the oscilloscope.

Surgical exposure of the artery (Fig. 87-6)

1. Palpate the artery and make a small (1.0 cm in infant, 2.0 cm in small children) skin incision perpendicular to the course of the artery.
2. Using the instruments on the umbilical arterial catheter tray, gingerly dissect out and identify the artery. *Be gentle.* Rough treatment of the vessel will cause spasm and make the procedure impossible.
3. Place 8- to 10-cm lengths of 4-0 silk suture around the artery at its proximal and distal points of exposure. *Do not tie the sutures.* Place hemostats around the loose ends so that the sutures can be used to control the artery if bleeding occurs.
4. Gently elevate the artery using a curved

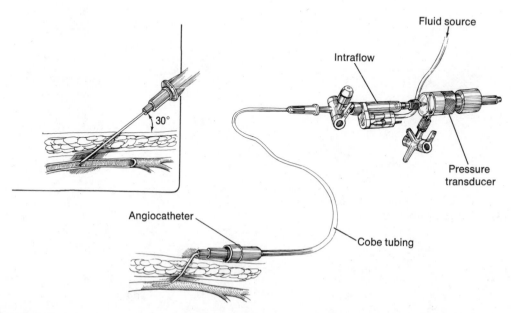

Fig. 87-5. Percutaneous peripheral artery catheterization. Thrust catheter through artery at a 30- to 45-degree angle to skin. Attach Cobe tubing to Intraflow and transducer.

hemostat or a curved eye-dressing forceps.
5. Apply gentle distal retraction using the distal suture.
6. Carefully introduce the catheter and stylet into the lumen of the vessel. Stop advancing the stylet as soon as the tip of the catheter is in the lumen. Hold the stylet and advance the catheter, applying gentle distal retraction with the suture.

7. Withdraw the stylet.
8. Observe blood in the hub of the catheter and attach the 4-inch Cobe tubing.
9. Aspirate blood and flush the tubing and catheter with heparinized 0.9% sodium chloride solution.
10. Never introduce air into the catheter.
11. Attach the Intraflow or Bentley disposable monitoring system, fluid source, and pressure transducer.
12. Check the arterial pressure waveform on the oscilloscope.

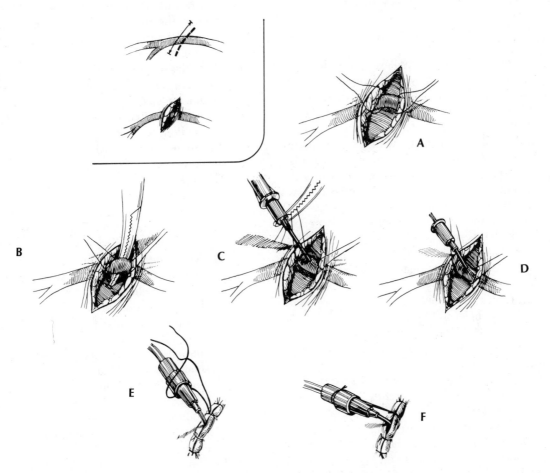

Fig. 87-6. Surgical exposure of peripheral artery: *inset,* make a small skin incision perpendicular to the course of the artery; **A,** place sutures around artery but do not tie them; **B,** gently elevate artery; **C** introduce catheter; and **D,** withdraw stylet. **E,** suture skin incision closed and, **F,** using long ends of suture, tie a knot around the plastic hub of the Cobe tubing connector.

13. Suture the skin together and, using the long ends of the suture, tie a knot around the white plastic hub of the Cobe tubing where it forms a Luer-Lok connection with the catheter hub (Fig. 87-6).
14. Suture the remainder of the skin incision closed and apply iodine ointment.
15. Tape the catheter in place.
16. If bleeding occurs, check all connections to assure proper fit. Bleeding may also be retrograde from a distal branch of the artery. A suture loosely applied and externalized through the incision may help control the bleeding.

Maintenance

1. Using the 3-ml/hr Intraflow or Bentley disposable monitoring system, keep the flow of heparinized solution into the catheter constant (0.9% sodium chloride solution in older children and 0.25% to 0.45% sodium chloride solution in infants, with 1 unit heparin per 1 ml fluid; glucose solutions may cause vasospasm, particularly in small arteries).
2. Frequently check the oscilloscopic display of the arterial blood pressure waveform. If the pressure tracing is damped or flattened or if the dicrotic notch is no longer visible:
   a. Check the patient to see that he is stable.
   b. Check to see that the stopcocks are turned correctly.
   c. Check the catheter system for loose connections or bubbles.
   d. Aspirate blood, check for small clots, discard if present, and gently flush the catheter system.
   e. Check to see that the catheter is not kinked or taped too tightly.
   f. Check the catheter for air bubbles and flush out any that are found.
3. Do not leave blood in the catheter for prolonged periods during sampling.
4. Check the skin or legs for signs of blanching, cyanosis, or induration.

5. *Do not infuse anything except the flush solution into a peripheral arterial catheter.* Papaverine as a continuous infusion or lidocaine, 0.5% or 1% (0.5 to 1 ml as a single dose), is sometimes instilled to decrease or prevent spasm.
6. Infection control concerning intravascular catheters and physiologic monitoring.
   a. A record should be kept to document the time and location of insertion of all catheters except percutaneous peripheral IV catheters.
   b. This record should be reviewed daily to evaluate the appropriateness of continued use of the catheter and the condition of the insertion site.
   c. Dressings on peripheral arterial catheters (as well as central venous catheters) should be changed on Mondays, Wednesdays, and Fridays. A dressing should be applied so that visualization of the skin immediately proximal to the insertion site is possible.
   d. The following procedure should be performed for all central and arterial catheters except for left atrial catheters.
      (1) Fluids infusing into the catheter should be changed every 24 hours.
      (2) The monitoring system down to the connector or short extension tubing should be changed Monday and Friday; this includes the Intraflow and the transducer dome.
      (3) When the monitoring device is discontinued, the transducer storage cap should be applied and the transducer gas-sterilized using ethylene oxide.
      (4) Immediately prior to assembling a monitoring system for use on a patient, the transducer should again be cleaned with Amphyl.
      (5) The transducer should never be stored with a used transducer dome in place.

(6) Any time back flow of blood occurs into the transducer dome, the system should be changed.

e. All unnecessary stopcocks should be eliminated from the catheter and transducer system.

Sampling arterial blood

1. Place a sterile 3×4 gauze pad under the stopcock closest to the arterial catheter.
2. Remove the injection cap from the sampling port of the stopcock and place the empty syringe in the stopcock port. If arterial blood gas tensions and pH are to be measured, the sampling syringe must initially be rinsed with a heparin solution. Be sure to leave no heparin solution in the syringe because large amounts of heparin mixed with the blood sample will alter the pH of the sample.
3. Turn the stopcock off to the fluid source.
4. Pull back gently on the syringe plunger and withdraw enough IV solution and blood to ensure that the catheter and stopcock are free of IV solution. The amount of blood it is necessary to withdraw varies with the volume of the catheter. When using a 22-gauge Angiocatheter and a 4-inch Cobe tubing, a minimum of 1 ml of blood must be withdrawn. In general, withdraw a volume equal to three times the volume of the system from the sampling port to the source of blood.
5. Turn the stopcock from the present position to halfway between this position and the syringe (45-degree angle, Fig. 87-7). This allows the syringe to be removed and replaced with a heparinized syringe without allowing blood to flow out of the stopcock or IV fluid to enter the catheter and mix with the patient's blood.
6. Remove the syringe with the blood and flush solution mixture, and place the syringe on the sterile 3×4 gauze pad.

7. Connect the heparinized tuberculin (1-ml) syringe to the stopcock sampling port.
8. Turn the stopcock off to the fluid source and withdraw 0.5 ml (or amount needed) of blood into the syringe.
9. Turn the stopcock to the 45-degree position.
10. Remove the syringe, cover it with a cap, and hold it upright, tapping it to expel any air bubbles. Avoid pulling room air into the syringe. The oxygen concentration in room air is usually higher and the carbon dioxide concentration lower than that in the blood sample. When the gases in the blood sample equilibrate with the room air bubble, the oxygen tension reading is usually higher and the carbon dioxide tension reading lower than the patient's true values.
11. Immediately place the sample in a cup of ice water and label the syringe with the patient's name, hospital number, sample time, and sample site.
12. Place the syringe with the blood and flush solution mixture into the stopcock sampling port and turn the stopcock off to the fluid source. Aspirate the catheter before returning blood to the patient, tapping any air bubbles up to the plunger end, and carefully return the blood from the syringe to the patient. Repeatedly discarding this volume of blood may contribute to anemia in patients, especially small babies.
13. After turning the stopcock to the 45-degree position, repeat step 12, using a small measured amount of flush solution to clear the catheter of blood.
14. Turn the stopcock off to the syringe, allowing the flow of IV fluid to the patient.
15. Remove the syringe and replace the sterile injection cap.
16. Record the amount of blood withdrawn and the amount of flush solution given to the patient. Record the respiratory support settings and the patient's temperature at the

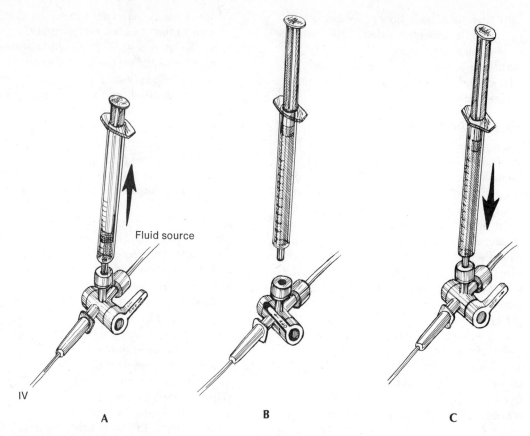

Fig. 87-7. Arterial blood sampling: **A,** turn stopcock off to fluid source and withdraw fluid and blood; **B,** turn stopcock to 45-degree angle and detach syringe; and **C,** after obtaining the blood sample, turn the stopcock off to fluid source and reinfuse the aspirated blood.

time of sampling (e.g., FI_{O_2} of 0.4, mechanical respirator at pressures of 20/4 cm H_2O and rate of 20/min, temperature 36.5° C).

Removal

1. Remove catheters when:
   a. The patient is stable and no longer requires frequent blood sampling or continous arterial blood pressure monitoring.
   b. The catheter is clotted.
   c. Any signs of infection occur at the catheter site.
   d. Any signs of vascular compromise occur in the area of or distal to the catheter.
   e. Most authors recommend removing umbilical arterial catheters after 1 week. Peripheral arterial catheters are also usually removed after 1 week but have been maintained for as long as 30 days without complication.
2. Umbilical arterial catheters should be removed slowly (1 cm every 3 to 5 minutes) over 20 to 30 minutes to allow the vessels to constrict and prevent bleeding.
3. Peripheral arterial catheters may be removed with gentle negative pressure applied at the stopcock to entrap and remove any clot that may be present at the tip.

4. Always inspect the catheter to see that the entire catheter was removed.

5. Always culture the tip of the catheter.

6. For peripheral arterial catheters, apply gentle, steady pressure to the arteriotomy site for 10 minutes after removal of the catheter.

7. Dress the site with a Band-Aid or gauze dressing and inspect it daily until healing has taken place.

RISKS AND COMPLICATIONS

Every indwelling catheter involves risk to the patient (Table 87-1). Although the bacterial colonization rate may be 25%, the septicemia rate may be as low as less than 1% for peripheral arterial catheters. Other major complications of peripheral arterial catheters are distinctly unusual when attention to the fluids infused and care of the catheter is appropriately given. Carefully assess the benefits of the information gained by the use of the catheter versus the risks to the patient. *Never infuse anything but the flush solution into a peripheral arterial catheter.* Used judiciously, arterial catheters supply a vast amount of critical information. Used recklessly, these catheters can be fatal.

ADDITIONAL READING

Adams, J.M., and Rudolph, A.J.: The use of indwelling radial artery catheters in neonates, Pediatrics **55**:261-265, 1975.

Adams, J.M., Speer, M.E., and Rudolph, A.J.: Bacterial colonization of radial artery catheters, Pediatrics **65**:94-97, 1980.

Barr, P.A., Sumners, J., Wirtschafter, D., and others: Percutaneous peripheral arterial cannulation in the neonate, Pediatrics **59**(suppl. 6, part 2):1058-1062, 1977.

Bauer, S.B., Feldman, S.M., Gellis, S.S., and Retick, A.B.: Neonatal hypertension: a complication of umbilical-artery catheterization, N. Engl. J. Med. **293**:1032-1033, 1975.

Book, L.S., and Herbst, J.J.: Intra-arterial infusions and intestinal necrosis in the rabbit: potential hazards of umbilical artery injections of ampicillin, glucose, and sodium bicarbonate, Pediatrics **65**:1145-1149, 1980.

Boros, S.J., Nystrom, J.F., Thompson, T.R., and others: Leg growth following umbilical artery catheter-associated thrombus formation: 4 year follow-up, J. Pediatr. **87**:973-976, 1975.

Boros, S.J., Thompson, T.R., Reynolds, J.N., and others: Reduced thrombus formation with silicone elastomere (Silastic) umbilical artery catheters, Pediatrics **56**:981-986, 1975.

Brown, D.R., Fenton, L.J., and Tsang, R.L.: Blood sampling through umbilical catheters, Pediatrics **55**:257-260, 1975.

Bull, M.J., Schreiner, R.L., Garg, B.P., and others: Neurologic complications following temporal artery catheterization, J. Pediatr. **96**:1071-1073, 1980.

Cartwright, G.W., and Schreiner, R.L.: Major complication secondary to percutaneous radial artery catheterization in the neonate, Pediatrics **65**:139-141, 1980.

Clark, J.M., and Jung, A.L.: Umbilical artery catheterization by a cutdown procedure, Pediatrics **59**(suppl. 6, part 2):1036-1040, 1977.

Cole, F.S., Todres, I.D., and Shannon, D.C.: Technique for percutaneous cannulation of the radial artery in the newborn infant, J. Pediatr. **92**:105-107, 1978.

Fan, L.L., Dellinger, K.T., Mills, A.L., and Howard, R.E.: Potential errors in neonatal blood gas measurements, J. Pediatr. **97**:650-652, 1980.

Ford, K.T., Teplick, S.K., and Clark, R.E.: Renal artery embolism causing neonatal hypertension, Pediatr. Radiol. **113**:169-170, 1974.

Galvis, A.G., Donahoo, J.S., and White, J.J.: An improved technique for prolonged arterial catheterization in infants and children, Crit. Care Med. **4**:166-169, 1976.

Goetzman, B.W., Stadolnik, R.C., Bogren, H.G., and others: Thrombotic complications of umbilical artery catheters, Pediatrics **56**:374-379, 1975.

Hecker, J.F.: Thrombogenicity of tips of umbilical catheters, Pediatrics **67**:467-471, 1981.

Henry, C.G., Gutierrez, F., Lee, J.T., and others: Aortic thrombosis presenting as congestive heart failure: an umbilical artery catheter complication, J. Pediatr. **98**:820-822, 1981.

Hoekstra, R.E., Semba, T., Fangman, J.J., and Strobel, J.L.: Intestinal perforation following withdrawal of umbilical artery catheter. J. Pediatr. **90**:290, 1977.

Kitterman, J.A., Phibbs, R.H., and Tooley, W.H.: Catheterization of umbilical vessels in newborn infants, Pediatr. Clin. North Am. **17**:895-912, 1970.

Krishnamoorthy, K.S., Fernandez, R.J., Todres, I.D., and DeLong, G.R.: Paraplegia associated with umbilical artery catheterization in the newborn, Pediatrics **58**:443-445, 1976.

Lehmiller, D.J., and Kanto, W.P., Jr.: Relationships of mesenteric thromboembolism, oral feeding, and necrotizing enterocolitis, J. Pediatr. **92**:96-100, 1978.

Malloy, M.H., and Nichols, M.M.: False abdominal aortic

aneurysm: an unusual complication of umbilical arterial catheterization for exchange transfusions, J. Pediatr. **90:** 285-286, 1977.

Mayer, T., Matlak, M.E., and Thompson, J.A.: Necrosis of the forearm following radial artery catheterization in a patient with Reye's syndrome, Pediatrics **65:**141-143, 1980.

Nagel, J.W., Sims, J.S., Aplin, C.E., II, and Westmark, E.R.: Refractory hypoglycemia associated with a malpositioned umbilical artery catheter, Pediatrics **64:**315-317, 1979.

Phibbs, R.H.: Supportive care of the premature and sick newborn infant. In Rudolph, A.M., editor: Pediatrics, ed. 16, New York, 1977, Appleton-Century-Crofts.

Plumer, B., Kaplan, G.W., and Mendoza, S.A.: Hypertension in infants: a complication of umbilical arterial catheterization, J. Pediatr. **89:**802-805, 1976.

Rajani, K., Goetzman, B.W., Wennberg, R.P., and others: Effect of heparinization of fluids infused through an umbilical artery catheter on catheter patency and frequency of complications, Pediatrics **63:**552-556, 1979.

Simmons, M.A., Levine, R.L., Lubchenco, L.O., and Guggenheim, M.A.: Warning serious sequelae of temporal artery catheterization, J. Pediatr. **92:**284, 1978.

Todres, I.D., Rogers, M.C., Shannon, D.C., and others: Percutaneous catheterization of the radial artery in the critically ill neonate, J. Pediatr. **82:**273-275, 1975.

Tooley, W.H.: What is the risk of an umbilical artery catheter? Pediatrics **50:**1-2, 1972.

Tooley, W.H., and Myerberg, D.A.: Should we put catheters in the umbilical artery? Pediatrics **62:**853-854, 1978.

Tyson, J.E., deSa, D.J., and Moore, S.: Thromboatheromatous complications of umbilical arterial catheterization in the newborn period: clinicopathological study, Arch. Dis. Child. **51:**744-754, 1976.

88 Pulmonary artery catheters

LAWRENCE J. MILLS

INDICATIONS

The ability to place catheters in the pulmonary artery allows determination of pulmonary arterial blood pressure and cardiac output as well as calculation of pulmonary vascular resistance. Pulmonary artery catheters are indicated for children with congenital heart disease who are undergoing surgery and in whom the pulmonary vascular resistance is elevated preoperatively (e.g., atrioventricular canal, VSD, truncus arteriosus). These catheters should also be used in patients with a variety of medical disorders including shock, congestive heart failure, and acute respiratory failure, particularly involving noncardiogenic pulmonary edema. Elevation of pulmonary arterial blood pressure is an indication for modification of pulmonary vascular resistance with drugs. With the use of a pulmonary artery catheter, the efficacy of this treatment by measurement of PAP, cardiac output, and mixed venous oxygen content can be immediately assessed.

TECHNIQUE
Surgical route of insertion

Two surgical routes of insertion are available.

1. Direct insertion of a small-gauge catheter or thermodilution probe can be accomplished through a pledgeted purse-string suture in the right ventricular infundibulum. The catheter tip can easily be advanced across the pulmonic valve. The other end of the catheter is passed out to the right of the lower portion of the sternotomy incision to avoid confusion if a left atrial catheter is also employed. These catheters can easily be removed in the early postoperative period with a minimal incidence of hemorrhage.

2. A second route is through a peripheral vein, with a catheter threaded into the right atrium before sternotomy. The tip of the catheter is retrieved through the atrium and threaded through the right ventricle into the pulmonary artery. The advantage of this technique is a somewhat safer removal postoperatively.

The care of pulmonary artery catheters is not as demanding as that for left atrial catheters. Drugs and blood can be administered through this route. Although the usual precautions are taken to eliminate air from the system, the danger of systemic embolism is remote, since the lungs provide an effective filtering action.

Percutaneous placement

Percutaneous placement of pulmonary artery catheters may be facilitated by the use of a wire guide (Desilets-Hoffman spring guide) and the Seldinger technique. The advantages of this technique include (1) avoiding a cutdown, (2) ability to use the internal jugular, external jugular, femoral, or subclavian vein and avoid the difficulties associated with catheterization of antecubital veins, and (3) ease of placement.

The flexible, usually Teflon, catheter may have three or four lumens. The lumen of the distal tip is the main catheter lumen and is used for measuring blood pressures, sampling blood, and infusing fluid; it extends from the tip to the catheter connector. A smaller lumen parallels the major one and terminates in a balloon located 1 mm from the distal tip. When inflated, the balloon assumes a concentric shape that protects the tip from impinging on vascular structures and promotes flow-directed movement of the catheter through the cardiac chambers. The third lumen ends proximal to the balloon and may be used for sampling or injecting or infusing fluid. The fourth lumen incorporates a thermistor. Sizes range from #3 to #8 French.

Placement technique

1. Prepare the skin antiseptically and infiltrate subcutaneously with 1% lidocaine. For the location of particular veins, see Venous cutdowns, p. 511. Sterile technique should be employed from this point.
2. If neck veins are used, place the patient in a slight Trendelenburg position to fill the vein and minimize the possibility of air embolization. Be certain a separate IV is available for giving antidysrhythmic medication.
3. Perform venipuncture with a syringe and needle or a plastic catheter over the needle unit to identify the appropriate large central vein.
   a. A small-gauge needle, usually 21 gauge, is used to minimize the size of puncture in the vessel wall.
   b. A thin-walled needle with a base plate for stabilization commonly used for roentgenographic procedures may be helpful.
4. Insert a flexible wire guide through the needle into the vein lumen and remove the introducing needle or IV catheter.
   a. The flexible-tipped guide minimizes the likelihood of perforating the posterior wall of the vein.
   b. The coiled outer wire over a semirigid central core facilitates insertion.
5. Thread the pulmonary artery catheter introducer sheath and dilator over the wire guide with a twisting motion, taking care not to dislodge the wire guide. To help place this larger catheter, the following techniques may be used:
   a. Enlarge the cutaneous puncture site slightly with a #11 scalpel blade.

   b. With a twisting motion, insert a tapered dilator and sheath over the wire guide into the vein lumen. Remove the dilator and wire guide. Sterile IV fluid should be flushed through the pulmonary artery catheter and it may then be threaded through the dilator sheath into the vein.
   c. Many catheter introduction kits include a sterile, transparent sleeve that fits into the introducer sheath. When the pulmonary artery catheter is threaded through this sleeve, a long segment of the catheter remains sterile and hence may be safely manipulated in or out at a later time (e.g., after chest roentgenogram).
6. Advance the catheter until the tip reaches the area of the superior vena cava or right atrium and inflate the balloon with the manufacturer's recommended volume. Do not use a large volume. The catheter is marked every 10 cm to facilitate estimation of length inserted.
   a. The integrity of the balloon should be ascertained before catheter insertion by inflating and deflating it with air while it is submerged in a sterile liquid.
   b. Carbon dioxide is preferred for balloon inflation because of its high blood solubility. Rupture of the balloon and subsequent embolization of gas are thus minimized. Air may also be used, but fluids or contrast media should not. Carbon dioxide will diffuse through the balloon at a rate of 0.5 ml/min, and the balloon should be deflated and reinflated every minute to ensure the catheter's flow-directed characteristics.
   c. If the balloon is intact, the syringe plunger will be forced backward after inflation. If there is no back pressure, remove the catheter and inspect the balloon.
7. Monitor the blood pressure tracing from

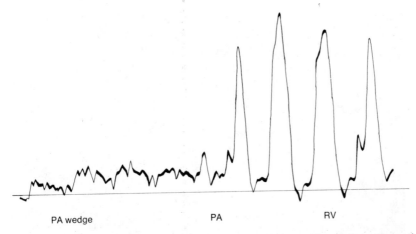

Fig. 88-1. Pressure tracing recorded during pullback of a Swan-Ganz catheter from the pulmonary artery to the right ventricle in a patient with residual right ventricular outflow tract obstruction.

the distal lumen port while advancing the catheter. With the balloon inflated, the flow of blood in the right atrium and ventricle will direct the catheter tip (being slowly advanced) into the pulmonary artery. Characteristic blood pressure waveforms for the right atrium, right ventricle, and pulmonary artery should be sequentially identified. (See Fig. 88-1).

   a. If the characteristic pressure tracing for the pulmonary artery is not identified, withdraw the catheter into the right atrium with the balloon deflated and repeat the advancement procedure.

   b. Deep inspiration by the patient during catheter advancement may be helpful.

   c. Direct fluoroscopy may be needed if catheter placement cannot be accomplished.

   d. Knotting of the catheter may occur within the ventricle, and estimation of the catheter length inserted may indicate an excess (Fig. 88-2).

8. In the wedge position, the characteristic pulmonary artery blood pressure tracing will be abolished (Fig. 88-1). Deflate the balloon and record the volume of air pres-

ent in the wedge position. Slowly reinflate the balloon to reconfirm the correct position. If the full inflation volume for the balloon is required to obtain a wedge pressure, advance the catheter 1 to 2 cm with the balloon deflated and recheck the position by reinflating the balloon. The catheter should not assume the wedge position and corresponding wedge pressure waveform without inflation of the balloon. If it does, this position is too peripheral.

9. Monitor blood pressures.

   a. Never inflate the balloon with a larger volume than that required to obtain a wedge pressure. Overdistention of a pulmonary artery branch can cause vessel rupture.

   b. Do not leave the balloon inflated for any amount of time (i.e., pulmonary wedge pressure should be measured on an intermittent, not a continuous, basis). Occlusion of the vessel by the balloon may lead to a pulmonary infarct.

   c. Monitor pulmonary arterial blood pressure continuously (with the balloon deflated); this is the only way to identify accurately the migration of the catheter

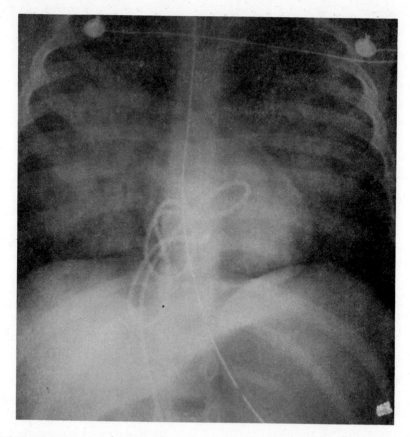

Fig. 88-2. Chest roentgenogram of a near-drowning patient during attempt at Swan-Ganz catheter placement. The catheter became knotted in the heart but could be withdrawn to the femoral vein and was removed using a venotomy.

tip into a more peripheral wedge position. If the waveform assumes the wedge configuration continuously, withdraw the catheter until the pulmonary arterial blood pressure waveform reappears.

10. Confirm the catheter position with a chest roentgenogram initially and daily thereafter.

11. Dress the insertion site with iodine ointment, sterile gauze, and tape after sewing the catheter sheath to skin. Note the total length of the catheter (in centimeters) that was introduced into the patient.

12. The catheter should be removed after 72 hours or when pulmonary arterial blood pressure monitoring is no longer needed.

RISKS AND COMPLICATIONS
Immediate

1. Dysrhythmias (self-limited PVCs in 19% of placement attempts; other, more severe dysrhythmias in 3%).
2. Inadvertent carotid artery puncture.
3. Hematoma formation.
4. Pneumothorax.
5. Removal of catheters placed directly through the pulmonary artery. These catheters may rarely manifest bleeding when removed.
6. Sampling errors.

Sampling errors can be significant. Recent studies have confirmed that eccentric balloon inflation can occur in catheters placed peripherally; removal of the catheter to a larger, less peripheral artery causes concentric inflation. Eccentric inflation due to peripheral position either may cause no change in the pressure waveform (catheter tip at vessel bifurcation) or may indicate a gradually increasing mean blood pressure, both of which are factitious. Eccentric inflation can be a cause of vessel rupture, especially if the catheter has been in place for some time so that multiple balloon inflations have occurred, causing erosion of the vessel wall. Another source of error is an inaccurate mixed venous oxygen determination ($P_{\bar{v}O_2}$ higher than normal) when the sample comes from the distal catheter sampling port. The catheter in the wedge position may sample pulmonary capillary blood (i.e., arterialized blood) rather than mixed venous blood, which should be obtained by withdrawing the catheter or sampling from a more peripheral lumen. Mechanical ventilation, particularly with high levels of CPAP (>12 cm H_2O) or inspiratory pressure may cause the correlation between PCWP and LAP to be poor because of changes in pulmonary vascular resistance. This error may be minimized by measuring PCWP at end-expiration with the ventilator disconnected momentarily or by averaging values obtained at end-expiration over several heart beats. The rate of ventilation must be slow enough to identify a stable period of end-expiration or the patient must hold his breath. Catheter migration over time may also account for changing values of pulmonary arterial and wedge pressure. For this reason, catheter tip location should be reconfirmed daily by a roentgenogram.

Long-term

The incidence of these complications, particularly infections, increases significantly after 72 hours.

1. Infection confirmed by positive blood culture occurs in 5% of patients; 4% show local inflammation at the site of the catheter introduction.
2. Pulmonary infarction and/or embolization occurs but may be minimized by strict attention to the details of catheter placement and wedge pressure determination. The recent introduction of catheters (Saf-T-Coat, USCI Cardiology and Radiology Products, Billerica, Mass) constructed of a polymer plastic with heparin bonded to the surface may reduce complications related to thrombus formation.
3. Aseptic right-sided endocarditis and endocardial mural thrombosis have been reported, especially when the catheter is left in place for long periods.
4. Rupture of a peripheral pulmonary vessel can occur with catheter placement that is too peripheral and/or with forced balloon inflation or overinflation, particularly in patients with pulmonary hypertension and vasoconstriction of pulmonary vessels.

Mechanical

1. Balloon rupture.
2. A coiled or knotted catheter, which occasionally occurs within a cardiac chamber (Fig. 88-2).
3. Failure of catheter to pass pulmonary valve (more common in children).

ADDITIONAL READING

Blitt, C.D., Wright, W.A., Petty, W.C., and others: Central venous catheterization via external jugular vein: a technique employing the J-wire, J.A.M.A. **229**:817-818, 1974.

Conahan, T.J., Schwartz, A.J., and Geer, R.T.: Percutaneous catheter introduction: the Seldinger technique, J.A.M.A. **237**:446-447, 1977.

Hoar, P.F., Wilson, R.M., Mangano, D.T. and others: Heparin bonding reduces thrombogenicity of pulmonary artery catheters, N. Engl. J. Med. **305**:993-995, 1981.

Katz, J.D., Cronhue, L.H., Barash, P.G., and others: Pulmonary artery flow-guided catheters in the post-operative period, J.A.M.A. **237**:2832-2834, 1977.

Pace, L.N.: A critique of flow-directed pulmonary arterial catheterization, Anesthesiology **47**:455-465, 1977.

Prince, S.R., Sullivan, R.L., and Hackel, A.: Percutaneous

catheterization of internal jugular vein in infants and children, Anesthesiology 44:170-174, 1976.

Shapiro, H.M., Smith, G., Prebble, A.H., and others: Errors in sampling pulmonary arterial blood with a Swan-Ganz catheter, Anesthesiology 40:291-296, 1974.

Shin, B., Ayella, R.J., and McAslon, T.C.: Pitfalls of Swan-Ganz catheterization, Crit. Care Med. 5:125-127, 1977.

Sise, M.J., Hollingsworth, P., Brimm, J.E., and others: Complications of the flow-directed pulmonary artery catheter: a prospective analysis of 219 patients, Crit. Care Med. 9:315-318, 1980.

Sorenson Research Corporation: Arterial wedge pressure catheter, pp. 1-4.

Swan, J.J.C., Ganz, W., Forrester, J., and others: Catheterization of the heart in man with use of a flow directed balloon-tipped catheter, N. Engl. J. Med. 283:447-451, 1970.

89 Venous catheters

DANIEL L. LEVIN

CATHERINE P. MAST

INDICATIONS

Venous catheters are used to measure central venous or right atrial pressure, to infuse large volumes of blood or fluid via a secure route, to infuse vasoactive drugs via a secure route, and to administer parenteral alimentation. In addition, venous catheters are used to administer routine solutions and drugs when percutaneous introduction of a needle or a catheter into a small vein is technically impossible. In the newborn, umbilical venous catheters are used for exchange transfusions.

TECHNIQUE
Site

1. In the newborn, the umbilical vein is occasionally catheterized for use in exchange transfusions. When the umbilical vein is used, the catheter tip should be placed in the inferior vena cava at its junction with the right atrium (Fig. 89-1).
2. Other veins used for catheters are the saphenous, antecubital, external and internal jugular, and rarely the axillary and superficial or deep femoral (Fig. 89-2).

Equipment

1. To catheterize the umbilical vein, prepare the same equipment used for umbilical artery catheterization (p. 490).
2. To catheterize peripheral veins, the following equipment is needed:
   a. Deseret catheters, 12 inches long in 22-, 19-, and 16-gauge sizes.
   b. A vein introducer (Becton-Dickinson) is helpful.

c. When venous pressure is measured, the remainder of the equipment necessary is similar to that described for arterial catheters (p. 490). When venous pressure is not being measured, only a fluid source with infusion pump is necessary.

Catheter insertion
Umbilical vein

1. Restrain the infant, clean and drape the area, and prepare the catheter as described for an umbilical artery catheter (p. 492). Do not place Dermick tape on the catheter.
2. Attach the catheter system to the fluid source and pressure transducer.
3. The umbilical vein is a single, large, thin-walled vessel on the cut surface of the umbilical cord, usually cephalad as one views the cut cord surface. Remove any clots from the orifice of the vein.
4. Introduce and advance the catheter until the pressure waveform indicates it is in the thorax. In the abdomen, there is little fluctuation of the pressure tracing and the pressure deflection is positive with inspiration (the diaphragm moving down). When the catheter moves through the ductus venosus into the inferior vena cava and the thoracic cavity, there is a recognizable atrial venous pressure wave with A and V waves and the deflection is negative with inspiration (negative intrapleural pressure). Do not open the catheter to atmospheric pressure. During deep inspiration, air can move through the catheter into the heart and kill the infant.
5. Apply the Dermick tape around the catheter

509

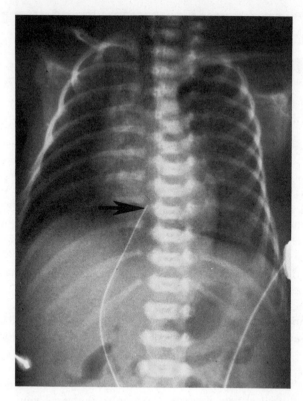

Fig. 89-1. Roentgenogram showing tip of umbilical venous catheter at inferior vena cava–right atrium junction.

at the umbilical cord surface, and secure the catheter in place as described for umbilical artery catheters (p. 494).

6. Obtain an anteroposterior roentgenogram of the chest and abdomen to confirm the location of the catheter tip.

Peripheral veins

1. Fig. 89-2 indicates the locations of the various veins.
2. Restrain the limb, clean the skin with an iodine solution, drape the area, and use lidocaine as with peripheral artery catheters (p. 495).
3. In small infants, use the instruments indicated for an umbilical artery tray (p. 490). In larger children, the larger-size instruments on a venous cutdown tray are more appropriate.

4. Prepare the catheter by attaching a Luer-Lok stopcock and flushing it with 0.9% sodium chloride solution.
5. Make a small (0.5 cm in infants, 1 to 2 cm in older children) incision perpendicular to the course of the vein (Fig. 89-3).
6. Gently dissect and identify the vein.
7. Place 8- to 10-cm lengths of 4-0 silk suture at the proximal and distal points of exposure of the vessel. Tie distal suture and clamp ends of sutures with hemostats.
8. Gently elevate the vein with a curved hemostat or curved eye-dressing forceps to maintain good visualization of the venotomy.
9. Apply gentle distal retraction using the distal suture.
10. Using a small scissors, make a small incision

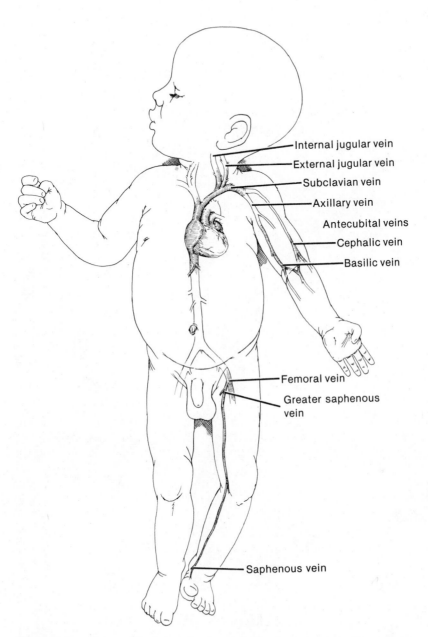

Internal jugular vein
External jugular vein
Subclavian vein
Axillary vein
Antecubital veins
Cephalic vein
Basilic vein

Femoral vein
Greater saphenous vein

Saphenous vein

Fig. 89-2. Locations of peripheral veins used for introduction of catheters.

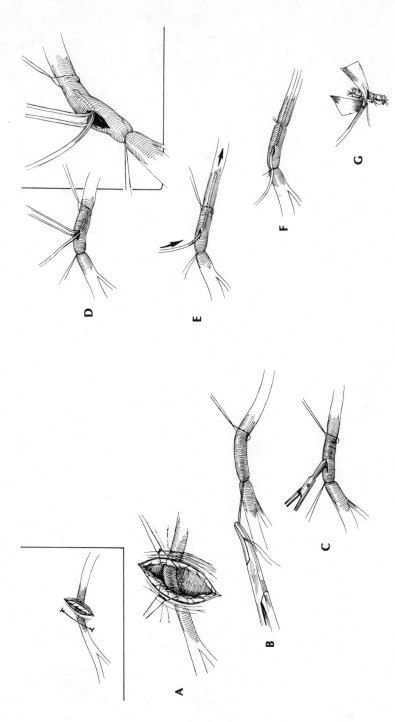

Fig. 89-3. Venous cutdown technique: *inset*, make a small skin incision perpendicular to the course of the vein; **A**, place suture around the vessel; **B**, tie the distal suture; **C**, make a small incision in the vessel; **D**, insert vein introducer and advance the catheter *(inset)*; **E**, remove vein introducer and advance the catheter; **F**, tie sutures around the catheter; and **G**, tape the catheter in place.

in the vein, being certain to cut into the lumen.

11. Insert the vein introducer into the lumen and advance the tip of the catheter under the introducer into the lumen.

12. Withdraw the introducer and advance the catheter.

13. When inserting the catheter into the thoracic cavity for pressure readings, note downward deflections of the pressure tracing with inspiration to confirm the location of the tip of the catheter.

14. Aspirate blood and flush the catheter.

15. Tie the proximal suture around the vein and the catheter. Tie the distal suture around the catheter.

16. Close the skin with sutures and apply iodine ointment.

17. Tape the catheter in place.

18. When introducing the tip of the catheter into the thoracic cavity for CVP readings or central parenteral alimentation, obtain a chest roentgenogram to confirm its location.

Maintenance

1. When obtaining pressure readings, attach the catheter to a 30-ml/hr Intraflow system and a constant infusion pump. If the catheter will also be used for fluid administration and the rate of infusion is to exceed 30 ml/hr, the continuous display of pressure by the Intraflow system cannot be used. Use 1 unit of sodium heparin per 1 ml of fluid in the solution.

2. When using the catheter for fluid administration, attach a simple fluid source or constant infusion pump.

Removal

1. Remove venous catheters when:
   a. The patient's condition no longer requires its use.
   b. Catheters have been in place for about 3 days (except those used for central parenteral alimentation). Use of this protocol may vary in some patients with limited venous access sites.
   c. When the catheter is clotted.
   d. Any signs of infection or phlebitis appear.
   e. Positive blood cultures are obtained with the catheter in place.

2. Always inspect the catheter to see that the entire catheter is removed.

3. Obtain a culture of the tip of the catheter.

4. Apply pressure to the umbilical stump or venotomy site for 5 to 10 minutes until no bleeding is observed.

5. Dress the site with a Band-Aid or gauze dressing and inspect every day until healing occurs.

RISKS AND COMPLICATIONS

As with arterial catheters, venous catheters are not without serious risk. The most prominent of these is local and systemic infection, followed by thrombus formation and the possibility of embolization. Infiltration with extravasation of fluid into the pleural space or subcutaneous tissue may occur, especially when increased concentrations of dextrose solutions are used, as in parenteral alimentation. With umbilical venous catheters, improper placement of the tip in the portal system or liver may result in necrotizing enterocolitis or in hepatic infarction or necrosis, respectively. Air embolism is also a risk. For fluid infusion it is generally preferable to use a percutaneously introduced needle or a short catheter rather than a cutdown for a venous catheter.

ADDITIONAL READING

Balagtas, R.C., Bell, C.E., Edwards, L.D., and Levin, S.: Risk of local and systemic infections associated with umbilical vein catheterization: a prospective study in 86 newborn patients, Pediatrics **48:**359-367, 1971.

Kitterman, J.A., Phibbs, R.H., and Tooley, W.H.: Catheterization of umbilical vessels in newborn infants, Pediatr. Clin. North Am. **17:**895-912, 1970.

Symchych, P.S., Krauss, A.N., and Winchester, P.: Endocarditis following intracardiac placement of umbilical venous catheters in neonates, J. Pediatr. **90:**287-289, 1977.

90 Left atrial catheters

LAWRENCE J. MILLS

INDICATIONS

The usefulness of measuring left ventricular filling pressure in the postoperative period has been well established (see Chapter 54). LAP is an accurate indication of left ventricular filling pressure, and pulmonary artery wedge pressure correlates reasonably well with LAP (correlation coefficient of 0.63) but is difficult to obtain in infants and small children. There is poor correlation between CVP and LAP, especially after open heart repair.

TECHNIQUE
Placement

LAP can be continuously measured in patients in the postoperative period by inserting the tip of the catheter directly into the left atrium through a purse-string suture in the left atrial appendage or right superior pulmonary vein. The other end of the catheter is brought out to the left of the midline in all cases to aid in identification when multiple catheters are used.

Management

1. The left atrial catheter is a direct route to the systemic circulation, and therefore extreme care must be taken to avoid gaseous or particulate emboli.
2. Identify the catheter by its position on the left side of the abdominal portion of the sternotomy incision.
3. The left atrial catheter is connected directly by high-pressure tubing to a three-way stopcock.
4. The three-way stopcock is connected to an Intraflow device that is connected to a pressure transducer and a flush bag pressurized to 300 mm Hg.
5. Flush solution should be degassed of all air bubbles by prior warming to body temperature.
6. No medications or blood products are infused via left atrial catheters except at the direct request of the responsible thoracic surgeon.
7. The catheter must be aspirated and observed for bubbles before flushing in all cases.
8. No attempt should ever be made to irrigate the system if blood cannot be freely aspirated. A clot is likely to have formed in the catheter, and the system must be removed by the surgeon.

RISKS AND COMPLICATIONS

1. The major hazard is sytemic gas or particulate embolism.
2. Bleeding may occur at the time of removal but rarely is a cause for surgical intervention.
3. Occasionally the catheter tip may shear off, leaving a foreign body in the thorax.

91 Measurement of cardiac output

Thermodilution technique

DAVID E. FIXLER

INDICATIONS

Measurement of cardiac output may provide an accurate evaluation of various therapeutic regimens used for cardiopulmonary support, such as the response to inotropic drugs or volume expansion in the neonate or child in the postoperative period. It can also be used to evaluate the effect of assisted ventilation on the circulation in children with heart failure or shock. Several different types of indicators have been successfully employed to measure cardiac output. The ideal indicator should be easily detectable, should be nontoxic, and should produce no cardiorespiratory changes. Thermal indicators meet these requirements. In the thermodilution technique, a known amount of liquid at room temperature or colder is introduced at one point in the circulation and the resultant change in intravascular temperature is measured downstream. In the clinical setting of the PICU, the indicator is usually cool saline or 5% dextrose solution, which is injected into a central venous or right atrial catheter and sampled downstream by a thermistor in the pulmonary artery. The cooler liquid bolus reduces the temperature of the blood flowing by the thermistor at the tip of the catheter. Commercially available instruments have the capability of inscribing a thermodilution curve, electronically integrating the area under the curve (the actual measurement), and calculating and digitally displaying the child's cardiac output in liters per minute. The advantages of the thermodilution technique that make it particularly attractive in the intensive care area are: (1) it does not require withdrawal and reinfusion of blood; (2) it does not require systemic arterial catheters; (3) the indicator has no significant effect on the circulation and is inexpensive; (4) recirculation is minimal, and therefore the primary curve is particularly suitable for electronic integration; and (5) multiple rapid-sequential measurements are possible.

TECHNIQUE
Sources of error

To obtain accurate cardiac output determinations with the thermodilution technique, several conditions must be met:

1. The indicator must be introduced as a bolus rapidly, without hesitation. The duration of the injection should be less than 2 seconds. With short catheters of moderate caliber, this can usually be accomplished by hand injection; however, with higher-resistance catheters, a pressure injector may be necessary.
2. The volume and temperature of the solution must be measured accurately. When calculating the volume of the injectate, one must correct for the volume of the dead space of the catheter, which has a different temperature from that of the injectate.
3. Thermal loss of the indicator must be pre-

vented. This loss may be reduced by using a solution at room temperature, but this requires larger volumes for accuracy, which may be a significant limitation in infants. When iced solutions are used, it is important to avoid handling the barrel of the syringe and to inject immediately after removing the syringe from ice.

4. The injectate must be mixed with the blood between the site of injection and the location of the thermistor. With central venous or right atrial injection catheters, mixing is usually accomplished within the right atrium and ventricle.

5. The thermistor must be positioned in the main pulmonary artery or the proximal branches. Proper placement of the injection and thermistor catheters is even more important in small children and infants, since complete mixing of the indicator must occur within a shorter distance.

6. A steady state must exist during the period of measurement. One may judge whether the child is in a steady state by observing for movement of the patient and changes in heart rate during the output determinations.

7. The thermodilution electronics must be accurately calibrated. All commercially available thermodilution devices have methods for electronic calibration. The device should be checked for precision several times before output determinations are performed.

8. The inscribed dilution curve must have an exponential downslope. Graphic display of the actual temperature-time curve should be obtained for quality control to be certain the dilution curve has an appropriate geometry.

Thermistor positioning

In patients undergoing cardiac surgery, a small #5F thermodilution catheter with a lumen may be inserted into the saphenous vein and advanced into the distal superior vena cava. Then, at the time of atriotomy the catheter can be manually manipulated through the right ven-

tricle into the pulmonary artery (see Chapter 88). These patients have central venous or Swan-Ganz catheters that can be used as injection sites. In nonsurgical patients, balloon flotation catheters are available that may be manipulated through the right heart into the pulmonary artery using fluoroscopy or blood pressure determinations. The advantage of using a thermistor catheter with a lumen is that it allows monitoring of pulmonary arterial blood pressure and documents proper catheter position. It is still necessary to obtain a chest roentgenogram to check on correct position of the catheter, since normal-appearing but unreliable thermodilution or pressure tracings may be obtained with the catheter tip in the right ventricular outflow tract.

Preparation of injectate

Solutions that are either iced or at room temperature may be used as injectates. Iced injectates reduce the volume required for accurate outputs but have the disadvantage of being prone to greater thermal loss. A solution is prepared by aspirating 5 to 10 ml of D_5W into plastic syringes under aseptic conditions. The syringes are capped, placed in a clear plastic sleeve, and stored in an ice bath. They must be capped airtight to prevent contamination of the injectate by the unsterile ice bath. Cooling to 0° C usually requires approximately 40 minutes. Most commercially available thermodilution equipment has an external thermistor to monitor the temperature of the injectate. One of the syringes should have the plunger removed and the external thermistor inserted into the barrel of the syringe while it is immersed in the ice bath. In this manner, the temperature of the injectate can be accurately measured and automatically inputted. When room-temperature solutions are used, two multiple-injection vials of D_5W are used. From one the required volume may be withdrawn just before injection. The external thermistor probe is inserted into the second vial for measuring injectate temperature. The dead space of the catheter varies, depending on whether an iced or a room-temperature injectate is used. If an iced solution is used, the dead space of the catheter includes the volume contained in the entire dead space of the catheter. Immediately before injection of iced solution, blood is withdrawn to fill the catheter with blood at body temperature; then the syringe containing iced solution is attached and rapidly injected. When room-temperature injectate is used, the dead space of the catheter includes only the catheter volume that is inserted into the patient. The syringe containing room-temperature injectate is attached to the catheter without prior flushing or withdrawal. The venous catheter used for injection of the indicator should not contain any medication, since bolus injection of a drug may cause a change in cardiac output or serious complications such as ventricular dysrhythmias.

Precision

Reproducibility of the cardiac output measurements should be checked by performing duplicate or triplicate determinations. The accuracy of cardiac output by thermodilution in children has been demonstrated. Cardiac outputs were simultaneously measured by the Fick technique and the thermodilution technique. The results of the study (Fig. 91-1) indicated a close correlation between the two methods when thermodilution measurements were done in duplicate or triplicate. The temperature-time curves should be closely inspected for evidence of artifact, which may be secondary to an irregular injection, poor mixing, or improper thermistor position. Fig. 91-2 demonstrates curves obtained at different thermistor locations. The individual performing the cardiac output determination must be responsible for quality control of the curves. With careful attention to detail,

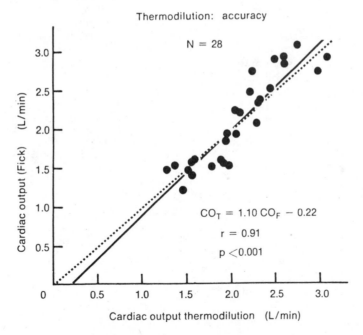

Thermodilution: accuracy

N = 28

$CO_T = 1.10 \, CO_F - 0.22$

$r = 0.91$

$p < 0.001$

Cardiac output (Fick)   (L/min)

Cardiac output thermodilution   (L/min)

Fig. 91-1. Mean value of cardiac output by thermodilution as compared with cardiac output by Fick technique in 28 studies. The dashed line is the line of identity. The solid line is the best fit for the least squares method. (Redrawn from Freed, M.D., and Keane, J.F.: J. Pediatr. **92:**40, 1978.)

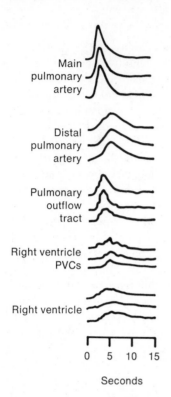

Main
pulmonary
artery

Distal
pulmonary
artery

Pulmonary
outflow
tract

Right ventricle
PVCs

Right ventricle

```
0   5  10  15
```

Seconds

Fig. 91-2. Thermodilution tracings from different catheter positions and during ventricular dysrhythmia. (Redrawn from Colgan, F.J., and Stewart, S.: Crit. Care Med. **5:**224, 1977.)

the thermodilution technique provides an accurate and relatively simple method for measuring cardiac output in the PICU.

RISKS AND COMPLICATIONS

See Chapters 88 and 89.

ADDITIONAL READING

Baskoff, J.D., and Maruschak, G.F.: Correction factor for thermodilution determination of cardiac output in children, Crit. Care Med. **9:**870-872, 1980.

Colgan, F.J., and Stewart, S.: An assessment of cardiac output by thermodilution in infants and children following cardiac surgery, Crit. Care Med. **5:**220-225, 1977.

Freed, M.D., and Keane, J.F.: Cardiac output measured by thermodilution in infants and children, J. Pediatr. **92:**39-42, 1978.

Kohanna, F.H., and Cunningham, J.N.: Monitoring of cardiac output by thermodilution after open heart surgery, J. Thorac. Cardiovasc. Surg. **73:**451-457, 1977.

Lawrie, G.M., Stacey, R.B., and Wright, J.S.: The perioperative measurement of cardiac output in infancy by the thermodilution technique, Anaesth. Intensive Care **3:**317-320, 1975.

Mathur, M., Harris, E.A., Yarrow, S., and Barratt-Boyes, B.G.: Measurement of cardiac output by thermodilution in infants and children after open heart operations, J. Thorac. Cardiovasc. Surg. **72:**221-225, 1976.

Meisner, H., Hagl, S., Heimisch, W., and others: Evaluation of the thermodilution method for measurement of cardiac output after open-heart surgery, Ann. Thorac. Surg. **18:**504-515, 1974.

Wyse, S.D., Pfitzner, J., Rees, A., and others: Measurement of cardiac output by thermodilution in infants and children, Thorax **30:**262-265, 1975.

92 Intracranial pressure measurements and ventricular taps

FREDERICK H. SKLAR
CINDY K. LYBARGER

INDICATIONS

ICP is monitored in the critically ill PICU patient who is symptomatic because of intracranial hypertension. Increased pressures are frequently seen in patients with intracranial neoplasm or head injury. Space-occupying lesions, hemorrhage, contusion, edema, and hydrocephalus are the usual underlying pathologic processes. Other conditions characterized by symptomatic cerebral edema include anoxic brain injury, infections, and metabolic disorders such as Reye's encephalopathy and lead poisoning. The PICU management of the child with increased ICP often necessitates direct ICP measurement. Frequently, ICP is measured prophylactically in certain neurosurgical patients who may be expected to have problems in the early postoperative period. For instance, after posterior fossa surgery in children, elevated pressure frequently develops because of hydrocephalus and may be avoided with simple ICP monitoring.

Rational therapeutic decisions can be based on the continuous assessment of this important physiologic variable. However, at the present time most techniques require invasive measures, and therefore the risks must be weighed against the benefits. Furthermore, ICP is sensitive to changes in numerous other physiologic variables. Changes in the cerebrovascular compartment, the CSF system, and edema bulk can all be expected to influence pressure. Thus, many factors must also be considered because of their direct and indirect effects on ICP. The physiology of ICP is discussed in Chapter 10. However, it is worth reemphasizing the sensitivity of the intracranial vascular bed, and of ICP indirectly, to changes in Pa_{CO_2}. Similarly, hypoxia can have deleterious effects on pressure.

Although isolated pressure measurements may be obtained during ventricular tap or lumbar puncture, they are of limited value. A single normal pressure measurement may not be indicative of the pressure minutes later. Children are often agitated and crying during these procedures, making pressure recording impractical. In addition, intracranial pathologic conditions that create pressure differences across the tentorium or at the foramen magnum may result in herniation when fluid is vented from the spine by lumbar puncture.

The ideal method of measuring ICP would be totally noninvasive. A few instruments have been described and are available for monitoring pressures through the fontanelle. Patients without fontanelles require implantation of some sort of telemetric or transducer device or use of a catheter system. Obviously, a self-contained system without wires or catheters violating the scalp is more desirable. Although numerous implantable devices have been described, the ideal device is not yet available for routine use. At present, ICP measurements are made with a ventricular catheter, subdural catheter, or a subarachnoid bolt device.

Occasionally it is not possible to tap the ventricle because the ventricles are very small or distorted by the intracranial pathologic condition. If ventricular tap is unsuccessful, the options are to position a subdural fluid-filled catheter for pressure monitoring or to place a subarachnoid screw through the original twist drill hole used for the unsuccessful ventricular tap. If the calvarial thickness is adequate to hold the threads of the pressure monitor bolt, this technique is a reasonable alternative to ventricular pressure monitoring.

A ventricular tap is important as an emergency procedure and occasionally as a diagnostic procedure. A discussion of the technical considerations is presented below.

TECHNIQUE
Ventricular tap

Preparation

Equipment. A sterile towel and gloves, antiseptic solution, 1% lidocaine, twist drill, 18-gauge and 20-gauge spinal needles, and 18-gauge and 20-gauge Cone needles (blunt-tipped needles with side openings and fitted with a stylet) should be available.

Patient. A generous area of the right frontal scalp is shaved, prepped, and draped with sterile towels. In older children, the scalp is infiltrated with lidocaine in the midpupillary line at or slightly anterior to the coronal suture. In infants, the scalp is infiltrated in the midpupillary line over the fontanelle or over the coronal suture if the fontanelle is small.

Procedure

Infants. A 20-gauge lumbar puncture needle is introduced through the scalp, fontanelle, and dura into the subdural space. As a routine, the stylet is removed to check for subdural fluid collections. The needle is then directed toward the medial canthus of the ipsilateral eye and the anterior aspect of the zygoma. These landmarks

are merely estimates, and adjustments are required when the puncture is made more anterior to the coronal suture. It is more appropriate to picture mentally the ventricular system in the lateral and anteroposterior planes and to direct the needle toward the frontal horn. After the needle is withdrawn, a scalp suture or collodion-soaked cotton is frequently needed to prevent CSF leakage.

Children. A small stab wound is made in the scalp with a knife blade, and a twist drill hole is made with one hand while countersupport is provided by the other to prevent accidental penetration of the dura and brain with the instrument. The dura is pierced with a short spinal needle, and the subdural space is checked. The needle is replaced by a blunt-tipped Cone needle, which is directed toward the frontal horn of the ventricle. After the procedure, a suture is placed for hemostasis and to prevent CSF leakage.

Children with shunts. For elective shunt taps, the scalp over the shunt pumping device or specially designed reservoir is shaved, prepped, and draped for needle aspiration. A 23-gauge butterfly is introduced through the dome of the pumping device (Pudenz) or Rickham reservoir (Holter system). The pressure can be measured; the fluid can be aspirated for laboratory analysis.

The child with shunted hydrocephalus who has a probable blocked shunt and who experiences cardiorespiratory arrest or decompensates suddenly requires emergency measures. The scalp over the shunt pumping device (Pudenz) or Rickham reservoir is shaved, prepped, and draped. An attempt is made to tap the shunt in the routine fashion, but if the ventricular catheter is not functioning, it will not be possible to aspirate fluid. Because of the urgency of the clinical situation, a lumbar puncture needle is then introduced through the shunt and directed toward the center of the head to tap the ventricle as a lifesaving procedure. Fortunately, under these circumstances such children frequently have large ventricles, which facilitate ventricular puncture. Such aggressive intervention can be lifesaving.

Risks and complications

Inability to tap the ventricle. Occasionally, despite several passes, one is unable to find the ventricle. Frequent checks by removing the stylet and introducing a drop of 0.9% sodium chloride solution meant for IV administration (without added preservatives) to the needle hub can facilitate finding the ventricle when the pressure is low. The fluid will pulsate and flow into the needle when the ventricle is entered. Failure is more frequent in infants because of their small size. Occasionally the ventricles are small because of the intracranial pathologic condition. They may be distorted, shifted, or collapsed as a result of associated diffuse brain swelling. If several attempts to tap the ventricle are unsuccessful, it may be unwise to persist.

Hemorrhage. It is possible to tear pial vessels or bridging veins and cause subdural bleeding. Intraparenchymal hemorrhage is also possible. These complications seem to be exceedingly uncommon.

Continued leak of CSF through the scalp wound after the procedure. This is uncommon when ICP is low. Cotton soaked in collodion will often seal the hole. In children with increased pressure, it is probably worthwhile to place a skin suture to prevent CSF leakage.

Infection. Sterile technique must be used to prevent introduction of pathogens into the ventricle.

Intraventricular pressure monitoring

Preparation

Equipment. Equipment is the same as for a ventricular tap plus a 36-inch #5F pediatric feeding tube or a commercially available intraventricular catheter, stopcocks, bile drainage bag, and pressure transducer. Sodium chloride solution (0.9%) intended for IV use (without preservatives) is used to fill the catheter and transducer system and for flushes.

Patient. Preparation is the same as for ventricular tap.

Procedure. The right frontal horn of the lateral ventricle is tapped with an 18-gauge Cone needle as described previously. The needle is left in place for a brief time and is then removed and replaced by a catheter previously filled with 0.9% sodium chloride solution. The solution should pulsate within the catheter and flow freely into the ventricle when the distal end of the catheter is elevated. Fluid is allowed to fill the catheter by lowering its exposed end, and the catheter is then capped with a double stopcock. The catheter is sutured to the scalp, and a sterile dressing is applied. A pressure transducer is attached to one stopcock port; when necessary, a bile bag for CSF drainage is attached to the other stopcock port (Fig. 92-1). A commercially available ventricular catheter is preferable to the feeding tube when the ventricles are small. These catheters generally have stylets and can be used to tap the ventricle directly. They require an additional stopcock and connection tube, however.

A transducer is calibrated and positioned at the level of the foramen of Monro (mid temple). A pulsatile waveform indicates that the catheter is patent (Fig. 21-1).

Intraventricular pressure is monitored with the stopcock open to the transducer. Should the pressure exceed safe limits, therapeutic measures to reduce it are instituted. These may include drainage of ventricular CSF into the bile bag for immediate ICP reduction. However, this is not practical if the ventricles are small, distorted, or compressed by diffuse brain edema or an intracranial space-occupying lesion. Ventricular drainage of CSF is the treatment of choice for postoperative intracranial hypertension secondary to hydrocephalus after posterior fossa surgery. The management of increased ICP is covered in Chapter 10.

Risks and complications

Inability to tap the ventricle. This occurs because of small or distorted ventricular anatomy.

Inability to thread the catheter through the needle tract into the ventricle. This is rarely a problem if it is possible to tap the ventricle.

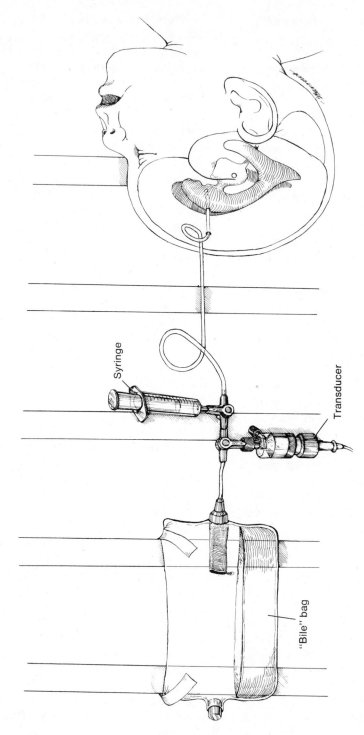

Fig. 92-1. Intraventricular pressure monitoring system utilizing a catheter in the frontal horn of the right lateral ventricle. The catheter is connected to a transducer, drainage bag, and syringe. System is "closed," minimizing contamination. Appropriate stopcock adjustments allow for measuring of intraventricular pressure, drainage of CSF, or flushing of ventricular catheter.

Syringe

Transducer

"Bile" bag

Alternatives to the #5F pediatric feeding tube are commercially available ventricular catheters or a Scott cannula. These have stylets and do not require a separate needle for introduction. The Scott cannula has a metal connector that must be sutured to the scalp in an infant, or the catheter will be easily dislodged. These systems may be considered less than ideal, since they require an extra connection where bacterial contamination may occur.

Blockage of the catheter by blood or brain tissue. A previously functioning catheter that has become obstructed can usually be cleared with 0.2 ml of sterile 0.9% sodium chloride solution meant for IV injection. The pressure response to a small volume flush is much greater in a patient with intracranial hypertension than in a patient with normal pressures. This is a physiologic feature of the pressure-volume function of brain elasticity. It is therefore desirable to avoid frequent or large flushes.

Infection. Large clinical studies report infection rates of 3% to 5% with the use of intraventricular catheters to monitor ICP. Head trauma patients with scalp injury may be more susceptible to infection. Prophylactic antibiotics are not routinely used unless an infection is strongly suspected. Under these circumstances the catheter is removed and replaced with another on the opposite side if pressure monitoring is absolutely necessary. In general, a catheter is removed within 5 days of its original placement. Occasionally, one can be left for a week. However, if continued pressure monitoring is needed, it is thought best to replace the original catheter with another one on the other side. IV infusions into veins of the scalp are contraindicated in patients with ICP monitoring devices because of increased risk of infection.

Subarachnoid bolt

Preparation
Equipment. Equipment is the same as for a ventricular tap plus a stainless steel hollow bolt device with a Luer-Lok connector on one end and threads for screwing into the skull on the other, #11 knife blade, and small curette.

Patient. Preparation is the same as for ventricular tap.

Procedure
Through the twist drill hole, the dura is incised in a cruciate fashion with a #11 knife blade, and the dural leaves are curetted to ensure an opening in the dura.

The bolt is screwed into the skull until it is secure, and the subarachnoid space (and probably the brain) is indented by the tip of the hollow bolt. A self-tapping screw device is easier to thread into the skull. Sterile 0.9% sodium chloride solution meant for IV injection is introduced into the bolt through a needle so that captured air is allowed to escape. The bolt is connected to a calibrated strain gauge by saline-filled pressure tubing (Fig. 92-2).

A waveform must be apparent and is generally an indication that the system is open and truly measuring ICP. Damping of the waveform may indicate that the tip of the bolt is clotted or plugged. If the waveform does not return after a small flush (0.1 ml) of sterile 0.9% sodium chloride solution, a spinal needle can be carefully introduced through the bolt in an attempt to dislodge the fibrin clot.

A sterile dressing is applied.

When the bolt is removed, the scalp incision is sutured.

Risks and complications
The bolt cannot be used on small children and infants because the skull is not thick enough to support this device. A subdural catheter is the alternative method of choice under these circumstances.

Persistent and repeated damping of the waveform is not uncommon with the bolt apparatus. Occasionally this can be improved by further tightening of the device into the skull (and brain). The system is less than ideal under these circumstances, since spurious measurements cannot be deciphered from actual changes in ICP.

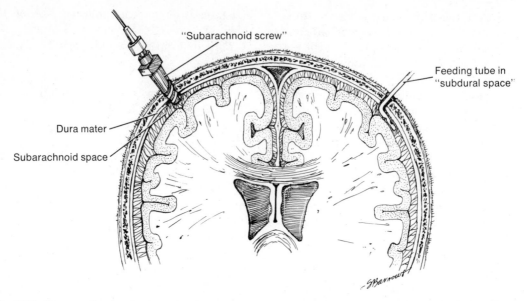

"Subarachnoid screw"

Feeding tube in "subdural space"

Dura mater

Subarachnoid space

Fig. 92-2. Two methods of measuring ICP. On the left is a hollow bolt that is screwed into the skull. The end of the bolt rests in the subarachnoid space. On the right is a pediatric feeding tube that measures pressure in the subdural space.

Infection is a risk as with ventricular catheters.

Subdural catheters

Preparation

Equipment. Equipment is the same as for ventricular tap plus a #5F pediatric feeding tube, small mastoid rongeur, #11 knife blade, and forceps.

Patient. Usually the patient who requires a subdural catheter to measure ICP is an infant whose ventricles cannot be tapped.

Procedure

In an infant, it is usually easier to make a small incision in the scalp adjacent to the fontanelle but over the frontal bone. A twist drill hole is made, and this is enlarged in a minimal fashion so that the dura can be visualized. The dura is incised under direct vision, and a #5F pediatric feeding tube filled with 0.9% sodium chloride solution is introduced into the subdural space. The scalp is sutured, and the catheter is secured to the scalp. The fluid-filled catheter is connected to a pressure transducer.

Pressure waveform pulsations must be present to indicate catheter patency. Small-volume flushes may improve the waveform recording.

Risks and complications

Risks and complications are the same as for a subarachnoid bolt.

ADDITIONAL READING

Kaktis, J.V.: An introduction to monitoring intracranial pressure in critically ill children, Crit. Care Q. 3:1-8, 1980.

Lundbert, N., Kjallquist, A., Kullberg, G., and others: Non-operative management of intracranial hypertension. In Krayenbuhl, H., editor: Advances and technical standards in neurosurgery, vol. 1, Heidelberg, 1974, Springer-Verlag.

McGraw, C.P.: Continuous intracranial pressure monitoring: review of techniques and presentation of method, Surg. Neurol. 6:149-155, 1976.

McGraw, C.P., and Alexander, E., Jr.: Durometer for measurement of intracranial pressure, Surg. Neurol. 7:293-295, 1977.

Mitchell, P.: Intracranial hypertension: implications of research for nursing care, J. Neurosurg. Nurs. **12:**145-154, 1980.

Raju, T.N.K., Vidysager, D., and Papazafiraton, C.: Intracranial pressure monitoring in the neonatal ICU, Crit. Care Med. **8:**575-581, 1980.

Robinson, R.O., Rolfe, P., and Sutton, P.: Non-invasive method for measuring intracranial pressure in normal newborn infants, Dev. Med. Child Neurol. **19:**305-308, 1977.

Vries, J.K., Becker, D.P., and Young, H.F.: A subarachnoid screw for monitoring intracranial pressure: technical note, J. Neurosurg. **39:**416-419, 1973.

Zeidelman, C.: Increased intracranial pressure in the pediatric patient: nursing assessment and intervention, J. Neurosurg. Nurs. **12:**7-10, 1980.

93 Echocardiography

W. PENNOCK LAIRD

INDICATIONS

Echocardiography has become a well-established diagnostic technique that is useful in patients suspected of having serious heart disease. The procedure provides valuable information about cardiac structure and function in a safe, noninvasive, and reproducible manner.

TECHNIQUE

Echo studies of the heart utilize high-frequency, pulsed sound waves to define cardiac anatomy. In pediatric work, frequencies of 2.25 to 7.5 MHz are generally used.

The patient should be examined in the supine position. The ultrasound transducer is placed along the left sternal border in the third or fourth intercostal space. Fig. 93-1 demonstrates an echo beam passing through the heart. As indicated in the diagram, different cardiac structures are visualized as the transducer beam is redirected.

Proper recording techniques are vital in order to achieve meaningful results. Generally a basic echo study of the heart includes identification and measurement of all four valves, both ventricles (including wall thickness and chamber size), the ventricular septum, the left atrium, the great arteries, and the pericardium. The anatomic relationships of these structures to one another should also be determined. A simultaneous ECG is always included for the timing of cardiac events within the cycle.

SELECTED EXAMPLES
Evaluation of congenital heart disease

Evaluation of possible congenital heart disease involves assessment of size and position of cardiac chambers, valves, and great arteries. Echocardiography can generally be used in place of cardiac catheterization to diagnose aortic atresia. In such instances, it is important to emphasize that all the anatomic features of this malformation must be present on the echogram. Fig. 93-2 is an ultrasound study from a patient with aortic atresia. All of the characteristic features are shown: an underdeveloped left ventricle, an enlarged right ventricle, a diminutive aortic root, and an absent or poorly visualized mitral valve echo. If these findings cannot be demonstrated on the echogram, another diagnosis should be considered and cardiac catheterization carried out.

Assessment of ventricular function

Recently there has been a great deal of interest in the use of ultrasound to evaluate cardiac function. Echocardiography has been used to estimate left ventricular stroke volume, ejection fraction, mean rate of circumferential fiber shortening (mean VCF), and relative change in minor axis with systole. In addition, both right and left heart systolic time intervals can be obtained from the echogram. This information is particularly useful in the management of pediatric patients with depressed ventricular function secondary to a variety of causes, including shock, sepsis, myocarditis, hypocalcemia, and hypoglycemia.

Recognition of pericardial effusion

The identification of a pericardial effusion is an extremely useful application of echocardiography. It is generally believed that an echogram

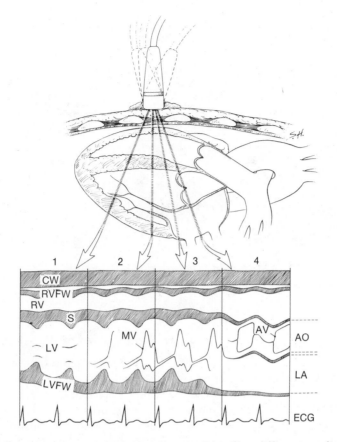

Fig. 93-1. Idealized sagittal section of the heart. One can visualize different cardiac structures by changing the direction of the echo beam. *CW,* Chest wall; *RVFW,* right ventricular free wall; *RV,* right ventricle; *S,* ventricular septum; *LV,* left ventricle; *LVFW,* left ventricular free wall; *MV,* mitral valve; *AV,* aortic valve; *AO,* aorta; *LA,* left atrium; *ECG,* electrocardiogram. (Reprinted from Applied Radiology, Vol. 5, No. 4. Copyright by Barrington Publications, Inc., 825 S. Barrington Ave., Los Angeles, Calif. 90049.)

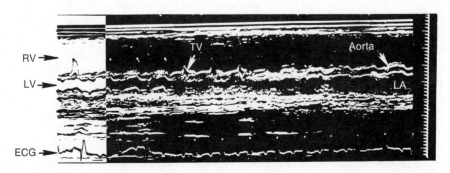

Fig. 93-2. Echogram illustrating aortic atresia. *TV,* Tricuspid valve. (Reprinted from Applied Radiology, Vol. 5, No. 4. Copyright by Barrington Publications, Inc., 825 S. Barrington Ave., Los Angeles, Calif. 90049.)

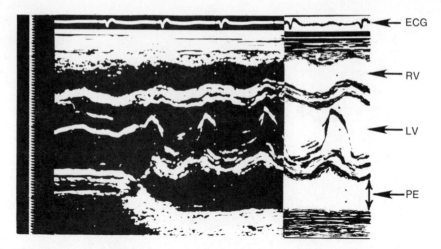

← ECG

← RV

← LV

←PE

Fig. 93-3. Echogram showing a large pericardial effusion *(PE)*. (Reprinted from Applied Radiology, Vol. 5, No. 4. Copyright by Barrington Publications, Inc., 825 S. Barrington Ave., Los Angeles, Calif. 90049.)

is the most sensitive method for detecting small amounts of fluid.

The patient is studied in either the supine or slight left lateral decubitus position. Occasionally it may be helpful to incline the patient's chest at a 30-degree angle. A complete echogram should be obtained. The pericardial space behind the left ventricular free wall is then carefully defined. To identify this space with confidence, all the usual left ventricular structures must be recorded. In particular, the endocardium and epicardium of the left ventricular free wall must be clearly shown. A pericardial effusion appears as an abnormal space separating the epicardium and the pericardium.

Fig. 93-3 illustrates a large pericardial effusion. A continuous sweep from the left ventricle to the aortic root shows another important diagnostic point. Generally, a pericardial effusion does not accumulate behind the left atrium. For this reason, the echo-free space should not persist behind the left atrium. As the sweep approaches the atrioventricular groove, the echo-free space abruptly disappears.

Evaluation of cardiac shunts

A major application of echocardiography in the pediatric age group has been the evaluation of the degree of L → R shunting through a PDA in newborns. Such information is extremely useful in premature infants with respiratory distress due to pulmonary disease and a coexisting PDA.

A large shunt through a ductus causes increased pulmonary blood flow, thereby producing an increase in both the left ventricular and left atrial size. The size of these chambers can be easily measured with ultrasound. Fig. 93-4 shows the echogram of a premature infant with lung disease and a large ductus. The left atrial diameter was nearly twice the diameter of the aortic root. After successful surgical ligation of the ductus, the left atrial size returned to normal (Fig. 93-5).

A large left atrium is not specific for a large ductus shunt. Other cardiac malformations with large L → R shunts may produce the same finding. In addition, heart failure from any cause may produce a large left atrium.

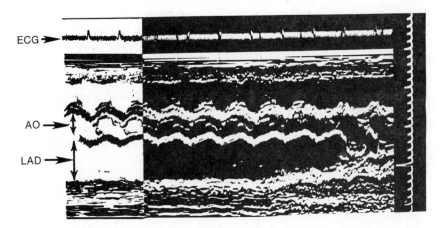

Pre-op.

Fig. 93-4. Preoperative echogram from a premature infant with a large PDA. The left atrial diameter *(LAD)* is nearly twice that of the aortic root. (Reprinted from Applied Radiology, Vol. 5, No. 4. Copyright by Barrington Publications, Inc., 825 S. Barrington Ave., Los Angeles, Calif. 90049.)

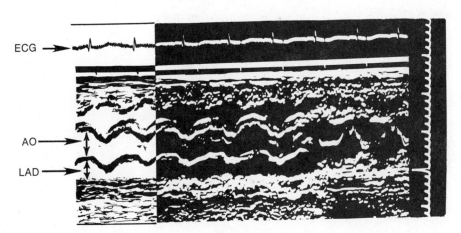

Post-op.

Fig. 93-5. Postoperative echogram from the infant referred to in Fig. 93-4. After ligation of a large PDA, the left atrial diameter returned to normal size. (Reprinted from Applied Radiology, Vol. 5, No. 4. Copyright by Barrington Publications, Inc., 825 S. Barrington Ave., Los Angeles, Calif. 90049.)

Echocardiography can also be used in combination with a simultaneous rapid injection of indocyanine green dye, 0.9% sodium chloride solution, or the patient's own blood to recognize intracardiac shunting. Such injections produce a cloud of reflective microcavitations that are detectable by ultrasound. Since echoes disappear after circulation through the pulmonary bed, selective right heart injections are useful in identifying the presence and level of R → L intracardiac shunts. Similarly, injection into the left heart chambers can be used to detect L → R shunts.

REAL-TIME ECHOCARDIOGRAPHY

The development of two-dimensional or real-time echocardiography has been a major advance in the diagnostic capability of echocardiography. The technique utilizes a transducer with either a moving crystal(s) or multiple crystals to image a two-dimensional sector of the heart. This enhanced visualization of the cardiac anatomy has proved to be extremely valuable in the initial evaluation of neonates with complex congenital heart disease. The technique is also particularly useful in identifying pericardial effusion, especially a loculated effusion, that may escape detection by the usual M-mode echo examination. Finally, since all cardiac chambers can be imaged simultaneously with two-dimensional echo, shunt studies utilizing an injected bolus of 0.9% sodium chloride solution (producing reflective microcavitations) readily demonstrate the location of intracardiac shunts.

94 Transcutaneous oxygen monitoring

PATRICIA WALTERS
GARY ELMORE
DONNA S. BURNS

INDICATIONS

Transcutaneous oxygen monitoring was first developed in the late 1960s for continuous evaluation of oxygenation in patients with neonatal respiratory disorders. Several models for such monitoring exist, and any model under consideration for use should be clinically demonstrated and evaluated within the hospital setting before a decision for purchase is made. Basic aspects for evaluation are: (1) ease of operation, (2) demonstrated clinical accuracy at both high and low values, (3) remedial maintenance procedures, (4) method of calibration, and (5) patient safety. A brief review of six transcutaneous oxygen monitors is presented in Table 94-1. Ptc_{O_2}, cP_{O_2}, and tcP_{O_2} are all scientific notations for transcutaneous oxygen tension, while TCOM, TCM, and tcP_{O_2} monitor are all popular abbreviations for the monitoring device itself. Transcutaneous carbon dioxide monitoring is now in the developmental phase; however, as of this writing, only a few prototypes have received FDA approval for clinical use in infants and/or adults.

While Ptc_{O_2} monitoring cannot replace arterial blood-gas and pH measurements, it is an important adjunct in the evaluation of hypoxemia and hyperoxemia. The assessment of patient oxygenation is immediate when Ptc_{O_2} monitors are utilized. Care givers can assess the effects of therapy and evaluate routine, yet potentially hazardous situations, such as suctioning, feeding, and physical manipulation of the patient. The frequency of blood sampling for arterial blood-gas and pH sampling is usually decreased; however, at this time such sampling, particularly from an indwelling arterial catheter, should not be replaced completely by transcutaneous oxygen monitoring. Definitive blood-gas and pH values used to assess and manage patients, particularly those on assisted ventilation, should be determined using arterial blood.

Indications for Ptc_{O_2} monitoring are subjective but may include those patients at high risk for debilitating Pa_{O_2} changes such as neonates (especially those susceptible to intracranial hemorrhage, retrolental fibroplasia, and/or persistent pulmonary hypertension of the newborn), some patients with cardiac disease (especially those with pulmonary hypertension), patients with chronic pulmonary disease on mechanical ventilation with supplemental oxygen therapy, patients suspected of sleep hypoxemia and/or apnea, and mothers in labor. The noninvasive technique of Ptc_{O_2} monitoring has obvious advantages and fewer patient hazards than the invasive indwelling polarographic or fiberoptic arterial catheters.

EQUIPMENT AND TECHNIQUE

The following features are important for proper equipment function: (1) functioning electrode and electrode membrane, (2) monitor

Table 94-1. Comparison of several PtC$_{O2}$ monitors

Model	Power source	Transport capability	Temperature range
Biochem-Lifespan 100	Electric	No	35°-45° C in 0.1° C increments
Kontron Medical* Cutan PO$_2$ Monitor 820	Two D-cell flashlight batteries or power pack (electric)	Yes	44°-45° C in 1° C increments
Litton Oxymonitor	Electric	No	37° and 43°-45° C in 1° C increments
Narco AirShields Transcutaneous PO$_2$ Monitor	Electric	No	38°-44.9° C in 0.1° C increments
Novametrix Tcomette "C" series	Electric or battery pack	Yes	40°-45° C in 0.5° C increments
Radiometer TCM2 TC Oxygen Monitor	Electric or battery pack	Yes	37° and 42°-45° in 0.5° C increments

*Formerly Roche.

calibration, (3) patient site selection and placement, (4) site change with regard to individual patient needs, and (5) quantitative and qualitative evaluation of clinical data.

1. The Ptc$_{O2}$ monitor contains a modified Clark electrode similar to the one utilized in blood-gas instruments (Fig. 94-1). A heater within the electrode generates a set temperature (usually 43° to 45° C) to produce localized hyperemia and vasodilation, which arterializes the capillary bed. Heating of the tissue increases the temperature of blood flowing under the electrode, and the increased blood temperature under the skin causes a shift of the oxyhemoglobin dissociation curve to the right (see Fig. 12-1), thus partially compensating for the amount of oxygen consumed by tissue metabolism. Heating of the skin slightly changes the lipid structure of the stratum corneum, possibly allowing oxygen to diffuse more rapidly through the epidermis to the electrode. When the electrode is exposed to oxygen, oxygen molecules flow through a semipermeable membrane and an electrochemical reaction occurs that causes electrical current to flow through the cathode. An amplifier connected to the cathode mea-

sures the current and converts it to a value proportional to the oxygen tension at the electrode/membrane interface, which in turn is displayed on the front of the monitoring system. The rate of reaction and the resulting current are directly and linearly proportional to the concentration of oxygen available for reduction at the cathode and they correlate significantly with Pa$_{O2}$ under certain conditions. A thermistor within the electrode housing maintains heat energy at a desired level.

Despite the similarity in membrane construction, the thickness and application of sensor membranes varies with the manufacturer. Specifications for storage, use, and care of the membrane should be followed carefully for proper functioning of the equipment. Different brands of membranes are not interchangeable between the different brands of sensors. Functioning membranes last between 2 to 14 days and the monitor must be removed from the patient for service for approximately 30 to 60 minutes when the membrane is changed. Many patient cables offer battery-controlled sensors so that polarity is not lost to the cable during storage. Membranes should be changed be-

Electrode construction	Membrane construction	Recorder integration
Platinum cathode/ silver anode	Teflon	Yes
Gold cathode/silver anode	Polyethylene	No
3 base platinum cathode/silver anode	Teflon	No
Platinum cathode/ silver anode	Polypropylene	Yes
3 base platinum cathode/silver anode	Teflon	Yes
Platinum cathode/ silver anode	Polypropylene	Yes

tween patients to prevent cross contamination.

When poor correlation exists between Ptc_{O_2} and Pa_{O_2} readings, the membrane may be at fault. Several monitors currently on the market offer electronic testing to evaluate the integrity of the membrane. Any membrane that contains a worn area, large air bubble, discoloration, or wrinkle should be replaced.

2. Monitor calibration is established for a high and a zero point. The procedure varies with the model; however, most units will convert to a dry room air high calibration and an electronic zero without sacrificing clinical accuracy. This technique is much simpler and less costly than wet calibration, gas calibration, thermal calibration, or zeroing solutions. While commonplace compounds, such as glycerin, may be used as a zeroing solution to reduce costs, care must be exercised so that these solutions do not decrease the integrity of the electrode or membrane. A drop of glycerin is placed on the membrane while the electrode is held in an upright position. Within 2 to 3 minutes the monitor should read zero or may be adjusted to the zero point. The high calibration point for dry room air calibration is determined by the barometric pressure in mm Hg minus water vapor pressure (relative humidity) multiplied by the fraction of inspired oxygen in room air at room temperature. A constant for this number may be established for the mean values of the variables. For example, in this area (Dallas) the accepted norm is 153 to 156 mm Hg. Given a barometric pressure of 750 mm Hg and a relative humidity of 40% (to produce a water vapor pressure of 19 mm Hg) at 21% oxygen (room air), the calibration point number becomes 153. Two to three minutes after the sensor has come in contact with room air, the monitor should read 153. If it does not, the calibration number may be achieved by turning the calibration knob located on the front of the unit. If this technique is used, care must be exercised not to calibrate the sensor under a radiant warmer or in an incubator, since these units alter the variables of the equation. An electronic zero may be accomplished simply by unplugging the patient cable from the monitor for a few seconds until a zero appears on the monitoring system.

3. A suitable site for transcutaneous monitoring is essential and should have the following features: (1) good capillary circulation, (2) location away from large surface blood vessels, (3) absence of hair and fatty deposits, (4) absence of bony prominences, since they may constrict the flow of blood between the electrode and capillary bed, and (5) a flat surface for a good airtight seal of the sensor to the skin surface (air leaks at this point will cause the electrode to sample ambient air). For monitoring in neonates the upper thorax, abdomen, and inner aspect of the thigh are used commonly. For monitoring in adults the neck, interclavicular area, upper thorax, and inner aspect of the upper arm are used commonly. In neonates with suspected right → left shunting via a PDA, such as in persistent pulmonary hypertension, place the electrode on a site, such as the upper arm or thorax, which will reflect most closely the better-oxygenated blood. Remember in such

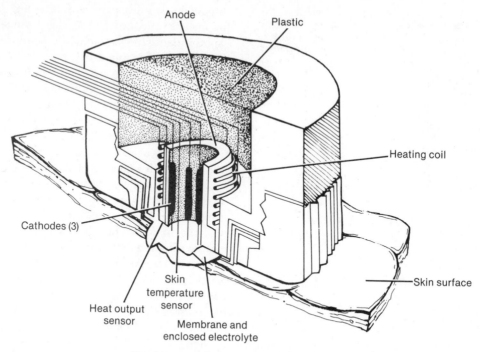

Fig. 94-1. Transcutaneous P_{O_2} electrode.

cases, the Ptc_{O_2} reading will be higher than a Pa_{O_2} in blood sampled from a site below the ductus arteriosus (e.g., from the abdominal aorta).

4. Prepare the patient's skin by scrubbing the area with an alcohol swab to remove oil and dead tissue. Excessively oily skin may require the use of Wisk or soap and water to cleanse the area for good contact. In adult patients the adhesive portion of tape may be used to skim away dead skin cells. The electrode or fixation ring for the electrode is self-adhesive for skin attachment. Exceptionally difficult skin attachment problems may be improved by using Benzoin at the interface site. Apply a small amount (1 to 3 drops) of contact gel or 0.9% sodium chloride solution to the sensor or fixation ring (depending on the model used) to provide a thin film between the skin and electrode inter-

face. After the electrode is in place, as much as 20 minutes may be required before the monitor reaches a stable reading; therefore, when the sensor site is changed, the Ptc_{O_2} reading will drop below normal and slowly rise to normal as the capillary bed dilates.

5. Site change should be made every 2 to 6 hours depending upon the patient's skin sensitivity to heat. Prolonged use of a single site will produce a burn. Best correlation of Ptc_{O_2} to Pa_{O_2} results from a skin temperature of 43° C for neonates and 44° C for adults. Since the electrode itself absorbs heat, the monitor temperature setting may be set at 44° C to produce a skin temperature of 43° C. Check temperature specifications for each model. The patient cable may be secured to the patient with tape to avoid extra pressure areas and burns. The sensor should never be placed beneath a patient.

6. Once the Ptc_{O_2} data are correlated and stabilized to Pa_{O_2} data by proper use of the equipment and individual patient considerations, a qualitative analysis may be charted with respect to ventilatory changes, circulatory changes, suctioning, and other events. Some units provide integration to a trend recorder. In the absence of such a device, meticulous observation and charting will suffice. Since peripheral perfusion is essential to good correlation, discretion should be exercised if Ptc_{O_2} values are to be used in patients with cardiac disease involving a peripheral circulatory impairment. Usually, the relatively immediate, accurate correlation of Ptc_{O_2} to Pa_{O_2} is valuable for changes in PEEP, FI_{O_2}, flow patterns, and other ventilatory settings.

RISKS AND COMPLICATIONS

The heat from the electrode routinely causes small areas of erythema that disappear in a few days. However, some patients, especially infants with fair skin, may develop a second-degree burn, which may become a source of infection and scarring. Contraindications to the use of transcutaneous monitoring are minimal but may include peripheral shunting, skin abrasions, rashes, petechiae and/or purpura, congenital skin diseases (e.g., ichthyosis), obesity, excessive skin edema, or deep hypothermia.

A monitoring system that cuts power to the patient cable in the event of an electronic problem or spontaneous voltage leak is incorporated into some currently marketed units. Some patient cables require a special wrap if used in the presence of phototherapy. In general, a well-maintained, well-placed monitor will give clinical data accurate to within ±5-6 mm Hg for low and ±10 mm Hg for high oxygen values. Erroneous data frequently occur when the unit

or patient is poorly prepared and when one fails to verify results by obtaining an arterial blood-gas sample. Those patients with suspected shock and $R \rightarrow L$ shunting (e.g., cardiac output less than 65% of predecompensated control value or necrotizing enterocolitis) as well as those receiving vasoactive agents (e.g., dopamine or tolazoline HCl) may produce inaccurate values for Ptc_{O_2} monitoring. Halothane is the only anesthetic gas known to affect the reliability of Ptc_{O_2} monitors. Thick- or dark-skinned patients and some adults may have decreased accuracy to 20% of normal Pa_{O_2} values, but that ratio generally remains constant for each patient. Ptc_{O_2} is theoretically lower than Pa_{O_2} due to partial compensatory metabolic and physiologic processes. If good clinical correlation does not exist in the absence of these patient-oriented problems, then one must reevaluate site placement, skin preparation, and mechanical maintenance of the monitor.

ADDITIONAL READING

Barr, P.A.: Transcutaneous measurement of oxygen tension in infants with hyaline membrane disease, Aust. Paediatr. J. **15**:3-6, 1979.

Enrico, J.: Transcutaneous oxygen monitoring in neonates, Respir. Care **24**:601-605, 1979.

Hill, D.: Making the most of tcO_2, Respir. Ther. **9**:33-36, 1981.

McDowell, J.W., Teasley, A., Vasconcelos, R., and others: Follow-up evaluation of transcutaneous PO_2 monitoring before and after adult exercise testing, Respir. Care **26**:963-965, 1981.

Tremper, K.K., and Shoemaker, W.C.: Continuous CPR monitoring with transcutaneous oxygen and carbon dioxide sensors, Crit. Care Med. **9**:417-418, 1981.

Tremper, K.K., Waxman, K., Bowman, R., and others: Continuous transcutaneous oxygen monitoring during respiratory failure, cardiac decompensation, cardiac arrest, and CPR, Crit. Care Med. **8**:377-381, 1980.

Tremper, K.K., Waxman, K., and Shoemaker, W.C.: Use of transcutaneous oxygen sensors to titrate PEEP, Ann. Surg. **193**:206-209, 1981.

95 Intubation

FRANCES C. MORRISS
DONNA S. BURNS
RICK VINSON

INDICATIONS

Although intubation is frequently considered an emergency procedure, there are few instances when endotracheal tube placement can be undertaken without some minimal planning. When a child is apneic for whatever reason, promptly establish a patent airway and use standard mouth-to-mouth or bag and mask techniques (see Chapter 5). Usually ventilation can be maintained adequately in this manner while preparations for intubation are made. The chance of inhalation of stomach contents or trauma to teeth, gums, or other oropharyngeal structures will be minimized if intubation is approached as a deliberate, planned procedure of an urgent rather than an emergent nature. Situations other than apnea that mandate tube placement are:

1. Respiratory failure (Pa_{O_2} less than 50 mm Hg with Fi_{O_2} greater than 0.8, Pa_{CO_2} greater than 55 mm Hg acutely).
2. Airway obstruction.
3. Control of ventilation, as in tetanus, deliberate hypocarbia, or status epilepticus.
4. Inadequate chest wall function such as may be seen with flail chest or Guillain-Barré syndrome.
5. Patient's inability to protect the airway because of inadequate reflex activity.

These situations are not always as emergent as apnea, and time for proper preparation is more easily available.

TECHNIQUE
Equipment

All necessary equipment should be at hand and functional before intubation is begun. Minimal equipment includes:

1. Laryngoscope and blades of several sizes and lengths (Check light source just before use.) Suggested blades may include:
   Neonate: Miller 0, 1
   Infant: Miller 1; Whis-Hipple 1½
   Child: Miller 2; MacIntosh 2
   Teenager: MacIntosh 3; Phillips

   In general, straight (Miller, Whis-Hipple) blades are recommended for use in infants and neonates because the rigidity of the epiglottis hampers use of a curved (MacIntosh) blade.

2. Oral endotracheal tubes of several sizes. The proper diameter of the tube may be estimated by the following formula:

$$\text{Tube size} = \frac{\text{Age in years}}{4} + 4.5$$

This formula does not apply to infants less than 2 years of age. In general, most premature infants require a 3.0-mm tube, term neonates to age 6 months a 3.5-mm tube, and infants 6 to 18 months a 4.0-mm tube. Compare tube diameter with that of the patient's fifth finger; they should be the same. Besides the proper-sized noncuffed tube, tubes a size larger and a size smaller should be available in case the expected tube will not pass or is too small. Tubes constructed of soft polyvinyl that mold to the airway at body temperature are preferred. *Oral tube placement is the preferred route in the urgent situation because it is technically an easier procedure.* If long-term tube maintenance is necessary, a nasal tube can be placed after the airway is secured orally and the patient is stabilized.

3. Proper-sized connectors for endotracheal tubes if the two are not packaged together.
4. A large-bore catheter or tonsil suction for the pharynx and a small-bore catheter for suctioning the artificial airway.
5. Bag, mask, and oxygen for maintaining ventilation between intubation attempts.
6. Atropine. Airway instrumentation frequently stimulates vagal receptors in and around the larynx, causing bradycardia. Though any bradycardia encountered during intubation attempts should be considered secondary to hypoxia and treated with oxygen, atropine may be useful in blocking vagal reflex activity.
7. If time allows, secure IV catheter for drugs.
8. Cardiac monitoring, preferably an ECG. If ECG monitoring is not feasible, a nurse should be assigned to monitor the pulse continuously during the procedure and to inform the intubator of acute changes.
9. Oral airway or bite block to place between the teeth after intubation to prevent the patient from biting the tube.

Insertion of the tube (Fig. 95-1)

1. Assemble all necessary equipment and obtain the aid of at least one other person to help position the patient and handle the suction, oxygen, etc.
2. Empty the stomach via the NG tube attached to the suction source. This is particularly important if the patient has had a recent meal or has gastric distention with air, a situation that is likely if the patient is being ventilated with a bag and mask. The NG tube may be removed if its presence interferes with intubation.
3. Hyperoxygenate the patient with 100% oxygen for several minutes; this fills the reserve volume of the lung with oxygen rather than room air and provides an added source of oxygen should the patient become apneic. If the patient is a premature infant, oxygenate with an inspired oxygen concentration 10% higher than he normally receives.
4. Consider giving atropine, 0.01 mg/kg IV or IM, to block the vagus. Allow 15 minutes if the IM route is selected.
5. Position the child with the intubator at his head. Remove the head of the bed if necessary. The patient's head should be in the sniffing position, that is, head slightly extended with the jaw thrust forward. A nurse or respiratory therapist should gently restrain the patient's arms, shoulder, and head. In the infant or older child, a roll placed between the shoulder blades to maintain head extension may be helpful. The neonate's occipital prominence will maintain the same position in lieu of a roll. Extreme extension of the head will obstruct the airway and interfere with visualization of the larynx. Ensure that oxygen is flowing over the patient's face.
6. Conditions that increase the difficulty of tube placement include:
   a. Normal anatomy of the neonate (anterior larynx with a more superior position in the neck, stiff epiglottis).
   b. Inability to open the mouth fully (broken or wired jaw).
   c. Inability to extend the neck fully, including cervical spine injuries.
   d. Dental curtain (missing or broken teeth) or dental appliances.
   e. Short, thick neck.
   f. Hypoplastic mandible.
   g. Cleft palate or other palatal or midfacial abnormalities.

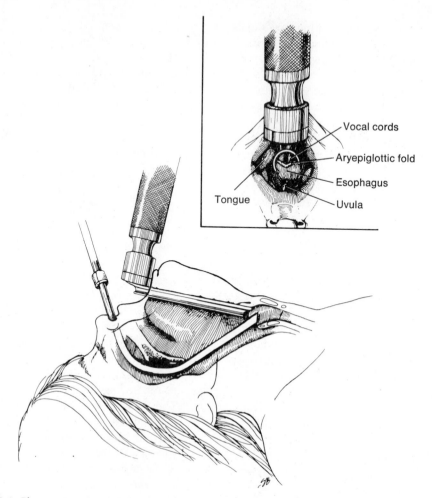

Fig. 95-1. Placement of nasotracheal tube with a straight laryngoscope blade. Note that the epiglottis is lifted out of the airway by the blade. *Inset,* Intubator's view of the airway.

h. Macroglossia.
i. Active bleeding in mouth or nose.
j. Epiglottitis, croup, or airway masses such as tonsillar hypertrophy or cystic hygroma.

If any of these conditions exist, plan to use the laryngoscope initially to assess the airway anatomy and to clear secretions without trying to place a tube. A styleted tube may be appropriate for these situations. Continue to oxygenate the patient between attempts to visualize the larynx.

7. Hold the laryngoscope in the left hand and insert the right thumb and forefinger into the mouth to open it widely. Insert the laryngoscope blade in the right side of the mouth and move the blade to the midline, keeping the tongue to the left of the blade. Place the blade in the vallecula. Lift the blade superiorly with a motion from the shoulder. Do not bend the wrist because this causes a levering motion, forcing the blade against the gum or teeth and pushing the larynx anteriorly out of line of vision. As the blade is

lifted and withdrawn slightly, the larynx should drop down into the line of vision. From the right side of the mouth, insert the tube under direct vision several centimeters through the vocal cords. Gentle pressure over the cricoid cartilage may be helpful in visualizing a larynx that seems anteriorly displaced. If the cords cannot be visualized, place the blade in front of the epiglottis and lift. This is often the easiest method to use in the neonate. If at any time the patient becomes bradycardic or cyanotic, cease efforts and ventilate the patient with bag and mask. Remember that the smallest diameter of the infant's airway is at the cricoid ring, and thus a tube may pass the cords and then meet resistance. Do not force the tube further if this occurs; try a tube with a smaller diameter. Should the patient vomit or regurgitate stomach contents at any time, place him in the lateral position with the head down and suction the pharynx with a tonsil suction or large-bore catheter.

8. Once a tube is placed, ventilate the patient using the bag and check him immediately for:

   a. Bilaterally equal breath sounds. Use a rapid rate of compression of the bag so that the person listening to the chest can easily distinguish this respiratory pattern from air movement in a spontaneously breathing but esophageally intubated patient. Louder or absent sounds on one side indicate that the tube may be in a mainstem bronchus and should be withdrawn until breath sounds are equal.

   b. Absence of breath sounds over the stomach. With an esophageal intubation, transmitted breath sounds may still be heard over the chest but will be much louder over the stomach. In addition, the child will still be able to phonate. Withdraw the tube, ventilate, and try again.

   c. Movement of the chest wall with pressure on the bag. Absence of chest movement may indicate an obstructed tube.

   d. If the child is breathing spontaneously, look for corresponding movement of the bag.

   e. If any doubt exists about tube position, laryngoscope the patient and check the tube position visually. If the patient's condition is deteriorating, remove tube, check for plugging or other mechanical problems, and reintubate after he is stabilized with bag and mask ventilation.

9. Continue to oxygenate the patient through the tube and remove airway secretions if necessary. Do not take your fingers off the tube until it is stabilized. Obtain a stat chest roentgenogram to check the tube position (the tip should be midway between clavicles and carina, i.e., midtrachea) and to ensure that there is no pneumothorax.

10. Once the child is stable, consider placing a nasotracheal tube if long-term respiratory support is anticipated. Choose a soft, uncuffed nasotracheal tube that will comfortably fit the nostril. Leaving the orotracheal tube in place, insert the tube into either nostril. A lubricant such as K-Y jelly may facilitate this. When the tube enters the posterior pharynx, move the untaped orotracheal tube, still connected to the oxygen source, to the left side of the patient's mouth and have the assistant hold it. Laryngoscope the patient and when the larynx and both tubes are visualized, have the assistant remove the orotracheal tube slowly. Advance the nasotracheal tube into the larynx either manually or by use of pediatric Magill forceps. If the latter are employed, hold them in the right hand, insert in the right side of the mouth, pick up the tip of the tube, and advance it into the laryngeal orifice. At this point a gentle push on the nasotracheal tube by the assistant will usually advance the tube through the vocal cords.

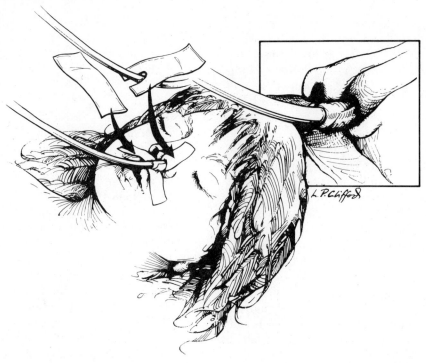

Fig. 95-2. Method of securing nasotracheal tube with tape reinforced by suture. The tape on the nose is necessary to prevent the tube from slipping out of the nose superiorly. *Inset,* Position of suture connecting tape on the tube with tape on the upper lip.

Tube stabilization (Fig. 95-2)

Many methods of tube stabilization exist. In general, the use of the following are helpful:

1. Use a bite block or oral airway to prevent kinking or obstruction from biting of an orotracheal tube. Oral airways will ulcerate the mouth after 24 hours.
2. Use benzoin on cheeks, upper lip, nose, and/ or tube to effect better tape adherence.
3. Use sturdy tape (Elastoplast, cloth).
4. Suture the tube to tape on lip or use a cuff of tape on the tube to tape onto the lip.
5. Reinforce with tape after suturing.

If the tube is excessively long, cut off the extra length to decrease anatomic dead space. If the tube position must be changed, reapply fresh benzoin and use fresh tape. Do not cover the junction between the tube and its connector with tape. The tube and connector may discon-

nect without being noticed. If the child is capable of moving, his hands should be restrained to prevent him from pulling out the tube. Restrain the patient's head using Montgomery straps made by placing two pieces of adhesive tape (sticky side to sticky side) together and securing with a tie. The patient may be further immobilized by placing his head between sandbags. Once an artificial airway is placed, the patient depends on its patency for adequate ventilation; thus, the presence of a tube requires constant, experienced nursing care for suctioning and observation of ventilatory variables.

RISKS AND COMPLICATIONS

The risks of endotracheal tube placement are related to the skill of the intubator and the conditions under which intubation is accomplished. Intubations performed in a deliberate manner with proper equipment and assistance carry a minimal risk. The most common and potentially most severe problem arising during intubation is hypoxia with bradycardia. Patients must be closely monitored during intubation attempts and the procedure discontinued until vital signs can be stabilized, usually by reinstituting ventilation with a bag, mask, and oxygen.

Inability to place an endotracheal tube is always a possibility, and failure to do so in a patient with a life-threatening airway obstruction can result in death. If assessment of the airway anatomy and the patient's clinical status indicates the likelihood of a difficult intubation, skilled help (e.g., anesthesiologist, otolaryngologist, or pediatric surgeon) should be obtained as quickly as possible. Under no circumstances should the unskilled intubator resort to the use of pharmacologic means (muscle relaxants or sedatives) without adequate, skilled support. Inability to intubate or ventilate the paralyzed or apneic patient can be rapidly fatal.

Long-term complications of intubation are outlined elsewhere (see Chapter 29). Early complications usually occur during the attempt to instrument the airway and are traumatic in nature. They include trauma to teeth; laceration of tongue, gums, or oropharynx; epistaxis; perforation of the esophagus or trachea; creation of an air leak (pneumothorax, pneumomediastinum); and dislocation of the arytenoid cartilages. In addition, a number of protective airway reflexes may be stimulated by direct contact with highly innervated structures of the posterior pharynx and larynx. The results may be laryngeal spasm (unremitting cord closure), bronchospasm, bradycardia with hypotension, cardiac dysrhythmias (asystole, PVCs, nodal rhythms), or apnea. The tachycardia and hypertension associated with awake intubation are known to increase ICP; patients in whom this rise is contraindicated must be handled in a different manner (see Chapter 10). Obtundation of protective airway reflexes, specifically absence of ability to gag, cough, or swallow, may be associated with inhalation of stomach contents, mucus, or blood present in the oropharynx at the time of intubation. Conditions other than CNS depression that predispose the patient to inhalation pneumonitis include (1) those that delay gastric emptying (pregnancy, ileus, gastrointestinal obstruction, pain or trauma, narcotics, abdominal masses including hepatomegaly), (2) bleeding in the pharynx, esophagus, or upper gastrointestinal tract, (3) esophageal disease with gastroesophageal incompetence (i.e., reflux), and (4) recent ingestion of food. If the patient displays one of the above and if time allows, 15 to 30 ml of an antacid (e.g., Maalox, milk of magnesia, etc.) may be given to neutralize gastric pH after the stomach is emptied. The morbidity and mortality of inhalation pneumonitis correlate with (1) introduction of acid material (pH <2.5) into the lungs, (2) inhalation of a large volume, and (3) inhalation of particulate matter. The resulting pneumonitis has characteristics of a pulmonary burn with edema and severe ventilation/perfusion defects combined with small-airway obstruction secondary to the particulate matter. It is difficult to treat and often fatal.

ADDITIONAL READING

Applebaum, B.: Tracheal intubation, Philadelphia, 1976, W.B. Saunders Co.

Blanc, V.R., and Tremblay, N.A.G.: The complications of tracheal intubation, Anesth. Analg. 53:203-210, 1974.

Bynum, L.J., and Pierce, A.D.: Pulmonary aspiration of gastric contents, Am. Rev. Respir. Dis. 114:1129-1136, 1976.

Cork, R.B., Woods, W., Vaughan, R.W., and Harris, T.: Oxygen supplementation during endotracheal intubation of infants (letter), Anesthesiology 51(2):186, 1979.

Emami, G.L., and Delbianco, L.M.: An improved technique for securing nasoendotracheal tubes, Matern. Child Nurs. J. 6:337-340, 1981.

Raju, T.N., Vidyasagar, D., Torres, C., and others: Intracranial pressure during intubation and anesthesia in infants, J. Pediatr. 96:860-862, 1980.

Salem, M.R., Mathrubhutham, M., and Bennett, E.J.: Difficult intubation, N. Engl. J. Med. 295:879-881, 1976.

White, A., and Kander, P.L.: Anatomical factors in difficult direct laryngoscopy, Br. J. Anaesth. 47:468-472, 1975.

96 Continuous positive airway pressure

GERALD C. MOORE

INDICATIONS

Continuous positive airway pressure (CPAP) is a technique for providing inspired gas with positive pressure in spontaneously breathing patients. This technique was first used successfully in the treatment of adult respiratory distress syndrome (ARDS) and has been adapted successfully for use in infants and children. The main effect of CPAP is to maintain an increased FRC. RV and therefore FRC are decreased in the presence of alveolar collapse, the result of which is intrapulmonary shunting of blood and loss of lung compliance. The hypoxemia that occurs with intrapulmonary shunting is partially a result of ventilation and perfusion mismatching. In addition, once the alveoli are collapsed, a much greater opening pressure is required to expand them, thus increasing the work of breathing. CPAP is an excellent means of improving oxygenation and lessening the requirements for exposure to high environmental oxygen concentrations in patients who are spontaneously breathing. CPAP may be useful in the following clinical situations:

1. Clinical hyaline membrane disease.
2. Inhalation or chemical pneumonitis.
3. Severe pneumonia.
4. Pulmonary edema with or without associated congestive heart failure.
5. Fluid overload.
6. Generalized atelectasis.
7. Infants with apnea of prematurity, occasionally.
8. Infants or children with ARDS.

Positive end-expiratory pressure (PEEP) is sometimes confused with CPAP. PEEP is similar but refers to the maintenance of a greater than atmospheric pressure, or positive end-expiratory pressure, in the airways of patients who are breathing with the assistance of a mechanical ventilator. Conditions that may require mechanical ventilation with PEEP are the same as those that may require CPAP alone.

There are several physiologic effects of CPAP and PEEP. The primary effect is to increase FRC, which may be beneficial or detrimental. When FRC is increased from abnormally low to optimal values, CPAP may be helpful in improving oxygenation. However, when used in a patient with optimal or high FRC values, CPAP may cause overdistention of the alveoli, exacerbate mismatching of ventilation and perfusion, and decrease lung elastic recoil. CPAP will reduce the subatmospheric intrathoracic pressure seen at end-expiration or even change it to positive values. This may exert profound effects on the circulation by increasing CVP and decreasing venous return to the heart (preload), thereby decreasing cardiac output. Impedance of venous return from the head may increase ICP. It is difficult, however, to predict accurately the effect of CPAP on the circulation, since venous blood pressure and cardiac output also depend on circulatory blood volume, myocardial performance, and acute factors such as hypoxemia and acidosis.

CPAP usually results in an increase in Pa_{O_2} and a decrease in the amount of physiologic

542

R → L shunting through the lungs. The increase in Pa_{O_2} is directly proportional to the decrease in the amount of the shunt, which in turn is inversely proportional to the FRC.

TECHNIQUE

CPAP may be effectively accomplished with nasal prongs, with an endotracheal tube, or through a large bag around the head fastened snugly around the neck. The last method is rarely used now because of the significant incidence of increased ICP secondary to the impedance of jugular venous return. In the most

widely used system (Gregory), a continuous supply of humidified fresh gas is introduced near the endotracheal tube and escapes through the tail end of a reservoir bag where the overall pressure in the system is adjusted by partial occlusion with a screw clamp. Another tube is placed in the system between the patient connector and the reservoir bag to connect a pressure gauge for monitoring the system pressure and to provide a safe pressure "pop-off" valve and thus avoid excessive pressure from developing within the system. Excessive pressure can prevent effective ventilation and can cause alveolar rupture. Another tube is connected to the circuit (not shown) for a low-pressure (about 2 cm H_2O) patient-disconnect alarm (Fig. 96-1). Most mechanical ventilators today have the

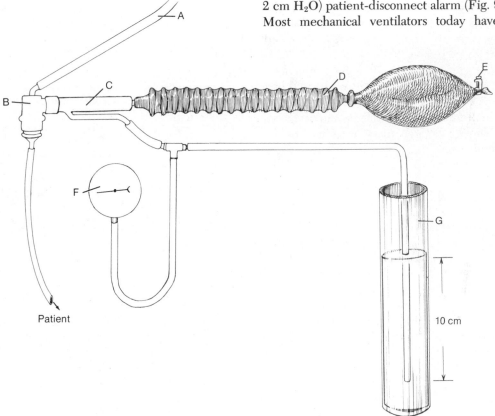

Fig. 96-1. Apparatus for administering CPAP: *A*, line from controlled humidified oxygen source; *B*, Norman elbow; *C*, Washington T-piece; *D*, flow tubing with rebreathing bag; *E*, bulldog clamp; *F*, pressure gauge; *G*, graduated cylinder for release of excessive pressure within the system.

capability of providing CPAP through the basic circuit. This allows for an easy method to wean a patient from assisted ventilation or to provide pressure in a spontaneously breathing patient who will likely require intermittent mechanical assistance.

RISKS AND COMPLICATIONS

In general, the complications of CPAP are related to barotrauma, oxygen toxicity (which may be unavoidable), cardiac output, and prolonged intubation. Physiologic complications associated with excessive reduction of cardiac output may be reflected by a decreased Pa_{O_2} and a widening of the arteriovenous O_2 difference without a proportionate decrease in the physiologic shunt fraction, and thus, there is more severe arterial hypoxemia than expected for any given shunt. Increased venous admixture due to aggravation of intrapulmonary shunting may also result in hypoxemia. When CPAP is transmitted preferentially to portions of the lung already well ventilated and perfused, blood flowing through these areas will be diverted to more diseased and therefore more poorly ventilated areas. Even if Pa_{O_2} increases with CPAP or PEEP, concomitant reductions in systemic arterial blood pressure, mixed venous oxygen tension ($P\bar{v}_{O_2}$), cardiac output, or urinary output should warn the physician that these abnormalities may reflect the effects of administering this form of therapy.

Anatomic complications include pneumothorax, pneumomediastinum, pneumopericardium, injury to the proximal airway by the endotracheal tube or prongs, and interstitial emphysema. Use of nasal prongs also increases gastric distention and may interfere with feeding. Impedance of intracranial venous return may exacerbate increased ICP, and CPAP must be used cautiously in patients with cerebral edema.

ADDITIONAL READING

Asbaugh, D.G., and Petty, T.L.: Positive end-expiratory pressure, J. Thorac. Cardiovasc. Surg. **65:**165-170, 1973.

Berman, L.S., Fox, W.W., Raphaely, R.C., and Downes, J.J., Jr.: Optimum levels of CPAP for tracheal extubation of newborn infants, J. Pediatr. **89:**109-112, 1976.

Greenbaum, D.M., Miller, E., Eross, B., and others: Continuous positive airway pressure without tracheal intubation in spontaneously breathing patients, Chest **69:**615-620, 1976.

Gregory, G.A., Kitterman, J.A., Phibbs, R.H., and others: Treatment of the idiopathic respiratory-distress syndrome with continuous positive airway pressure, N. Engl. J. Med. **284:**1333-1340, 1971.

Kattwinkel, J., Fleming, D., Cha, C.C., and others: A device for administration of continuous positive airway pressure by the nasal route, Pediatrics **52:**131-133, 1973.

Kumar, A., Falke, K.J., Geffin, B., and others: Continuous positive-pressure ventilation in acute respiratory failure: effects on hemodynamics and lung function, N. Engl. J. Med. **283:**1430-1436, 1970.

Stevens, P.S.: Positive end expiratory pressure breathing, Basics of RD **5:**1-6, 1977.

97 Assisted ventilation

GERALD C. MOORE
RONALD M. PERKIN

INDICATIONS

Assisted ventilation is supplied when a patient is unable to sustain adequate spontaneous ventilation as defined by Pa_{O_2} and Pa_{CO_2} and by clinical criteria that vary with the condition being treated (see Chapter 12). Patients with chronic obstructive lung disease and clinical deterioration as assessed by the presence of coma, agitation, or inability to cooperate and by marked worsening of arterial blood-gas measurement fulfill the criteria for airway intervention and assisted ventilation. Other indications for mechanical ventilation include reduced ventilatory capacity (as measured by abnormalities in pulmonary function), increasing atelectasis, instability of the chest wall secondary to trauma

or surgery, and the early treatment of patients at high risk for developing ARDS (see Chapter 14). Chapter 95 outlines the procedures for intubation. Common medical indications for the institution of assisted ventilation for certain conditions in which respiratory failure may occur are listed in Table 97-1. Surgical indications are listed in Table 97-2. Some of these indications are relative and prophylactic in nature, but others are based on the immediate need to sustain ventilation. An example of the former is a patient with cerebral edema who may require assisted ventilation to deliberately lower Pa_{CO_2} and cause cerebral vascular constriction, thus reducing one of the major space-occupying compartments in the cranium. Examples of pa-

Table 97-1. Common medical indications for the insertion of an endotracheal tube and/or the institution of assisted ventilation

Newborn
1. Prematurity and clinical hyaline membrane disease
2. Apnea
3. Asphyxia
4. Inhalation pneumonia
5. Sepsis with pneumonia
6. CNS abnormalities

Less than 2 years of age
1. Pneumonia
2. Acute severe asthma
3. Croup
4. Congenital heart disease
5. Foreign body inhalation
6. Congenital abnormalities of the airway (e.g., tracheal webs, cysts, lobar emphysema)

7. Nasopharyngeal obstruction due to large tonsils or adenoids
8. CNS abnormalities

Greater than 2 years of age
1. Epiglottitis
2. Acute severe asthma
3. Cystic fibrosis
4. Peripheral polyneuritis
5. Poisoning
6. Near-drowning
7. Encephalitis
8. Early treatment of patients at high risk for ARDS
9. Trauma
10. Myasthenia gravis

Table 97-2. Common surgical indications for the institution of assisted ventilation in children

General surgery	Cardiac surgery
1. Prolonged operations (more than 8 hours)	1. Patients with large L → R shunts in whom there is an elevation of pulmonary vascular resistance: VSD, common atrioventricular canal, transposition of the great vessels
2. Intraoperative trauma to the lung or airway	
3. Interference with the integrity of the chest wall	
4. Biochemical disturbances that may result in muscle weakness: hypokalemia, hypocalcemia, hypoglycemia	2. Patients with pulmonary oligemia: tetralogy of Fallot, pulmonary valvar stenosis or atresia with intact ventricular septum, tricuspid atresia
5. Need for analgesics in doses that would produce respiratory depression	3. Anomalies that when corrected produce an increase in pulmonary venous pressure during the postoperative period: total anomalous pulmonary venous drainage, transposition of the great vessels
6. Acquired or congenital malformations that may limit respiratory reserve	

tients in whom the need is immediate and life sustaining include those with ARDS that may occur secondary to massive trauma and hemorrhagic shock, overwhelming inhalation pneumonia, severe viral pneumonia, narcotic overdose, and fluid overload.

TECHNIQUE
Principles

Most ventilators in use today are positive-pressure generators. Negative-pressure devices are logical extensions of the normal physiologic method of breathing but have limited application, primarily because of equipment size and because the negative-pressure device necessitates that the patient be enclosed so that a negative pressure surrounding the chest wall can be created to effect ventilation. Positive-pressure devices are of two general types: pressure- and volume-controlled. The pressure-controlled ventilators provide flow into the lungs at rates determined by the flexibility of the machine until a desired preset peak inspiratory pressure is achieved or until a preset maximum pressure safety limit is generated in the ventilatory circuit. In this type of flow-generated pressure device, the delivered TV changes with lung compliance and with changes in the degree of

airway obstruction. Commonly used pressure ventilators are the Bennett PR-2; Bird Mark 7, 8, and 14; Baby-Bird; Bourns P200 infant ventilator; and the Sechrist IV-100B infant ventilator. Volume-controlled ventilators deliver a preset volume from a cylinder that is usually driven by a piston or by a chain-driven bellows. The pressure delivered varies with lung compliance and the degree of obstruction, but the volume delivered remains the same, provided that a maximum allowable preset pressure is not exceeded. Actually, with most ventilators, exhaled volume is measured, so that allowances must be made for compliance of the ventilator tubing and for air leaks around the endotracheal tube when the preset inspired volume is calculated. Commonly used volume ventilators are the Bennett MA-1, Ohio 560, Siemens 900C, and Bourns LS104-150. All of these devices are adaptable to infants and children, but the most efficient ventilators for infants are those specifically designed for them, e.g., the Baby-Bird, Bourns P200, Bourns LS104-150, and Sechrist IV-100B.

Characteristics of an ideal infant and pediatric ventilator include the following:

1. Accurate measurement of the pressure of proximal airways.

2. Reliable delivery of preset TV.
3. Accurate blending of gases.
4. Delivery of gas at rapid rates.
5. Alarm systems sensitive to both high- and low-pressure abnormalities and system malfunction.
6. Mode flexibility: control, assist, assist/control, IMV, spontaneous breathing.
7. Variable inspiratory and expiratory ratio settings (controls rate).
8. Reliable maximum-pressure setting.
9. System for providing warm humidified gas.
10. Ability to provide an intermittent sigh volume.
11. Inspiratory hold.
12. Ability to deliver CPAP and PEEP.

Physiologic effects of positive-pressure ventilation

During spontaneous ventilation, peripheral alveoli are ventilated first because they are closer to the expanding chest wall. Since the process is reversed in positive-pressure ventilation, central alveoli are ventilated before peripheral alveoli. Also, during positive-pressure ventilation there is a slight increase in anatomic dead space because small bronchi are expanded more than they would be with spontaneous breathing from the positive pressure during the inspiratory phase of ventilation and because preferential ventilation occurs in areas that are more compliant. This has clinical significance when one is trying to expand a lung with localized atelectasis, in which slower inspiratory rates and inspiratory holds are useful to ensure delivery of gas to less compliant airways.

Venous return is decreased during IPPV, particularly if high pressures are being used. Significant embarrassment to venous return may be corrected by short inspiratory times, a slowly rising peak inspiratory pressure curve, and prompt termination of positive pressure at end-inspiration. The pulmonary circulation is usually not affected by mechanical ventilation as long as the intrapleural pressures are not excessive and higher degrees of end-pressure are not required. Because of the slight decrease in venous return, the intracranial circulating volume is slightly increased, and this may be reflected by increased ICP measurements, especially in patients with abnormally increased ICP.

Ventilator modes

Several modes for delivering assisted ventilation are available.

In the control mode of ventilation, the patient takes no active role in the ventilatory cycle. The machine initiates inspiration, provides the power for inspiration, and determines the rate of ventilation and TV. The advantage of this method is that one knows the total amount of support provided to the patient. This mode is particularly useful in critically ill patients who do not have the ability to initiate spontaneous respiration, who are comatose, or who may require sedation and/or muscle relaxants. The primary disadvantage of this type of ventilation is in the spontaneously breathing patient. For example, if the patient is awake, he may try to initiate breathing if the machine is not delivering adequate ventilation. Since there is no continuous air flow to the patient when the ventilator is not cycling, it is impossible for the patient to receive a self-initiated breath, a stressful and dangerous situation.

A second mode of ventilation is the assist mode in which the ventilator begins inspiration in response to a patient-initiated breath. The patient generates a negative (subatmospheric) pressure that triggers the machine to deliver the preset volume or pressure. The disadvantages are: (1) the patient may not be alert enough for one reason or another to initiate an inspiratory breath, and (2) the machine may be insensitive to small amounts of negative pressure initiated by a patient who is critically ill.

To circumvent these problems, a combination assist and control mode may be used in which the patient receives a mandatory number of breaths at a preset volume or pressure and rate and he may intermittently initiate his own inspiratory effort and receive the same preset volume or pressure. This offers a definite overall advantage when compared with the strict assist mode, but there is danger of overventilation and the consequences of respiratory alkalosis, which include decreased cardiac output, decreased cerebral blood flow, transient leftward shift of the oxyhemoglobin dissociation curve, and increased oxygen consumption.

Intermittent mandatory ventilation (IMV) is a modification of the assist and control modes of ventilation which provides a solution to many of the problems encountered with the other types of ventilation. If a continuous flow of gas (rather than the intermittent flow that occurs during the conventional type of ventilation described above) passes through a ventilator circuit, the problem of asynchronous breathing is minimized. IMV is a mode in which the patient is allowed to breathe on his own and, at certain intervals, a mandatory inspiration is provided by the ventilator. This mandatory breath is completely independent of the patient's own ventilatory pattern and may be determined by either a preset pressure or volume limit. Should the patient breathe spontaneously, he will receive fresh gas at a predetermined oxygen concentration at his own TV. This type of ventilation is more physiologic than either the assist or control mode of ventilation in most instances.

Institution of assisted ventilation

The following variables must be specified when assisted ventilation is initiated:
1. Equipment to be used (Baby-Bird, Siemens 900C, etc.).
2. FI_{O_2}.
3. Humidification of gases (heated or not).
4. Minute ventilation (TV × rate/min).
   a. Ventilator rate: 15 to 20 assisted breaths per minute if the patient is totally con-

trolled, or 5 to 15 breaths per minute if on IMV or assist modes.
   b. TV: 7 to 15 cc/kg per assisted breath if on volume-controlled machine, or a peak inspiratory pressure of 20 to 30 cm H_2O in a normally compliant lung on a pressure-controlled device. (A small premature infant may require less than 20 cm H_2O peak inspiratory pressure; see Chapter 34.)
   c. Mode: control, assist, assist/control, IMV, CPAP.
   d. PEEP/CPAP (in cm H_2O).
   e. Special instructions: sigh, inspiratory hold, I:E ratio, flow rate, etc.

Once the initial settings are determined, check the patient for adequacy of breath sounds, chest wall movement, color, and peripheral perfusion. Obtain arterial blood-gas tensions within 15 minutes of initiation of assisted ventilation. If the patient deteriorates, disconnect him from the device and sustain him with bag and tube ventilation. Changes in the above variables may be necessary before a satisfactory clinical status is achieved.

Measurement

Ventilation

1. Measure the patient's TV (volume-controlled ventilator), which should be approximately 10 cc of delivered volume per kg. Most machines allow for the measurement of expiratory volume, which is a reasonable estimate of the volume delivered if no significant air leak is present. Ventilator rates and pressures or volumes should be adjusted to achieve adequate minute ventilation (TV times the rate of breathing in 1 minute), which is readily assessed by measuring Pa_{CO_2}.
2. Monitor inspiratory pressures frequently when a volume ventilator is used. With improving compliance, the inspiratory pressures will decrease. With obstruction of the

endotracheal tube or ventilator circuit, the pressure will suddenly increase to a very high value.

3. If one has the ability to measure expired gases, V_D/V_T may be measured.
4. Measure respiratory rates of the machine and the patient every hour.

Gas exchange

1. Measurement of Pa_{O_2} and Pa_{CO_2} provides the most readily available assessment of pulmonary gas exchange. These should be measured frequently, preferably through an indwelling peripheral arterial catheter to ensure that a stable-state specimen is obtained.
2. Pet_{CO_2} can be measured and continuously displayed. This is a valuable adjunct to intermittent arterial blood gas determinations.
3. $P(A - a)O_2$ may also be measured.
4. Tissue gas exchange can be measured by monitoring organ function (e.g., urine output, level of consciousness, metabolic acidosis).

Chest roentgenograms

Obtain chest roentgenograms every day during the acute phase and whenever pneumothorax, tube malposition or obstruction, or infection is suspected.

Weaning procedure

Criteria for weaning patients from assisted ventilation are listed in Table 97-3.

RISKS AND COMPLICATIONS

Positive-pressure ventilation is associated with numerous physiologic and mechanical complications (Table 97-4). In order to prevent these complications, it is imperative to comprehend not only how and when to apply airway pressure therapy, but also how and when the therapy may be detrimental or contraindicated. The clinical goal of positive-pressure ventilation is to optimize ventilatory mechanics and gas exchange while minimizing impairment of the central and peripheral circulations.

Table 97-3. Criteria for weaning from assisted ventilation

1. Pa_{O_2}, Pa_{CO_2}, pH, and base deficit improved as much as can be expected considering the clinical course
2. Resolution or adequate improvement of the condition that necessitated airway intervention
3. Metabolic, cardiovascular, and CNS stability
4. Physiologic measurements
   a. Simple:
      (1) TV greater than 5 cc/kg
      (2) VC greater than 10 cc/kg
      (3) MIF of −20 cm H_2O
   b. More sophisticated:
      (1) $P(A - a)O_2$ in 100% oxygen less than 350 mm Hg
      (2) V_D/V_T less than 0.5
      (3) FRC more than 50% predicted

Table 97-4. Complications of positive-pressure ventilation

Positive mean airway pressure
1. Decreased cardiac filling and output
2. Altered distribution of ventilation and pulmonary blood flow
3. Extravascular water accumulation
4. Pulmonary parenchymal damage
5. Gastrointestinal malfunction
6. Cerebral ischemia and/or intracranial hypertension
7. Alveolar hypoventilation or hyperventilation
8. Alveolar rupture with extra-alveolar free air

Endotracheal or tracheostomy tubes
1. Mucosal damage
2. Accidental malposition or extubation
3. Partial or complete tube obstruction
4. Pneumonia

Operation of ventilator
1. Mechanical failure
2. Alarm failure
3. Inadequate nebulization or humidification

Most adverse physiologic responses to positive-pressure ventilation result from inappropriately high mean airway pressure. Elevation of the mean airway pressure may detrimentally affect cardiac filling and output. Depressed cardiac output and changes in peripheral vascular resistance and blood flow can lead to hypotension, oliguria, and fluid retention, all of which tend to aggravate pulmonary pathology and decrease systemic oxygen transport. Hemodynamic monitoring, IV fluid therapy, and cardiovascular pharmacologic therapy are inseparable from positive-airway-pressure therapy.

Positive-pressure ventilation may also adversely affect the distribution of ventilation and pulmonary perfusion. Inappropriately high levels of mean airway pressure can lead to over-inflation of alveoli, increased dead space, decreased compliance, fluid accumulation in the lungs, and increased intrapulmonary shunt. The beneficial effects and optimum level of positive mean airway pressure depend on the underlying pulmonary pathology.

Alveolar rupture and its sequelae constitute the most frequent life-threatening complication of ventilatory assistance. The capacity for instant recognition, evaluation, and relief of these disorders is a primary requisite for PICU personnel.

The occurrence of mechanical failure is more often due to personal errors than defective equipment. The common mechanical misadventures such as disconnected tubes, extubation, endotracheal tube obstruction, and apparatus malfunction are largely preventable and underscore the need for continuous electrical and human monitoring of both the machine and the patient.

ADDITIONAL READING

Daily, W.J.R., and Smith, P.C.: Mechanical ventilation of the newborn infant, Parts I and II, Clin. Probl. Pediatr., June-July, 1971.

Fox, W.W., Berman, L.S., Dinwiddie, R., and Shaffer, T.H.: Tracheal extubation of the neonate at 2 to 3 cm H_2O continuous positive airway pressure, Pediatrics **59**: 257-261, 1977.

Kirby, R.R.: Intermittent mandatory ventilation in the neonate, Crit. Care Med. **5**:18-22, 1977.

Mushin, W.W., Rendell-Baker, L., Thompson, P.W., and Mapplawn, W.W.: Automatic ventilation of the lungs, ed. 3, Oxford, Eng., 1980, Blackwell Scientific Publications.

Perkin, R.M., and Levin, D.L.: Adverse effects of positive-pressure ventilation in children. In Gregory, G.A., editor: Respiratory failure in the child, New York, 1981, Churchill Livingstone, pp. 163-187.

Petty, T.L.: IMV vs IMC, Chest **67**:630-631, 1975.

Sahn, S.A., Lakshminarayan, S., and Petty, T.L.: Weaning from mechanical ventilation, J.A.M.A. **235**:2208-2212, 1976.

Zwillich, C.W., Pierson, O.J., Creagh, C.E., and others: Complications of assisted ventilation, Am. J. Med. **57**: 161-170, 1974.

98 Oxygen administration

PATRICIA WALTERS
GARY ELMORE
MARY E. GRANDY

INDICATIONS

The indications for oxygen administration are (1) to relieve hypoxemia, (2) to decrease the work of breathing, and (3) to decrease myocardial work. There are many devices available for pediatric use that supply various concentrations of oxygen. The efficiency of any system used with children depends on the child's acceptance of the treatment or device. Children require special attention and reassurance when a continuous oxygen device is employed.

TECHNIQUE

Hoods (Fig. 98-1). A hood is a Plexiglas encasement for the head of an infant. With adequate flow rates from an oxygen source, an FI_{O_2} of 1.0, or 100% oxygen, may be achieved. There are several different designs available in various sizes. Two important distinctions exist between the Oxyhood and the halo. The large-bore connection on the Oxyhood is perpendicular to and several inches above the base. This produces a turbulent flow that makes it difficult to maintain a stable FI_{O_2} Therefore, an extension and/or lid is required to establish a stable oxygen concentration. The Plexiglas lid can absorb much of the heat from a radiant heating system. When an Oxyhood is used, nothing should be placed around the infant's neck that would restrict the flow of carbon dioxide from the system. Alternatively, the large-bore connection on a halo is connected to a T-bar that is parallel to the base of the system. This produces a vortex flow that helps stabilize the oxygen con-

centration and at the same time allows carbon dioxide to escape through the top of the halo. A diaper or other pad may be placed around the neck opening to protect the infant's skin when a halo is used; however, the top must never be occluded. A mist device will help stabilize oxygen concentration; but if a humidifier is used with an Oxyhood, a lid must be used to maintain

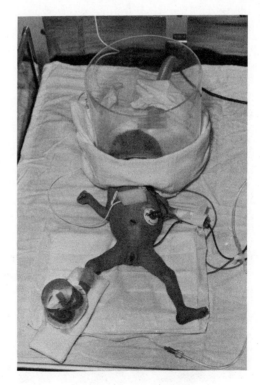

Fig. 98-1. Infant in halo.

a constant $F_{I_{O_2}}$. Twelve inches has been shown to be the optimal height of a hood to produce efficient oxygen delivery. Any hood requires a minimum of 8 to 12 L of flow to flush the system properly. The oxygen concentration will then be equal to that of the source gas.

Closed incubators (Fig. 98-2). Closed incubators can provide a means of oxygen administration and can produce a neutral thermal environment. On the side or back of most closed incubators is a small-bore connection that may be attached to an oxygen flowmeter to provide an $F_{I_{O_2}}$ up to 0.40. Some incubators have a popoff device that restricts high oxygen flows. When the red flag located on the back of the incubator is placed in a vertical position, the Venturi ports inside the incubator will close and prevent room air entrainment. However, because of the construction of the incubator, the highest $F_{I_{O_2}}$ attainable is approximately 0.85 (Table 98-1). Hoods are frequently used inside closed incubators when a stable $F_{I_{O_2}}$ is impor-

tant. A fan, heating coil, and water reservoir provide for the circulation of warm humidified gas. Only distilled water should be used in any nebulizer attached to a closed incubator. Saline will cause salt deposits to build up on the fan and motor damaging the unit. This system limits access to the patient, since gas escapes whenever the ports are opened unless flexible sleeves are present on the ports.

Tents. Mist tents are being used less frequently because they are cumbersome and difficult to maintain, patient access is limited, the canopies have to be kept tightly sealed around the patient, and they are frequently frightening to the patient. The gas supply to tents may be either refrigerated or heated, with closed or open canopies. Refrigeration is not required with an open-top tent, since heat rises and the mist employed in the unit produces an environment slightly below room temperature. A dense mist will help stabilize the oxygen concentration. The environmental temperature should be maintained 6° to 8° F lower than room air for patient comfort. At least 10 to 12 L of flow are required to flush an open-top tent and to provide a stable oxygen concentration. A wide range of oxygen concentrations may be ob-

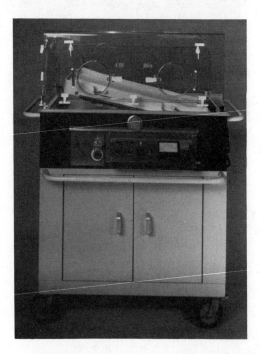

Fig. 98-2. Vicker's closed incubator.

Table 98-1. Incubator oxygen therapy

Flow of oxygen (L/minute)	Concentration of oxygen
Red reminder flag in horizontal position	
4	28%-31%
6	32%-36%
8	37%-40%
Red reminder flag in vertical position	
4-6	Flow not sufficient for high concentration
8	70%-75%
10	75%-80%
12	80%-85%

Adapted from Lough, M.D., and Doershuk, C.F.: Respiratory therapy. In Lough, M.D., Doershuk, C.F., and Stern, R.C., editors: Pediatric respiratory therapy, Chicago, 1974, Year Book Medical Publishers, Inc., p. 106.

tained. However, tents require frequent monitoring to determine actual $F_{I_{O_2}}$, particularly if the patient is very active.

Masks. Different types of masks are manufactured in adult, pediatric, and infant sizes to produce different ranges of oxygen concentration. An aerosol mask will deliver a 100% source gas if the flow used is high enough to meet minute volume requirements and a good seal is established. A simple mask will deliver a low to moderate concentration at a specific liter flow and room air entrainment value. Venturi masks will deliver a precise concentration and are manufactured in 24%, 28%, 30%, 35%, 40%, and 45% oxygen-delivery levels. A nonrebreathing mask with a reservoir bag that partially collapses during inspiration will deliver moderate to high concentrations of oxygen. All masks should be constructed of clear, soft vinyl for better comfort and visibility. Masks afford easy patient accessibility but should be used with caution in patients prone to vomiting and inhaling secretions. The $F_{I_{O_2}}$ being delivered is that which reaches the mask, and this may not accurately reflect that which is reaching the patient's lungs (Table 98-2).

Face tents. Face tents combine the good qualities of both aerosol masks and mist tents and are generally accepted by children. The large, soft vinyl contour fits loosely around the patient's face and is held in place by elastic straps. The straps may be cushioned with cotton pads for extra comfort. The patient is accessible

Table 98-2. Oxygen flow required to achieve desired oxygen concentration in mask therapy

Oxygen flow required L/minute	Oxygen concentration desired	
	Nonrebreathing oxygen mask	Pediatric medium-concentration oxygen mask
6-8	40-50%	35-45%
8-10	50-60%	45-55%
10-12	60-95%	55-60%

Reproduced with permission from Lough, M.D., and Doershuk, C.F.: Respiratory therapy. In Lough, M.D., Doershuk, C.F., and Stern, R.C., editors: Pediatric respiratory therapy. Copyright © 1974 by Year Book Medical Publishers, Inc., Chicago.

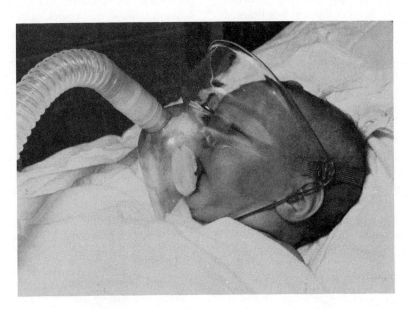

Fig. 98-3. Inverted adult face tent used on an infant.

and may continue to play without feeling confined. Presently, face tents are manufactured in the adult size only; however, they may be inverted to create a smaller reservoir and a better fit for the smaller patient (Fig. 98-3). At least 8 to 10 L of flow should be used to flush the system and provide a stable oxygen concentration. Larger patients will require higher flows to meet their minute-volume requirements and inspiratory flow rates. Face tents, when set properly, will provide an oxygen concentration equal to the source gas.

Nasal cannulae and catheters. Cannulae fit just proximal to the opening of the nares and will deliver a low, nonspecific oxygen concentration if the nares are patent. Oxygen flow through cannulae provides the patient with continuous oxygen while he is eating. Catheters may be inserted nasally to the level of the uvula. This may prove uncomfortable and is rarely tolerated by a child. Since most catheters occlude more of the nasal passage than is practical for proper ventilation in infants, the tip of the catheter, which may be a small feeding tube, may be positioned at the base of the nostril and taped in place for delivering a low oxygen concentration. Both devices require oxygen flows of 1 to 6 L/min. The nasopharynx acts as a reservoir, providing an oxygen-enriched atmosphere for both nose and mouth breathers.

T-bars and tracheostomy masks. Both devices are used to deliver oxygen to intubated patients and require adequate flows to meet the minute-volume requirements of the patient and to provide 100% source gas. T-bars require a short, flexible tube on the distal end to act as a reservoir and prevent room air entrainment.

Bag/mask devices. An anesthesia bag with a nonrebreathing pressure-relieving elbow, C-clamp, and mask can be used to deliver oxygen when other devices must be interrupted; however, the concentration of oxygen delivered is approximate.

Aerosol units. Aerosol units designed to deliver medication as well as gas should have an optimal particle size range of less than 5 μ with an output of at least 2 ml/min. Large-bore hoses should be kept free of excess water from aerosol rain out. High aerosol outputs (6 ml/min) may cause fluid retention in infants. Aerosolized oxygen mixtures are a source of nosocomial infection.

Endotracheal tube with CPAP or assisted ventilation. No special devices other than standard tubing and a 16-mm connector are needed to deliver humidified gas to an airway tube.

RISKS AND COMPLICATIONS

Oxygen should be regarded as a drug, and toxicity is possible in children as well as in infants. Systemic oxygen toxicity (e.g., retrolental fibroplasia) is in part the result of excessive Pa_{O_2} delivered to the retinal artery. Pulmonary oxygen toxicity is in part the result of excessive inhaled oxygen tensions and is manifested by cessation of mucociliary activity, a decrease in production of surface-active material, atelectasis, and ventilation/perfusion abnormalities. Pulmonary and systemic oxygen toxicity depends on the level of oxygen concentration and the duration of administration and varies from individual to individual. In an effort to establish safe guidelines, the American Academy of Pediatrics has issued the following statements concerning oxygen therapy in the newborn:

1. Pa_{O_2} should not exceed 100 mm Hg and should be maintained between 60 and 80 mm Hg.
2. Relatively high concentrations of inspired oxygen may be necessary to maintain Pa_{O_2} within a normal range.
3. If blood-gas measurements are not available, a full-term, mature infant who is not apneic but who exhibits generalized cyanosis may be given oxygen in a concentration just high enough to abolish the cyanosis.
4. The recommended blood sampling sites for Pa_{O_2} studies are the radial or temporal arteries. In most circumstances, however, a blood sample from an arterial catheter located in the descending aorta will be satisfactory.
5. When an infant is placed in an oxygen-en-

riched atmosphere, the oxygen concentration should be measured at least every 2 hours. The oxygen analyzer itself should be calibrated daily on both room air and 100% oxygen.

6. Mixtures of oxygen and room air should be warmed and humidified when delivered to an infant.
7. As the patient's condition improves, FI_{O_2} should be lowered in 10% increments as guided by arterial blood-gas measurements.
8. It should be appreciated that oxygen is toxic to organs, particularly the lungs, which may be damaged even if the above criteria are adhered to.
9. A person experienced in recognizing retrolental fibroplasia should examine the eyes of all infants born at less than 36 weeks' gestation or weighing less than 2,000 g who have received oxygen therapy. This examination should be made at the time of discharge and also at 3 to 6 months of age.

A general rule is to give only enough oxygen to achieve the desired results, bearing in mind that cyanosis is usually not an accurate method of evaluating hypoxia. Caution should be used any time an oxygen-enriched environment is interrupted for various hospital procedures. Periodic monitoring of oxygen environment should be charted for future reference. If constant oxygen monitoring is employed, the analyzer should be adapted to prevent erroneous readings due to moisture.

Sudden decreases in inspired oxygen concentrations may occur secondary to inadvertent withdrawal of oxygen (e.g., due to plugged or kinked endotracheal tubes, CPT, suctioning and disconnection from the oxygen source) and may result in serious clinical problems, such as:

1. Pulmonary arterial hypertension with R → L shunting of blood through a PDA or foramen ovale in an infant.
2. Significant hypoxemia, pulmonary vasospasm, acute right heart dilation, decreased cardiac output, shock, and death in a child with preexisting pulmonary arterial hypertension.
3. Intracranial hemorrhage.
4. Renal damage.
5. Necrotizing enterocolitis.

ADDITIONAL READING

American Academy of Pediatrics: Standards and recommendations for hospital care of newborn infants, ed. 6, Evanston, Ill., 1977.

Korones, S.B.: High-risk newborn infants, ed. 3, St. Louis, 1981, The C.V. Mosby Co.

Lough, M.D., Doershuk, C.F., and Stern, R.C., editors: Pediatric respiratory therapy, Chicago, 1974, Year Book Medical Publishers, Inc., pp. 100-115.

Shapiro, B.A.: Clinical application of blood gases, Chicago, 1976, Year Book Medical Publishers, Inc.

Slonim, N.B., Schneider, S.N., Weng, T.R., and others: Pediatric respiratory therapy; an introductory text, Sarasota, Fla., 1974. Glenn Educational Medical Services, Inc.

Young, J.A., and Crocker, D., editors: Principles and practice of respiratory therapy, ed. 2, Chicago, 1976, Year Book Medical Publishers, Inc., pp. 668-673.

99 Chest physiotherapy

DONNA BADGETT

CAROLINE CASSELBERRY

INDICATIONS

Chest physiotherapy (CPT) is one of the most used forms of therapy to treat acute and chronic respiratory disease. Though seemingly unsophisticated, it can be most effective in mobilizing secretions and improving ventilation/perfusion imbalances in patients whose normal pulmonary mechanisms are impaired. This procedure consists of four different physical modalities: postural drainage, percussion, vibration, and secretion removal. Each modality may be used singly or combined, to be tailored to the patient's individual need.

Pulmonary toilet utilizing CPT should be considered for any patient with retained and/or excessive secretions, or with limited ventilatory capacity. It may be employed both therapeutically and prophylactically in patients with medical, surgical, and neurologic diseases. Some specific medical conditions requiring the use of CPT are hyaline membrane disease, pneumonia, drained lung abscess, bronchiectasis, cystic fibrosis, treated foreign body inhalation, acute atelectasis, or presence of an artificial airway. Acute pulmonary problems need 24-hour therapy, whereas prophylactic treatments are done during the usual waking hours only.

TECHNIQUE
Postural drainage and percussion

The technique for postural drainage requires a functional knowledge of pediatric pulmonary anatomy. The principle of gravity is used by placing segmental bronchi in a vertical position, permitting downward flow of secretions out of the segment into larger airways, thus promoting better secretion removal. Percussion aids postural drainage in that the vibrations over the previously positioned lobe assist the downward flow of the secretions by loosening them from the bronchial walls. Used simultaneously, postural drainage and percussion are excellent tools for pulmonary hygiene.

Infants can be positioned for postural drainage while in an incubator, a crib, or the lap of the therapist. The lap technique and a gentle rocking motion will sometimes soothe an irritated infant; however, extra precaution must be taken to keep the infant from falling. Children may be positioned in bed or on a tiltboard with pillows, towels, or sandbags for support. The patient should be in a relaxed, comfortable position with knees flexed to reduce any muscle tension that would decrease the effectiveness of the therapy. The prone and head-down positions are the most uncomfortable because of diaphragmatic displacement by abdominal viscera, and these positions should be modified for unstable patients. Basic positions for the child and infant are the same (Fig. 99-1), using modifications as indicated. More time is spent on the affected area first, after which the rest of the lung is treated prophylactically. Patients are encouraged to cough after each position. After a vigorous coughing spell, the patient should be allowed to sit up and rest, with added oxygen if necessary, before continuing.

To prevent inhalation of stomach contents,

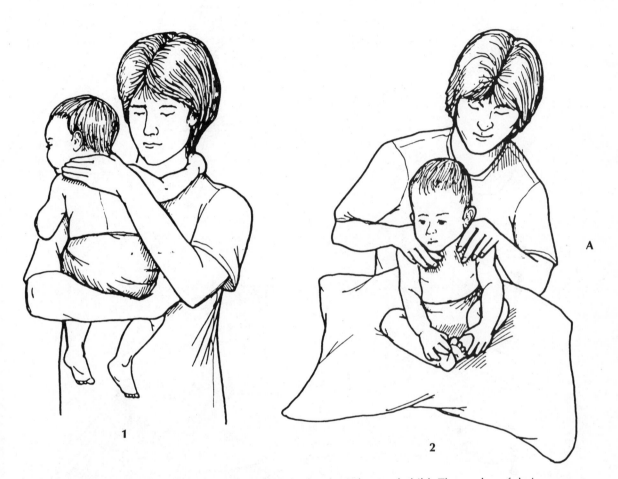

Fig. 99-1. Postural drainage and percussion position for the infant and child. The angles of drainage for the infant are not as obtuse as those for the child. **A,** Position *1:* The posterior segments of the right and left upper lobes are drained with the patient in an upright position at a 30-degree angle forward. Percuss over the upper posterior thorax, above the bottom of the scapula. Position *2:* The apical segments of the right and left upper lobes are drained with the patient in an upright position, leaning forward 30 degrees. Percuss over the area between the clavicle and the top of the scapula on each side.

Continued.

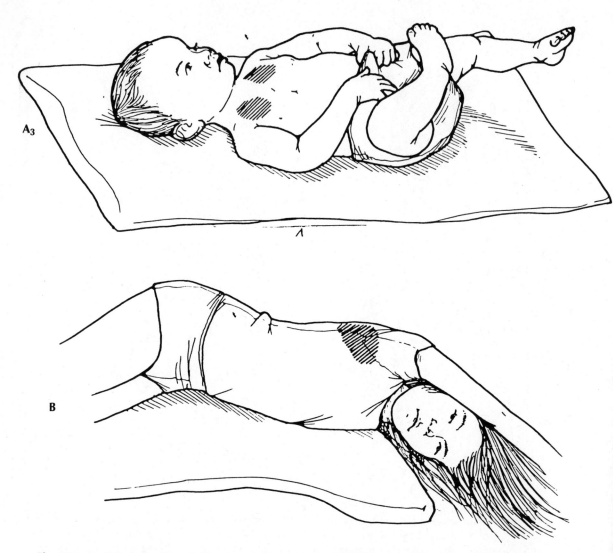

Fig. 99-1, cont'd. A, Position 3: The anterior segments of the right and left upper lobes are drained with the patient in a flat, supine position. Percuss the anterior chest directly under the clavicles to around the nipple area (shaded). Avoid direct pressure on the sternum. **B,** The right middle lobe, medial and lateral segments, is drained at 15 degrees Trendelenburg with the patient lying on the left side and at a 45-degree rotation backwards. The lingula of the left upper lobe, superior or inferior segments, is drained at 15 degrees Trendelenburg with the patient lying on the right side and at a 45-degree rotation backwards. Percuss above the anterior lower margin of the ribs.

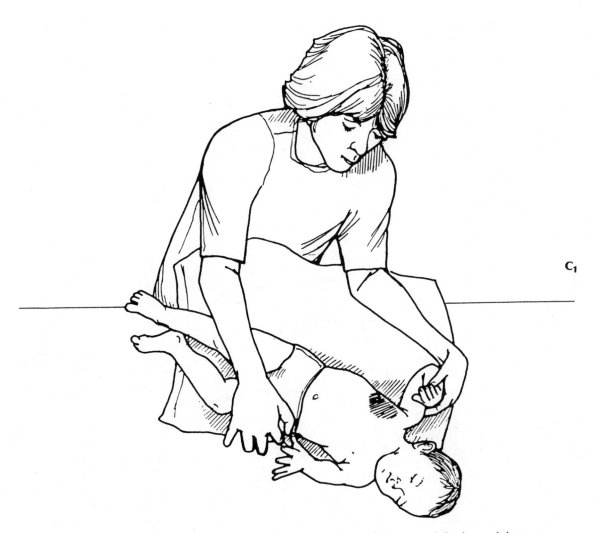

C₁

Fig. 99-1, cont'd. C, Position *1:* The right and left anterior basal segments of the lower lobes are drained at 30 degrees Trendelenburg. The patient lies on the appropriate side with a 30-degree turn backwards. Percuss above the anterior lower margin of the ribs.

Continued.

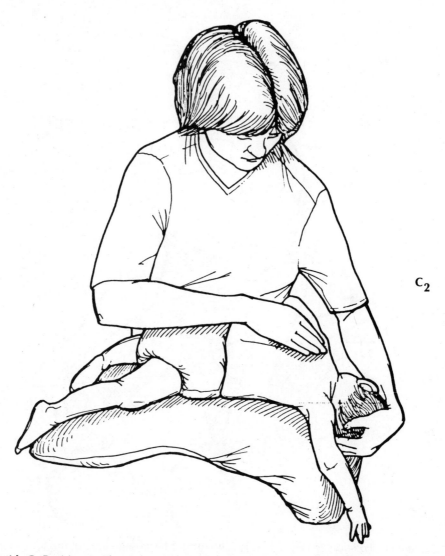

C₂

Fig. 99-1, cont'd. C, Position 2: The right and left lateral basal segments of the lower lobes are drained at 30 degrees Trendelenburg. The patient lies on the appropriate side, rotated 30 degrees forward. Percuss over the uppermost portions of the lower ribs.

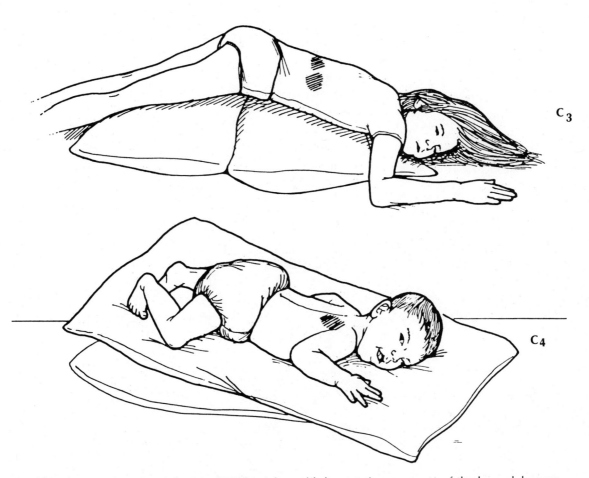

C_3

C_4

Fig. 99-1, C₃ and C₄. cont'd. Position *3:* The right and left posterior segments of the lower lobes are drained at 30 degrees Trendelenburg with the patient in the prone position. Percuss just above the lower margin of the ribs. Position *4:* The right and left superior segments of the lower lobes are drained at 15 degrees Trendelenburg with the patient in the prone position. Percuss below the scapula in the midback area.

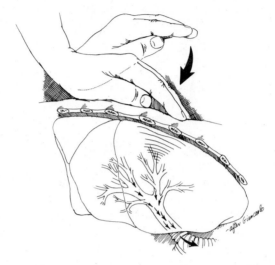

Fig. 99-2. Principle of therapeutic chest percussion. The cupped hands create air vibrations that are transmitted to lung tissue.

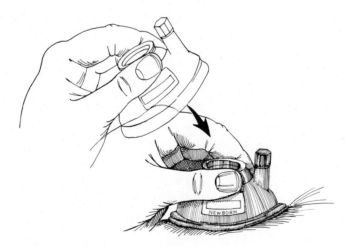

Fig. 99-3. Cuffed Ohio mask with plug in premature and infant sizes used in percussion of the infant.

therapy is done 30 minutes before or at least an hour after an oral feeding.

Percussion (Fig. 99-2) is accomplished with a cupped hand and flexed wrist clapping against the rib cage. It is important to produce a pop sound, since it is the sound generated by properly cupped air and not the actual contact of the hand, which causes the vibration. If the pop is too forceful it may injure skin and lung tissue. The pop ensures that a cushion exists, which protects the patient from being slapped. A T-shirt, cloth diaper, or sheet over the skin will provide further protection from stinging when laid upon the area being percussed. The therapist's jewelry should be removed. Percussion is done only over the ribs at the segmental area in drainage positions. Bony prominences, such as spine, sternum, clavicle, or fractured ribs, are avoided to prevent bruising and unnecessary discomfort. CPT should not be done on the floating ribs, since they are not connected to the sternum and may cause internal organ contusion. Premature and infant IPPB masks, with the opening plugged (Fig. 99-3), or finger percussion can achieve the same results as the hand in those patients too small for the hand. Finger percussion is accomplished by curving three or four fingers, slightly elevating the middle finger, and percussing over the contour of the thorax. Small electric percussors may also be used unless the patient is in an oxygen-enriched environment. If a patient starts coughing with percussion, stop and assist the cough with vibration.

Vibration

Vibration is a fine, shaking motion applied during exhalation. It is used after postural drainage and percussion to help move secretions from peripheral airways toward the trachea. This may be done with the hands, palms, or fingers, depending on the size of the patient. Electric vibrators are easier to use on small infants but should be used cautiously in oxygen-enriched environments.

To apply vibration, the therapist first observes the patient for exhalation, then stiffens the upper arm, extends the wrist with fingers spread-eagle, and gently shakes the hand on the patient's chest. The larger the patient, the more force is applied. Older patients should be instructed to inhale deeply and exhale through pursed lips for this procedure. It is generally easier to vibrate rapidly breathing infants every second or third exhalation rather than each breath. Vibration may also be applied effectively during crying or cooing. A tussive squeeze may be combined with this vibration technique by pushing in and up on the patient's chest while giving a vibrating motion.

Secretion removal

Adequate secretion removal is an integral part of CPT. Mobilization of secretions may occur and result in increased respiratory distress, hypoxia, or hypercarbia. Efforts must be made to reverse those effects.

It is extremely difficult to teach critically ill children proper coughing techniques and impossible with infants. However, the therapist should be as instructive as possible with the patient, offering assistance and demonstrating attempts that the patient can mimic. The patient is asked to breathe in slowly and as deeply as possible and then forcibly exhale. A cough should arise due to irritation of pulmonary sensory nerve receptors. The patient is encouraged to expectorate secretions.

There are several ways to facilitate cough effort and/or to induce a cough. A tussive squeeze maneuver is used to mimic the cough action by quickly applying pressure on the area of drainage throughout the cough attempt and/or exhalation. If the patient is uncooperative or has an ineffective cough, a tracheal tickle is especially effective. This is accomplished by applying gentle pressure and sideward motion across the trachea at the sternal notch with an index finger or thumb. Often, deep pharyngeal suctioning will elicit a cough or the catheter will enter the glottic orifice, allowing secretion removal.

A quick check of breath sounds will determine if the cough is effective. Patients with suppressed, ineffective coughs or artificial airways are to be suctioned routinely.

Evaluation

Throughout each therapy session the therapist should take vital signs (pulse and respiratory rate) and observe and evaluate available monitors, color changes, level of consciousness, secretion color and amount (volume in milliliters), and patient's level of tolerance. Auscultation is to be done before and after therapy to evaluate therapy effectiveness. All observations should be charted accurately in the patient's records. Intolerance of therapy, respiratory distress, or significant changes in vital signs should be reported to the patient's physician so that modifications in therapy can be planned.

Special considerations

Patient comfort and confidence are important to achieve maximum results of therapy. Understanding of and patience with the patient's fear and the therapist's reassurance of the therapy's purpose will help achieve cooperation and relaxation of all involved.

Special thermal- and oxygen-controlled environments should not be interrupted, but maintained as much as possible during therapy. Equipment used will be affected by the environment. For instance, electrical devices may not be used safely in oxygen-enriched environments due to potential electrical sparks and/or leakage. In such situations, pneumatically operated equipment is preferred.

RISKS AND COMPLICATIONS

All patients are to be carefully watched during therapy for signs of increased respiratory distress and levels of intolerance (fatigue, cyanosis, unstable vital signs, pain, alteration in level of consciousness). Some patients should be identified by the therapist as at high risk for complications because of their medical state or condition. Patients needing extra caution and modification of positions are those with cardiac disease, increased ICP, open wounds or recent incisions, orthopedic or muscular limitations, compromised diaphragmatic action, abdominal distension, bruises, fractured ribs, trauma to internal organs, chest tubes, and artificial airways. Careful management of each condition allows the use of CPT to be beneficial and effective rather than hazardous. Head-down positions may produce dysrhythmias and cyanosis, especially in patients with heart disease. New surgical incisions may bleed or induce pain; therefore, stress of CPT on healing tissue is to be avoided. Percussion done below the costal margin may cause contusion of internal organs, and over bony prominences it may cause pain and bruising. Too vigorous percussion can fracture ribs in very young or fragile patients.

ADDITIONAL READING

Lough, M.D., Doershuk, C.F., and Stern, R.C., editors: Pediatric respiratory therapy, Chicago, 1974, Year Book Medical Publishers, Inc., pp. 137-148.

Rarey, K.P., and Youtsey, J.W.: Respiratory patient care, Englewood Cliffs, N.J., 1981, Prentice-Hall, Inc., pp. 128-144.

Shapiro, A., Harrison, R.A., and Trout, C.A., editors: Clinical applications of respiratory care, Chicago, 1976, Year Book Medical Publishers, Inc., pp. 199-209.

Slonim, N., Schneider, S.N., Weng, T.R., and others: Pediatric respiratory therapy: an introductory text, Sarasota, Fla., 1974, Glenn Educational Medical Services, Inc.

100 Suctioning

NANCY HATFIELD
TERRY RAUSCHUBER

INDICATIONS

Sputum is produced by the mucosal and submucosal glands in the lungs and may consist of several substances, including cellular debris, mucus, blood, inflammatory cells, microorganisms, water, glycoproteins, and immunoglobulins. The amount and character of the sputum can be an important diagnostic aid. Normal mobilization of secretions may become greatly impaired or impossible in certain pathologic conditions. Suctioning of secretions should be performed for any patient who has (1) an inability to mobilize an accumulation of secretions in the tracheobronchial tree, (2) obstruction of the airways by secretions or edema, (3) an inability to cough effectively, (4) an inability to swallow, or (5) an endotracheal or tracheostomy tube. Frequency of suctioning will be determined by the nature and amount of airway secretions as well as by the patient's general medical condition.

TECHNIQUE
Equipment

The vacuum canister setup (Fig. 100-1) should include a manometer to measure the amount of vacuum applied, a vacuum wall outlet, supply tubing to connect to the collection bottle, a ring mount to hold the collection bottle, and enough extra supply tubing to reach readily from the suction setup to the patient's bed (3 to 5 feet). This setup should be replaced with sterile equipment every 24 hours.

Sterile disposable suction packets (Fig. 100-2) are now available at minimal cost. Each

should contain a peel-back sterile wrap, an unpowdered glove, and an appropriate-size catheter (Table 100-1). A good suction catheter should be constructed of as pliable a material as possible to prevent trauma and yet not collapse with negative pressure. It must pass easily

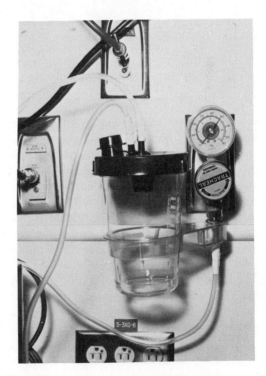

Fig. 100-1. Vacuum canister setup: wall vacuum, outlet, manometer, connective tubing, collection bottle, and connection tubing. Setup should be replaced every 24 hours with sterile equipment.

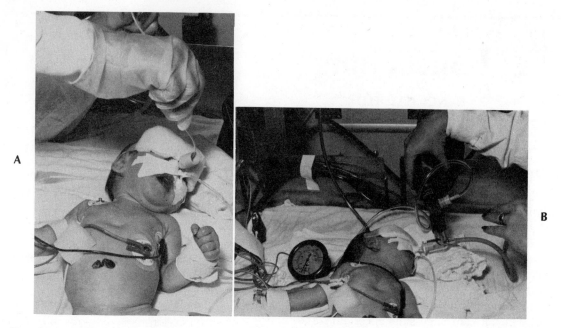

Fig. 100-2. A, Suctioning with sterile glove and catheter (use each only once). **B,** Hand ventilate the patient with an anesthesia bag with pressure manometer before and after each suctioning attempt.

through the artificial airway, be long enough to pass the tip of the artificial airway, have smooth ends to avoid mucosal trauma, and have side holes to minimize mucosal trauma. The proximal end must have a thumb hole that allows room air to enter and neutralize the negative pressure within the suction catheter. The hole may be occluded to produce suction, and it should be larger than the internal diameter of the catheter to prevent creation of negative pressure within the distal portion of the catheter. The use of sterile technique is essential. Gloves should be worn to protect both the patient and the nurse or therapist. Viscid secretions will not be drawn through a narrow suction catheter. In adults, it is a general rule to use a suction catheter with an outer diameter of at least one-half the inner diameter of the tracheal tube. Endotracheal tubes for infants and children are too small for this rule to apply. The flow of a dense fluid through a tube is directly proportional to the fourth or fifth power of

the tube's radius; therefore, increasing the diameter of the suction catheter increases the flow of secretions by an exponential factor of four or five. For infants and children, the largest suction catheter that will easily pass through the tracheal tube should be used. In some cases a sterile feeding tube may be used in place of a suction catheter. All catheters should be discarded after a single use.

Sterile single-use packets of 0.9% sodium chloride solution should be used to irrigate endotracheal and tracheostomy tubes in an effort to liquify and mobilize secretions. Sodium chloride solution comes in disposable packs that offer the added benefit of being free of bacteriostatic and preservative agents and are small enough to prevent reuse of the vial. In an effort to reduce trauma, a water-soluble jelly should be used to lubricate any catheter used for nasotracheal suctioning.

A bag and mask device is essential to good suctioning technique. This device is used to

Table 100-1. A guide to tube sizes and appropriate suction catheters

French gauge*	Tracheal tubes		Suction catheters, French gauge*
	Internal diameter, mm	Outer diameter,* mm	
12	2.5	4.0	
12-14	3.0	4.5	
14-16	3.5	5.0	5
16-18	4.0	5.5	5
18-20	4.5	6.0	6
20-22	5.0	6.5	6
22	5.5	7.0	8
24	6.0	7.5	8-10
26	6.5	8.0	10
28	7.0	8.5	12
30	7.5	9.0	12
32	8.0	9.5	12-14
34	8.5	11.5	14
36	9.0	12.0	14
38	9.5	12.5	14
40	10.0	13.0	16
42	10.5	14.5	18

Reproduced with permission from Stackpole, I.: Airway management. In Young, J.A., and Crocker, D., editors: Principles and practices of respiratory therapy, ed. 2. Copyright© 1976 by Year Book Medical Publishers, Inc., Chicago.
*Some tracheal tubes are constructed with thicker walls than others; therefore, outer diameter and French gauge may not correspond exactly from one style to another.

administer oxygen or to ventilate the patient when necessary.

Endotracheal and tracheostomy suctioning

1. Wash hands thoroughly with povidone-iodine complex (Betadine) or Septisol.
2. Assemble the equipment.
3. Explain the procedure to the patient if indicated. Place the patient in a modified Fowler's position, which offers the best results using a rotation of head up, head to left side, head to right side, and head up with successive suctioning maneuvers. Turning the patient's head to the left should

allow the catheter to enter the right mainstem bronchus. It is unlikely that an unangulated catheter will enter the left mainstem bronchus; however, if it occurs at all, it will happen in the head-right position with the left shoulder slightly elevated.

4. Set wall suction at 50 to 95 mm Hg for infants or at 90 to 115 mm Hg for children.
5. Open the catheter packet and, using sterile technique, place the wrap near the patient's T-adapter, put on the glove, grasp the catheter with the gloved hand, and connect the catheter to the supply tubing with the ungloved hand.
6. With the ungloved hand, remove the patient's T-adapter and place it on the sterile wrapping.
7. Using a bag device, hyperventilate the patient for 10 breaths with an Fio_2 0.1 higher than the maintenance concentration. In premature infants, use the same Fio_2 as the maintenance concentration. In patients with pulmonary arterial hypertension use an Fio_2 of 1.0. Care is essential in this maneuver. Lack of attention to assisting or controlling ventilation may asphyxiate the patient, and excessive pressures generated by the bag device may produce a pneumothorax. A pressure gauge may be attached to the bag to regulate the inflating pressure delivered to the patient.
8. Instill into the endotracheal tube 0.5 to 1 ml of 0.9% sodium chloride solution for infants or 1 to 5 ml for children. Repeat step 7.
9. Hold the catheter so that its natural curve is aligned with the endotracheal or tracheostomy tube. Without applying suction, quickly and *gently* insert the catheter through the tube until the patient coughs or a slight obstruction is felt. Never force a catheter further if an obstruction is met. Withdraw the catheter 0.5 cm and apply suction while rotating the catheter between the thumb and forefinger. *Never suction for longer than 5 seconds.* Repeat step 7.

10. Rotate the head position and repeat steps 8 and 9 as indicated. Monitor the patient's heart rate and color throughout the procedure; if any irregularity occurs, discontinue suctioning and ventilate the patient.
11. Return to the previous oxygen setting.
12. The same catheter may be used to suction the oropharynx and nose.
13. Discard the entire suction packet.
14. Record on the patient's chart the color, consistency, odor, and amount of secretions, as well as any change in characteristics from previous procedures.
15. Wash hands thoroughly.

Blind nasotracheal suctioning

1. Wash hands thoroughly with povidone-iodine complex (Betadine) or Septisol.
2. Assemble the equipment.
3. Explain the procedure to the patient if indicated. Position the patient: use the sniffing position for infants, with the chin up, head slightly flexed, and shoulders straight and slightly elevated; use a more hyperextended head position for older children. Remember that an infant's larynx is more cephalad than an adult's.
4. Set wall suction at 50 to 95 mm Hg for infants or at 95 to 115 mm Hg for children.
5. Open the catheter packet using sterile technique, put on the glove, grasp the catheter with the gloved hand, and connect the catheter to the supply tubing.
6. Using a bag and mask device, hyperoxygenate the patient for approximately 1 minute with an Fio_2 0.1 higher than the maintenance level, with the assistance of another nurse or therapist if possible. In premature infants, use the same Fio_2 as maintenance concentration. In patients with pulmonary arterial hypertension, use an Fio_2 of 1.0.
7. Lubricate the catheter tip with a water-soluble jelly to facilitate passage and decrease trauma.
8. Hold the catheter so that its natural curve is aligned with the patient's trachea. Gently insert the catheter into one of the patient's external nares, using an upward motion until the nasal septum is passed and then using a downward motion until the epiglottis is felt. Attempt to enter the trachea carefully and on inspiration only. Tracheal tickle may be applied at this point to stimulate coughing and ease the passage of the catheter into the trachea. Gentle pressure at the level of the vocal cords may also be helpful. Rotate the catheter and apply suction during withdrawal. *Never suction longer than 5 seconds.* Repeat step 6. Repeat the procedure as indicated. Monitor the patient's heart rate and color throughout the procedure; if any irregularity occurs, discontinue suctioning and ventilate the patient.
9. Return to the previous oxygen setting.
10. Record the procedure and chart the color, consistency, odor, and amount of secretions, as well as any change in characteristics from previous procedures.
12. Wash hands thoroughly.
13. Especially active children may require a two-person technique to ensure a sterile and efficient procedure.
14. Blind nasotracheal suctioning is contraindicated in patients during the first 4 to 6 hours after extubation or decannulation (tracheostomy tube), since it may cause laryngospasm.
15. See Chapter 58 for use of marked catheters when suctioning patients with tracheal or esophageal suture lines.

RISKS AND COMPLICATIONS

Mucosal damage. Mucosal hemorrhage and erosion occur frequently in the suctioned patient. Suction catheters may elevate the mucosa when suction is applied, invaginating the mucosa into the catheter holes; this immediately produces areas of hemorrhage and a nidus for infection. Continued trauma of this type such as may occur with a permanent artificial airway predisposes the patient to the development of granulation tissue and even bronchial stenosis. Proper catheter design and sterile technique minimize airway trauma.

Hypoxemia. When a suction catheter is introduced into an airway, tracheal gases as well as secretions are evacuated when suction is applied. This gas is replaced by room air that enters around the catheter as the patient is breathing spontaneously. Patients requiring added oxygen are especially deprived of it during this procedure, and significant hypoxemia may result. Acute hypoxemia may produce cardiac abnormalities. Frequently, the initial response is tachycardia, which is relieved with oxygenation; however, bradycardia and other dysrhythmias may occur and should be presumed to be due to hypoxemia. The patient should be ventilated immediately if these dysrhythmias occur. Careful oxygenation and ventilation of the patient during suctioning will help prevent hypoxemia.

Dysrhythmias. Significant dysrhythmias due to hypoxemia and/or vagal stimulation from direct tracheal irritation may result during suctioning. Be aware of the patient's state of health and lability. A patient should never be allowed to become stressed during suctioning, and appropriate technique can prevent this complication. If ECG monitoring leads have been removed for CPT, be certain that they are reconnected and the alarm system is functional before beginning to suction.

Hypotension. Hypotension during suctioning may result from vagal stimulation and profound bradycardia or prolonged coughing. Reflexes initiated in the trachea can interrupt ventilation and significantly reduce venous return and cardiac output (Table 100-2). Limiting the suction process to 5 seconds or less and close cardiac monitoring will help prevent this complication.

Table 100-2. Respiratory reflexes that may occur during suctioning

Reflex	Area stimulated
Spasm	Larynx, bronchi
Gag	Pharynx
Cough	Pharynx, larynx, trachea, bronchi
Sneeze	Nasopharynx
Swallow	Pharynx
Apnea	Pharynx, larynx

Lung collapse. Too large a suction catheter in too small an airway will prevent room air from entering around the catheter during suctioning, and lung collapse may occur. This may be prevented by using the appropriate-sized catheter.

Epistaxis. Epistaxis may occur with passage of a nasal catheter.

ADDITIONAL READING

Burton, G.G., Gee, G.N., and Hodgkin, J.E.: editors: Respiratory care, Philadelphia, 1977, J.B. Lippincott Co., pp. 523-527.

Hunsinger, D.L., Lisnerski, K.J., Maurizi, J.J., and others: Respiratory technology, Reston, Va., 1973, Reston Publishing Co.

Jemison, P.: The art and science of secretion extraction, Respir. Ther. **6:**23-25, 1976.

Levin, R.M.: Pediatric respiratory intensive care handbook, Flushing, N.Y., 1976, Medical Examination Publishing Co., Inc.

Shapiro, B.A., Harrison, R.A., and Trout, C.A.: Clinical application of respiratory care, Chicago, 1976, Year Book Medical Publishers, Inc.

Storm, W.P.: Transient bacteremia following ETT suctioning in ventilated newborns, J. Pediatr. **65:**487-490, 1964.

Williams, J., and Hill, J.W., editors: Handbook of neonatal respiratory care, Riverside, Calif., 1975, Bourns, Inc., pp. 105-110.

Young, J.A., and Crocker, D., editors: Principles and practice of respiratory therapy, ed. 2, Chicago, 1976, Year Book Medical Publishers, Inc., pp. 390-395.

101 Inhaled medications

GERALD C. MOORE

INDICATIONS

There are a number of agents capable of modifying airway caliber by changing bronchial smooth-muscle tone, decreasing mucosal and submucosal edema secondary to vasoconstriction, and liquifying retained secretions either chemically or by increasing humidity. Since the effects of agents on airway smooth muscle can be quantitated by measuring changes in lung function after their administration, the last two components, edema and secretions, are occasionally not considered when the various forms of therapy available are evaluted.

Sympathetic agents

Sympathetic agents have in common five actions that are termed "adrenergic." The actions are generalized and not directed toward any specific organ system and are most readily measured by changes in cardiopulmonary dynamics.

1. Peripheral excitatory action causes an increase in smooth-muscle tone, resulting in arterial and venous constriction that causes an increase in blood pressure proximal to and a decrease in flow distal to the arterial constriction (alpha-receptor system).
2. Peripheral inhibitory action causes relaxation of smooth muscle within the bronchi and bronchioles, resulting in an increase in lumen size and a decrease in resistance to air flow through the bronchial tree. The peripheral inhibitory effects also cause a decrease in peripheral smooth-muscle tone that tends to lower systemic arterial blood pressure and to increase blood flow distal to the relaxation (beta-receptor system).

3. Cardiac excitatory action may be divided into two types: a stimulatory action on the force of contraction (inotropic) and an increase in the rate of contraction (chronotropic).
4. Metabolic actions are best characterized by increased oxygen consumption and mobilization of glucose from the liver.
5. CNS actions are characterized by increased awareness or alertness, dizziness, agitation, or a generalized feeling of impending doom. Beyond the point of increased awareness, these symptoms are generally considered to be adverse reactions.

Receptors, which are divided into alpha and beta types, mediate the five general actions. Stimulation of the alpha receptors is associated with vasoconstriction and intestinal relaxation as well as contraction of the uterus, ureter, and dilator pupillae muscle. Beta receptors have been divided into two types, and their actions are listed in Table 101-1. Naturally occurring sympathetic agents, or the catecholamines (epinephrine, norepinephrine), have both alpha- and beta-adrenergic stimulation properties. The basic catecholamine molecule is phenylethylamine (Fig. 101-1), whose pharmacologic properties may be altered by replacement or manipulation of the N-alkyl moiety. The size of the substituted group determines the relative alpha- and beta-adrenergic stimulating activity: the smaller the group, the greater the alpha stimulation; the larger the group, the greater the beta stimulation. Multiple agents are thus available with varying degrees of alpha and beta activity. Whether the compounds are endogenously produced or given to the patient, they are metabolized by the enzyme catechol-*O*-methyltransferase (COMT).

The following catecholamines or derivatives have proved useful.

Epinephrine. Epinephrine is a naturally occurring catecholamine that stimulates the alpha- and beta-adrenergic receptors equally. The onset of action is immediate and effective when given parenterally or by inhalation. The half-life is less than 10 minutes, and when given by inhalation, systemic reactions are minimized. The dextrorotary (D-) form of epinephrine found in racemic epinephrine (a mixture of equal amounts of the D- and L-, or levorotary, forms) is not significantly active biologically; hence,

Table 101-1. Lands' classification of beta-adrenergic receptors in mammalian tissues

Responses mediated by beta-1 adrenergic receptors
1. Increased force and rate of contraction of cardiac muscles
2. Dilation of coronary blood vessels
3. Relaxation of smooth muscles in the alimentary tract
4. Lipolysis

Responses mediated by beta-2 adrenergic receptors
1. Relaxation of smooth muscle in bronchi, uterus, and arteries that supply skeletal muscles
2. Decreased twitch tension in skeletal muscle
3. Glycolysis
4. Glycogenolysis

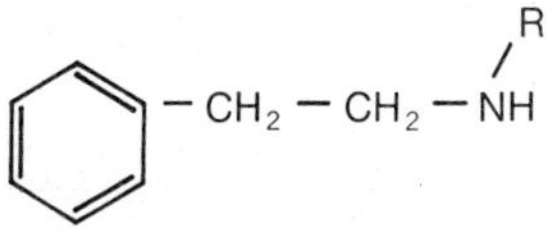

Phenylethylamine

Fig. 101-1. Basic catecholamine molecule. *R* indicates the most common substitution site.

fewer side effects are noted with the use of racemic epinephrine.

Isoproterenol. Isoproterenol (Isuprel), the synthetic prototype beta-adrenergic stimulant, results in powerful bronchial dilation when given by aerosol (beta-2 stimulus, Table 101-1). Unfortunately, because the drug is so readily absorbed when given parenterally or by aerosol, all beta-adrenergic receptors are activated, resulting in considerable cardiovascular effects. When given orally, the drug is degraded in the stomach before absorption, and this is not a recommended route of administration. The onset of action is immediate, and isoproterenol has a half-life of approximately 1 minute because of the rapid metabolism by COMT. Isoproterenol is the most thoroughly studied inhaled bronchodilator in terms of its dose-response characteristics. It is routinely used before CPT in patients with acute asthma in lieu of subcutaneous epinephrine when treatment of acute bronchospasm is necessary. In children with bronchial pneumonia, inhalation pneumonitis, or cystic fibrosis and in newborns with lung disease, isoproterenol is frequently used to dilate the airways to facilitate the removal of secretions during CPT.

Isoetharine. Isoetharine (Bronkosol) was developed in an attempt to maintain beta-2 adrenergic properties while decreasing the cardiovascular side effects. Isoetharine has not only an *N*-alkyl substitution but also alpha substituents on the phenylethylamine side chain. Introduction of the beta-ethyl group on the side chain reduces bronchodilator activity by a factor of about 10 and cardiovascular activity by about 300 when compared with isoproterenol. Thus, the agent displays selective preference for bronchial smooth muscle (beta-2 receptor) over cardiac muscle (beta-1 receptor). Isoetharine is administered by inhalation. The half-life is not known.

Metaproterenol. Metaproterenol (Alupent, Metaprel), a resorcinol, differs slightly in structure from isoproterenol. It is 10 to 40 times less active than isoproterenol in all of its beta-adrenergic actions. When given by inhalation or orally, the duration of action is up to 4 hours.

Terbutaline. Terbutaline (Bricanyl, Brethine), a tertiary-butyl derivative of metaproterenol, is about twice as potent as its parent compound on bronchial muscle (beta-2) but one fourth as active on heart muscle (beta-1). It has a relatively long duration of action. Terbutaline is currently available for oral and subcutaneous use. The frequent and unpleasant tremor observed after oral administration in children apparently does not occur when it is administered by inhalation.

Fenoterol. Fenoterol, a hydroxyphenyl derivative of metaproterenol, is a more potent and selective bronchodilator than its parent compound, but it is not yet available for use in this country.

Albuterol. Albuterol (Ventolin, Proventil), a saligenin, has undergone extensive experimental and clinical investigation. It is a potent beta agonist, and when given to experimental animals by inhalation it is 10 times more active than isoproterenol and 100 times more active than metaproterenol. Doses of 100 to 200 μg cause significant and immediate bronchodilation that persists for several hours. Bronchodilation may be of longer duration after inhalation than after oral administration, possibly because albuterol is so well absorbed from the intestinal tract and rapidly excreted in the urine, whereas after inhalation its absorption is slower.

Phenylephrine. Phenylephrine (Neo-Synephrine) differs from epinephrine in that it lacks a hydroxyl group in the "4" position on the benzene ring. It is a potent systemic arterial constrictor but when given by inhalation causes local vasoconstriction or decongestion of the respiratory mucosa. Given in this manner, it exerts little systemic effect.

Parasympathetic agents

Atropine produces bronchodilation in humans that may persist for as long as 300 minutes. This compound may be effective in reversing bronchospasm caused by agents that precipitate large-airway hyperreactivity (exercise, irritants, coughing, infection).

Wetting agents

Although numerous agents have been used to enhance removal of retained secretions, the most efficient way to liquify airway secretions continues to be adequate systemic hydration given either orally or parenterally.

1. The most widely used wetting agent is 0.9% sodium chloride solution administered in an ultrasonic particle size.
2. Pharmacologically active compounds such as L-acetylcysteine (Mucomyst), which liquifies mucus, and DNA (the component of pus responsible for its viscosity), act directly on mucoproteins to open disulfide bonds and lower viscosity. The clinical effectiveness of acetylcysteine remains to be established. Furthermore, its administration results in increased airway resistance thought to be bronchospasm secondary to direct airway irritation.
3. The administration of distilled water by aerosol also results in a decrease in airway caliber as measured by an increase in resistance. This may be the result of bronchoconstriction or edema due to cellular uptake of the water.

TECHNIQUE

There are several considerations involved in delivery of medication to the airways. These include particle size, timing of delivery, physical state and carrier agent of the drug, and method of delivery. Fig. 101-2 depicts the size of particles deposited in the different parts of the respiratory tract. Smaller particles reach a more peripheral site of deposition when they are taken beginning at FRC and slowly inhaling to TLC. If, however, the particles are contained in a small bolus of gas delivered from a pressurized dispenser, the site of particle deposition

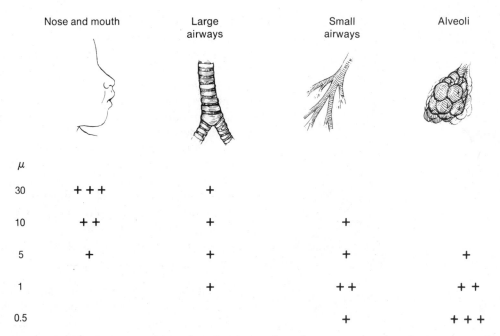

μ	Nose and mouth	Large airways	Small airways	Alveoli
30	+ + +	+		
10	+ +	+	+	
5	+	+	+	+
1		+	+ +	+ +
0.5			+	+ + +

Fig. 101-2. Site of deposition of various-sized particles when aerosolized and administered to spontaneously breathing subjects.

depends on the point at which the bolus enters the inhaled airstream. Patients should hold their breath at TLC for 4 seconds after inhaling the medication to obtain efficient deposition of particles in the lung.

The size of the particles, not their physical state, is closely related to their deposition in the airways. For example, wet or dry aerosols do not behave differently, but any changes in the size of the particles during breathing may have profound effects on their deposition in the lung. Aqueous droplets are an example of this phenomenon, since they equilibrate their osmotic pressure until it is the same as the body fluids and by this mechanism change their size rapidly (enlarge) as they move down the airways. The addition of a hygroscopic carrying agent such as propylene glycol to nebulizer solutions may therefore have unexpected effects on the apparent pharmacologic actions of the inhaled drug.

The method of delivery of inhaled medication has received much attention. The central issue involves the relative efficiency of delivering medication of proper particle size in situations where the amount of medication delivered depends on the patient's spontaneous inspiratory breath as compared with delivery of medication of the same particle size by externally applied positive pressure. There are several studies showing that medications given by aerosol during spontaneous breathing are delivered as efficiently as those given by IPPB devices. Freon-propelled medication is delivered as efficiently as the above methods. All three methods are equally safe as long as the condition being treated is not associated with abnormally high intrapleural pressures, such as those observed in patients with asthma. Increasing already dangerously high levels of intrapleural pressure may be associated with pneumothoraces and progressive airway obstruction by fur-

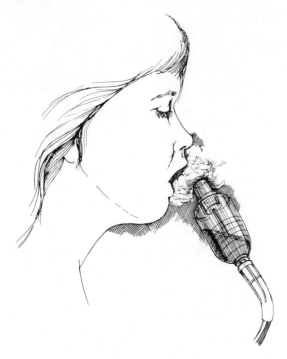

Fig. 101-3. Acorn nebulizer.

ther impaction of mucus in the small airways. Therefore, IPPB should be avoided as a mode of delivery of medication in patients with asthma and functionally similar conditions.

Despite the extensive pharmacologic and clinical knowledge of agents that act directly on the bronchial tree, the dosage of most of these medicines has not been critically evaluated. Dose-response characteristics have been evaluated for isoproterenol and atropine. Because atropine has such limited usefulness, it will not be discussed here, except that if it is to be given by inhalation, pure atropine sulfate powder should be diluted with 0.9% sodium chloride solution. Acidic compounds with preservatives (such as the parenteral solution) should not be inhaled. Isoproterenol aerosol solution is commercially available in a solution of 1:200 or 5-mg/ml concentration. It is administered through a nebulizer in a dose of 0.005 ml/kg in 1 to 2 ml of 0.9% sodium chloride solution

(Fig. 101-3). A Y-connector is placed in the aerosol tubing so that the agent is administered only during inspiration. Each inhalation should be taken from FRC to TLC with a period of breath-holding at TLC for 2 to 4 seconds. In children too young to cooperate, the dose should be doubled, and the agent may then be continuously nebulized.

Acetylcysteine (Mucomyst) is usually given with the aerosol bronchodilator as a 10% solution. Sodium chloride solution (0.9%) delivered by an ultrasonic device is frequently given before and/or after administration of the aerosol. These procedures are routinely followed by CPT and suctioning (see Chapters 99 and 100).

RISKS AND COMPLICATIONS

Untoward effects of the bronchodilators are usually excessive responses of desired effects. Side effects are generally due to overdosage, idiosyncratic responses, or an unusually sensitive autonomic nervous system because of the nature of the illness. Adverse reactions include:

1. CNS: fear, anxiety, tenseness, restlessness, throbbing, headache, tremor, weakness, dizziness, pallor, emesis.
2. Cardiovascular: palpitations, tachycardia, dysrhythmias, hypotension, hypertension.

ADDITIONAL READING

Ahlquist, R.P.: A study of the adrenotropic receptors, Am. J. Physiol. **153:**586-600, 1948.

Assem, E.S.K.: Inhibition of allergic reactions by beta-adrenergic stimulants, Postgrad. Med. J. **47**(March suppl): 31-33, 1971.

Avner, S.E.: β-Adrenergic bronchodilators, Pediatr. Clin. North Am. **22:**129-139, 1975.

Brittain, R.T., Jack, D., and Ritchie, A.C.: Recent β-adrenoreceptor stimulants, Adv. Drug Res. **5:**197-253, 1970.

Cavanaugh, M.J., and Cooper, D.M.: Inhaled atropine sulfate: dose response characteristics, Am. Rev. Respir. Dis. **114:**517-524, 1976.

Davies, D.S.: Metabolism of isoprenaline and other bronchodilator drugs in man and dog, Bull. Physiopathol. Respir. **8:**679-682, 1972.

Gold, W.M., Kessler, G.F., and Yu, D.Y.C.: Role of vagus nerves in experimental asthma in allergic dogs, J. Appl. Physiol. **33:**719-725, 1972.

Goodman, L.S., and Gilman, A., editors: The pharmacological basis of therapeutics, ed. 5, New York, 1975, Macmillan, Inc., Chapters 19 and 24.

Jenne, J.W.: The clinical pharmacology of bronchodilators, Basics of RD **6:**1-6, 1977.

Kennedy, M.C.S., and Simpson, W.T.: Human pharmacological and clinical studies on salbutamol: a specific β-adrenergic bronchodilator, Br. J. Dis. Chest **63:**165-174, 1969.

Lands, A.M., Arnold, A., McAuliff, J.P., and others: Differentiation of receptor systems activated by sympathomimetic amines, Nature **214:**597-598, 1967.

Watanabe, S., Turner, W.G., Renzetti, A.D., and others: Bronchodilator effects of nebulized fenoterol: a comparison with isoproterenol, Chest **80:**292-299, 1981.

102 Thoracentesis and chest tube insertion

GERALD C. MOORE
LAWRENCE J. MILLS
CATHERINE P. MAST

INDICATIONS
Pleural effusion

Diagnostic thoracentesis should be performed on all patients with pleural effusions of unknown cause. The amount of pleural fluid, normally present in small quantities, depends on the opposing hydrostatic and omsotic pressures present in the visceral and parietal pleural membranes (Fig. 102-1). Pleural fluid is formed at the parietal pleural surface and absorbed through the visceral pleura. A net hydrostatic pressure of +35 cm H_2O, consisting of +30 cm H_2O of hydrostatic pressure produced by the systemic capillaries and −5 cm H_2O of intrapleural pressure, tends to force fluids from the parietal pleural capillaries into the pleural space. The colloid osmotic pressure in the systemic capillaries is +34 cm H_2O and that of the fluid in the pleural cavity +8 cm H_2O, resulting in a net opposing force of +26 cm H_2O of colloid osmotic pressure. The difference between these forces is 9 cm H_2O, which tends to force fluid from the parietal pleura into the pleural cavity. The visceral pleura is supplied by the pulmonary arterial capillaries, which have a hydrostatic pressure of approximately +11 cm H_2O. The net hydrostatic pressure difference between the visceral pleura and the parietal pleural cavity therefore is +16 cm H_2O. The colloid osmotic pressure of the visceral pleural capillaries is also approximately +26 cm H_2O,

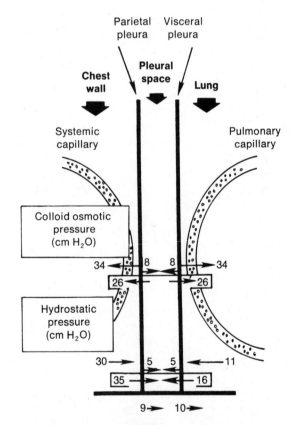

Fig. 102-1. Diagrammatic representation of the pressures involved in the formation and absorption of pleural fluid. (From Fraser, R.G., and Paré, J.A.P.: Diagnosis of diseases of the chest, Philadelphia, 1970, W.B. Saunders Co.)

which creates a net effect of +10 cm H_2O pressure and tends to force fluids toward the visceral pleural capillaries.

Knowledge of these pressure differences will allow one to understand the conditions under which excessive pleural fluid accumulates (e.g., increased hydrostatic pressure, decreased colloid oncotic pressure, increased intrapleural pressure, capillary damage). In patients with congestive heart failure, pleural fluid accumulation results from an overall increase in hydrostatic pressure. In contrast, the decrease in colloid osmotic pressure seen in hypoalbuminemia may result in a pleural effusion. Increases in capillary permeability occur with inflammatory and neoplastic lesions. With significant atelectasis, an increased negative intrapleural pressure may occur and result in the accumulation of fluid.

Pleural effusions are often recognized radiographically before they are suspected clinically. Inflammatory lesions of the pleura are frequently characterized by signs of pleurisy (e.g., fever, chest pain, cough) in the absence of a demonstrable collection of fluid. Large effusions usually cause asymmetry in chest expansion. A dull percussion note will be found directly over areas of fluid density, and sound transmission through a layer of fluid is decreased. Fremitus is decreased over the area of fluid. If the accumulation is excessive, a shift of the mediastinal structures may occur, with ipsilateral atelectasis. It is frequently impossible to visualize pleural effusions on routine posteroanterior chest roentgenograms; however, a lateral decubitus chest roentgenogram with the affected side in the dependent position may demonstrate even small effusions.

Causes of pleural effusions are listed in Table 102-1. Differentiation between a transudate and an exudate is helpful when the diagnosis is not obvious clinically. Criteria that were thought to be specific in the past have not stood up to critical evaluation. An exudate was believed to be present if the protein concentration of the fluid was greater than 3 g/dl or if the fluid had a specific gravity greater than 1.016. A white cell count of greater than 1,000 cells/mm^3 was also used as a criterion to define an exudative process. A ratio of pleural fluid to serum proteins of greater than 0.5, a pleural fluid LDH concentration of greater than 200 IU, and a pleural fluid to serum ratio of LDH of greater than 0.6 are new criteria which have

Table 102-1. Causes of pleural effusions

Transudates
1. Congestive heart failure
2. Cirrhosis
3. Nephrotic syndrome
4. Acute glomerulonephritis
5. Myxedema
6. Peritoneal dialysis
7. Sarcoidosis

Exudates
1. Pulmonary infarction
2. Neoplasms
3. Infections
   a. Viral (adenovirus)
   b. Bacterial (Staphylococcus, Streptococcus, Haemophilus influenzae)

Exudates—cont'd
   c. Tuberculosis
   d. Fungal
   e. Rickettsial
4. Parasites
5. Collagen vascular disease
6. Gastrointestinal disease (pancreatitis, subphrenic abscesses)
7. Drug reactions
8. Trapped lung
9. Postmyocardial infarction
10. Lymphatic abnormalities
11. Trauma

been found useful in defining an exudative effusion; otherwise the effusion is considered a transudate. An effusion with more than 25,000 WBCs, which are predominantly polymorphonuclear leukocytes, is considered an empyema. This diagnosis has specific bearing on therapy, whereas the differentiation between transudate and exudate may not. Neutrophils are generally found in effusions caused by pneumonia, pulmonary infarction, early tuberculosis, and pancreatitis. Lymphocytes are predominant in tuberculous effusions, lymphomas, and other malignancies; they are also usually the predominant cell type of transudates. A hemorrhagic pleural effusion with more than 5,000 RBCs/mm^3 can be the result of either trauma during thoracentesis or marked inflammation due to infection or pancreatitis. The presence of more than 100,000 RBCs/mm^3 suggests a malignancy, trauma, or pulmonary infarction.

Various chemical analyses of pleural fluid may be helpful in establishing the cause of the effusion. There does not appear to be a consistent relationship between pleural fluid glucose and blood glucose during a glucose tolerance test. If the pleural fluid glucose level is less than 30 mg/dl, rheumatoid pleuritis should be strongly suspected. Tuberculous, malignant, and empyematous effusions frequently have glucose concentrations of less than 60 mg/dl. Ten percent of patients with pancreatitis have associated pleural effusions. Simultaneous serum and pleural fluid amylase determinations may be helpful in diagnosing this condition. If the supernatant lipid content appears high, it is probably a chylous effusion, whether due to a severed thoracic duct or to a lymphoreticular malignancy. Chyloform effusions accompany long-standing or loculated effusions due to tuberculosis, malignancies, trapped lung, and rheumatoid pleuritis. A pH of less than 7.3 is consistent with infection. Cytology should be interpreted with caution because mesothelial cells, the pleura lining cell type, are frequently confused with malignant cells.

A large transudate or exudate need not be completely removed unless a clinical indication such as respiratory distress or progressive atelectasis exists. Once the diagnosis of an empyema is made by the aspiration of either grossly purulent material or material that has a cell count greater than 25,000 WBC/mm^3, a chest tube should be inserted for closed drainage.

Pneumothorax

A pneumothorax occurs when air enters the pleural space through either a rent in the lung or a hole in the chest wall. Air in the pleural space may cause the lung to collapse, and if the air is under pressure, the mediastinum may be shifted, causing compromise of the contralateral lung. Tension pneumothorax is most likely to occur in a patient on a positive pressure mechanical ventilator.

The chest roentgenogram diagnoses a pneumothorax most reliably. In most instances, an anteroposterior view will be sufficient, but an upright expiratory, lateral decubitus, or cross-table lateral view may be needed. Physical findings are usually unreliable but may include:

1. Decreased breath sounds on the affected side.
2. Unequal thoracic wall motion with decreased movement on the affected side.
3. Shift of the trachea toward the unaffected side.
4. Subcutaneous emphysema.
5. Hyperresonance to percussion on the affected side.

A small, stable pneumothorax in a nonintubated, spontaneously breathing patient can be observed with serial chest roentgenograms. A pneumothorax that is greater than 20% of the thoracic volume or that is under tension should be treated by closed-system drainage through an intercostal space. A single attempt at aspiration using a plastic IV catheter may be made in a stable patient, but a chest tube should be placed if aspiration is unsuccessful.

TECHNIQUE
Preparation of the patient

The complication rate of a diagnostic or therapeutic thoracentesis should be less than 0.5% if the patient is relatively stable and is properly prepared as follows:

1. Premedicate patients older than 12 months with IM meperidine (Demerol), 2 mg/kg, and promethazine (Phenergan), 0.5 mg/kg, 30 minutes before beginning the procedure. Since respiratory depression may occur as long as 8 hours after this sedation, cardiorespiratory monitoring should be considered for this period.
2. Infants and children too young to cooperate should be physically restrained. A squirming child significantly increases the risk of injury to the lung during the procedure.
3. An older child may straddle a chair, holding his arms in front of him in order to position the tips of the scapulae laterally in the posterior axillary line. The seventh intercostal space should be directly below the scapular tip.

Equipment

1. Iodine scrub solution.
2. Surgical gloves.
3. Sterile gowns, cap, and mask.
4. Sterile drapes.
5. Syringes: 5-ml, 10-ml, and 50-ml.
6. Disposable needles: 22-gauge and 25-gauge.
7. Sponges: 4 × 4 inches, 6 packages.
8. Plastic IV catheters (Intracath, Angiocath): 16-gauge, 18-gauge, and 20-gauge.
9. Stopcock, plastic, two-way.
10. Extension tubing.
11. Sterile basin, 250-ml.
12. Cultures tubes: aerobic and anaerobic.
13. Microscopic slides.
14. Tubes for laboratory analysis of fluid: with and without anticoagulant.
15. Lidocaine, 1%, without epinephrine.
16. Intercostal tube placement set.

17. Chest tube appropriate for the size of the child: #8 to #10 French for premature infants and up to #28 French for adolescents.
18. A 2-0 silk suture on a cutting needle, straight or curved.
19. Surgical blades: #11 and #15.
20. Tincture of benzoin.
21. Tape.
22. High-intensity operating light.
23. Double-glass bottle suction set or disposable system (Pleur-Evac) (Fig. 102-2).
24. Crate to hold bottles.
25. Large clamp to keep at bedside.
26. Emergency cart.
27. Marking pen.

Procedure

1. Locate fluid level, if present, by marking the point at which tactile fremitus disappears and the percussion note becomes dull.
2. Prepare the skin with the iodine solution.
3. Drape the area.
4. Use 1 to 3 ml of 1% lidocaine to achieve analgesia to the pleura and adjacent periosteum. Infiltrate from the skin through the intercostal muscle to the rib.
5. Insert a #11 surgical blade through the skin to make an incision slightly larger than the outside diameter of the needle to be inserted. The incision is made in the intercostal space immediately below the scapula in the posterior axillary line. Since the neurovascular bundle associated with each rib is located along the inferior margin, the needle should pass just above the superior rib margin.
6. The IV catheter needle is introduced through the skin until the pleural pop is felt. The catheter is then advanced approximately 2 mm to ensure insertion past the tip of the catheter.
7. Remove the needle.
8. Attach a 50-ml syringe with a two-way stopcock to the catheter.

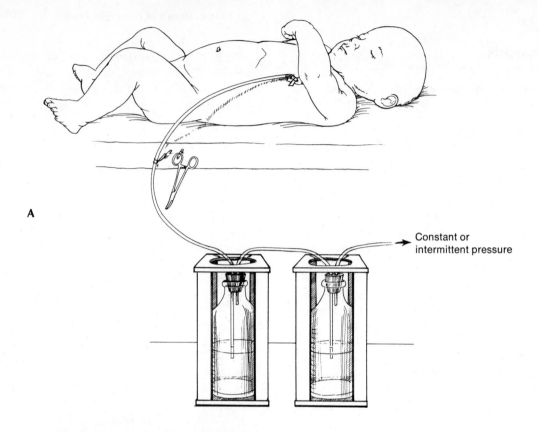

A

Constant or
intermittent pressure

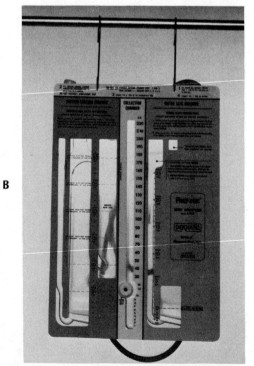

B

Fig. 102-2. A, Double-bottle suction set. The left
bottle will collect fluid from the patient. The right
bottle acts as an extra reservoir and should be
partially filled with water. **B,** Pleur-Evac disposable
system.

9. If fluid is anticipated and not obtained, the catheter may be advanced to 1 to 2 mm while constant negative pressure is applied on the syringe. If still unsuccessful, the catheter may be directed medially and laterally in a search for the effusion. If no fluid is obtained, the catheter should be withdrawn and the patient reexamined for insertion at another site. It is occasionally necessary to reinsert the needle one interspace caudal and medial to the previous insertion site. If a diagnostic tap is done, no more than 10 to 20 ml needs to be withdrawn. When thoracentesis is complete, remove the needle and dress the site with a Band-Aid.

10. If a pneumothorax is anticipated, aspirate the site of planned tube placement to confirm the presence of air.

11. If possible, completely evacuate the pneumothorax before inserting the chest tube.

12. The sites for chest tube placement to evacuate a pneumothorax are, in order of preference (Fig. 102-3):
    a. The axilla behind the head of the pectoralis major muscle in the second or third intercostal space for ease of insertion into the thoracic apex and for the best cosmetic result.
    b. The anterior second or third intercostal space in the midclavicular line.
    c. Other locations specifically indicated by loculation of a pneumothorax, prior tube placements, or operative incisions.

13. A small skin incision is made. Use blunt dissection to enter the thoracic cavity *over* the top of a rib to avoid the intercostal neurovascular bundle.

14. Place the tip of the catheter between the tips of an appropriate-sized curved hemostat and gently insert the catheter into the pleural space. Be certain to advance the catheter so that all side holes are within the pleural space.

15. Connect the catheter to the chest drainage system. If more than one chest tube is necessary, they may be connected by a Y-connector to a single drainage system.

16. Observe for respiratory fluctuations in the water seal chamber to confirm tube patency.

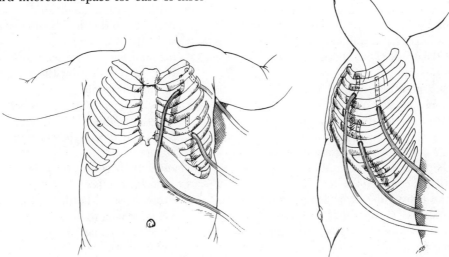

Fig. 102-3. Preferred sites for insertion of chest tubes for evacuation of pneumothorax.

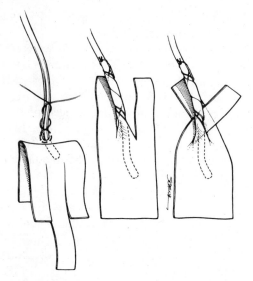

Fig. 102-4. Method for securing tube to the chest. The tails of the purse-string suture should be sufficiently long to extend under the section of tape to be wrapped around the tube.

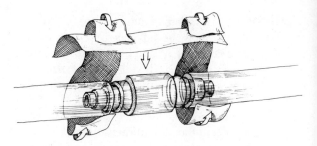

Fig. 102-5. Method for taping connections.

A chest roentgenogram should be obtained 2 to 3 hours after the suction is turned off or the tube is clamped and 2 to 3 hours after removal of the chest tube. An upright expiratory or lateral decubitus roentgenogram will demonstrate free air or reaccumulated fluid.

Care of chest tube

1. Secure the tubing to the bed with a hemostat to avoid tension and kinks.
2. Strip the chest tubes every hour to maintain patency and facilitate drainage.
   a. Pinch the chest tube near the insertion site.
   b. Lubricate fingers of the other hand.
   c. With the other hand, firmly compress the tubing with the thumb and forefinger and slide them down the tube 20 to 25 cm, maintaining compression of the tubing.
   d. Release pressure on the hand closest to the insertion site.
   e. Repeat steps b to d, progressing along the length of tubing.
   f. Mark and record the chest drainage after stripping.
3. Change the bottle when it is approximately three-fourths full.
   a. Prepare a new bottle or Pleur-Evac.
   b. While changing the bottle, clamp the chest tube using a Kelly clamp in two locations with the teeth covered to avoid damage to the tube.

17. Suture the tube in place by a purse-string suture, which will be tied to close the skin when the tube is removed.
18. Tape the tube to the chest as shown in Fig. 102-4. Note that use of large, bulky dressings in neonates may prevent adequate observation of chest wall movement and increase the work of breathing secondary to excess weight.
19. Tape all connections (Fig. 102-5).
20. Continuous suction at 20 to 40 cm H_2O is adequate to evacuate fluid or air from the chest.
21. Obtain a chest roentgenogram immediately after the tube is secure or after the needle aspiration is completed.

Once the chest tube is no longer deemed necessary, suction should be discontinued for 12 to 24 hours before removal. If the tube was inserted to drain blood or an effusion, it should be clamped for 12 to 24 hours before removal.

Transportation of patient with chest tube

1. Clamp the tube with a large hemostat if the drainage system is to be elevated above the insertion site (this prevents entry of water into the chest).
2. Drainage systems other than Pleur-Evac should be protected by metal or wood cases firmly attached to the bed.
3. Some patients with tension pneumothorax may need a portable suction device to maintain air evacuation during transportation.

Removal of chest tube

1. Position and restrain the patient as needed.
2. Rapidly remove the chest tube during expiration (in a spontaneously breathing patient) and cover the insertion site with petroleum-jelly gauze and 4 × 3 plain gauze. If a purse-string suture was placed at the time of chest tube insertion, draw the ends tightly as the chest tube is being removed. A physician usually removes the tube.
3. Apply a sterile dressing.
4. Obtain a chest roentgenogram 1 to 2 hours after removal to look for reaccumulation of fluid or free air.

RISKS AND COMPLICATIONS

1. The lung may be punctured during needle or tube placement, which could result in an air leak or hemorrhage.
2. Placement too low may cause injury to the liver, spleen, or kidney.
3. Placement of the tube with the tip impinging on the aorta may cause hypotension in small or hypovolemic patients.
4. If the most proximal fenestration of the tube is not within the chest, subcutaneous emphysema, persistent pneumothorax, or extension of the infection into the subcutaneous tissues may occur.
5. Empyema may develop if sterile technique is not employed.
6. Trauma to the intercostal neuromuscular bundle may cause significant bleeding.
7. Incorrect connection of the suction system may cause air to remain in the chest under tension.
8. Inadequate placement of the tube in the posterior chest cavity for tension pneumothorax may not relieve the tamponade.

ADDITIONAL READING

Agostini, E., and D'Angelo, E.: Thickness and pressure of the pleural liquid at various heights and with various hydrothoraces, Respir. Physiol. 6:330-342, 1969.

Allen, R.W., Jung, A.L., and Lester, P.D.: Effectiveness of chest tube evacuation of pneumothoraces in neonates, J. Pediatr. 99:629-634, 1981.

Banagale, R.C., Outerbridge, E.W., and Aranda, J.V.: Lung perforation: a complication of chest tube insertion in neonatal pneumothoraces, J. Pediatr. 94:973-975, 1979.

Cope, C.: New pleural biopsy needle, J.A.M.A. 167:1107-1108, 1958.

Funahashi, A., Sarkar, T.K., and Kory, R.C.: Measurements of respiratory gases and pH of pleural fluid, Am. Rev. Respir. Dis. 108:1266-1268, 1973.

Gooding, L.A., Kerlan, R.K., and Brasch, R.C.: Partial aortic obstruction produced by a thoracostomy tube, J. Pediatr. 98:471-473, 1981.

Light, R.W., Erozan, Y.S., and Ball, W.C., Jr.: Cells in pleural fluid, Arch. Intern. Med. 132:854-860, 1973.

Light, R.W., Macgregor, M.I., Luchsinger, P.C., and others: Pleural effusions: the diagnostic separation of transudates and exudates, Ann. Intern. Med. 77:507-513, 1972.

Paddock, F.: The relationship between the specific gravity and the protein content in human serous effusions, Am. J. Med. Sci. 201:569-574, 1941.

Russakoff, A., LeMaistre, C., and Dewleth, H.: An evaluation of the pleural fluid glucose determination, Am. Rev. Respir. Dis. 85:220-223, 1962.

103 Extubation

FRANCES C. MORRISS
DONNA S. BURNS
RICK VINSON

INDICATIONS

The primary requirement for withdrawing ventilatory support of any sort is resolution or improvement of the process that necessitated support. This is especially true for extubation. Before removal of an endotracheal or tracheostomy tube, these points must be considered.

Pulmonary stability

There should be a trend toward resolution, and the absence of acute change just before extubation needs to be documented. There should also be documentation of the absence of hypoxemia and hypercarbia, with the inspired oxygen concentration usually 0.4 or less. There should be no acute change in pulmonary secretions, since increasing quantity, discoloration, or increasing viscosity of secretions may herald a new infection that might cause extubation to be unsuccessful. It is assumed that the patient's only form of ventilatory support at this point is an endotracheal tube, oxygen, and minimal CPAP (see Chapter 96).

Oxygen-carrying capacity

Hematocrit should be greater than 30% in children and greater than 40% in neonates. Low hematocrits (low oxygen-carrying capacity) may cause extra work for the cardiovascular system and indirectly contribute to a failed attempt at extubation.

Cardiovascular stability

Cardiac output should be judged adequate either by clinical signs (good peripheral perfusion, adequate urine output, normal systemic arterial blood pressure) or by specific determination if such is available. Output should *not* be supported artificially at the time of extubation, i.e., no vasoactive infusions. Congestive heart failure should be under control, and dysrhythmias should be absent. This does not imply that the patient is not receiving cardiac medications, only that life-threatening cardiovascular instabilities are controlled. Even though the pulmonary status may be normal, the possibility of obstruction or hypoxia after extubation exists, and either of these conditions combined with a highly unstable cardiac status might be fatal.

Central nervous system stability

Any seizure disorder present should be under good control. Physical examination before extubation should document absence of apnea, presence of reflexes that protect the airway (intact swallow, gag, and cough), and presence of good muscle strength.

Inspiratory pressures (>22 cm H_2O negative pressure) and VC (10 to 15 ml/kg body weight) measurements may be useful in older patients, particularly if the initial condition was associated with muscle weakness or dysfunction, such as Guillain-Barré syndrome or tetanus. Some assessment of how easily the patient tires with respiratory effort needs to be made, and this is usually done by observing the patient for 12 to 24 hours without ventilatory support other than an endotracheal tube. Since minimal amounts of CPAP are physiologic, CPAP need not be decreased to less than 2 to 3 cm H_2O.

Metabolic stability

The presence of hypermetabolic state will increase oxygen consumption and the work of breathing; therefore, the patient should be afebrile. In addition, abnormalities of serum sodium, potassium, calcium and glucose should be corrected, particularly in the neonate in whom apnea may be associated with metabolic imbalance. Since the patient will be without oral intake for at least 8 hours, good hydration must be assured small infants and neonates must have IV fluids to avoid dehydration and hypoglycemia and to ensure that pulmonary secretions remain liquid.

Summary of patient needs before extubation

1. Recent chest roentgenogram.
2. Arterial blood-gas tensions and pH.
3. Hct.
4. Normal systemic arterial blood pressure and cardiac rhythm.
5. Good urine output.
6. Normal neurologic examination for protective reflexes.
7. Absence of acute infection, as manifested by normal temperature and thin, clear pulmonary secretions. Consider a peripheral WBC count or a tracheal aspirate for smear and Gram stain if doubt exists.
8. Normal metabolic status. Consider serum Na, K, Cl, Ca, and glucose determinations.
9. For patients who have been intubated for long periods of time or who are known to have had traumatic intubations, pre-extubation laryngoscopy or bronchoscopy may be prudent.

Preparation for extubation

1. The patient should have all oral intake withheld for 4 hours before extubation. Protection of the airway will be imperfect for 6 to 8 hours after extubation because of glottic and supraglottic edema, and inhalation of stomach contents is much more likely during this period. In addition, should reintubation be required, it can be accomplished in a safer manner if the patient's stomach is empty.
2. Resuscitation equipment must be available, including oxygen, suction, bag and mask, and equipment for intubation (see Chapter 95).
3. Any drug that depresses respiratory effort (such as narcotics or sedatives) should be discontinued, with the exception of anticonvulsants. Muscle relaxants should not be given for 12 to 24 hours before extubation, or their effects *must* be adequately reversed.
4. Consider placing the patient on apnea and ECG monitors. Also consider giving CPT 1 to 2 hours before the extubation attempt; however, the degree of the patient's fatigability must be considered if CPT is given.

TECHNIQUE

1. Empty the stomach and withdraw the NG tube.
2. Suction the airway, being careful to clear both the tube and the oropharynx of excess secretions.
3. Remove the tape and sutures that are securing the endotracheal tube.
4. Hyperventilate the patient manually with a bag for five to ten deep breaths at the patient's inspired oxygen concentration.
5. Remove the tube at the peak of an inspiratory effort while maintaining positive pressure on the bag. This will induce the patient to cough as the tube comes out, thus expelling any secretions remaining in the airway. Be sure to deflate the cuff on a cuffed tube.
6. Most patients are placed in an inspired oxygen concentration 0.05 to 0.1 higher than they received before removal of the tube. If the patient is breathing oxygen at a concentration of 60% or greater, the inspired

oxygen concentration should always be increased. If he is receiving a concentration of less than 40%, the inspired oxygen concentration need not be increased. Patient comfort should determine the oxygen delivery system (mask, halo, etc.) (see Chapter 98).
7. Auscultate for bilaterally equal breath sounds.
8. The mouth and nose may require suctioning again, but deep tracheal suction, which can induce apnea and/or bradycardia, should be avoided until it is determined that the patient is not suffering from postextubation croup.

Postextubation monitoring

The most common problems necessitating reintubation are:
1. Obstruction, usually secondary to edema but sometimes secondary to viscid secretions.
2. Fatigue with the development of hypercarbia.
3. Apnea.
4. Cardiovascular instability induced by the increased work of breathing.
   The following regimen may be helpful:
1. Close observation should be maintained for at least 24 hours in an intensive care unit or by a trained nurse at the bedside.
2. The presence of increasing tachypnea or tachycardia, retractions, anxiety, stridor, increasing hoarseness, or signs of poor peripheral perfusion must be brought to a physician's attention immediately. The physician should probably remain at the bedside for the first 10 to 15 minutes after extubation to observe the patient's ability to breathe without an artificial airway.
3. Oral fluids should still be withheld for a minimum of 4 hours because glottic closure (and hence airway protection) is incomplete in the immediate postextubation period. If the patient is croupy, hoarse, or showing signs of stress, oral fluids should be withheld until improvement occurs or the patient is reintubated.
4. Sedative medication should be withheld. The treatment of restlessness and anxiety (air hunger) is reintubation, not depression of respiratory drive.
5. Measurement of arterial blood-gas tensions and pH 30 to 60 minutes after extubation can be helpful in ascertaining oxygenation (cyanosis is a late sign of respiratory distress).
6. A chest roentgenogram 12 to 24 hours after extubation should show any acute change, the most common being some type of atelectasis.
7. CPT for the underlying condition should be continued, but not within the first 2 hours after extubation.

RISKS AND COMPLICATIONS

The risks and complications occurring after extubation are outlined in Chapter 29; in the immediate postextubation period the main problem is the possibility of airway obstruction with the development of hypoxia and hypercarbia.

At present, steroids are not given routinely with the first attempt at extubation, nor is bronchoscopy or extubation with the patient under anesthesia recommended. With second attempts or specifically identified airway problems, such as subglottic stenosis or airway granuloma formation, a variety of additional measures as well as consultation with specialty services may be considered.

If postextubation obstruction (croup) requires therapy, nebulized racemic epinephrine may be used (see Chapter 29).

Obstructive symptoms requiring therapy within the first 2 hours of extubation warrant close observation by a physician, and reintubation may be necessary.

ADDITIONAL READING

Fagraeus, L.: Difficult extubation following nasotracheal intubation, Anesthesiology **49:**43-44, 1978.
Fox, W.W., Berman, L.S., Dinwiddie, R., and Shaffer, T.H.: Tracheal extubation of the neonate at 2 to 3 cm H_2O continuous positive airway pressure, Pediatrics **59:** 257-261, 1977.

104 Tracheostomy

WILLIAM DAMMERT
MARY E. GRANDY

INDICATIONS

The creation of a relatively permanent communication from the skin to the trachea via a neck incision for the purpose of establishing an airway is called a tracheostomy. With better understanding and care of endotracheal tubes and ready availability of skilled intubators to establish endotracheal airways, the necessity for tracheostomy has decreased markedly. The main indications are (1) relief of upper airway obstruction (60% of patients), (2) management of secretions (30%), and (3) facilitation of long-term ventilatory assistance (7%); approximately 80% of tracheostomies are performed in children less than 5 years of age. The following are the most common conditions associated with the need for establishing a permanent artificial airway:

1. In newborns (30% of procedures):
   a. Congenital malformations and neoplasms of the upper airway (e.g., hemangiomas, congenital vocal cord paralysis, Pierre Robin syndrome, cystic hygroma.)
   b. Long-term ventilatory support in respiratory distress syndrome or chronic neurologic conditions. Even though a neonate can tolerate intubation for longer periods than an adult, subglottic stenosis does occur.
2. In infants and children (1 to 5 years of age—50%; 6 to 12 years of age—20%:
   a. Airway obstruction. The most usual indication for a tracheostomy is failure to extubate a patient after provision of airway support for croup or rarely epiglottitis. This is the case in 40% of all tracheostomies. Other, less frequent causes include diphtheria, juvenile laryngeal papilloma, burns or trauma to the upper airway, neoplasms, and caustic ingestions.
   b. Problems requiring long-term ventilation, including Guillain-Barré syndrome, tetanus, postoperative respiratory failure (most often associated with correction of congenital heart defects), postoperative management of craniofacial repairs, and management of head trauma.

TECHNIQUE

1. If at all possible, tracheostomy should be performed in the operating room, where the surgeon has access to excellent lighting, proper instruments, and the assistance of trained personnel.
2. In most cases, an endotracheal airway can be established before initiation of the procedure. Particularly in the small child who cannot lie still or cooperate with verbal requests, tracheostomy under local anesthesia can be extremely difficult and even hazardous. With a secure airway in place, surgery can be done deliberately. Delivery of a general anesthetic, usually by an inhalation technique, and tube placement should be accomplished by an anesthesiologist skilled in pediatric techniques.
3. The patient should be supine with the neck hyperextended to facilitate easy palpation of the trachea (place a small roll or sandbag

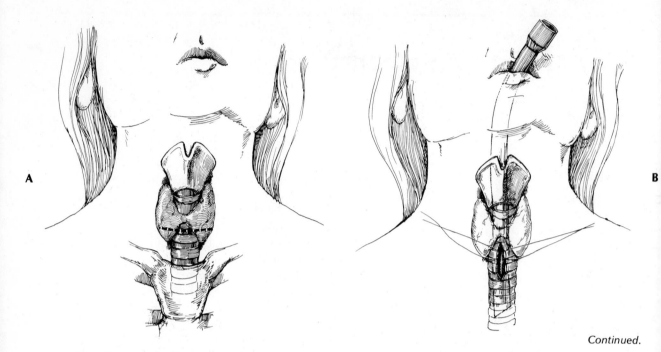

A

B

Continued.

Fig. 104-1. A, Site of skin incision for tracheostomy. Note proximity of the thyroid isthmus to the incision. **B,** Tracheal incision through third and fourth tracheal rings. Note the Prolene stay sutures on either side of the incision. **C,** Insertion of tracheostomy tube and repositioning of endotracheal tube.

beneath the shoulders). Avoid lateral tracheal deviation by maintaining the head in a midline position.

4. Prepare and drape the neck in a standard sterile fashion.

5. Choose an appropriate tube, check cuff function if applicable, and make certain that the tube will connect to the ventilating system. Cuffed tubes are almost always inappropriate for use in infants and children.

6. Incise the neck transversely at the level of the thyroid isthmus after identifying the trachea (Fig. 104-1, *A*).

7. Spread the strap muscles vertically, taking care to stay in the midline and thus avoid vascular structures in the neck. Dissection should be precise and hemostasis meticulous. Identify the pretracheal fascia and the

tracheal rings to be incised. The isthmus of the thyroid may have to be divided.

8. Place stay sutures of 3-0 Prolene suture around the second and third (or third and fourth) tracheal cartilages. Make a vertical incision in the trachea in the midline between the stay sutures (Fig. 104-1, *B*). Never excise tracheal tissue or create tracheal flaps.

9. Withdraw the endotracheal tube just enough to allow a tracheostomy tube to be inserted (Fig. 104-1, *C*). The endotracheal tube should remain in the upper airway above the tracheostomy until the procedure is completed and the tracheostomy tube is tied in place. In the event of intraoperative problems, the patient can still be ventilated via the endotracheal tube.

10. Connect the tracheostomy tube to the ven-

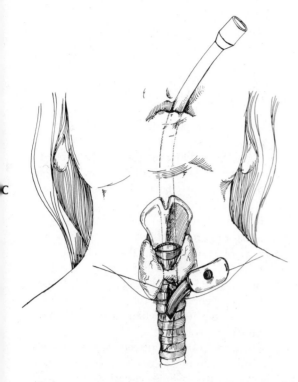

C

Fig. 104-1, cont'd. For legend see opposite page.

tilating system and auscultate the chest to ensure the presence of bilaterally equal breath sounds. Suction and culture tracheal secretions if necessary.

11. Remove the shoulder roll to place the neck in a normal position and securely tie the tube in place. It should be possible to insert only one finger between tie and neck. Tape the long stay sutures to the upper chest.

12. Obtain a chest roentgenogram to check tube position and ensure that there is no pneumothorax or infiltrate.

13. It is preferable to nurse the patient in a PICU setting for at least 24 hours to ensure tube patency, particularly if subcutaneous emphysema is present. If the tube is accidentally dislodged, an open airway can be quickly reestablished by lateral traction on the stay sutures. Before healing occurs,

the skin incision will not overlie the tracheal incision when the neck assumes a normal position. Traction on stay sutures approximates these two orifices and allows insertion of a tube. Should edema or subcutaneous air prevent reinsertion of the tracheostomy tube, replace it with a smaller tracheostomy or endotracheal tube.

14. The stay sutures can be removed a week after surgery when a fibrous tract between skin and trachea has been established. The tracheostomy tube should not be changed during this period.

Care of tubes

The following equipment must be available:
1. Suction setup with appropriate-sized suction catheters.
2. Stethoscope.
3. Oxygen source; ventilator if necessary.
4. Hydrogen peroxide.
5. Cotton-tipped swabs.
6. Tracheostomy dressing.
7. Tracheostomy ties.
8. Bag and mask.
9. Extra tracheostomy tube.

Care of patient

Suctioning

Immediately after tracheostomy, suctioning may be necessary every 10 to 15 minutes, then every 30 minutes to 1 hour. Blood-tinged secretions are common; frank hemorrhage is not usual.

Moisture and oxygen requirements

1. Continuous humidification is essential because the normal humidification mechanism in the upper airway has been bypassed.
2. Oxygen should be administered by whatever system tht patient's needs require (e.g., ventilator, T-bar, tracheostomy mask).

Tracheostomy care

1. Frequency of care should be once a shift.
2. The extent of tracheostomy care to be performed within the first 24 hours after the

procedure should be at the physician's discretion.

3. The tracheostomy site should be cleansed, using sterile cotton-tipped swabs, with hydrogen peroxide diluted with an equal volume of water.

4. Tracheostomy ties and dressings should be changed every shift. The knot should be at the back of the neck so that an infant cannot reach it to untie it. Two nurses should be involved in changing the tracheostomy ties to prevent the tracheostomy tube from slipping out.

5. If there is an inner cannula, it should be removed and cleaned of debris every 8 hours.

6. Extra tubes should be kept at the bedside.

Communication

1. If the patient's condition permits and the patient is capable of writing, a pad and pencil should be made available.

2. The older patient must have a means of alerting the nurse when he is in distress or needs something; a bell is useful for this purpose.

Nutrition

1. NG feedings may be instituted before oral fluids are tried. Check carefully for NG position before beginning feeding, and place the patient in the sitting or semisitting position. Observe for signs of possible inhalation of stomach contents (choking, coughing, return of liquid from the tracheostomy tube).

2. Begin oral fluids and feeding with small amounts of clear liquids, and progress as tolerated. The patient should be in a sitting position.

Special problems

1. Head position should be closely observed to ensure that the tracheostomy tube does not become occluded by the chin; placing a roll beneath the patient's shoulders during sleep may help to prevent hyperflexion of the neck and tube occlusion.

2. Patients with short, fat necks (neonates) tend to develop rashes and macerated skin beneath the tracheostomy ties. Such problems can be eliminated only by close observation, good skin cleansing, and frequent changes of ties.

3. If the tracheostomy tube should accidentally come out, the following procedure should be instituted:

   a. Observe the patient. Do not leave him alone.

   b. Place the child on his back with the head hyperextended and direct the flow of oxygen toward the tracheostomy stoma.

   c. If the child is distressed, insert a clean tracheostomy tube and auscultate for equal breath sounds.

   d. Use of stay sutures, the tracheostomy tube stylet, or a small suction catheter placed into the stoma and over which the larger tracheostomy tube can be slipped may all be helpful when the tube cannot be easily replaced.

   e. Once the tube is replaced, obtain a chest roentgenogram to confirm tube position.

4. Changes in the volume, viscosity, or color of secretions obtained from the tube may herald an acute infection and should be noted on the chart.

5. A fenestrated tube has a hole in the greater curve of the tube so that the opening is in line with the tracheal air column. Air can flow from the tube to the upper airway on expiration and move through the vocal cords, encouraging vocalization and preventing a fixed larynx. Inhalation of feedings is more likely with this type of tube.

6. Standard tracheostomy tubes may be too long for small premature infants, so that with changes in head or neck position the tip of the tube occludes the airway. If this is the case, the tube end may be cut to an appropriate length; the cut edges must be beveled to prevent trauma from rough edges. Alternatively, padding may be placed over the skin at the stoma site, under the flared connector site of the tracheostomy tube, to re-

move the tip from its distal position. A new type of shorter tracheostomy is now commercially available.

TRACHEOSTOMY TUBES: TYPES AND SIZES (Fig. 104-2)

There is a variety of metal and plastic tracheostomy tubes available, the most common being the Hollinger, Jackson, Aberdeen, and Shiley tubes. The Hollinger and Jackson tubes are metal, usually silver, and consist of three parts: the tracheostomy tube, an inner cannula, and a stylet used for introducing the tube. Of the two, the shorter, less curved Hollinger tube is more appropriate for small infants. The Aberdeen and Shiley tubes are made of polyvinyl chloride; the major difference between the two is the presence of a standard 6-mm adapter on the Shiley tube. Cuffed, plastic tubes (Shiley or Portex) are available for older children. Metal tubes are nonreactive, easy to keep clean, fit flush with the neck, and generally have thinner walls than comparably sized plastic tubes. Many surgeons prefer them for long-term home-care situations. All synthetic tubes should be marked with the Initials ITT or Z$^{.79}$ to indicate that standard tissue testing for irritability has been done by the Anesthesia Equipment Committee of the U.S. Standards Institute. Of the tubes mentioned, only the Shiley and Portex are suitable for long-term mechanical ventilation.

The proper tube size can be estimated visually from examination of the trachea and from the size of the previously placed endotracheal tube. Usually the tracheostomy tube will have an internal diameter 0.5 mm larger than the endotracheal tube, because the endotracheal tube must pass the smallest diameter of the airway (cricoid cartilage) but the tracheostomy tube does not. The tube should never be forced into the trachea; a smaller tube should be placed instead.

PHYSIOLOGIC CONSEQUENCES OF TRACHEOSTOMY

There are certain consequences of placing a tube in the trachea, including:
1. Placement of a foreign body in the airway, which produces an inflammatory response.
2. Bypass the natural mechanism for filtration

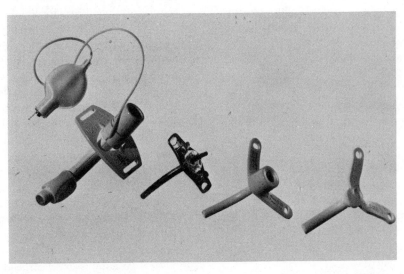

Fig. 104-2. Types of tracheostomy tubes *(left to right):* cuffed tube for older children, metal tube, Shiley tube with standard 6-mm connector, and Aberdeen tube.

and humidification of incoming gas with subsequent increase in viscosity of secretions.
3. Introduction of infection.
4. Cessation of air flow through the larynx (vocal cords assume the cadaveric position).
5. Loss of dead space by about 50%.

These expected responses to tracheostomy can augment complications of the procedure.

RISKS AND COMPLICATIONS
Operative

Operative complications increase substantially when tracheostomy is performed in a suboptimal manner. The most recent review of emergency pediatric tracheostomy indicates a mortality of 1% to 4% from the procedure itself (done in large centers where good surgical, nursing, and anesthetic experitise is available). The single most common fatal complication is pneumothorax, to which the struggling, anoxic, obstructed child is particularly prone. The incidence of pneumothorax has been shown to decrease significantly when the technique is modified to include prior establishment of an airway. General anesthesia adds only a negligible risk to the overall operative mortality. Other operative complications include hemorrhage, recurrent laryngeal nerve injury, esophageal injury, mediastinal tube insertion, and mediastinal or subcutaneous emphysema.

Immediate postoperative

Immediate postoperative problems are related to improper surgical technique, inadequate nursing, and physiologic changes inherent in the procedure.

Improper placement of the tube may result in innominate artery erosion with rupture (too low placement) or subglottic stenosis (too high placement). Occasionally in small infants, persistent endobronchial tube placement with atelectasis can occur. Tracheomalacia can result from excision of cartilage.

Inattention to proper nursing technique may result in mucous plugging (viscid secretions,

increased amounts of secretions), accidental or inapparent extubation, irritation and/or maceration of skin beneath the ties, and secondary infection.

Long-term

Long-term complications include:
1. Difficult decannulation (9% to 20%), which is defined as inability to remove the airway within 30 days.
2. Erosion into vital structures (less than 1%).
3. Persistence of a fistulous tract after decannulation (less than 1%).

The problem of difficult decannulation is related to one of the following conditions: (1) presence of granuloma in the trachea at the tip of the tube or on the anterior tracheal wall at the level of the stoma, (2) presence of excessive tissue reaction, causing subglottic stenosis or more peripheral obstructions, (3) absence of air movement through the cords, resulting in fixed larynx, and (4) tracheomalacia secondary to tracheal damage from the surgery or the tube. The first two appear to be related to airway infection, particularly preexisting viral processes such as croup that enhance the inflammatory response produced by a foreign body (the tube). Subglottic stenosis will develop in 3% to 20% of children less than 5 years of age who require some form of airway support (intubation or tracheostomy). The histologic changes associated with tracheostomy are similar to those seen with long-term intubation (see Chapter 29). Daily cleansing of the stoma, frequent tube changes, and meticulous suctioning technique cannot be overemphasized in minimizing the long-term complications noted above.

Many methods of decannulation have been devised; the criteria for tube removal are the same as those for removing endotracheal tubes (see Chapter 103). If the airway has been in place longer than 3 to 4 weeks, bronchoscopy and laryngoscopy should precede decannulation to identify the presence of stenosis or granuloma. Decannulation usually entails a period of several days to weeks during which time the child is gradually transferred from tube breathing to upper airway breathing by use of a fenestrated tube, replacement of the tracheostomy tube with a series of tubes with successively smaller diameters, or gradual restriction of the tube orifice with plugs. Sudden restoration of dead space or of air flow through a relatively immobile larynx may increase the work of breathing and retard weaning, particularly if combined with problems with secretions. Tracheomalacia can sometimes be treated with a nasotracheal tube for several days to weeks so that the tracheal wall can strengthen. Some prefer to remove the tube with the patient awake; others prefer extubation under general anesthesia. The specific technique chosen should depend on the experience of the surgeon and intensivist handling the problem; decannulation using any method should be accomplished in a PICU setting, where constant observation and monitoring are available should airway obstruction develop.

ADDITIONAL READING

Aberdeen, E.: Tracheostomy and tracheostomy care in infants, Proc. R. Soc. Med. **58**:42-44, 1965.

Bush, G.H.: The management of the retained tracheostomy tube, Anaesth. Intensive Care **4**:113-117, 1976.

Fairshter, R.D., Liff, M.O., and Wilson, A.F.: Complications of long tracheostomy tubes, Crit. Care Med. **5**:271-273, 1976.

Filston, H.C., Johnson, D.G., and Crumrine, R.S.: Infant tracheostomy: a new look with a solution to the difficult cannulation problem, Am. J. Dis. Child. **132**:1172-1176, 1978.

Friedberg, S.A., Griffith, T.E., and Haas, G.M.: Histologic changes in trachea following tracheotomy, Ann. Otolaryngol. **74**:785-798, 1965.

Greenberg, L.M., Davenport, H.T., and Shimo, G.: Method for difficult decannulations in children, Arch. Otolaryngol. **81**:72-76, 1965.

Hazards of prolonged intubation and tracheostomy equipment (editorial,), J.A.M.A. **204**:624-625, 1968.

Levinger, L.: Safer tracheostomy tube reinsertion, Am. J. Surg. **136**:284, 1978.

Mendez-Picon, G., Ehrlich, F.E., and Salzberg, D.M.: The effect of tracheostomy incisions on tracheal growth, J. Pediatr. Surg. **11**:681-685, 1976.

Oliver, P., Richardson, J.R., Blubb, R.W., and others: Tracheotomy in children, N. Engl. J. Med. **267**:632-637, 1972.

Perrotta, R.J., and Schley, W.S.: Pediatric tracheotomy: a five year comparison study, Arch. Otolaryngol. **104**:318-321, 1978.

Sasaki, C.T., Gaudet, P.T., and Peerless, A.: Tracheostomy decannulation, Am. J. Dis. Child. **132**:266-269, 1978.

Symthe, P.M.: The problem of detubating an infant with a tracheostomy, J. Pediatr. **65**:446-453, 1964.

Stool, S.E., and Beebe, J.K.: Tracheotomy in infants and children, Curr. Probl. Pediatr. **3**:1035, 1973.

Tucker, J.A., and Silberman, H.D.: Tracheotomy in pediatrics, Ann. Otolaryngol. **81**:818-824, 1972.

Von Schulthess, G.: Tracheotomy: complications and late sequelae, Arch. Otolaryngol. **82**:405-408, 1965.

105 Sending a patient home from the PICU

ANNETTE MUSSELMAN

INDICATIONS

When should one consider sending a patient home from PICU? How does one prepare the parents or caretakers to handle emergency situations or even just the routine daily care needs of their child? How can one assess their abilities before actually sending the patient home? These are just a few of the questions that must be answered with regard to the child who is hospitalized but stable, requires extra ventilatory support or artificial airway maintenance, and may be considered ready for discharge to the home.

The patient who is stable and in good condition but requires continuous oxygen and/or CPAP could be a candidate for home care. Such a patient may or may not have a tracheostomy. At this point, parental education about life support systems and basic airway maintenance could be started. This frees expensive PICU beds sooner and allows the child to have the benefit of a more normal home environment and family life.

When determining if a family situation is appropriate for home ventilatory care, one must take into consideration the family's psychological, intellectual, and financial resources. An assessment of the family's capability by a social worker may help to decide whether home care will be feasible. The parents must have a desire to care for their child at home and have enough family support to provide 24-hour care. They also need to be able to learn and perform any necessary skills that pertain to their child's

needs, as well as have an understanding of the disease process and its treatment, including equipment and drugs.

Financial resources are important. After the patient has been hospitalized for a period of time, there will be major financial strain on the family. Will the parents be able to afford the cost of necessary equipment? Will insurance cover the purchase or rental of home care equipment? Since medical equipment is expensive, the stress of dealing with these costs may not be worth it to the family. It is important that doctors, nurses, therapists, and equipment dealers work together to determine the approximate length of time the patient will require any equipment. This will help to make a decision about whether rental or purchase is more cost-effective. Table 105-1 gives a price estimate of the equipment necessary for a child sent home on CPAP.

TECHNIQUE

Parental instruction should begin as soon as there is a possibility of the parents being able to take the child home. It is imperative that the parents be given every opportunity and as much time as possible in the hospital to learn care skills and to ask questions. Therapists and nurses should recognize the lack of medical sophistication in most parents. Information and teaching sessions should be numerous, brief, and repetitive. The information given should be on a level the parents can understand and easily assimilate. Encourage parents to ask questions,

Table 105-1. Cost estimate of equipment

Item	Approximate cost of purchase ($)	Approximate cost of rental ($)
Suction machine	212	35/mo
Apnea monitor	1,495	195/mo
CPAP compressor	415	60/mo
Simple compressor	150	35/mo
Bunn disconnect alarm	200	40/mo
Oxygen concentrator	2,000-3,000	250-300/mo
Compressed oxygen H cylinders with regulator deposit and tank stand	—	160/first mo, then 40/mo
H refill exchange	—	18 each tank
Liquid oxygen	—	90-150/mo
Refills on 75-lb reservoir	—	.90-1.30/lb

even if they feel that the questions are silly or something they should already know. In addition to instruction in treatment modalities and equipment care, parents should be taught basic CPR. Hazards of smoking in the home should be carefully explained to all family members.

A respiratory therapist and a nurse who have definitive prepared teaching programs should be responsible for the educational process. They may be assisted by other therapists and nurses, but the primary responsibility should lie with one therapist and one nurse. Unprepared individuals should not be casually or haphazardly assigned to do such instruction.

A reputable medical equipment supplier should be used, preferably one who is willing to work with the family on financial matters or who will handle insurance paperwork for the family. Equipment should be ordered as soon as possible, since some items may require special ordering and may take several weeks to arrive. The teachers should be responsible for making certain that all necessary equipment is ordered and that the proper items arrive. Table 105-1 also lists the individual pieces of equipment that are needed but often forgotten.

The doctor should write individual prescriptions for each piece of equipment. These may be required in duplicate for insurance purposes. A letter stating the patient's prognosis and need for the ordered equipment may be required by some insurance companies.

The use of oxygen at home requires a method of delivery. Oxygen delivery can be accomplished by the use of one of three methods. The oxygen concentrator is an electrical compressor that makes use of molecular sieves or filters to separate the oxygen from the other gases in room air. The Fi_{O_2} delivery range varies with the different brands. The size and cost of the units are also widely varied. Oxygen can also be delivered by tanks of compressed oxygen or by the liquid oxygen system, similar to the ones used by most hospitals. These last two methods deliver an Fi_{O_2} of 1.0 at any liter flow.

The choice of delivery method is made by cost analysis, comparing the patient's oxygen needs and the cost of each method. Generally, tanks of compressed oxygen or oxygen concentrators are more widely available. Oxygen concentrators have limited liter flow capabilities, which make them difficult to use with the higher oxygen concentrations necessary with tracheostomy collars, CPAP, or mist tents. Oxygen tanks must be changed frequently if the child is on a continuous oxygen device. The cost of the frequent changes can be considerable. Liquid oxygen, while less available, offers the best capabilities of high liter flow with high Fi_{O_2}, along with portability from shoulder pack units that the parents fill themselves from the main reservoir in the home. The medical equipment supplier must refill this reservoir an average of 2½ times a month, as opposed to 2 changes per week with oxygen tanks.

Before the patient goes home on oxygen, a qualified electrician should check the home's wiring and observe for any electrical hazards that could make the use of oxygen dangerous to the family. The electrician should also check for the necessity of new or changed circuits in the house's wiring if the patient will be on any kind of electrical support systems. This will reduce the fire hazard and reduce the possibility of circuit overload from all the patient's equipment operating simultaneously. Electrical equipment includes mechanical ventilators, compressors, suction machines, and delivery pumps for NG feedings or TPN. For sections on suctioning, TPN, and NG feedings, see Chapters 100, 111, and 112.

Mechanical ventilators for children are not widely available for home use. The LP4 by Life Products, Inc., offers volume ventilation capabilities of 0-3,000 cc. The peak inspiratory pressure can be adjusted up to 100 cm H_2O, although there are no mechanisms for PEEP or for CPAP alone. It is made to use room air. Increased Fi_{O_2} concentrations require bleeding

oxygen into the intake ports on the back panel. The LP_4 is extremely portable and can run off 100 VAC or automobile-type batteries or its own internal battery.

CPAP can be delivered via a heavy-duty electric air compressor and a circuit setup similar to that used in the hospital. Oxygen can be bled in until the desired Fi_{O_2} is achieved. The compressor CPAP circuit can be easily changed to a simple tracheostomy collar setup by the parents if the CPAP is not a 24-hour-a-day necessity. See the schematics in Fig. 105-1 for the organization of equipment.

A smaller compressor is needed for any nebulized bronchodilator therapy. A suction machine should be ordered for any patient with a tracheostomy or one who cannot easily clear his own airway adequately. (See Chapters 100 and 104.)

The family should also be taught how to clean the equipment and should have enough spare equipment so that they can clean one circuit while the patient is on another. The need for clean equipment cannot be overemphasized to the family. Instruction on cleaning should include the risks of infection that they take by using dirty equipment on their child.

It is usually adequate to wash the equipment in detergent once a day followed by a 30-minute soak in 1 part acetic acid to 2 parts water. If the equipment requires the use of

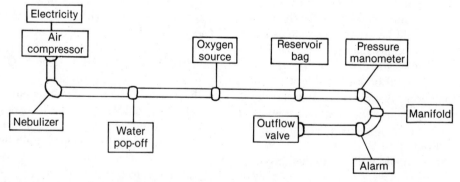

Fig. 105-1. Block diagram of a continuous positive airway pressure circuit for home use.

0.9% sodium chloride solution, the family should be instructed on making this themselves by adding ¼ teaspoon uniodized table salt per 1 cup boiled water. The solution should be kept in the refrigerator in a clean covered container and made fresh every 2 days.

It is always a good idea to put the child with the parents in an accessible, but isolated room prior to hospital discharge so that the parents can assume total care while remaining in the hospital setting. Any equipment that will be used at home should be checked for proper grounding by the hospital's Biomedical Department and should be used by the parents in this room. Once parents have indicated that they are comfortable with total care of the patient, they should be left entirely in charge of their child for a period of time. They should be able to do all procedures without supervision before the child is discharged. A reasonable trial period is 72 hours. This allows the parents to see just how they will have to organize their days and nights around the child's care. Staff should be readily available to offer assistance in case problems or questions arise. Continuing interviews by the social worker help to ensure that the parents are coping well with the stress of giving total care and are not ex-

periencing any unforeseen emotional, financial, or physical difficulties in handling their child.

The day and approximate time of discharge should be planned in advance. Last-minute checks of all equipment should be made by the instructors and parents together. It is helpful for the parents to have a folder with all their instructional pamphlets, notes, and diagrams. This can be quickly reviewed by the parents and instructors to make certain that all points are clear.

It is a good idea for the medical equipment supplier to move any equipment from hospital to home. A nurse and/or therapist should accompany the family home and help set up the equipment. A list of parent instructors, therapists, nurses, and doctors that the family is familiar with should be provided, including phone numbers and backup emergency numbers. The family should have a definite plan of action for an emergency situation.

Close follow-up on a weekly basis helps ensure that procedures are being done smoothly and properly so that the patient receives adequate care. This follow-up may include routine telephone contact by hospital personnel as well as home visits by a public health nurse.

106 Blood product transfusions

GEORGE R. BUCHANAN
MARY E. GRANDY

INDICATIONS

Children receiving care in the PICU often require transfusions of blood products to correct deficiencies of RBCs, clotting factors, and platelets or to replace intravascular fluid volume. Component therapy is now the preferred mode of treatment of practically all disorders that require blood replacement. Most blood banks are able to divide a unit of freshly drawn whole blood into three or four separate components so that the child can receive only that in which he is deficient. Physicians caring for ill children must often make their requests for transfusions in terms of ml/kg of body weight, since a single unit of packed RBCs or plasma contains a volume equal to the entire blood volume of many small infants.

Use of specific blood products

Whole blood. Whole blood is used only for treatment of acute hemorrhage and for purposes of exchange transfusion, although in both circumstances the combination of packed RBCs and FFP is just as effective. The amount of fresh whole blood to be used varies tremendously from child to child, depending on the extent of blood loss that needs to be replaced. There is much confusion regarding the term fresh whole blood. One must specify what is the key desired component before one can determine how fresh the whole blood must be in order for this component to be present and functional. For instance, platelets are functional in a unit of blood for only a few hours, and the labile clotting factors (factors V and VIII) begin

to decrease precipitously within 24 to 36 hours. However, blood remains fresh for purposes of exchange transfusion for as long as 4 or 5 days since it is not until then that the potassium level increases (because of RBC breakdown) and oxygen affinity increases because of depletion of 2,3-diphosphoglycerate (2,3-DPG). The major use of whole blood in neonates is for exchange transfusion. Either citrated (acid citrate dextrose [ACD] or citrate phosphate dextrose [CPD]) or heparinized whole blood can be used, although the latter must be administered within 48 hours after collection.

Packed RBCs. Sedimented or centrifuged whole blood can be easily separated into concentrated RBCs and plasma. The former usually has a hemoglobin concentration of 18 to 25 g/dl and is the treatment of choice for children with acute or chronic anemia who require replacement of red cell mass to increase oxygen-carrying capacity. The usual recommended dose is 10 ml/kg administered over 2 to 4 hours. This generally results in a rise in the hemoglobin concentration of 3 g/dl and a rise in the hematocrit by 10%. In those children who have severe anemia (less than 5 g/dl), congestive heart failure, or hypertension, the transfusion should be given in a smaller volume (4 to 5 ml/kg) and administered extremely slowly, i.e., over 4 to 6 hours. More rapid administration of a large bolus of blood may precipitate congestive heart failure or an extreme and life-threatening hypertensive episode.

Packed RBCs can be further washed of plasma and other cellular elements so that a more pure product of red cells is obtained. This is achieved by multiple saline washes, passage through nylon filters, or freezing of washed RBCs. The last maneuver permits the storage of blood (particularly cells possessing rare surface antigens) for prolonged periods, removes most of the foreign non-RBC antigens, and theoretically lessens the risk of hepatitis. Frozen or washed packed RBCs are particularly useful in the chronically transfused patient in whom transfusion reactions (see below) are common or in the child in whom a transplant of bone marrow is anticipated in the future. However, these products are more expensive than packed RBCs and should not be used for routine purposes.

Plasma. Outdated plasma obtained from units of whole blood which have served their 21- to 28-day shelf-life is still sometimes used for volume replacement. However, it is markedly depleted of labile clotting factors and may have increased amounts of fibrin split products and other potentially toxic substances. Therefore its use is not generally recommended. The major plasma product in current use is FFP, which is separated from anticoagulated whole blood within 6 hours after drawing and then rapidly frozen. Its use as a source of colloid in patients requiring volume replacement is discouraged because of the significant risk of hepatitis. Albumin or plasma-protein fraction (Plasmanate) is preferred in such circumstances. However, FFP is indicated to replace depleted clotting factors in patients with congenital or acquired bleeding disorders such as hemophilia, liver disease, or DIC. It is administered in a dose of 10 to 15 ml/kg over 30 to 120 minutes and can be repeated as often as two to three times daily as necessary. However, frequent use is accompanied by congestive heart failure secondary to volume overload.

Platelet concentrates. Concentrates of platelets containing as many as 10^{11} platelets per unit are separated from whole blood by differential centrifugation immediately after drawing and

can be used immediately or stored for up to 72 hours. The volume of each platelet concentrate (obtained from a single donor) ranges from 10 to 60 ml, depending on the amount of supernatant plasma in which the platelets are suspended. A large volume of plasma is required to maintain platelet integrity when storage is carried out at room temperature. Indications for transfusion of platelet concentrates are actually quite limited. They should be administered only to children who have marked thrombocytopenia (i.e., platelet count of less than $20,000/\mu l$) and who are hemorrhaging or thought to be at great risk of bleeding. Transfusions are particularly indicated in those children whose thrombocytopenia is due to decreased platelet production (such as leukemia or aplastic anemia), but in life-threatening situations they can be useful even in patients who have destructive thrombocytopenia (e.g., children with DIC). It should be remembered that even though the normal platelet count is 175,000 to $400,000/\mu l$, bleeding seldom occurs when the platelet count is greater than $75,000/\mu l$ and severe life-threatening hemorrhage rarely occurs unless the platelet count is less than $10,000/\mu l$ in the absence of other coagulation abnormalities. Surgical procedures can usually be safely undertaken when the platelet count is greater than $50,000/\mu l$. In rare circumstances platelet concentrates are necessary for treatment of abnormalities of platelet function. No attempt should be made to increase the platelet count to normal when platelet concentrates are being administered. The usual recommended dose is 1 unit of platelets per 6 to 8 kg of body weight. Hence, most neonates require only a single unit.

Factor concentrates. Concentrated forms of clotting factors are rarely indicated in the PICU setting but mainly are of use for patients with congenital deficiencies of single coagulation factors. These concentrates are:

1. Cryoprecipitate, a noncommercial product prepared by blood banks, contains large quantities of fibrinogen, factor VIII coagu-

lant activity, and von Willebrand factor activity. Although there is great variability, it can be assumed for practical purposes that approximately 75 units of factor VIII are present in each bag of cryoprecipitate. Its use should be reserved for patients with hemophilia A, von Willebrand's disease, or afibrinogenemia and rarely for children with DIC.

2. Factor VIII concentrates are commercial preparations of factor VIII that contain a variable but known number of units of factor VIII activity in each vial. They are not always efficacious in von Willebrand's disease, but their indications are otherwise the same as those of cryoprecipitate.

3. Factor IX concentrates (Proplex and Konyne) are mainly reserved for patients with Christmas disease (hemophilia B), although they have also been found to benefit patients with hemophilia A with inhibitors. They are rarely needed for subjects with vitamin K deficiency and are not recommended at all for children with liver disease or DIC, since their infusion is followed by great danger of accelerated thrombosis.

TECHNIQUE

1. All of the blood products discussed above should be administered to the patient as soon as possible after they are obtained from the blood bank, since the risk of bacterial contamination and degradation or inactivation of the blood components often occurs within hours. If the blood products cannot be administered shortly after they are received, they should be returned promptly to the blood bank, since refrigerators on hospital wards usually do not maintain proper temperature control for safe storage.

2. Check in blood according to hospital procedure which should include the patient's name, hospital number, and blood type. This is the single most important procedure in preventing administration of mismatched blood and resultant disastrous sequelae.

3. Select an appropriate blood filter. The woven-nylon clot filter (mesh size 170 μm) found in routine blood administration sets allows passage of RBCs and microaggregates less than 150 μm in size. Such microaggregates may embolize to the pulmonary circulation and contribute to a respiratory insufficiency syndrome. Micropore filters, such as Intrasept (Johnson and Johnson), Bently PFS-127, Fenwall 4C2417, and Ultipore (Pall Corporation), can reduce the number of such microaggregates that enter the bloodstream.

   a. Use a double-filter setup for postoperative cardiac patients and for patients in whom massive transfusion is likely (e.g., for acute gastrointestinal hemorrhage or exchange transfusion).

   b. Platelets come from the blood bank with a special administration set because use of the regular blood administration set may filter out the platelets.

   c. With factor VIII and IX concentrates, a small filter needle is usually provided through which the preparation is withdrawn into a syringe from the vial.

4. Flush the IV line with 0.9% sodium chloride solution, since dextrose can hemolyze RBCs and induce agglutination of RBCs and platelets.

   a. Intermittent flushing with small volumes of 0.9% sodium chloride solution may be required to keep IV lines patent. A new Y tubing is now available specifically to accommodate blood in one arm of the Y and an IV bottle in the other. This avoids multiple injections in line and hence decreases chance contamination.

   b. An alternate method to ensure patency of the vein is to administer blood with a constant infusion pump.

5. Regulate the rate. For infants and small

children, use a Metriset to measure volumes precisely.

6. Children in whom temperature control is a problem should receive blood warmed to body temperature by immersion in a water bath or by some other suitable device. Cold blood should never be given through a right atrial catheter, since this may cause dysrhythmias.

7. Blood products open for more than 6 hours are considered contaminated and should be discarded.

8. When a neonate has only one fluid source, observe him closely for signs of hypoglycemia while blood is being infused, since his only source of glucose is being intermittently interrupted to infuse blood.

9. When possible, blood should be administered through a second IV line with as large a needle as possible to minimize hemolysis, although transfusions can be given through needles as small as 27 gauge. Do not force the blood through a peripheral arterial catheter.

10. In the event that a second IV line is not feasible, it may be necessary to push small volumes of blood (1 to 3 ml) every 15 to 30 minutes, depending on the size of the infant. It is important to clear the line with 0.9% sodium chloride solution before and after blood infusion.

RISKS AND COMPLICATIONS
Immediate side effects

During a blood transfusion or within minutes to hours afterward, the major risks are volume overload and transfusion reactions. Even children with normal cardiovascular status cannot acutely receive more than 15 to 20 ml of colloid volume per kg without developing pulmonary edema. Children with congestive heart failure, hypertension, or renal failure usually cannot tolerate more than 10 ml/kg over 1 to 2 hours unless active hemorrhage is occurring.

Transfusion reactions are of several types. By far the most common are allergic, febrile, or cutaneous reactions. These episodes, which occur particularly in children who have previously received numerous blood product transfusions, consist of fever (often as high as 39° to 40° C) and urticaria. Less common are angioneurotic edema and bronchospasm. The symptoms are usually benign and transient and are managed by temporarily stopping the transfusion and administering acetaminophen and an antihistamine (e.g., diphenhydramine, 1 mg/kg). After the symptoms have abated, the transfusion can usually be carefully continued. Children with frequent transfusion reactions should be premedicated with an antihistamine and an antipyretic. Most of these reactions are probably secondary to circulating antibodies in the recipient directed against alloantigens on transfused WBCs or platelets or against foreign plasma proteins.

A more serious type of transfusion reaction is the hemolytic transfusion reaction secondary to infusion of mismatched blood. These episodes, usually due to clerical error, are fortunately rare but can be catastrophic. They usually occur during a transfusion of whole blood or packed RBCs. The reactions are heralded by high spiking fever, back and abdominal pain, chills, and passage of dark urine. Jaundice and a bleeding diathesis secondary to DIC (see Chapter 20) may occur in the most severe reactions. The affected patient has hemoglobinemia, hemoglobinuria, and a positive direct Coombs' test as well as spherocytes on the peripheral blood smear, and rapidly progressive anemia. The transfusion must be stopped immediately and the suspected offending unit of blood returned to the blood bank with a blood specimen from the patient for re-crossmatching. The child must be vigorously hydrated and should receive an osmotic diuretic to maintain urinary output and to avoid acute tubular necrosis, the major serious complication of a hemolytic transfusion reaction.

Delayed side effects

The major delayed side effect of transfusion therapy is hepatitis. This still occurs, at a variable frequency (generally considered 1% per unit of blood transfused), despite the fact that most blood banks carefully check all donor units for hepatitis B surface antigen by radioimmunoassay or similar sensitive tests. Unfortunately, screening is not totally effective in diagnosing infected blood. Moreover, 80% to 90% of cases of posttransfusion hepatitis are due to non-A, non-B hepatitis virus(es). The incubation period, signs and symptoms, and natural history of posttransfusion hepatitis are extremely variable.

ADDITIONAL READING

Herrera, A.J., and Corless, J.: Blood transfusions: effects of speed of infusion and of needle gauge on hemolysis, J. Pediatr. **99:**757-758, 1981.

Marshall, B.E., Wurzel, H.A., Newfeld, G.R., and others: Effects of Intrasept micropore filtration of blood on microaggregates and other constituents, Anesthesiology **44:**525-534, 1976.

Nathan, D.G., and Oshi, F.A., editors: Hematology of infancy and childhood, ed. 2, Philadelphia, 1981, W.B. Saunders Co., pp. 1491-1551.

Urbanick, S.J., and Cash, J.D.: Blood replacement therapy, Br. Med. Bull. **33:**273-282, 1977.

Wallace, J.: Blood transfusion for clinicians, New York, 1977, Churchill-Livingstone, Inc.

107 Exchange transfusions

DANIEL L. LEVIN
TERRY RAUSCHUBER
CATHERINE P. MAST

INDICATIONS

Exchange transfusions are usually done in newborns for hyperbilirubinemia (see Chapter 64); however, they are also occasionally used in newborns and older patients to remove endogenous or exogenous toxic substances (see Chapters 19, 21, and 66). An exchange transfusion is a major undertaking and should be performed with the utmost caution.

TECHNIQUE
Personnel

The exchange transfusion team should consist of two physicians, one to do the exchange and one to record its progress, and a nurse to observe the patient and provide materials.

Locale

An exchange transfusion should be performed in an intensive care unit or an operating room (in emergencies, in the delivery room) with proper lighting, heating, monitoring devices, and maintenance of sterility.

Route

In the newborn, the routes in order of preference are:
1. Umbilical artery and vein. This allows isovolumetric exchange with withdrawal from the artery and infusion into the vein. The tip of the umbilical arterial catheter should be at L4 (just cephalad to the aortic bifurcation) and the tip of the umbilical venous catheter should be cephalad to the diaphragm (in the

inferior vena cava [IVC] or the right atrium) (see Chapters 87 and 89 for placement).
2. Umbilical artery alone
3. Umbilical vein with the tip of the catheter in the inferior vena cava
4. Venous catheter introduced into the inferior or superior vena cava in the thoracic cavity via a cutdown. This is necessary in some infants, especially those with omphalitis.
5. Peripheral arterial catheter (out) and peripheral vein catheter or needle (in)
6. Umbilical vein with the tip of the catheter in the portal system

In older children, the preferred routes are:
1. A systemic arterial catheter (out) and a venous catheter (in) in the superior or inferior vena cava in the thoracic cavity for an isovolumetric exchange transfusion
2. A venous catheter in the superior or inferior vena cava in the thoracic cavity

Preparation

1. Place the patient in a warm, well-lighted environment. For newborns use a radiant warmer and restrain all four extremities. Aspirate the stomach contents. Place the patient on a cardiorespiratory monitor. Have the emergency cart for CPR immediately available.
2. In all patients, before exchange transfusion measure:
   a. Hct and Hb.
   b. Platelet count.
   c. Arterial blood-gas tensions and pH.

603

d. Heart rate.
e. Respiratory rate.
f. Serum Na, K, Cl, and Ca.
g. Temperature.
h. Dextrostix.
i. Systemic arterial blood pressure.
j. CVP when available.
3. In newborns with hyperbilirubinemia, before exchange transfusion also measure:
a. TSP.
b. Serum bilirubin, total and direct.
c. Reticulocyte count.
d. Coombs' test.
4. In patients undergoing exchange transfusion for endogenous (e.g., ammonia) or exogenous (e.g., carbon monoxide) toxins, measure the blood level of the toxin before and after the procedure.

Method

1. In newborns with hemolytic disease, use donor blood that is compatible with the mother's blood. For example, if the mother is ORh$^-$ and the infant ORh$^+$, use ORh$^-$ blood so that antibodies to the Rh positive factor that remain in the infant after the exchange will not destroy donor cells.
2. Use the freshest blood possible, preferably less than 1 day old.
3. In infants with thrombocytopenia ($<100,000/mm^3$), use fresh heparinized blood when available.
4. Warm blood to 35° to 37° C using coiled tubing and blood warmer. Use micropore filter.
5. Intermittently agitate the donor unit so that the cells do not sink, leaving RBC-poor blood at the end of the exchange.
6. Calculate the volume to be exchanged. Usually a two-volume exchange will remove 83% of the patient's RBCs.
7. If the push-pull method is used, use volumes of 5 ml for infants weighing less than 2000 g and 10 ml for infants weighing more than 2000 g. In older children use 15 ml/kg.

8. The exchange should not be completed in less than 45 to 60 minutes in a vigorous patient and should be slower in a patient with unstable systemic arterial blood pressure, ventilatory status, or temperature.
9. Give 1 ml of 10% calcium gluconate for every 100 ml of ACD or CPD (citrated) donor blood when the serum calcium level is low (less than 7.5 mg/dl) at the beginning of the procedure. It is probably unnecessary to give calcium to infants who have a normal serum calcium level before exchange transfusion.
10. Observe the patient and the monitor for signs of distress. Stop the exchange transfusion if the patient's condition is unstable.
11. If the patient's condition is unstable but the exchange transfusion must proceed, measure the systemic arterial blood pressure and arterial blood-gas tensions and pH after every 100 ml exchanged.
12. After the exchange transfusion, continue to monitor the patient, especially the Dextrostix, since hypoglycemia is common 20 to 60 minutes after the exchange transfusion if glucose is suddenly withdrawn. Maintain IV glucose until the patient is feeding again.
13. Consider giving new doses of any medications whose serum concentrations are lowered by exchange transfusions (e.g., digitalis, antibiotics, anticonvulsants).
14. If the catheters malfunction, do not force blood through them. They are probably clotted, and application of force will dislodge clots, which can have disastrous results (see Chapters 87 and 89). Change the catheters immediately.
15. After the exchange transfusion measure:
a. Heart rate.
b. Respiratory rate.
c. Temperature.
d. Dextrostix.
e. Systemic arterial blood pressure.
f. Arterial blood-gas tensions and pH.
g. Hct and Hb.

h. Platelet count.

i. Serum Na, K, Cl, and Ca.

j. Blood level of substance exchanged (e.g., bilirubin, ammonia); continue to determine blood levels of this substance until the post–exchange transfusion trend is established.

RISKS AND COMPLICATIONS

Patients can become hypotensive, cold, hypoglycemic, hypocalcemic, bradycardic, acidotic, hypoxic, and hypovolemic or hypervolemic during or shortly after an exchange transfusion. The possibility of transfusion reactions and the introduction of infection is always present.

Use of old (more than 4 days) or damaged (hemolyzed due to mechanical or thermal injury) RBCs may introduce a large potassium load into the patient. In small and unstable patients this can result in hyperkalemia and cardiac dysrhythmias terminating in cardiac arrest. In some infants hypernatremia occurs after an exchange transfusion. This is probably due to excessive sodium in the donor blood. An increased incidence of intracranial hemorrhage in infants undergoing exchange transfusions has been noted and could be due to hypernatremia. Alternatively, a reproducible decrease in ICP during the withdrawal of blood and an increase in ICP during infusion of blood has been noted; since cerebral blood flow is directly related to systemic arterial blood pressure in infants, these rapid, alternating changes may be etiologically related to the occurrence of intracranial hemorrhage.

There is an association between exchange transfusions and the development of necrotizing enterocolitis. When exchange transfusions are performed via the umbilical artery, the necrotizing enterocolitis may be caused by emboli to the mesenteric arteries or by decreases in arterial perfusion pressure to the gut with excessively large and/or rapid withdrawal of blood. When exchange transfusions are performed using the umbilical vein with the catheter tip in the portal venous system, the development of necrotizing enterocolitis may be caused by emboli or thrombosis and collapse of veins due to excessively large and/or rapid withdrawal of blood.

Aortic perforations and injuries may occur during an exchange transfusion. Exchange transfusion is a major undertaking, and these risks should be carefully considered in the decision to perform the procedure.

ADDITIONAL READING

Adamkin, D.H.: New uses for exchange transfusion, Pediatr. Clin. North Am. 24:599-604, 1977.

Aranda, J.V., and Sweet, A.Y.: Alterations in blood pressure during exchange transfusion, Arch. Dis. Child. 52:545-548, 1977.

Bada, H.S., Chua, C., Salmon, J.H., and Hajjar, W.: Changes in intracranial pressure during exchange transfusion, J. Pediatr. 94:129-132, 1979.

Berman, B., Krieger, A., and Naiman, J.L.: A new method for calculating volumes of blood required for partial exchange transfusion, J. Pediatr. 94:86-89, 1979.

Brunner, L.S., Suddarth, D.S., and Faries, B.B.: Jaundice in the newborn. In Brunner, L.S., and Suddarth, D.S., editors: The Lippincott manual of nursing practice, Philadelphia, 1974, J.B. Lippincott Co.

Campbell, N., and Stewart, I.: Exchange transfusion in ill newborn infants using peripheral arteries and veins, J. Pediatr. 94:820-822, 1979.

Doyle, P.E., Eidelman, A.I., Lee, K., and others: Exchange transfusion and hypernatremia: possible role in intracranial hemorrhage in very-low-birth-weight infants, J. Pediatr. 92:548-549, 1978.

Gregory, G.A., Hoffman, J.I.E., Kitterman, J.A., and others: House officers manual of neonatal intensive care, 1974, San Francisco, Section of Neonatology, University of California, pp. 71-75.

Hilliard, J., Schreiner, R.L., and Priest, J.: Hemoperitoneum associated with exchange transfusion through an umbilical arterial catheter, Am. J. Dis. Child. 133:216, 1979.

Malloy, M.H., and Nichols, M.M.: False abdominal aortic aneurysm: an unusual complication of umbilical arterial catheterization for exchange transfusion, J. Pediatr. 90:285-286, 1977.

108 Pericardiocentesis

LAWRENCE J. MILLS

INDICATIONS

Pericardiocentesis, or aspiration of the contents of the pericardium, is of considerable diagnostic and therapeutic value in conditions where an accumulation of pericardial fluid is likely. Proper technique is essential to minimize hazards. Echocardiography has greatly aided in the precise diagnosis of pericardial effusions and has replaced more invasive procedures (see Chapter 93). Pericardiocentesis is indicated for diagnosis when pericardial effusion is associated with signs of systemic infection, tuberculosis, or uremia or in instances where a clear cause, such as hypoparathyroidism or chronic congestive heart failure, does not exist.

Acute accumulation of pericardial fluid leads to impaired cardiac filling and tamponade. The most common causes are penetrating trauma, uremic pericarditis, acute purulent pericarditis, or bleeding immediately after open heart surgery. Relief of pericardial pressure may be an emergency and lifesaving procedure (see Chapter 54).

TECHNIQUE
Equipment

1. A 20-gauge needle, preferably with a metal hub (reusable spinal needle), 1½ inch for infants, 2 inches for children greater than 8 kg or obese.
2. A 19-gauge Intracath.
3. Cutdown tray.
4. Iodophor prep solution and sterile drapes.
5. Local anesthetic.
6. Several plastic syringes, 5 to 30 ml.

7. Sterile culture tubes and specimen tubes for cell count, glucose, and protein and a plain glass tube to observe clotting of bloody fluid.
8. A sterile alligator clip, which may be obtained from the cardiac catheterization laboratory.

Method

1. Check PT, PTT, and platelet count. Consult a thoracic surgeon if these are abnormal.
2. Place the patient in a supine position with approximately 10 to 15 degrees of reverse Trendelenburg position.
3. Attach the limb leads of an ECG machine and adjust for continuous display (oscilloscopic on paper).
4. Prepare a sterile field from the nipples to the umbilicus.
5. Inject local anesthetic just to the left of the midline at the level of the xiphoid cartilage.
6. Attach the spinal needle to a 5-ml syringe, and attach the alligator clip to the hub of the needle.
7. Attach the other end of the alligator clip to the V lead of the ECG machine.
8. Select the V position on the ECG machine for recording.
9. Insert the needle 45 degrees from the horizontal and 45 degrees to the left (toward the left midscapular region through a skin wheal) (Fig. 108-1).
10. Aspirate intermittently until fluid is obtained or an injury current is obtained on ECG.

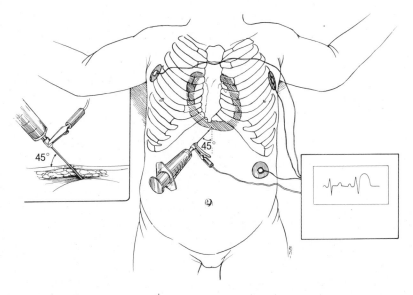

Fig. 108-1. Technique of pericardiocentesis. The needle is attached to the V lead of the ECG monitor and inserted beneath the xiphoid 45 degrees to horizontal and 45 degrees toward the left shoulder. The inset at right shows a typical injury current recorded from a needle in contact with the epicardium.

Interpretation of results

1. If no fluid is obtained, fluid is loculated, usually anteriorly.
   a. Consult a thoracic surgeon.
   b. Review the echocardiogram for precise location of fluid.
2. Bloody fluid is obtained.
   a. It does not clot in a glass tube.
      (1) If aspiration was performed for trauma, remove the needle and replace it with a 19-gauge Intracath for continuous aspiration through a three-way stopcock.
      (2) Consult a thoracic surgeon.
   b. It clots in a glass tube.
      (1) The sample is almost certainly intracardiac blood.
      (2) Remove the needle and observe carefully for development of tamponade.
         (a) Check systemic arterial blood pressure every 5 minutes, observing for paradoxical pulse.

      (b) Check CVP if available.
      (c) Obtain a chest roentgenogram initially and repeat again in 1 hour.
3. If serous or serosanguineous fluid is obtained, perform:
   a. Culture and Gram stain.
   b. Glucose, protein, and cell count.
   c. Tests appropriate for suspected diagnoses.

RISKS AND COMPLICATIONS

The major complications are failure to aspirate fluid when significant fluid is present and bleeding from ventricular puncture or laceration of a coronary vessel. Impaired coagulation may be present, especially in uremic patients or patients with sepsis, exacerbating bleeding problems. If intrapericardial bleeding is suspected after pericardiocentesis as indicated by development of hypotension, paradoxical pulse, and venous hypertension, a repeat aspiration with a catheter left in place is indicated. Unless the bleeding stops within a few minutes of reaspiration, surgical exploration should be rapidly performed.

All patients who have undergone pericardiocentesis should be monitored for a period of 4 to 6 hours. A full ECG should be obtained. An injury current pattern should not persist. Acute changes in ST segments can indicate coronary artery injury. Observation and frequent systemic arterial blood pressure determinations will detect those patients with continued accumulation of pericardial fluid.

109 Abdominal paracentesis

WILLIAM DAMMERT

INDICATIONS

Paracentesis is a procedure by which the abdominal cavity is entered percutaneously (1) to obtain diagnostic information for the differential diagnosis of ascites, peritonitis, and intraperitoneal hemorrhage, including culture or analysis of intraperitoneal fluid, or (2) to institute therapeutic measures such as dialysis (see Chapter 110), abdominal decompression to relieve respiratory compromise secondary to diminished diaphragmatic excursions from large amounts of gas or fluid in the abdomen, decompression of chylous ascites, and internal cooling.

There are no absolute contraindications to paracentesis; however, bleeding disorders, extensive disruption of the abdominal wall integrity (burns, widespread cutaneous infection), and marked distention of the bowel which predisposes the bowel to puncture and leakage because of elevated intraluminal pressure, require some planning before the procedure is initiated.

TECHNIQUE (see also Chapter 110)

1. Place the patient in a supine position with the head slightly raised; leg and arm restraints may be needed.
2. Prepare the area to be punctured with a standard antiseptic solution (e.g., povidone-iodine complex [Betadine], hexachlorophene [pHisoHex]).
3. Infiltrate the area chosen with 1% lidocaine.
4. Empty the bladder, using an in-and-out catheter technique.
5. Introduce a 20- or 22-gauge Intracath needle and catheter set perpendicular to the skin in either flank in line with the nipples and below or at the level of the umbilicus (or lower than the umbilicus in the midline if the bladder is empty) (see Fig. 110-1). Puncture through a scar or other points of possible fixation of bowel to the abdominal wall should be avoided.
6. Advance the set until the peritoneum is entered, withdraw the needle, and advance the catheter. During advancement, apply suction via a syringe.
7. Sample the contents of the abdomen, using sterile technique. Analysis of the specimen should include culture, Gram stain, TSP determination, and cell count with differential analysis. Chemical determinations, such as glucose or amylase, or cellular morphology may be desired as well. The volume of fluid withdrawn should be measured and recorded.
8. Do not manipulate the needle once it is inside the abdomen. If the tap is unsuccessful, withdraw the Intracath set and relocate.
9. Peritoneal lavage can be used to diagnose an intra-abdominal hemorrhage or other trauma. Insert a standard dialysis catheter instead of an Intracath, and infuse lactated Ringer's solution, 20 ml/kg. The fluid should then be withdrawn and analyzed for RBCs, WBCs, bile, amylase, and fecal material.
10. Apply a sterile dressing, and affix the catheter to the skin with 4-0 silk suture. Otherwise, withdraw the catheter and affix a ster-

609

ile dressing. If ascites is present, leakage of peritoneal fluid through the puncture site may occur.

RISKS AND COMPLICATIONS

Complications of paracentesis may be intraperitoneal or extraperitoneal.

Intraperitoneal

Intraperitoneal problems include:

1. Perforation of a hollow viscus; the lumen usually seals off quickly without leakage unless needle manipulation has produced a laceration or intraluminal pressure is increased.
2. Perforation of a blood vessel, which usually seals off quickly.
3. Introduction of contaminants (bacteria, chemicals, etc.), which is minimized by strict attention to aseptic technique.

Extraperitoneal

Extraperitoneal problems are usually confined to hematoma formation secondary to trauma of the deep epigastric vessels in the lateral aspect of the recti muscles; usually the rectus sheath can be avoided by proper needle placement.

If a large volume of fluid is suddenly removed from the abdominal cavity, profound fluid shifts in the intravascular and extracellular fluid compartments with resultant hypotension can occur. Cardiovascular variables (systemic arterial blood pressure, heart rate, peripheral perfusion, and level of consciousness) need to be monitored closely during and after the procedure.

ADDITIONAL READING

Drapanas, T., and McDonald, J.: Peritoneal tap in abdominal trauma, Surgery 100:22-26, 1960.

110 Acute peritoneal dialysis

RONALD J. HOGG

When body homeostasis is severely disturbed as a result of the accumulation of toxic quantities of endogenous or exogenous substances, an attempt should be made to increase the renal, metabolic, or intestinal clearance rates of these substances. If, however, such measures do not quickly correct the existing abnormalities or if there is evidence of increasing toxicity, it is necessary to employ maneuvers that provide alternative routes of excretion. The most efficient techniques currently available for this purpose are (1) sorbent hemoperfusion, or the passage of blood directly over an absorbing surface, which is a relatively new procedure that is proving to be extremely effective in removing exogenous poisons, (2) hemodialysis, a well-established technique that permits the simultaneous removal of toxins and restoration of normal body homeostasis in an efficient manner, and (3) peritoneal dialysis, a somewhat less efficient technique that continues to be extremely important in many disease states, particularly in infants and children.

INDICATIONS FOR DIALYSIS

Specific indications for hemoperfusion and hemodialysis are discussed below, but consideration is first given to the relative merits of peritoneal dialysis in the pediatric age group.

1. Peritoneal dialysis is much simpler to perform, can be instituted quickly, and does not require the sophisticated equipment that is necessary for hemodialysis.
2. The insertion of a peritoneal catheter is usually much easier than establishing vascular access in small children.
3. Rapid fluid and electrolyte shifts are rare in peritoneal dialysis, provided that extremely hypertonic solutions are not used continuously. In children undergoing acute hemodialysis, complications resulting from rapid fluid and electrolyte changes are quite common, particularly when the procedure is carried out by physicians who are inexperienced with this age group.
4. Peritoneal dialysis is more efficient in infants and children than it is in adults. This is because the relative size of the peritoneal membrane area in young children is two to three times as large as it is in adults (383 cm^2/kg in infants; 177 cm^2/kg in adults). Therefore, although hemodialysis remains more efficient than peritoneal dialysis in the pediatric age group, the difference in efficiency between the two procedures is much less than in adults.
5. If hemodialysis is considered to be the optimal therapy for a child who is cared for in a hospital that does not have immediate access to hemodialysis equipment, two problems may arise:
   a. It may be necessary to transfer the child to an adult facility that is serviced by physicians lacking expertise in pediatric intensive care.
   b. Such a move will involve further delay before dialysis can be instituted.

This final consideration is often of paramount importance because of the limited number of pediatric units that are able to offer acute hemodialysis or hemoperfusion. The majority of pediatric centers therefore have relied primarily on peritoneal dialysis in children with acute renal failure and acute exogenous poisoning.

611

However, to obtain significant peritoneal clearance of any substances, certain criteria must be met. The substance must possess (1) high water solubility, (2) low serum protein binding, and (3) efficient dialyzability.

There are certain situations in which sorbent hemoperfusion appears to be the only procedure that is able to achieve significant toxin removal. This occurs in cases of exogenous poisoning with substances that are lipid soluble and/or show high protein binding. Peritoneal dialysis is generally not useful in such cases, nor is it the preferred treatment when endogenous toxin accumulation occurs at a rate that is greater than the peritoneal clearance rate. Such a situation may be seen when acute renal failure is superimposed on a severe crush injury, since in this situation there will be rapid tissue breakdown and peritoneal dialysis may not remove the endogenous toxins quickly enough. With these reservations in mind it can be stated that the following situations may be successfully treated with peritoneal dialysis:

1. Acute renal failure. Specific indications are given below.
2. Acute exogenous poisonings with certain compounds, as listed in Table 66-4.
3. Salt intoxication.
4. Congenital lactic acidosis.
5. Other rare inborn errors of metabolism, including those that lead to excessive accumulation of organic acids, particularly in young infants (e.g., maple syrup urine disease).
6. Severe hyperbilirubinemia, usually in older infants and children with inborn errors of bilirubin clearance. Peritoneal clearance of bilirubin is poor because of the high plasma protein binding of bilirubin. Attempts to improve this clearance rate by addition of albumin to the dialysate have only effected a small improvement.
7. Reye's syndrome. The use of peritoneal dialysis in this disorder is controversial, al-

though there is certainly efficient peritoneal clearance of ammonia. Acute hepatic failure from other causes is also regarded as an indication for peritoneal dialysis by some authorities.

8. Ornithine transcarbamylase deficiency and other disorders of the urea cycle that lead to hyperammonemia.
9. Hydrops fetalis. Peritoneal dialysis has been used successfully in the treatment of a number of infants with severe hydrops fetalis in order to remove excess fluid.
10. Hyperuricemia. A high level of uric acid may complicate the clinical course in children with leukemia or malignant lymphoma, particularly when appropriate prophylactic measures are not taken at the time remission is induced. If urate nephropathy develops, peritoneal dialysis may be used to reduce the serum uric acid levels. The peritoneal clearance is most efficient at uric acid levels greater than 20 mg/dl, and peritoneal dialysis should not be used when lower levels are present. Improved clearance of uric acid has been achieved by increasing the alkalinity of the dialysis fluid, a procedure that causes trapping of urate ions in the dialysis fluid.

INDICATIONS FOR PERITONEAL DIALYSIS
Acute renal failure

Acute renal failure is by far the most common indication for peritoneal dialysis in children. The specific indications for dialysis in such cases may be considered under three categories.

Prophylactic indications. When acute renal failure develops in circumstances where experience has shown early dialysis to be beneficial, dialysis should be started before significant derangements of clinical or biochemical variables occur. This approach is appropriate in acute renal failure associated with (1) crush injuries, (2) exertional rhabdomyolysis, and (3) poor myocardial reserve, as in the acute renal failure seen after cardiac surgery.

Clinical indications. Clinical deterioration provides the most common indication for dialysis in acute renal failure. The clinical abnormalities are often associated with worsening of biochemical or hemodynamic variables, but there are some cases in which the overall clinical picture is much worse than would be expected from the laboratory data. This appears to occur in a number of patients with hemolytic-uremic syndrome. Specific clinical abnormalities that indicate the need for dialysis are:
1. Deteriorating neurologic state in the absence of medically correctable abnormalities
2. Volume overload and/or hypertension leading to congestive cardiac failure, pulmonary edema, and/or hypertensive encephalopathy
3. Gastrointestinal bleeding resulting from uremic platelet dysfunction
4. Metastatic calcification resulting from a high calcium-phosphate product that is unresponsive to medical therapy

Biochemical indications. Although it is customary to list absolute serum levels of urea, creatinine, potassium, bicarbonate, etc. as the prime indicators of the need for dialysis, biochemical determinants should remain secondary to clinical indications in terms of importance, and dialysis should not be postponed just because the patient has not satisfied certain set biochemical criteria. Medical measures are often successful in controlling the serum levels of the presently measurable endogenous toxins that accumulate in acute renal failure. Laboratory values do, however, provide a guideline before the patient shows significant clinical deterioration. The need for dialysis should be considered imminent when the following values are obtained:
1. BUN, 125 to 150 mg/dl.
2. Serum K $\geq$6.5 mEq/L despite ion exchange therapy.

3. Persistent metabolic acidosis ($HCO_3 < 12$ mEq/L), particularly in the presence of volume overload, a situation that restricts the amount of sodium bicarbonate that can be administered.
4. Severe metabolic alkalosis ($HCO_3 > 35$ mEq/L, pH >7.6), an unusual situation but one that may be managed by peritoneal dialysis using a high chloride (120 mEq/L), low acetate (20 mEq/L) dialysis fluid.
5. Serum uric acid >20 mg/dl.
6. Serum Na >160 mEq/L.
7. Serum Ca >12 mg/dl.

Acute poisonings

The role of dialysis has diminished in most cases of drug intoxication because improvements in intensive supportive care have enabled patients to be managed conservatively until the offending drugs have been metabolized or excreted. Dialysis remains the treatment of choice in patients with severely compromised renal function in whom the toxic agent is usually cleared by the kidney (see Chapter 66).

TECHNIQUE
Preparation

See also Chapter 109.
1. If time permits, patients who are conscious should be sedated while preparations for the procedure are in progress. This can be accomplished with meperidine (Demerol), 1 mg/kg, and promethazine (Phenergan), 0.5 mg/kg IM. This will improve the patient's tolerance of the procedure and make the insertion of the catheter easier for both patient and pediatrician. Additional sedation during the dialysis procedure is usually unnecessary except in very restless patients.
2. Empty the bladder, by catheterization if necessary, and weigh the patient. The patient should be placed in the supine position, and measures should be taken to immobilize the arms and legs when necessary.

3. Prepare the abdomen. Use sterile technique.
4. Initial fluid instillation is optional. The chosen puncture site is infiltrated with 1% lidocaine (Xylocaine) (skin and subcutaneous tissues). Optimal puncture sites (Fig. 110-1, *A*) are in the midline 2 to 3 cm below the umbilicus (*a*) or lateral to the rectus muscle in the left lower quadrant (*b*). Puncture the skin and muscle and inject dialysis fluid, 10 ml/kg, (warmed to 37° C) through a 14-gauge needle. This maneuver distends the abdomen and makes the subsequent catheter insertion easier. If the patient's abdomen is distended with ascitic fluid, the initial fluid instillation is not performed.
5. Skin incision. A stab wound (approximately 5 mm long and 1 cm deep) is made with a #11 blade. Do not make a larger incision, since this may later give problems with regard to leaking of dialysis fluid.

Catheter insertion

Pediatric and adult sizes of multipuncture catheters are available (Fig. 110-1, *inset*). The catheter is inserted, with the stylet intact, into the peritoneal cavity. This is achieved by the operator pushing the catheter and stylet through the abdominal wall into the peritoneal cavity with the catheter held perpendicular to the abdominal wall (Fig. 110-1, *B*). Considerable force is often needed, especially in larger children, and this usually alarms a physician who is performing his or her first catheter insertion. Fear of perforation of a viscus results in one of the most common early problems encountered in peritoneal dialysis, namely, failure to reach the peritoneal cavity, a situation that results in the catheter lying in a preperitoneal position. When the catheter is being pushed into the peritoneal cavity, it is usually helpful to use a twisting motion. Successful entry into the peritoneal cavity is evidenced by a sudden decrease in resistance, often associated with a rapid rush of peritoneal fluid up

and around the catheter and stylet. The stylet is then removed (Fig. 110-1, *C*), and the catheter is "threaded" into the left pelvic gutter (Fig. 110-1, *D*). The catheter should be sutured to the skin at the puncture point. It is cut to an appropriate length and attached to the dialysis administration set (Fig. 110-1, *E*). A sterile dressing is then applied around the catheter insertion site and firmly secured.

The introduction of pediatric-sized catheters has been of considerable help. These catheters have the same internal diameter as the adult size, but the drainage holes are limited to the distal 4.2 cm. In the standard adult catheters the holes extend for 8.4 cm from the tip of the catheter. The peritoneal cavity of small children and infants may not be able to accommodate all the holes in such catheters.

The choice of catheter size is important because all the holes must be inside the peritoneal cavity to prevent problems with leakage, infection, and inaccurate recording of dialysis fluid volume.

Dialysis fluid infusion

1. Before infusion, dialysate should be warmed to body temperature by an infrared lamp or by prewarming the bottles in a warm water bath.
2. Initial runs should consist of 20 to 30 ml/kg. During the first few cycles the dialysis fluid should be allowed to drain out within a few minutes of being introduced, in order to determine catheter patency and to check for bleeding. The volume is then progressively increased until runs of 50 to 100 ml/kg, as tolerated, are achieved (maximum 2 L).
3. Add the following to the dialysis fluid when appropriate:
   a. Heparin: 500 units/L of dialysate until the returns are clear of blood
   b. Potassium chloride: none until serum K is less than 4 mEq/L; then add 4 mEq/L to the dialysate. Particular attention should be paid to the serum K if the patient is

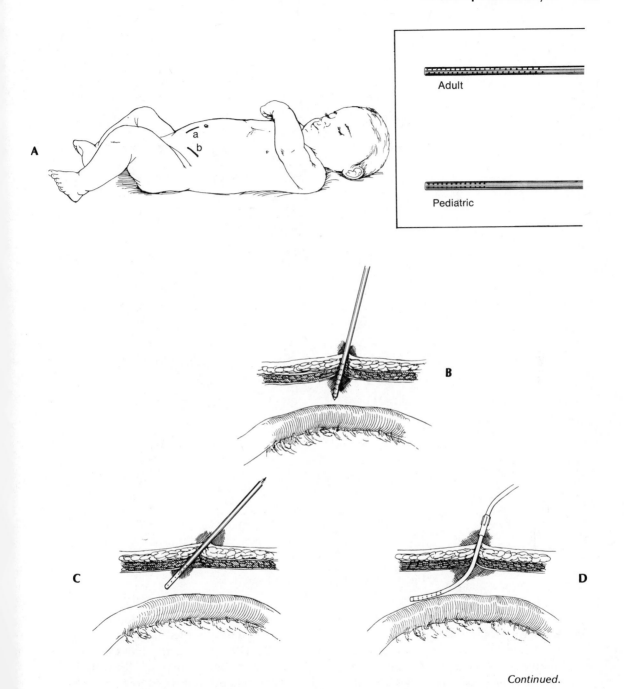

Adult

Pediatric

A

B

C

D

Continued.

Fig. 110-1. *Inset,* Choice of peritoneal catheter: comparison of lengths of distal perforated portion. **A,** Optimal sites for peritoneal catheter insertion. **B,** Insertion of catheter and stylet into the peritoneal cavity. **C,** Removal of stylet. **D,** Peritoneal catheter in situ. **E,** Peritoneal dialysis in progress.

E

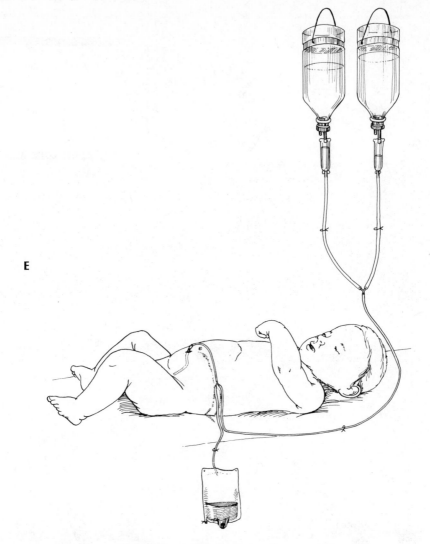

Fig. 110-1, cont'd. For legend see p. 615.

digitalized. Prolonged dialysis with K-deficient fluid may induce digitalis toxicity if the serum K level falls too low.

c. Antibiotics: none in the absence of peritonitis. If peritoneal infection is diagnosed, appropriate antibiotics should be added to the dialysate after a specimen of fluid has been sent for culture (see Risks and complications, p. 720).

4. The composition of the dialysis fluid that should be used in an individual patient depends on the disorder that is to be corrected. Table 110-1 depicts the types of situations that might be encountered, the dialysis fluid that would be most appropriate in each case, and the potential problems that may occur.

5. When the appropriate volume of dialysis

Table 110-1. Suitable dialysis fluid for specific clinical disorders

Clinical disorder	Principal objectives of dialysis	Dialysis fluid recommended
1. Acute renal failure a. Without volume overload	Removal of uremic toxins Restoration of biochemical status toward normal	1.5% standard dialysis solutions* (containing dextrose, 1.5 g/dl) (osmolality = 340-360 mOsm/kg)
b. With volume overload	Fluid depletion	4.25% dialysis solution NOTE: In 4.25% solutions, the Na should not exceed 132 mEq/L (osmolality = 480-500 mOsm/kg)
2. Severe congestive cardiac failure (e.g., hydrops fetalis)	Fluid depletion	As in 1b
3. Salt intoxication	Removal of excess sodium chloride from the body and restoration of serum Na to normal	Dextrose in water, 8 g/dl (water that is removed by osmosis should be replaced IV)
4. Lactic acidosis a. With normal acetate metabolism	Removal of lactate, correction of acidosis	Standard 1.5% dialysate containing acetate
b. With abnormal acetate metabolism	Removal of lactate, correction of acidosis	Use sodium bicarbonate (40 mEq/L dialysate) as base; add just before fluid is instilled; maintain serum Ca with IV calcium gluconate
5. Removal of highly protein-bound compounds (salicylates, barbiturates, bilirubin)	Removal of toxic compound	Addition of albumin (4 g/dl dialysate) to standard dialysis solution will increase clearance rates to variable extent
6. Metabolic alkalosis with renal insufficiency	Restoration of normal acid-base balance	High chloride, low acetate dialysis fluid

*Standard solutions should contain: Na, 130-135 mEq/L; K, none; Cl, 95-105 mEq/L; Ca, 3.5 mEq/L; Mg, 1.5 mEq/L; pH, 5.1; lactate or acetate, 35 mEq/L; dextrose, 1.5 g/dl.

fluid has been determined, the following sequence should be instituted.
a. Run the fluid in as rapidly as the patient can tolerate.
b. Allow an equilibration time of 30 minutes (dwell time).
c. Allow the fluid to run out rapidly. The entire cycle should last no more than 1 hour. Initial runs may produce a positive fluid balance for the patient in terms of the volume of dialysis fluid recovered as compared with the amount run in. This

situation is acceptable initially but should not continue after the first few runs, since by this time a sufficient reservoir will have been established in the peritoneal cavity.

Recording and monitoring

1. Maintain an accurate record of the exchange volumes and the start and finish times of each run. This can best be accomplished with a standard flow sheet such as the one shown in Fig. 110-2.

Cycle number	Dialysis fluid composition	Medication added to fluid	Time inflow complete	Time outflow started	Peritoneal contact time	Fluid volume run-in	Fluid volume drained	Single cycle balance	Cumulative fluid balance	Additional comments

Date:

Fig. 110-2. Peritoneal dialysis flow sheet.

2. Routine monitoring should include:
   a. Pulse, respiratory rate, and systemic arterial blood pressure every hour.
   b. Temperature every 6 hours.
   c. Body weight every 12 hours.
   d. Serum Na, K, Cl, HCO_3, Ca, BUN, glucose, Hb, and Hct every 12 hours (or more often if necessary). Serum Cr and PO_4 every 24 hours.
   e. Send a specimen of dialysate for culture daily or if peritonitis is suspected (see Risks and complications below for signs of peritonitis).
   f. ECG (continuously) for postoperative cardiac patients or those receiving digitalis.

Factors that improve peritoneal dialysis efficiency

1. Increased dialysate volume may be achieved by increasing the volume of each run and/or increasing the frequency of the cycle (reducing dwell times).
2. A good dialysate flow rate reduces the drainage time, which in turn increases the amount of time that the peritoneal cavity is filled with dialysis fluid. Good flow depends on good catheter placement.
3. If the dialysis-fluid temperature is maintained at 37° C (by infrared lamps, heater coils, and preimmersion of sealed bottles in warm water), urea clearance may be increased by 30% as compared with dialysis fluid at room temperature.
4. Use of hyperosmotic solutions (dialysis fluid containing 4.25% dextrose) is indicated when rapid fluid removal is important. The use of this solution is also associated with increased solute clearances, particularly of urea, sodium, and creatinine. This occurs as a result of solvent drag and increased peritoneal mem-

brane permeability. Increased solute clearance without rapid water removal can be achieved by incorporating runs of hypertonic dialysis fluid between cycles using 1.5% dialysis solution.

5. Certain vasodilating agents and diuretics (e.g., furosemide and ethacrynic acid) have also been shown to improve solute clearance rates, but experience with these agents in clinical circumstances is limited and they are not recommended for routine clinical use at this time.

Factors that reduce peritoneal dialysis efficiency

1. Systemic diseases affecting the peripheral vasculature (e.g., systemic lupus erythematosus, diabetes mellitus) reduce the plasma solute clearance achieved by peritoneal dialysis.

2. Systemic hypotension and shock reduce the splanchnic blood flow, but experimental data in dogs suggest that the plasma clearance rates of solutes across the peritoneal membranes are not greatly affected by such disturbances.

RISKS AND COMPLICATIONS

In pediatric patients the most common complication is peritoneal infection. The incidence of peritonitis has been reported to be as high as 68% in children less than 2 years of age and 30% in older children. It is recommended that the following precautions be taken to reduce the incidence of peritoneal infections:

1. Use strict aseptic technique during catheter insertion.

2. Ensure that the perforated portion of the catheter is entirely within the peritoneal cavity.

3. Place sterile dressings over the catheter to prevent introduction of infection by the patient.

4. Remove peritoneal catheters after 48 hours.

5. Avoid using prostheses that keep access to the peritoneal cavity open between dialyses.

6. Avoid using prophylactic antibiotics, a practice that increases the potential for *Candida* peritonitis.

7. Maintain the drainage receptacle below the level of the peritoneum to avoid backflow of dialysate.

8. Obtain cultures and Gram stains of the dialysis fluid returns every 24 hours and whenever there are clinical findings that might be attributable to early peritoneal infection (e.g., pain, cloudy returns, fever).

9. Ensure that fecal material is not allowed to contaminate the patient's bed.

10. Use automated, closed dialysate delivery systems when available. These systems are capable of delivering preset volumes of dialysate to the patient for variable dwell periods. Hopefully the recent development of pediatric-sized delivery systems will result in a reduced incidence of peritonitis in patients treated by peritoneal dialysis.

11. Soft Silastic dialysis catheters (Tenckhoff catheters) may be used in children with acute renal failure who are probable candidates for multiple peritoneal dialysis procedures. Placement of such catheters usually requires general anesthesia, but once inserted they may be left in place for prolonged periods, enabling repeated dialysis procedures to be performed without repeated catheter placements.

Minor and major problems that may complicate peritoneal dialysis are listed in Table 110-2 to enable the reader to troubleshoot when problems arise. Table 110-3 lists the antibiotic treatment for those patients who develop peritonitis.

There are few absolute contraindications to peritoneal dialysis. As stated earlier, there are some situations in which the relative inefficiency of peritoneal solute transfer results in hemodialysis or hemoperfusion being the preferred

Table 110-2. Complications of peritoneal dialysis

Problems	Causes	Preventive measures	Management
Technical			
1. Complications arising from catheter insertion (other than transient bleeding, an occurrence that is rarely significant)	a. Perforation of bladder	Empty bladder before insertion; use bladder catheter if necessary	Supportive measures and/or surgical repair
	b. Perforation of other viscera or blood vessels	Instill dialysis fluid, 10-20 ml/kg, into the peritoneal cavity through a large-bore needle before catheter insertion unless the abdomen is already distended by ascitic fluid	Surgical repair
2. Leakage of dialysate	a. Part of the perforated tip of the catheter may be preperitoneal	Use a catheter that is the appropriate size for the patient; when inserting the catheter, make sure that all holes are within the peritoneal cavity	If recognized while sterile conditions prevail, insert the catheter deeper or use a smaller catheter as indicated
	b. Large stab wound inadequately sutured	Stab wound should admit catheter with a snug fit; if it has been made too large, a purse-string suture should be used	Purse-string suture
	c. Overdistended abdomen	Do not exceed 100 ml of dialysis fluid per kg; reduce appropriately if organomegaly is present	Reduce dialysis fluid volumes; may achieve same clearance with small volumes and short dwell times
3. Inadequate dialysate flow rate	a. Preperitoneal catheter position	Make sure that catheter is in peritoneum and ensure a rapid drainage flow initially	Insert catheter deeper (as in 2a)
	b. Catheter blockage by fibrin, omentum, or an air-block	Add heparin to the initial runs; make sure that the catheter tip is in the pelvis; make sure that all catheter holes are within the peritoneum	Irrigate catheter with heparinized saline solution; withdraw catheter slightly; if these measures fail, replace catheter
	c. Inadequate reservoir of dialysate in the peritoneal cavity	Do not expect to recover all dialysate volume in early runs; stop drainage of early runs when flow becomes intermittent; allow a positive balance up to 10-20 ml/kg	Build up a reservoir of 10-20 ml/kg
	d. Fluid loculation within the peritoneal cavity		Reposition patient

Complication	Cause	Management	
4. Abdominal pain associated with the dialysis runs (note that diaphragmatic pain may be referred to the shoulder tip)	a. Catheter placement against a viscus; usually the pain is mainly associated with inflow	Reposition catheter if initial infusion of dialysate causes severe pain	Withdraw catheter slightly
	b. Cold dialysate	Warm dialysis fluid to 37° C	Warm dialysis fluid to 37° C
	c. Hyperosmotic dialysis solution; peritoneal inflammation	Use hyperosmotic fluid intermittently	Reduce number of runs of hyperosmotic fluid
	d. Dialysate flow too rapid	Increase rate of dialysate flow gradually when starting dialysis	Reduce rate of flow; then increase gradually as tolerated by patient
	e. Overdistention of peritoneal cavity as a result of excess dialysate volumes	Commence with 20-30 ml/kg; observe carefully as dialysis volume is increased	Reduce dialysis volume
	f. Peritoneal infection	See p. 720	Antibiotics as indicated (Table 110-3)
	g. Undetermined; anxiety ± lowered pain threshold	Allay anxiety as much as possible; sedate if very anxious	Sedation, analgesics; local treatment with infusion of 1-5 ml 1% lidocaine (Xylocaine) may be useful in some cases; should only be given when other causes of pain have been excluded
5. Cardiopulmonary embarrassment	a. Basilar atelectasis b. Pneumonia c. Pleural effusion d. Restriction of respiratory excursion by distended abdomen	Use small dialysate volumes and short dwell times when cardiopulmonary problems exist	Revert to smaller dialysate volumes; respiratory therapy; antibiotics rarely necessary

Continued.

Table 110-2. Complications of peritoneal dialysis—cont'd

Problems	Causes	Preventive measures	Management
Abnormalities in plasma composition that may complicate peritoneal dialysis			
1. Hypokalemia	Continued use of K-free dialysate after serum K has returned to normal	Add potassium chloride to dialysis fluid (4 mEq/L) when serum K is less than 4 mEq/L	Measures other than this preventive measure usually unnecessary; exception may occur when hypokalemia develops in patient taking digoxin, when it may be necessary to add oral or parenteral potassium chloride
2. Hypernatremia	Usually a complication of prolonged use of hyperosmotic dialysate (particularly those solutions with $[Na^+] \geq 140$ mEq/L)	Avoid 7% dialysis solution except in salt poisoning; avoid 4.25% dialysis solutions containing $[Na] \geq 140$ mEq/L, i.e., should be 120-132 mEq/L; replace free water when 4.25% dialysis fluid is used for prolonged period	Replace free water if patient is volume depleted (almost always the case); reduce [Na] in dialysate; use 1.5% dialysate if possible
3. Hyperglycemia	a. Prolonged use of hyperosmotic solutions b. Dialysis in diabetic patients	a. Avoid prolonged use of hyperosmotic solutions b. Additional insulin may be required in diabetics	Discontinue hyperosmotic solutions if possible; avoid insulin if hyperglycemia results from use of 4.25% dialysate to relieve volume overload; insulin may potentiate cellular edema in such cases
4. Metabolic alkalosis	High sodium bicarbonate levels resulting from metabolic conversion of acetate or lactate in absence of renal mechanism for bicarbonate excretion; usually associated with hypernatremia and dehydration following use of 4.25% dialysate	Avoid unnecessary and prolonged use of hyperosmotic solutions; avoid 4.25% dialysate containing $[Na^+]$ greater than 132 mEq/L	Active treatment usually unnecessary; if severe, hyperchloremic dialysate can be used
5. Hypoproteinemia	Prolonged peritoneal dialysis	Maintain protein intake of 1-2 g/kg/day	Increase protein intake

Table 110-3. Antimicrobial therapy for peritonitis in children on peritoneal dialysis*

Antimicrobial	Systemic loading dose	Dialysis fluid concentrations
Bacterial peritonitis		
Ampicillin	50 mg/kg	25-50 mg/L
Carbenicillin	100 mg/kg	50-100 mg/L
Cephalothin	20 mg/kg	25-50 mg/L
Gentamicin	2.5 mg/kg	5-10 mg/L
Kanamycin	7.5 mg/kg	10-20 mg/L
Penicillin	50,000 units/kg	50,000 units/L
Candida peritonitis (isolated reports of successful treatment)		
Amphotericin B	None	1 mg/L instilled for 2 hours twice a day for 10 days
	None	5 mg/L given with each cycle of dialysis
5-Fluorocytosine	None	100 mg given intraperitoneally as single dose before catheter removal

*The doses recommended are intended to be used as guidelines. There is no substitute for serial serum concentration measurements.

treatment. Certain intra-abdominal lesions represent relative contraindications to peritoneal dialysis and often necessitate surgical insertion of the catheter. These include intestinal adhesions, recent abdominal surgery or major trauma, bowel distention, colostomy, significant organomegaly, and undiagnosed abdominal disease. Care should also be taken to ensure that the patient's coagulation status is normal before insertion of the catheter. If abnormalities of the clotting studies are found, as in some cases of renal failure after cardiac surgery, appropriate measures should be taken to correct the abnormalities before placement of the catheter.

ADDITIONAL READING

Anand, S.K., Northway, J.D., and Gresham, E.L.: Peritoneal dialysis catheter for small infants, J. Pediatr. **86**:985, 1975.

Bortolussi, R.A., MacDonald, M.R.A., Bannatyne, R.M., and Arbus, G.S.: Treatment of candida peritonitis by peritoneal lavage with amphotericin B, J. Pediatr. **87:**987, 1975.

Day, R.E., and White, R.H.R.: Peritoneal dialysis in children, Arch. Dis. Child. **52:**56-61, 1977.

Esperanca, M.J., and Collins, D.L.: Peritoneal dialysis efficiency in relation to body weight, J. Pediatr. Surg. **1:**162-169, 1966.

Goldschmidt, Z.H., Pote, H.H., Katz, M.A., and Shear, L.: Effect of dialysate volume on peritoneal dialysis kinetics, Kidney Int. **5:**240-245, 1974.

Siegel, N.J., and Brown, R.S.: Peritoneal clearance of ammonia and creatinine in a neonate, J. Pediatr. **82:**1044-1046, 1973.

Vidt, D.G.: Recommendations on choice of peritoneal dialysis solutions, Ann. Intern. Med. **78:**144-146, 1973.

Winchester, J.F., Gelfand, M.C., Knepshield, J.H., and Schreiner, G.E.: Dialysis and hemoperfusion of poisons and drugs—update, Trans. Am. Soc. Artif. Intern. Organs **23:**762-808, 1977.

111 Total parenteral nutrition

CHARLES E. MIZE
BETSY COHEN TEITELL

INDICATIONS

The primary purpose of complete intravenous or total parenteral nutrition (TPN) is major augmentation of caloric support and access to positive nitrogen balance in patients not capable of receiving sufficient nutrient support by enteral means alone. It is also possible concomitantly to control a patient's vitamin and mineral metabolism during caloric and nitrogen supplementation. The specific goals of TPN thus encompass maintenance of positive nitrogen balance and homeostatic control of fluid, electrolyte, and metabolic function. Clinical indications of positive nitrogen balance will include wound healing, nonfluid weight gain, and progressive brain growth.

Any PICU patient may be considered for TPN if his feeding mechanisms and/or gastrointestinal tract are not capable of supporting adequate nutrition for metabolic maintenance, growth, and tissue repair. In surgical conditions expected to create difficulties for nutritional intake, TPN can be initiated presurgically and continued from the immediate postoperative period for any length of time necessary. An anticipated duration of 10 to 30 days for TPN is not unusual for situations requiring its use; shorter times may be considered, although time-effectiveness may not be best served with only brief use.

TPN requires maximal cooperation from the separate supporting services necessary to provide the successful technology for TPN. The ultimate success of TPN requires interactive decisions and prearranged commitment from these services: pharmacy, central supply, infection control, metabolic, nutrition support, surgical, nursing.

EQUIPMENT AND TECHNIQUE
Types of parenteral nutrition: site

Two types of TPN, central and peripheral, based on the physical site of the infusate tubing (peripheral or central), are recognized. TPN metabolic monitoring and choice of nitrogen source can be identical for both types, but they are separated here by virtue of (1) potential restriction on maximal infusate glucose concentration in peripheral-catheter TPN and (2) the complications and risks of the two types.

Central-catheter TPN. Central-catheter TPN refers to nutrient infusion after placement of an indwelling catheter in one of the large veins entering the heart. This is performed by the surgical service, generally with subcutaneous tunneling of the catheter from the large vein entry site to the chest wall, where daily care of the exit site can be expedited.

A high concentration of infused glucose can be achieved, generally 20 to 30 g/dl. Higher concentrations (up to 45 g/dl) can be employed for selective regimens, during which lower fluid volume infusion is coupled with these concentrations of glucose. Depending on the patient's endogenous regulation of carbohydrate utilization, the addition of supplemental insulin to the infusate can be considered without interfering with metabolic control and monitoring variables. Intravenous lipid may be utilized in central-catheter or peripheral-catheter infusions simultaneously with glucose infusions, unless contraindications for lipid infusion exist.

Peripheral-catheter TPN. Peripheral-catheter TPN involves infusion after placement of a simple infusion needle or infusion catheter in a peripheral vein, generally of the scalp or extremities. A peripheral vein cutdown infusion site may also be used for peripheral-catheter TPN.

Preservation of the integrity of the peripheral veins generally limits the infused glucose concentration to 10 to 12 g/dl. The source of nonprotein calories, however, can be both glucose and IV lipid (lipid range of 1 to 3 g/kg/24 hr). For short periods with a well-placed catheter, higher glucose concentrations may be used with concomitant lipid infusion.

Types of parenteral nutrition: content

Protein, glucose, minerals, vitamins. Parenteral nitrogen sources are available in the form of protein hydrolysates or as crystalline amino acid solutions (complete or essential amino acids only). Glucose is presently used almost exclusively as the carbohydrate source for TPN. Major, and some minor, minerals are available parenterally in the form of aqueous salt solutions of the respective ions. A multivitamin source (e.g., MVI-Pediatric) can supply a combination of water- and lipid-soluble vitamins, although not all vitamins desired are presently available in a single preparation. Biotin is also available parenterally as part of a multiple-vitamin solution (Berocca-C). Folate, vitamin B_{12}, and vitamin K will be required as separate supplements if these are not compatible with the chosen parenteral multiple-vitamin infusion mixture. Iron can be given enterally or parenterally.

Heparin. Heparin can be used directly in TPN solutions. A final concentration of 1 to 3 units heparin/ml may aid in preventing catheter clotting and will normally not affect hemostatic mechanisms.

Table 111-1. Essential fatty acid caloric yield from IV lipid (10%)

Lipid	Total calories/dl	EFA calories/dl
Intralipid	110	57
Liposyn	110	68

Lipid. Parenteral lipid is available as an emulsion of triglyceride with carrier phospholipid (Intralipid, Liposyn). It may be used as a separate daily source of calories, or on an intermittent basis to meet essential fatty acid (EFA) requirements to provide at least 4% of total daily calories (as EFA specifically) over the desired interval (see Table 111-1). These lipid preparations provide polyunsaturated fatty acid for peripheral tissues after endogenous hydrolysis by lipoprotein lipase.

Water. The water of oxidation of infused substrate in pediatric patients should be considered when net water balance is of critical importance (see Table 111-2). With successful tissue utilization and complete oxidation of substrate, net water is formed. In central TPN the generally larger amount of glucose infused, compared to the amounts of lipid infused, focuses attention clinically on the calculated grams of glucose received (Table 111-2). Under conditions in which glucose is provided in excess of oxidative energy needs, however, and the extra glucose is converted to fat rather than to carbon dioxide and water, the net water is considerably less.

Carbon dioxide. Similarly, net carbon dioxide is formed by the complete oxidation of glucose and fatty acid (see Table 111-2). With respiratory conditions in which retention of carbon dioxide is a significant clinical problem, the addition of large amounts of glucose to the parenteral regimen may worsen the carbon dioxide retention. For an equivalent caloric input in these cases, fewer grams of carbohydrate relative to lipid can be infused to reduce the carbon dioxide of oxidation and hence reduce the carbon dioxide respiratory burden.

Table 111-2. Substrate oxidation yields

Substrate	mmol CO_2 per g substrate	g water per g substrate
$C_6H_{12}O_6 + 6\,O_2 \rightarrow 6\,CO_2 + 6\,H_2O$ (glucose)	33.3	0.60
$9\,C_6H_{12}O_6 + 54\,NAD + 46\,NADPH \rightarrow \; 2\,C_{18}H_{36}O_2 + 18\,CO_2 + 14\,H_2O +$ (glucose) (stearic acid) $54\,NADH + 46\,NADP$	11.1	0.16
$C_{57}H_{104}O_6 + 80\,O_2 \rightarrow 57\,CO_2 + 52\,H_2O$ (triolein)	64.5	1.06

Procedure

Notify the pharmacy for activation of a sterile hood unit (class 100 laminar flow). Using aseptic technique, the pharmacy should prepare all solutions for TPN and can attach basic infusion tubing and appropriate filter(s) for the solutions. Key details include:

1. A bacterial filter (0.22 μ) is placed into the infusion tubing.
2. Bacterial filters are changed when infusion sets are changed.
3. Once the solution leaves the pharmacy, addition of other parenteral materials to the TPN infusion must be avoided. This specifically excludes blood or blood products and antibiotics.
4. If a central catheter is to be used as venous access for other infusions, scrupulously *avoid* infusion of blood products or antibiotics simultaneously with the TPN solution or until the TPN solution has been adequately flushed out of the infusion catheter. For resumption of TPN, similarly flush out completely the other solutions.
5. Use constant infusion pumps that are appropriate for the coupled infusion tubing sets prepared by the pharmacy, central supply, or nursing services.
6. The surgical service will perform central catheter placement under sterile conditions, generally in the operating suite.
7. Percutaneous subclavian line placement should be done under strict aseptic conditions; remember to mask all personnel, including the patient.
8. Peripheral-catheter sites and needle or catheter placements may be managed in the PICU by the surgical, medical, or nursing services.
9. Maintenance of central catheter insertion sites must include sterile dressing changes, with appropriate local antiseptic care (e.g., Betadine or Hibiclens), by the PICU surgical and medical staffs at 2-day intervals.
10. Defined-interval local care of peripheral catheter sites must be performed frequently to avoid infiltration and vascular inflammation (at least hourly).
11. With central catheters, a chest roentgenogram must be obtained initially and at regular intervals to verify catheter tip location.
12. TPN solutions, filters, and all tubing should be changed every day.
    a. With central catheters, make certain to remove all air from new tubing before connecting it to the patient, since the catheter tip is generally in the superior vena cava or right atrium.
    b. Cleanse all connection sites with povidone-iodine (Betadine) solution, dry with sterile 2 × 2 gauze pads, and wrap connection with adhesive to secure junctions.

Order initial and subsequent daily infusates through the pharmacy, using either stock solutions (Table 111-3) or order forms that allow for

Table 111-3. Suggested guidelines for stock TPN solutions for pediatric patients

Item (concentration)	Starter strength (ml)	Full strength (ml)
Amino acid (10%)	85	140
50% glucose	125	220
NaCl (2.5 mEq/ml)	5	5
KPO_4 (4.4 mEq K; 5.4 mEq P_i/ml)	1	1.5
KCl (2 mEq/ml)	3	2
Ca gluconate (0.45 mEq/ml)	9	13
$MgSO_4$ (4 mEq/ml)	2	2
MVI-Pediatric	10	10
Sterile water	259	106
$ZnCl_2$ (1 mg/ml)	0.5	0.5
$CuCl_2$ (0.4 mg/ml)	0.2	0.2
$CrCl_3$ (4 μgm/ml)	0.2	0.2
$MnCl_2$ (0.1 mg/ml)	0.1	0.1
TOTAL	500	500.5
Nonprotein calories* (kcal/ml)		0.75
Total calories (kcal/ml)		0.86
Glucose concentration (g/dl)	12.5	22.0
Protein concentration (g/dl)	1.7	2.8

*Glucose monohydrate = 3.4 cal/g; amino acid mixture = 4 cal/g.

detailed formulation of individual needs on a daily basis (Fig. 111-1). The initial infusion begins with adequate daily fluid and electrolyte needs (see Chapter 16) but contains less than the optimal calorie and nitrogen input, e.g., 60 to 80 calories/kg/24 hr and 1.5-2.5 g amino acids/kg/24 hr initially (see Chapter 17 for nitrogen requirements in renal diseases). TPN solutions containing 10% to 12% glucose may generally be started at a maintenance fluid rate. Higher-concentration glucose solutions should be initiated slowly to avoid extreme hyperglycemia. Adjust the input rate of the TPN fluid to 300 to 500 mg glucose/kg/hr and increase the rate gradually (by 15% to 20% increments every 2 hours) to the desired fluid volume maintenance rate. If glucosuria greater than 1+ occurs, increase the rate more slowly or return to a lower rate for 1 to 2 hours before increasing it again in order to achieve a final desired infusion rate without urinary glucose spillage. If fluid reduction for several hours is undesirable, specific glucose solutions of increasing concentrations can be mixed and changed at 2 to 4 hr intervals in order to reach the final equivalent concentration of the TPN solution, which is then directly infused at the continuing fluid volume input rate. The estimated daily needs for protein, calories, minerals, and cofactors are listed in Table 111-4.

During central TPN catheter flushes, when other infused materials (such as antibiotics) must be given by the same access, it is reasonable to flush with a glucose solution of the same concentration as that in the TPN solution, in order to avoid significant hypoglycemia. Confirm with the pharmacy the compatibility of all infused materials with even simple electrolyte and glucose solutions.

The desired TPN volume containing protein, glucose, minerals, and vitamins is infused over 24 hours at a constant rate via infusion pump and also monitored by visual inspection of the dispensing units (e.g., Volutrol readings).

CONSULTATION

PARENTERAL ALIMENTATION

Mth day	DATE			
Wt	Weight		kg	
P	Protein Desired		gm/kg, gm	
PV	Protein Volume	FreAmine 0.085, Travasol 0.085, Aminosyn 0.100 gm/cc	cc	$\dfrac{P}{conc}$
L	Lipid Desired		gm/kg, gm	
LV	Lipid Volume	Intralipid 10%, Liposyn 10%	cc	$\dfrac{L}{0.1}$
C	Calories Desired		Cal/kg, Cal	
PC	Protein Calories	4.0 cal/gm	Cal	P×4
LC	Lipid Calories	11 Cal/gm	Cal	L×11.0
GC	Glucose Calories		Cal	C-PC-LC
G	Glucose Monohydrate	3.4 Cal/gm	gm	$\dfrac{GC}{3.4}$
V	Volume Desired		cc/kg, cc	
MWF	Metabolic H$_2$O—Fat	$\dfrac{1.04\ cc\ H_2O}{gmTG}$	cc	L×1.04
MWG	Metabolic H$_2$O—Glucose	$\dfrac{0.545\ cc\ H_2O}{gm\ Glucose \cdot H_2O}$	cc	G×0.545
LW	Water in Lipid Solution	$\dfrac{0.864\ cc}{cc\ Fat}$	cc	LV×0.864
SAVE	Volume SAVE		cc	V-MWF-MWG-LW
CGC	Calculated Glucose Conc		gm/cc	G/SAVE
DGC	Desired Glucose Conc	Max: Perip—0.12, Central—0.26	gm/cc	Lower of: Max or CGC
DGV	Desired Glucose Volume	$\dfrac{0.5\ gm\ glucose \cdot H_2O}{cc}$	cc	(DGC) × (SAVE) × 2
RMWG	Revised Metabolic Water—Glucose	$\dfrac{0.545\ cc\ H_2O}{gm\ Gluc \cdot H_2O}$	cc	DGV × 0.5 × .545
RSAVE	Revised Volume SAVE		cc	V-MWF-RMWG-LW
SF	Supplement Factor			$\dfrac{RSAVE+100}{RSAVE}$
Pharm I	Pharm. Lipid		cc	LV+20
Pharm II	Pharm. SAVE		cc	(RSAVE)×(SF)
Pharm III	Pharm. Amino Acid		cc	(PV)×(SF)
IV	Pharm. Glucose		cc	(DGV)×(SF)× RSAVE/SAVE
V	Ca Gluc. $\dfrac{0.46\ mEq}{cc}$	1-2 mEq Ca/kg	mEq/kg, cc	$\dfrac{(wt)\times(SF)\ (mEq/kg)}{0.46}$
VI	KPhosphate $\dfrac{5.4\ mEq\ P}{cc}$	1-3 mEq Phos/kg	mEq/kg, cc	$\dfrac{(wt)\times(SF)\ (mEq/kg)}{5.4}$
VII	KCl $\dfrac{2mEq}{cc}$	2-4 mEq K/kg	mEq/kg, cc	$\dfrac{(wt)\times(SF)\ (mEq/kg) - (4.4\times VI)}{2}$
VIII	NaCl $\dfrac{2.5mEq}{cc}$	3-5 mEq Na/kg	mEq/kg, cc	$\dfrac{(wt)\times(SF)\ (mEq/kg)}{2.5}$
IX	MgSO$_4$ $\dfrac{4.06\ mEq}{cc}$	1-3 mEq Mg/kg	mEq/kg, cc	$\dfrac{(wt)\times(SF)\ (mEq/kg)}{4.06}$
X	ZnCl$_2$ $\dfrac{1\ mg}{cc}$	.15—.30 mg/kg	mg/kg, cc	$\dfrac{(wt)\times(SF)\ (mg/kg)}{1}$
XI	CuCl$_2$ $\dfrac{0.4\ mg}{cc}$	.02 mg/kg	mg/kg, cc	$\dfrac{(wt)\times(SF)\ (mg/kg)}{0.4}$
XII	MnCl$_2$ $\dfrac{0.1\ mg}{cc}$	0.002—0.01 mg/kg	mg/kg, cc	$\dfrac{(wt)\times(SF)\ (mg/kg)}{0.1}$
XIII	CrCl$_3$ $\dfrac{4\ mcg}{cc}$	0.2 mcg/kg	mcg/kg, cc	$\dfrac{(wt)\times(SF)\ (mcg/kg)}{4}$
XIV	MVI Pediatric / Berocca-C		cc / cc	SF × 1.0 / SF × 10.0
XV	Heparin $\dfrac{1000U}{cc}$		cc	Pharm II × 0.001
XVI	Sterile Water		cc	Pharm II—(III to XV)
CD	Caloric Density		Cal/cc	$\dfrac{(DGV\times0.5\times3.4)+PC}{RSAVE}$
	Infusion Rates — Lipid		cc/hr	LV/24
	SAVE		cc/hr	RSAVE/24
	Actual Cal Received		Cal	(RSAVE) × (CD) + (1.1×LV)

CMC 18099/05220

Fig. 111-1. Order form for individualized parenteral nutrition. Each column will provide data for one 24-hour period. The supplement factor (SF) is designed to provide sufficient extra final solution for filling of connecting tubings, unexpected equipment changes, etc.

Table 111-4. Estimated daily TPN needs for metabolic maintenance, growth, and tissue repair of infants

Protein	1.5-4.5 g/kg
Calories	120-200/kg
Water	120-180 ml/kg
Sodium	3-8 mEq/kg
Potassium	2-4 mEq/kg
Chloride	2-4 mEq/kg
Calcium	1-2 mEq/kg
Phosphorus	1-3 mEq/kg
Magnesium	1-3 mEq/kg
Zinc	150-300 μg/kg
Copper	20 μg/kg
Chromium	200 ng/kg
Manganese	2-10 μg/kg
Vitamins	
A	600 μg
B_1	0.5-5 mg
B_2	0.5-2 mg
B_6	0.5-2 mg
B_{12}	1 μg
C	75-100 mg
D	10-15 μg
E	3-5 mg
K	50-100 μg
Folic acid	35-50 μg
Niacin	10-30 mg
Biotin	50-300 μg
Pantothenate	5-10 mg
Essential fatty acid	0.5-1.0 g/kg

When intravenous lipid is used, it may be infused over a 24-hour period.

When lipid is being given simultaneously with peripheral TPN by means of a Y-connector (which is provided with infusate tubing by the pharmacy), the lipid side of the Y-connector should be on top to prevent backflow up the other side, since the lipid infusion is less dense than the aqueous solution.

Antibiotics should not be used in catheters through which lipid has run, to avoid possible drug absorption or inactivation interactions. Filters cannot be used on tubing through which the lipid is infused, since the emulsified particles would not pass.

Table 111-5. Suggested routine clinical laboratory blood studies during TPN

Day of the week	Laboratory studies
Tuesday	NH_3, PO_4, SGPT, bilirubin (direct and total), protein electrophoresis, CBC
Friday	Ca, PO_4, BUN, bilirubin (direct and total), Na, K

MONITORING

See also Chapter 4.
1. Body weight daily; head circumference and length weekly; triceps skinfold thickness and mid–upper arm circumference weekly, if possible
2. Complete input and output recorded every hour
3. Check every urine for glucose (e.g., Tes-Tape, Chemstrip). Check Dextrostix frequently when initiating TPN. Occasionally, exogenous regular insulin (1 unit per 6 to 12 g of glucose infused) is administered to counteract hyperglycemia when the reduction of the infusion rate is not possible or effective. This can be given by a separate IV, or prepared with the TPN solution by the pharmacy. Insulin, as a protein, is subject to denaturation; ambient room temperature may cause this to occur gradually. The pharmacy can prepare insulin-containing bottles of smaller total volume for shorter infusions if this is a problem.
4. Obtain clinical laboratory studies prior to starting TPN. These include serum Na, K, Cl, CO_2, Ca, Mg, PO_4, glucose, albumin, globulin, BUN, creatinine, SGPT, bilirubin (direct and total), prealbumin, NH_3 and CBC. Initiate a minimal weekly routine schedule of studies, an example of which is shown in Table 111-5, plus serum triglyceride measurements, outlined below.
5. During lipid infusions, a serum triglyceride measurement should be done to assess physiologic tolerance of the infused emul-

sion (less than 200 mg/dl is acceptable). A serum turbidity test drawn 3 to 4 hours after the lipid infusion can help indicate the adequacy of triglyceride clearing but is not as accurate a monitor; the serum should be nonturbid at that time.

Discontinuing TPN

TPN infusions should be discontinued gradually, optimally over 1 to 3 days. More rapid reduction can be handled by progressive decrements over 1 to 4 hours, depending upon the level of blood glucose and/or other sources of parenteral or enteral glucose being provided. If an infusion is stopped suddenly:

1. A new peripheral infusion containing glucose (8 to 10 g/dl) should be started immediately.
2. Frequent blood glucose estimations at the bedside (e.g., by Chemstrip bG, Dextrostix, or chemical laboratory determination) are done to monitor for significant hypoglycemia every 15 to 20 minutes for 4 to 6 hours and/or until blood glucose is stable.

RISKS AND COMPLICATIONS
Infection

The most significant risk involved in TPN is systemic infection. It may result from seeding due to:

1. A local contaminated or infected insertion site or a remote site
2. Systemically acquired bacteremia from the urinary tract or gut
3. Contaminated infusate solutions
4. Hospital-associated infectious sources

The extended period over which TPN occurs enhances the likelihood of systemic infection, and every effort must be made to forestall clinical septicemia by rigorous attention to the details of technical management and infection control.

The unexpected occurrence of glucosuria, when the IV glucose has not been increased concomitantly, may be an early clinical indicator that incipient bacteremia and/or septicemia has altered peripheral-tissue glucose uptake by increasing peripheral insulin resistance. Decreasing the rate of glucose infusion or supplementing TPN with regular insulin may resolve the glucosuria, but extraordinary attention must be given to excluding an infectious process.

A positive blood culture for *Candida* necessitates catheter removal. Bacteremia and associated septicemia may be initially treated with antibiotics while a TPN infusion schedule continues, but catheter removal is essential if clinical improvement does not occur promptly.

Technical problems

1. Catheter blockage may occur with fibrin clots intraluminally or surrounding the catheter tip, particularly at low infusion rates; with central-catheter TPN, a superior vena caval syndrome can occur if there is associated major vessel thrombosis. It is therefore important to maintain an adequate flow in the TPN catheter. If the catheter is not infusing fluid:
   a. Undress the site quickly to relieve possible catheter coiling or kinking.
   b. Clamp the catheter with a special TPN toothless clamp, followed by sterile connection of the catheter to a 3-ml syringe containing 0.9% sodium chloride solution with heparin (1:1000) for modest irrigation attempts.
   c. If a significant fibrin clot is likely, success with fibrinolysis in situ may be possible using urokinase injection of the line (2 ml of urokinase, 3500 units/ml, placed into the catheter for 2 hours, then gently aspirated out, with subsequent irrigation with 0.9% sodium chloride solution).
   d. Catheter removal is indicated if flow cannot be established.
2. For catheter breakage or leakage, clamp with special TPN clamps on the patient side of the catheter, and follow, using absolute sterile technique, with either:

a. temporary repair: blunt needle insertion into the catheter after excising the damaged catheter section, and/or

b. permanent repair (for Broviac catheters): excising the damaged catheter, followed by placement of a new catheter section (provided in the appropriate lumen-sized Broviac Repair Kit), which is then bonded with sterile glue

3. If there is air in the Silastic tubing, clamp the tubing proximal to the air, and try thumping the air back up the Silastic tubing to the connector with the blunt needle; then remove the air by aspiration. If this is not successful, cut the tubing proximal to the air and insert a new blunt needle, using sterile technique. If only a small quantity of air is present, one may elect to do nothing and allow it to be infused.

4. Dislodgement of the catheter, with the potential for unrecognized hypoglycemia in central-catheter TPN or for rapid fluid extravasation into tissue spaces with either type of TPN, occasionally occurs. Most often the catheter must be completely removed. The risk of significant postinfusion hypoglycemia is small but demands close monitoring initially. In peripheral-catheter TPN, fluid extravasation can occasionally produce a severe subcutaneous reaction and/or necrosis, which can result in tissue sloughing and scarring (Fig. 111-2).

5. A high concentration of infused glucose in peripheral-catheter TPN may lead to significant phlebitis. Local vascular inflammation at infusion entry sites may predispose the patient to thrombophlebitis.

6. Excessive calcium and/or phosphorus concentration in the TPN solution may lead to precipitation in either the main solution or the infusion catheter. New solution must be prepared once precipitation has occurred, and the infusion tubing must be changed.

7. Rare complications include lymphatic duct

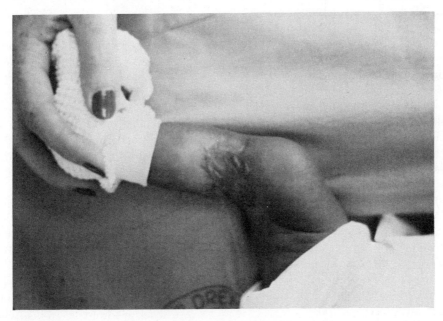

Fig. 111-2. Moderately severe skin scarring secondary to infiltration of peripheral TPN solution.

perforation, nerve injury, pneumothorax, hemothorax, cardiac dysrhythmias resulting from catheter tip placement in the ventricle, perforation of the great vessel, arteriovenous fistula after arterial perforation, catheter embolization, atrial perforation, and thoracic accumulation of infusate fluid through central site leakage.

Metabolic risks

Carbohydrates. Hyperosmolar nonketotic dehydration, and the resulting coma, may reflect uncontrolled hyperglycemia (blood glucose level of 400 to 1000 mg/dl) with massive glucosuria and accompanying osmotic diuresis. This may be a consequence of (1) excessively vigorous or rapid advancement of infused glucose quantities and/or (2) inability of peripheral tissues to couple regulation of endogenous insulin and glucagon output to glucose concentration and utilization. However, the underlying possibility of deteriorating pancreatic and hepatic function in severely compromised patients must be recognized.

Nitrogen. Moderate hyperammonemia (1.5 to 2.5 times normal values) and/or rising blood transaminase levels occur not infrequently in the first 7 to 10 days of gradually increasing central or peripheral TPN (in the absence of IV lipid) but usually decline thereafter to normal or mildly elevated levels with no apparent significant sequelae. Persistent elevations must be viewed with caution and attention should be given to reduction of the concentration of nitrogen in the infusate, at least temporarily.

The possibility of amino acid imbalances continues to be investigated, e.g., amino acid–related cholestasis. Use of currently available synthetic amino acid solutions has not produced recognized serious nitrogen disorders. The occurrence of metabolic acidosis and prerenal azotemia during TPN is rare when the presently available amino acid mixtures are used at recommended levels (Table 111-4).

Lipid

1. Use of IV lipid has occasionally been associated with acute chills, fever, and local allergic skin reactions within the first 12 hours after infusion was begun. Anemia and/or thrombocytopenia occur uncommonly; eosinophilia, although more common, has no clinical correlates presently.
2. Hepatic reticuloendothelial cells may accumulate a brownish pigment, the clinical significance of which, particularly with conjugated hyperbilirubinemia, is not established. Diverse biliary alterations may occur, i.e., cholestasis, biliary tract dilatation, or cholecystitis (acalculous or with radiotransparent stones). Oral feedings may modulate such changes.
3. Abnormal pulmonary diffusion has been observed in humans receiving IV lipid, and the presence of parenchymal fat accumulation in pulmonary alveolar cells and reticuloendothelial cells in experimental animal studies indicates a potential problem in infants, particularly those at risk for pulmonary dysfunction.
4. Rarely, an overloading syndrome characterized by fever, jaundice, splenomegaly, gastrointestinal bleeding, diffuse pulmonary infiltrates, focal seizures, and shock has been associated with IV lipid–supplemented TPN.
5. The metabolism of IV triglyceride to free fatty acids and glycerol may provide a source of fatty acids that can displace bilirubin from albumin-binding sites. Hence, such IV glyceride must be used cautiously in neonates with jaundice who have significant unconjugated hyperbilirubinemia.
6. IV lipid should not be infused in the same catheter as additive drugs or antibiotics.

Minerals and vitamins

1. Unrecognized hypophosphatemia in association with TPN has been associated with severe shock syndrome as well as with anemia

secondary to reduced red cell 2,3-DPG. Serum phosphate levels should be maintained at 4 to 5 mg/dl. Parenteral phosphate is available in the form of aqueous potassium phosphate or sodium phosphate.

2. Iron deficiency may occur with prolonged TPN if iron is not provided separately at appropriate intervals. Similarly, deficiencies of trace minerals and certain vitamins may occur with long-term TPN or as a consequence of increased needs during recovery from malnutrition or hypercatabolic states. Iodine and selenium, for example, are not generally included presently in routine TPN formulations. Trace metal excess may produce morbidity rarely.

3. Vitamin deficiencies will not be a complication of TPN if daily water-soluble and fat-soluble vitamins are provided as indicated above. Vitamin D and E supplementation may be required individually in special situations of expected high need. Hypervitaminosis A or D are a theoretical risk when using multi-component vitamin products; restriction to recommended fat-soluble vitamins input in these preparations will avoid this potential problem.

ADDITIONAL READING

Barness, L.A., Dallman, P.R., Anderson, H., and others: (AAP Committee on Nutrition): Use of intravenous fat emulsions in pediatric patients, Pediatrics **68:**738-743, 1981.

Bernstein, J., Chang, C.H., Braugh, A.J., and others: Conjugated hyperbilirubinemia in infancy associated with parenteral alimentation, J. Pediatr. **90:**361-367, 1977.

Binstadt, B.R., and L'heureux, P.R.: Rickets as a complication of intravenous hyperalimentation in infants, Pediatr. Radiol. **7:**211-214, 1978.

Filler, R.M.: Parenteral support of the surgically ill child. In Suskind, R.M., editor: Textbook of pediatric nutrition, New York, 1981, Raven Press, pp. 341-355, 1981.

Ricour, C., Navarro, J., and Duhamel, J.F.: Trace elements and vitamin requirements in infants on total parenteral nutrition, Acta Chir. Scand. [Suppl.]**498:**67-69, 1980.

Winters, R.W., and Hasselmeyer, E.G.: Intravenous nutrition in the high risk infant, New York, 1975, John Wiley & Sons, Inc.

112 Total enteral nutrition
Special feeding techniques and formula selection

CHARLES E. MIZE
BETSY COHEN TEITELL
CYNTHIA CUNNINGHAM

INDICATIONS

When patients are not capable of taking formula or food routinely in sufficient amounts to maintain positive caloric and nitrogen balance, controlled enteral feeding techniques, often designated total enteral nutrition (TEN), are preferred methods of providing nutrition. These techniques rely on a gastrointestinal tract capable of accepting and absorbing nutrients. Utilization of TEN generally represents a significantly lower cost than TPN.

Those conditions for which TEN can be successfully employed include presurgical and postsurgical gastrointestinal obstructions or anomalies, protracted or recurrent diarrhea, intractable gastroesophageal reflux, presurgical and postsurgical cardiac lesions, recovery phases of necrotizing enterocolitis, complex oncology treatment and recovery programs, predialysis and postdialysis renal dysfunction, chronic hepatic disease, and conditions requiring artificial ventilatory and/or tracheostomy tubes for extended periods. Low-birth-weight infants with limited endogenous energy stores frequently demand special enteral feeding plans. Infants with congenital heart disease or others whose sucking reflex is normal but in whom the energy required exhausts them before adequate nutrition is ingested can benefit from selected TEN.

EQUIPMENT AND TECHNIQUES
Types of TEN delivery

Per os (PO). In infants who have adequate swallowing function but poor sucking reflex, cross-cutting of nipples, or the use of premature or lambs' nipples can lessen sucking demand considerably. Such nipples can be successful in patients with oral-facial abnormalities, e.g,. Pierre Robin anomalies.

Tube feeding. Enteral formulations are administered by a variety of feeding tubes and in one of two modes: bolus or continuous drip. Bolus feedings provide intermittent amounts of predesignated volumes. Continuous-drip feedings provide constant infusion of formula at a specified administration rate. Continuous-drip infusions are usually controlled by infusion pumps, rather than gravity flow, for accuracy of delivery. For both nursing care and for choice of enteral formula, feeding tubes are classified according to tube location and method of placement.

Method of placement
1. Nonsurgically placed feeding tubes
   a. Nasogastric (NG): a tube placed via the nostril into the fundus of the stomach. This can be placed easily and repeatedly, at the bedside, without ancillary personnel or roentgenographic support.
   b. Nasoduodenal (ND) or gastroduodenal

(GD): a tube placed into the duodenum via the naris, or occasionally through a gastrostomy opening. This may require placement under direct fluoroscopic observation, for correct positioning, and is inconvenient for repeated placement. A pediatric flexible tube can be guided into the duodenum, with the aid of a soft, blunt internal-lumen guide wire, but this technique is less consistently successful when done at the bedside than placement using fluoroscopy.

c. Nasojejunal (NJ) or gastrojejunal (GJ): a tube placed into the jejunum via the nostril, or occasionally through a gastrostomy opening. This allows delivery of nutrients directly into the absorptive upper small intestine and may be particularly useful in early postoperative management. If not placed surgically, this tube is the most difficult tube to insert, entailing fluoroscopic placement by a skilled radiologist or many hours to allow a mercury-weighted tube to pass to the jejunum.

2. Surgically placed feeding tubes

a. Gastrostomy: a tube placed directly into the fundus of the stomach, exiting percutaneously through a fistula tract. This is useful for long-term enteral feeding.

b. Jejunostomy: a tube threaded through the intestinal serosal surface, along the subserosal space, and into the jejunal lumen. The tube is sutured to the peritoneal reflection beneath the skin exit site or anchored at the exit site if placed retroperitoneally. This is useful when simple nutrient absorption is required and has functioned successfully in immediate postoperative periods under conditions of postoperative ileus.

Types of tubes

1. The standard polyvinyl chloride tube, #5 through #18 French, is excellent for short-term feedings. This tube is semirigid and therefore relatively easy to guide (without a guide wire), but it stiffens after 48 to 72 hours upon exposure to intestinal secretions, thereby increasing the risk of mechanical complications.

2. The polyurethane or silicone tube, #5 through #8 French, with mercury weighting enclosed in the tip of the tube and exit ports proximal to the mercury, is useful for long-term feedings (e.g., Nutriflex, Enteriflex, Keofeed). It is somewhat less rigid than a polyvinyl chloride tube, and an accompanying stylet guide wire allows more easily directed placement. A radiopaque line along the tube length allows evaluation of tube location. It does not stiffen over long periods in the intestinal tract.

3. The polyurethane tube, #5 through #8 French, without mercury weighting but designed especially for small infants (Argyle Indwell), is extremely pliable and soft, has a radiopaque line for location identification (by roentgenogram), and does not stiffen over long periods in the intestinal tract. Placement distal to the stomach requires special wire construction and skilled fluoroscopic technique.

Infusion pumps. Accuracy of formula delivery by feeding tube is accomplished by controlled pump infusion. Pumps designed specifically for enteral formula use (Kangaroo, Flexiflow, Keofeed) are accurate and less expensive than standard IV pumps (which will also handle enteral solutions). Several enteral pumps have minimum flow rates that may be too high for neonates. When increments of 1 ml/hr or less are desired, selective enteral or IV pumps should be utilized.

Tube placement

1. Estimate the correct maximum tube length to be inserted. For nasal feeding tubes, measure the distance from nose to ear to xiphoid process; then mark the tube with an indelible ink pen at the tape site so that if the tube slips out of the tape, the mark

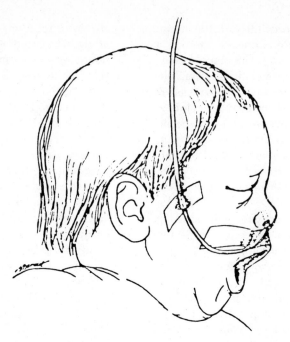

Fig. 112-1. Proper taping of an NG tube. Note that the tube is not pulled up in a way that would distort the nares and that the other nostril is not covered by tape.

will change position and alert the staff that this has occurred. A position between the xiphoid and the umbilicus is recommended for this measurement in infants.

2. Lubricate the tube with standard water-soluble lubricant. For tubes with a special polymer coating that becomes slippery upon contact with liquid, simple moistening of the tubes with water is sufficient.

3. If possible for gastric tubes, place the child in the upright position, leaning forward slightly. Gently push the tube through the nostril until it reaches the desired adhesive tape marking. Allowing the infant to suck on a pacifier during the tube insertion may aid esophageal peristaltic movement and avoid tracheal misdirection. Do not force the tube or continue if the child experiences distress. Secure the tube with non-irritating tape to avoid irritation or pressure on the nasal tip; Opsite is useful in small

infants, to avoid skin and cheek irritation (see Fig. 112-1).

4. For duodenal tubes, position the child on his right side. In order to help guide the tube tip directly to the pylorus, have a colleague apply gentle upward (cephalad) pressure beneath the stomach continuously while the tube is being moved forward. Maintain this posture for 5 to 15 minutes, gently pushing at the pylorus to allow pyloric junction contracture to capture the tube. Gently advance thereafter to the distance marked on the tube (at the nose) for desired duodenal location.

5. Check the location of the tube tip. For gastric tubes, inject 5 to 10 ml of air through the tube, listening over the fundus of the stomach with a stethoscope for air movement. Gastric juice may also be found on gentle aspiration. A chest/abdominal roentgenogram can verify location and is neces-

sary for all tubes placed distal to the stomach.

6. Frequent attention is necessary to determine tube tip location before feedings. Major repositioning generally requires removal of the old tube and insertion of a new tube, rather than manipulation of the malpositioned tube. Less risk is involved in pulling back a tube than in pushing forward.

7. Short-term gastric feeding tubes for bolus feedings may be placed at the time of each feeding and removed immediately thereafter. Use the smallest diameter lumen through which the formula will pass. If there is increased risk of mucosal trauma, the tubes for bolus feedings can be left in place between feedings, but for less than 48 hours to avoid tube stiffening. Polyurethane tubes may be left in place for long periods (4 weeks or even longer).

8. Inspect the entry sites of tubes frequently (hourly for nasal tubes, every 8 hours for gastrostomy or jejunostomy sites) for dermatitis or erosions.

9. Elevate the head of bed or maintain neonates in a slightly head-up position (in an infant seat) if possible.

10. For a tube with a distal mercury weight, obtain an abdominal roentgenogram to confirm that the location of the formula exit ports (several millimeters proximal to the mercury) rests in the desired position.

Formula selection (Table 112-1 and 112-2). Knowledge of specific patient metabolic demands and intestinal physiologic state and maturation, and basic knowledge of enteral formula characteristics, will allow proper formula selection. When selecting an enteral formulation, consider:

1. Completeness of the formula. Note the degree to which there is a complete complement of protein, carbohydrate, fat, vitamins, and minerals.

2. Electrolyte content. Enteral feedings designed for adults have a highly variable content.

3. Osmolality. Generally, in pediatric illness gastrointestinal tolerance is increased with lower osmolal formulations.

4. Individual substrate composition, particularly protein, carbohydrate, and fat. Gastrointestinal function and pathophysiology will largely determine whether hydrolyzed or simpler components, individual unique supplements, entirely modular formulations, or chemically defined diets are necessary.

5. Lactose content. Acquired or relative lactose intolerance may occur in a variety of gastrointestinal disorders.

While standard infant formulas are easily administered by special feeding techniques, there are a variety of commercially available specialized materials (Table 112-1).

Formula infusion

1. Begin infusion at slow rates, initially with a glucose-electrolyte solution (e.g., Pedialyte, Lytren), to be followed by formula (usually at dilute concentration initially, and gradually increased).

2. Administer formula at room temperature.

3. Monitoring during infusion:
   a. Keep accurate records of hourly input and output.
   b. Measure abdominal girth once each shift and more frequently if girth is increasing.
   c. Check gastric residuals every 2 hours during initiation of constant infusions and just prior to feeding a bolus of formula.
   d. Check Dextrostix values every 4 hours.
   e. Monitor urine glucose level every 4 hours and specific gravity every 8 hours.
   f. Check the liquid portion of stool or ostomy output every 4 hours for glucose concentration (e.g., Tes-Tape strips) and every 8 hours for blood (e.g., Hematest).
   g. Check serum glucose, electrolytes, se-

Table 112-1. Formula selection

Category	Product	100 ml				Composition (%)			mEq/dl			mg/dl			Renal solute load (mOsm/L)	Osmolality (mOsm/kg H₂O)
		kcal	CHO (g)	Fat (g)	Protein (g)	CHO	Fat	Protein	Na	K	Cl	Ca	P	Fe		
Casein	Cow milk*	66	4.9	3.7	3.5	Lactose	Butterfat	Casein (82) Whey (18)	2.2	3.5	2.9	117	92	.05	226	270
	Human milk†	71	6.8	3.8	1.1	Lactose	Breast milk fat	Whey (60) Casein (40)	0.7	1.3	1.1	34	14	.05	75	273
	Enfamil 20 with Fe (M-J)	67	7.0	3.7	1.5	Lactose	Soy (80) Coconut (20)	Skim milk	1.0	1.7	1.3	52	44	.15 1.3	100	278
	Enfamil Premature Formula 24 kcal (M-J)	80	8.9	4.1	2.4	Corn syrup solids (60) Lactose (40)	Corn (40) MCT (40) Coconut (20)	Whey (60) Casein (40)	1.4	2.3	1.9	94	47	.13	208‡	300
	Evaporated milk 13:19:1	67	7.2	3.4	2.9	Lactose (51) Dextrins (24) Maltose (15) Dextrose (5) Sucrose (5)	Butterfat	Cow milk	2.1	3.2		104	84			300
	Similac 20 with Fe (Ross)	67	7.2	3.6	1.6	Lactose	Coconut (60) Soy (40)	Skim milk	1.1	2.0	1.5	51	39	.15 1.2	108	290
	Similac PM 60/40 (Ross)	67	6.9	3.8	1.6	Lactose	Coconut (60) Corn (40)	Demineralized whey (60) Casein (40)	0.7	1.5	0.7	40	20	.30	93	260
	Similac 24 Special care (Ross)	80	8.6	4.4	2.2	Lactose (50) Corn syrup solids (50)	MCT (50) Corn (30) Coconut (20)	Whey (60) Casein (40)	1.5	2.6	1.8	144	72	.30	208‡	300
	SMA (Wyeth)	67	7.2	3.6	1.5	Lactose	Oleo (33) Coconut (27) Soy (15) Safflower (25)	Demineralized whey (60) Casein (40)	0.7	1.4	1.0	44	33	1.3	91	300
Soy	Isomil (Ross)	67	6.9	3.6	2.0	Corn syrup solids (54) Sucrose (46)	Coconut (60) Soy (40)	Soy isolate	1.3	1.8	1.5	70	50	1.2	126	250
	Isomil SF (Ross)	67	6.8	3.6	2.0	Corn syrup solids	Coconut (60) Soy (40)	Soy isolate	1.3	1.8	1.5	70	50	1.2	126	150
	ProSoBEE (M-J)	67	6.9	3.6	2.0	Corn syrup solids	Soy (80) Coconut (20)	Soy isolate	1.2	2.1	1.5	63	49	1.3	128	194‖
Protein hydrolysate	Nutramigen (M-J)	67	8.8	2.6	2.2	Sucrose (72) Modified tapioca (28)	Corn	Hydrolyzed casein	1.4	1.7	1.3	63	47	1.3	132	547‖
	Pregestimil (M-J)	67	9.1	2.7	1.9	Corn syrup solids (84) Modified tapioca (16)	Corn (58) MCT (42)	Hydrolyzed casein	1.4	1.9	1.6	63	42	1.3	124	348

Category	Product					Protein source	Fat source	Carbohydrate source								
Others	Meatbase (Gerber)	68	6.7	3.4	2.8	Beef heart	Sesame (81) Animal fat (19)	Sucrose (70) Modified tapioca (30)	0.8	1.0	0.6	98	65	1.4	135	284‖
	Portagen (M-J)	67	7.8	3.2	2.4	Na caseinate	MCT (66) Corn (11) Lecithin (3)	Corn syrup solids (74) Sucrose (25) Lactose (trace)	1.4	2.2	1.6	63	47	1.3	148	217‖
	RCF (Ross)	40		3.6	2.0	Soy isolate	Coconut (90) Soy (10)	To be added	1.3	1.8	1.5	70	50	.15	126	(d)§
Electrolyte solutions	Lytren (M-J)	29	7.6	0	0			Glucose polymers (90) Dextrose (10)	3.0	2.5	2.5	8	8.9	0	80	290
	Pedialyte (Ross)	19	5.0	0				Dextrose	3.0	2.0	3.0	8		0	80	390
Specialized enteral feedings	CIB & Homo (3.5% fat) (Carnation)	105	13.1	3.0	5.6	Cow milk Soy isolate Ca caseinate	Butterfat	Sucrose Corn syrup solids Lactose	4.0	6.8		153	145	1.7		615 van. 649 choc. malt 650
	Criticare HN (M-J)	106	22.2	0.3	3.8	Hydrolyzed casein: amino acids (70) small peptides (30)	Safflower	Maltodextrin (89) Modified cornstarch (6) Citrates (5)	2.7	3.4	3.0	53	53	1.0	243	450
	Ensure (Ross)	106	14.3	3.7	3.7	Na and Ca caseinate (88) Soy isolate (12)	Corn	Glucose polymers (74) Sucrose (26)	3.7	4.1	4.0	53	53	1.0	266	450
	Ensure Plus (Ross)	150	20	5.3	5.5	Na and Ca caseinate (88) Soy isolate (12)	Corn	Glucose polymers (74) Sucrose (26)	5.0	5.9	5.6	63	63	1.4	385	600
	Formula 2 (Cutter)	100	12.3	4.0	3.8	Skim milk (67) Beef (22) Egg yolk (4) Other (3)	Beef Corn Egg yolk	Sucrose Fructose Lactose Wheat starch	2.6	4.5	5.4	72	56	1.3	273	435-510
	Isocal (M-J)	106	13.2	4.4	3.4	Na and Ca caseinate (79) Soy isolate (21)	Soy (75) MCT (20) Lecithin (5)	Maltodextrins	2.3	3.4	3.0	63	53	1.0	220	300
	Isocal HCN (M-J)	200	22.5	9.1	7.5	Na and Ca caseinate	Soy (70) MCT (30)	Corn syrup solids	3.5	3.6	3.4	67	67	1.2	404	740
	Magnacal (Organon)	200	25	8	7	Na and Ca caseinate	Soy (partially hydrogenated) Lecithin	Maltodextrins (95) Sucrose (5)	4.3	3.2	2.7	100	100	1.8	382	590
	Osmolite (Ross)	106	14.5	3.8	3.7	Na and Ca caseinate (88) Soy isolate (12)	MCT (50) Corn (40) Soy (10)	Corn syrup solids	2.4	2.6	2.4	55	55	0.9	222	300

Continued.

%	Dextrose	Sucrose	Polycose
2%	202	141	93
3%	267	175	106
4%	332	209	120
5%	397	243	134
6%	463	277	147
7%	515	304	158

*Not recommended under 1 year of age.
†Fomon, S.J.: Infant nutrition, ed. 2, Philadelphia, 1974, W.B. Saunders Co.
‡Ziegler, E., and Ryu, J.: Renal solute load and diet in growing premature infants, J. Pediatr. 89:609, 1976.
‖Children's Medical Center (Dallas) laboratory.

Table 112-1. Formula selection—cont'd

Product	100 ml kcal	100 ml CHO (g)	100 ml Fat (g)	100 ml Protein (g)	Composition (%) CHO	Composition (%) Fat	Composition (%) Protein	mEq/dl Na	mEq/dl K	mEq/dl Cl	mg/dl Ca	mg/dl P	mg/dl Fe	Renal solute load (mOsm/L)	Osmolality (mOsm/kg H2O)
Sustacal (M-J)	100	14.0	2.3	6.1	Sucrose (71) Corn syrup solids (29)	Soy (partially hydrogenated)	Ca caseinate (75) Soy isolate (25)	4.0	5.3	4.4	100	92	1.7	381	625-van. 697-choc.
Sustacal HC (M-J)	150	19.0	5.8	6.1	Corn syrup solids (73) Sucrose (27)	Soy (partially hydrogenated)	Na and Ca caseinate	3.6	3.8	3.6	84	84	1.5	354	650
Vital (Ross)	100	18.8	1.1	4.2	Glucose polymers (83) Sucrose (17)	Safflower (55) MCT (45)	Partially hydrolysed whey, meat, and soy (87)	1.7	3.0	1.9	67	67	1.2	234	460
Vivonex (Eaton)	100	23.1	0.1	2.2	Glucose polymers	Safflower	Amino acids	2.0	3.0	2.0	56	55	1.0	158	550 (596-610 flavored)
Vivonex HN (Eaton)	100	21.0	<0.1	4.6	Glucose polymers	Safflower	Amino acids	2.3	3.0	2.3	33	33	0.6	260	810 (850-855 flavored)

Defined formulas for special metabolic indications

Product	100 ml kcal	100 ml CHO (g)	100 ml Fat (g)	100 ml Protein (g)	Composition (%) CHO	Composition (%) Fat	Composition (%) Protein	mEq/dl Na	mEq/dl K	mEq/dl Cl	mg/dl Ca	mg/dl P	mg/dl Fe	Renal solute load (mOsm/L)	Osmolality (mOsm/kg H2O)
Amin Aid# (McGraw)	200	36.5	4.6	1.9	Malto-dextrins (67) Sucrose (33)	Partially hydrogenated soy oil (98) Lecithin (2)	L-amino acids	<0.5	<0.5	<0.5				<91	1050
3% Protein Mineral Module (Baylor Core)# (Ross)				2.2			Na and Ca caseinate	1.3	2.1	1.4	57	39	0.5	136	1%-29‖ 2%-68 3%-103
Lofenalac (M-J)	71	9.2	2.8	2.3	Corn syrup solids (84) Tapioca (16)	Corn	Casein hydrolysate; low phenylalanine	1.4	1.8	1.3	63	48	1.3	129	654
MSUD (M-J)	68	9.0	2.9	1.2	Corn syrup solids (84) Tapioca (16)	Corn	L-amino acids; no branched-chain amino acids	1.4	1.2	1.5	70	38	1.3	89	358
Phenyl-Free (M-J)	84	13.7	1.4	4.2	Sucrose (66.8) Corn syrup solids (22.5) Tapioca (6.6)	Corn	L-amino acids; no phenylalanine	2.3	3.8	3.0	127	95	2.5	259	893
3200AB (M-J)	68	8.7	2.6	2.2	Corn syrup solids (84) Tapioca (16)	Corn	Casein hydrolysate; low phenylalanine and tyrosine	1.4	1.8	1.3	63	48	1.3	133	454
3200K (M-J)	68	6.7	3.7	2.1	Corn syrup solids	Corn (45-50) Coconut (50-55)	Soy isolate; low methionine	1.1	1.5	1.2	63	42	1.3	122	200
3232A (M-J)	44	2.5	2.9	2.2	Tapioca	MCT (88) Corn (12)	Casein hydrolysate	1.4	1.8	1.3	63	48	1.3	133	626

	100 ml				Modular components Composition (%)			mEq/dl			mg/dl			Renal solute load (mOsm/L)	Osmolality (mOsm/kg H₂O)
Product	kcal	CHO (g)	Fat (g)	Protein (g)	CHO	Fat	Protein	Na	K	Cl	Ca	P	Fe		
CHO															
Corn Syrup (Karo)	287	74			Polysaccharide (48) Glucose (26) Maltose (13) Trisaccharide (11) Fructose (3)			5		5	46	16	4.1		
Moducal Powder (M-J)	380	95			Maltodextrin			2.4	0.2	4.4					
Polycose Powder (Ross)	380	94			Corn starch hydrolysate			<5.0	<1.0	<6.0	<60	<13			
Fat															
Corn oil	900		100			Fatty acids: saturated—14%, 16:1—2%, 18:1—50%, 18:2—34%									
Safflower oil	900		100			Fatty acids: saturated—7%, 18:1—19%, 18:2—70%, 18:3—3%									
MCT oil (M-J)	830		100			Fatty acids: <C₈ <6% C₈ 67% C₁₀ 23% >C₁₀ <4%									
Microlipid (Organon)	450 per 100 ml		50 per 100 ml			Safflower									80
Protein															
Casec Powder (M-J)	370		2	88		Butterfat	Ca caseinate	6.5			1600	800			
Other															
80056 Powder (M-J)	445	65.3	20.4		Glucose polymers (84) Cornstarch (16)	Corn	To be added (provides vitamins and minerals)	2.8	7.8	3.5	491	270	10		

#Supplement with vitamins.

Table 112-2. Essential fatty acid content of various oils and fat

Product	Density 15°	Essential fatty acid (g/100 g total)	
		Linoleic (18:2)	Linolenic (18:3)
Coconut oil	0.924	Trace	—
Corn oil	0.922	34	—
Peanut oil	0.914	26	—
Safflower oil		70	3
Soybean oil	0.927	51	7
Sunflower seed oil	0.923	66	—
Wheat germ oil		52	4
Butterfat	0.911	3	1
Medium-Chain Triglyceride Oil (M-J)	0.928	—	—
Partially Hydrogenated Soy Oil (M-J)		37	2
Depot Fat (Homo Sapiens)		10	—

Data from Sober, H.A., editor: Handbook of biochemistry, ed. 2, Cleveland, 1970, Chemical Rubber Co., pp. E20-E21.

rum osmolality initially and then daily until a satisfactory feeding regimen is established. More frequent determinations are necessary if vomiting, diarrhea, or other intolerance occurs.

h. Weigh the patient daily, at approximately the same time.

4. If residuals are equal to the volume given in a bolus feeding or the hourly rate by continuous-drip feedings, then an adjustment in the volume rate of feeding or temporary cessation of feeding is necessary.

5. Do not increase the rate and concentration of infusate simultaneously.

6. In the absence of glucosuria or evident gastrointestinal distress, gradually increase the rate or concentration of the infusate.

7. Formula adjustments are generally required for evidence of glucose malabsorption in stool i.e., ≥2+ glucose spillage.

8. Hang commercially prepared or terminally sterilized formulas for no more than 8 hours. Hang modular-prepared formulas for no more than 4 hours.

9. Consider a cotton-backed nipple for suck-

ling stimulation during tube infusion feedings. Nipple feedings may be interspersed with tube feedings as early as possible. Decrease the number of tube feedings as the number of nipple feedings is increased.

RISKS AND COMPLICATIONS

Nasogastric tube feedings in infants with respiratory distress may precipitate regurgitation, inhalation of formula and secretions, apnea, or pneumonitis. Maintenance of a tube in or beyond the stomach artificially maintains a relatively open sphincter between the esophagus, stomach, or duodenum, and normal reflex closure cannot occur to prevent reflux. The problem may be more acute in low-birth-weight infants. Too large a feeding tube can distort stomach anatomy, produce abnormal fluid movements, and increase the risk of viscus perforation. To avoid mucosal damage or perforation stylet must not migrate through a lower exit site.

Polyvinyl feeding tubes that are left in place for longer than 72 hours may stiffen sufficiently to enhance the risk of mucosal irritation, bleeding, perforation, or fistulous tract formation (e.g., tracheoesophageal fistula).

Malpositioned tubes may allow the delivery of high-osmotic formula to luminal surfaces that may be injured, leading to diarrhea, dehydration, and possibly significant enteritis or colitis. Duodenal tubes may easily return to the stomach by repeated coughing or other Valsalva maneuvers by the child.

Prepared formulas hanging at the bedside for prolonged periods are at risk for bacterial contamination. Following strict guidelines for hang times will avoid such contamination. Bolus feedings may result in decreased gastric emptying in some patients and occasionally may be associated with significant osmotic diarrhea. These feedings also distend the stomach, elevate the diaphragm, and decrease FRC, which increases intrapulmonary R $\rightarrow$ L shunting. In patients with abnormal or compressed lung function, this can cause significant hypoxemia and apnea.

ADDITIONAL READING

Andrassy, R.J.: Pediatric nutrition: alternatives to central venous cannulation, Contemp. Surg. 14:23-27, 1979.

Andrassy, R.J., Mahour, G.H., Harrison, M.R., and others: The role and safety of early postoperative feeding in the pediatric surgical patient, J. Pediatr. Surg. 14:381-385, 1979.

Benda, G.I.: Modes of feeding low–birth weight infants, Semin. Perinatol. 3:407-415, 1979.

Boros, S., and Reynolds, S.W.: Duodenal perforation: a complication of neonatal nasojejunal feeding, J. Pediatr. 85:107-108, 1974.

Coln, D.: Simultaneous drainage gastrostomy and feeding jejunostomy in the newborn, Surg. Gynecol. Obstet. 145:594-595, 1977.

Dryburgh, E.: Transpyloric feeding in 49 infants undergoing intensive care, Arch. Dis. Child. 55:878-882, 1980.

Hanson, R.L.: Predictive criteria for length of nasogastric tube insertion for tube feeding, J. Par. Ent. Nutr. 3:160-163, 1979.

Pereira, G.R., and Lemons, J.A.: Controlled study of transpyloric and intermittent lavage feeding in the small preterm infant, Pediatrics 67:68-72, 1981.

Robbins, S., Thorp, T.W., and Wadsworth, C.: Tube feeding of infants and children, A.S.P.E.N. Monograph, Washington, D.C., 1981, American Society of Parenteral and Enteral Nutrition.

APPENDIXES

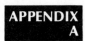

Abbreviations

ACD	Acid citrate dextrose	COMT	Catechol-O-methyltransferase
ACTH	Adrenocorticotropic hormone	CPAP	Continuous positive airway pressure
ADH	Antidiuretic hormone		
AG	Abdominal girth	CPD	Citrate phosphate dextrose
A/G	Albumin/globulin ratio	CPK	Creatinine phosphokinase
AI	Apnea of infancy	CPP	Cerebral perfusion pressure
ALT	Alanine amino transferase	CPR	Cardiopulmonary resuscitation
AMP	Adenosine monophosphate	CPT	Chest physiotherapy
ARDS	Adult respiratory distress syndrome	CSF	Cerebrospinal fluid
		CT scan	Computerized tomography scan
ASD	Atrial septal defect	Cvo_2	Content of oxygen in mixed venous blood
AST	Aspartate amino transferase		
ATP	Adenosine triphosphate	CVP	Central venous pressure
BUN	Blood urea nitrogen	DIC	Disseminated intravascular coagulation
C	Chest circumference		
°C	Degree(s) Celsius	DKA	Diabetic ketoacidosis
Ca	Calcium	2,3-DPG	2,3-diphosphoglycerate
Cao_2	Content of oxygen in arterial blood	DTPA	Diethylenetriaminepentaacetic acid
CBC	Complete blood count		
Cco_2	Content of oxygen in pulmonary capillary blood	$D_5W, D_{10}W$	5% dextrose in water solution, 10% dextrose in water solution
CDC	Centers for Disease Control	ECF	Extracellular fluid
CDI	Central diabetes insipidus	ECG	Electrocardiogram
CI	Cardiac index	EDTA	Ethylenediaminetetraacetic acid
CIE	Counterimmunoelectrophoresis	EEG	Electroencephalogram
C_L	Lung compliance	EFA	Essential fatty acid
Cl	Chloride	ESR	Erythrocyte sedimentation rate
cm H_2O	Centimeter(s) water	°F	Degree(s) Fahrenheit
CMV	Cytomegalovirus	FEF_{25-75}	Mid-maximal forced expired flow
CNS	Central nervous system	$FEV_{1.0}$	Forced expired volume in 1 second
CO	Cardiac output	FFA	Free fatty acid
CoHb	Carboxyhemoglobin	FFP	Fresh-frozen plasma

F_{IO_2}	Fraction of oxygen in inspired gas
FOC	Frontal-occipital circumference
FRC	Functional residual capacity
FVC	Forced vital capacity
g	Gram(s)
GD	Gastroduodenal
GER	Gastroesophageal reflux
GJ	Gastrojejunal
H^+	Hydrogen ion
Hb	Hemoglobin
HAAb (IgM)	Hepatitis A antibody (IgM)
HBcAb	Hepatitis B core antibody
HBsAg	Hepatitis B surface antigen
HC	Heel-crown
HCl	Hydrochloride
HCO_3	Bicarbonate
Hct	Hematocrit
Hz	Hertz
IC	Intracardiac
ICF	Intracellular fluid
ICP	Intracranial pressure
I-E	Inspiratory-expiratory ratio
IM	Intramuscular
IMV	Intermittent mandatory ventilation
IPPB	Intermittent positive-pressure breathing
IPPV	Intermittent positive-pressure ventilation
ISADH	Inappropriate secretion of antidiuretic hormone
IU	International units
IV	Intravenous
IVC	Inferior vena cava
IVH	Intraventricular hemorrhage
K	Potassium
kc	Kilocycle(s)
kg	Kilogram(s)
L	Liter(s)
LAD	Left axis deviation
LAP	Left atrial pressure
LDH	Lactic dehydrogenase
LES	Lower esophageal sphincter
LP	Lumbar puncture
L → R	Left-to-right shunt
LTB	Laryngotracheobronchitis
LVH	Left ventricular hypertrophy
m^2	Square meter(s)
ma	Milliampere(s)
MAP	Mean aortic pressure

mEq	Milliequivalent(s)
mg	Milligram(s)
Mg	Magnesium
MHz	Megahertz
MIF	Maximal inspiratory force
Min	Minute
ml	Milliliter(s)
mm	Millimeter(s)
mm^3	Cubic millimeter(s)
mm Hg	Millimeter(s) of mercury
mmol	Millimole(s)
mOsm	Milliosmol(s)
msec	Milliseconds
mU	Milliunit(s)
mV	Millivolt(s)
μ	Micron(s)
μg	Microgram(s)
μl	Microliter(s)
μV	Microvolt(s)
Na	Sodium
NDI	Nephrogenic diabetes insipidus
ND	Nasoduodenal
NG	Nasogastric
NJ	Nasojejunal
NH_3	Ammonia
nm	Nanometer(s)
N_2O	Nitrous oxide
NPO	Nothing per os
OR	Operating room
P	Phosphorus
P_{50}	Partial pressure of oxygen at which hemoglobin is 50% saturated
$P(A - a)O_2$	Alveolar-arterial oxygen tension difference
Pa_{CO_2}	Tension of carbon dioxide in arterial blood (mm Hg)
Pa_{O_2}	Tension of oxygen in arterial blood (mm Hg)
PAP	Pulmonary arterial blood pressure
PCWP	Pulmonary capillary wedge pressure
PDA	Patent ductus arteriosus
PE_{CO_2}	Pressure of carbon dioxide in expired gas
PEEP	Positive end-expiratory pressure
PEFR	Peak expiratory flow rate
PE_{O_2}	Pressure of oxygen in expired gas
$PetCO_2$	Pressure end-tidal carbon dioxide

PGD_2	Prostaglandin D_2	RVH	Right ventricular hypertrophy
PGE_1	Prostaglandin E_1	RVSTI	Right ventricular systolic time intervals
PGE_2	Prostaglandin E_2	S_1	First heart sound
$PGF_{2\alpha}$	Prostaglandin $F_{2\alpha}$	S_2	Second heart sound
PGI_2	Prostaglandin I_2	SAD	Sugar and acetone determination
pH	Hydrogen ion concentration	SAP	Systemic arterial blood pressure
PICU	Pediatric intensive care unit	SC	Subcutaneously
PO	Per os (by mouth)	SC disease	Sickle cell disease
PO_4	Phosphate	SGOT	Serum glutamic-oxaloacetic transaminase (equivalent to AST)
P_{pa}	Pulmonary arterial blood pressure	SGPT	Serum glutamic-pyruvic transaminase (equivalent to ALT)
PPHN	Persistent pulmonary hypertension of the newborn	SIDS	Sudden infant death syndrome
PR	Per rectum	SL	Sublingual
P_{sa}	Systemic arterial blood pressure	SU	Shoulder-umbilicus
psi	Pounds per square inch	SVR	Systemic vascular resistance
PtC_{O_2}	Tension of oxygen measured transcutaneously	TEN	Total enteral nutrition
PT	Prothrombin time	TLC	Total lung capacity
PTT	Partial thromboplastin time	TORCH	Toxoplasmosis, other, rubella, cytomegalic inclusion disease, *Herpes-virus hominis*
PVC	Premature ventricular contraction		
Pv_{O_2}	Partial pressure of oxygen in mixed venous blood	TPN	Total parenteral nutrition
PVR	Pulmonary vascular resistance	TSH	Thyroid stimulating hormone
qh	Every hour	TSP	Total serum protein(s)
qHs	Every hour before sleep (bedtime)	TT	Thrombin time
Q_S/Q_T	Ratio of shunted blood flow to total blood flow (shunt fraction)	TV	Tidal volume
		TxA_2	Thromboxane A_2
RAD	Right axis deviation	UDPG	Uridine diphosphoglucose
RAH	Right atrial hypertrophy	UTI	Urinary tract infection
R_{aw}	Airway resistance	UUN	Urine urea nitrogen
RBC	Red blood cell	VC	Vital capacity
RDA	Required daily allowance	VCF	Mean rate of circumferential fiber shortening
REM	Rapid eye movement		
$R \rightarrow L$	Right-to-left shunt	V_D/V_T	Dead space–to–tidal volume ratio
RPEP/RVET	Right preejection period/right ventricular ejection time	VSD	Ventricular septal defect
RV	Residual volume	WBC	White blood cell

Normal values

BLOOD

Na	135-144 mEq/L
K	4.0-5.5 mEq/L
Cl	100-105 mEq/L
Ca	9-11 mg/dl
Mg	1.2-1.8 mEq/L
PO_4	4-8 mo, 4.5-6.8 mg/dl
	1-2 yr, 4.6-5.7 mg/dl
	6 yr, 4.2-6.7 mg/dl
	10 yr, 4.0-5.5 mg/dl
CO_2 content	Premature, 18-26 mmole/L
	Full term, 20-26 mmole/L
	1 wk-2 yr, 20-25 mmole/L
	>2 yr, 23-27 mmole/L
Glucose	Newborn, 20-80 mg/dl
	Adult, 60-110 mg/dl
Bilirubin	0.25-0.8 mg/dl (total)
BUN	4-8 mg/dl
Creatinine	0.5-1.3 mg/dl
Osmolality	275-295 mOsm/kg serum water
TSP	4 mo,4.7-6.2 mg/dl
	4 yr, 6.2-8.1 mg/dl
	Adult, 6.6-8.3 mg/dl
A/G	4 mo, 1.56-4.0
	4 yr, 3.7-5.5
	Adult, 3.3-5.7
NH_3	Newborn, 90-150 μg/dl
	Child, 45-80 μg/dl
	Adult, 18-48 μg/dl
Alkaline phos-	<19 yr, 30-205 IU/L
phatase	>19 yr, 25-80 IU/L
CPK	0-70 IU/L

LDH	Birth, 290-501 IU/L
	1 day, 185-404 IU/L
	1 mo-2 yr, 110-244 IU/L
	3-17 yr, 80-165 IU/L
SGOT (AST)	5-20 IU/L
SGPT (ALT)	4-25 IU/L
Amylase	60-160 Caraway units
Sedimentation	Newborn, 0-2 mm/hr
rate	1 wk-puberty 3-13 mm/hr
	Adult male 0-20 mm/hr
	Adult female 0-15 mm/hr
Uric acid	Male, 3-7 mg/dl
	Female, 2-6 mg/dl

URINE

Volume	Infant, >0.5 ml/kg/hr
	Child, >1.0 ml/kg/hr
Osmolality	50-1200 mOsm/kg urine water
Specific	1.002-1.045
gravity	

HEMATOLOGY

Hct	Birth, 44%-64%
	14-90 days, 35%-49%
	6 mo-1 yr, 30%-40%
	4-10 yr, 31%-43%
Hb	Birth, 14-24 g/dl
	1 mo, 11-17 g/dl
	1 yr, 11-15 g/dl
	9-13 yr, 13-15.5 g/dl

For coagulation studies, see Table 20-1

PRESSURES

For systemic arterial blood pressure, see Table C-1

Central venous blood pressure	1-5 mm Hg (mean)
Left atrial blood pressure	5-10 mm Hg (mean)
Right atrial blood pressure	1-5 mm Hg (mean)
Pulmonary arterial blood pressure (higher during the first few days of life)	15-30 mm Hg (systolic) 5-10 mm Hg (diastolic)
Pulmonary capillary wedge pressure	5-10 mm Hg (mean)
Intracranial pressure	<15 mm Hg
Cerebral perfusion pressure	40-50 mm Hg

PULMONARY

	Newborn				
	1-4 hr	12-24 hr	24-48 hr	96 hr	Child
Pa_{O_2} mm Hg	62 ± 13.8	68	63-87		100
Pa_{CO_2} mm Hg	39	33	34	36	35-45
pH_a	7.30	7.30	7.39	7.39	7.38-7.42

OTHER

Temperature	36°-37.5° C (96.5°-99.5° F) rectally
Heart rate	Normal full-term infant, 130 beats/min (range, 70-180 beats/min) Child, declines to 70 beats/min by 16 years of age
Cardiac output	See Fig. B-1.
CSF	See Table 43-2

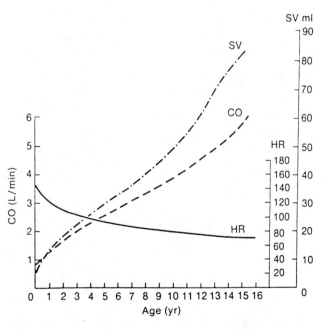

Fig. B-1. Diagrammatic representation of changes in cardiac output *(CO)*, heart rate *(HR)*, and stroke volume *(SV)* from birth to 16 years. (From Rudolph, A.M.: Congenital diseases of the heart. Copyright © 1974 by Year Book Medical Publishers, Inc., Chicago. Used by permission.)

Tables

Table C-1. Normal blood pressure for various ages (Adapted from data in the literature. Figures have been rounded off to nearest decimal place.)

Ages	Mean systolic ±2 S.D.	Mean diastolic ±2 S.D.	Ages	Mean systolic ±2 S.D.	Mean diastolic ±2 S.D.
Newborn*	80 ± 16	46 ± 16	7-8 years	102 ± 15	56 ± 8
6 mos-1 year	89 ± 29	60 ± 10*	8-9 years	105 ± 16	57 ± 9
1 year	96 ± 30	66 ± 25*	9-10 years	107 ± 16	57 ± 9
2 years	99 ± 25	64 ± 25*	10-11 years	111 ± 17	58 ± 10
3 years	100 ± 25	67 ± 23*	11-12 years	113 ± 18	59 ± 10
4 years	99 ± 20	65 ± 20*	12-13 years	115 ± 19	59 ± 10
5-6 years	94 ± 14	55 ± 9	13-14 years	118 ± 19	60 ± 10
6-7 years	100 ± 15	56 ± 8			

From Nadas, A.S., and Fyler, D.C.: Pediatric cardiology, ed. 3, Philadelphia, 1972, W.B. Saunders Co.
*See Fig. C-1.
†In this study the point of muffling was taken as the diastolic pressure.

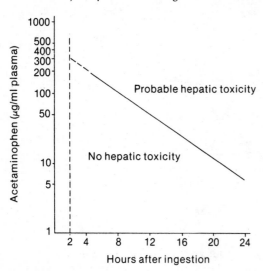

Fig. C-1. Semilogarithmic plot of plasma acetaminophen levels versus time. (From Rumack, B.H., and Matthew, H.: Acetaminophen poisoning and toxicity, Pediatrics **55**:871-876, 1975. Copyright 1975. Reproduced by permission of Pediatrics.)

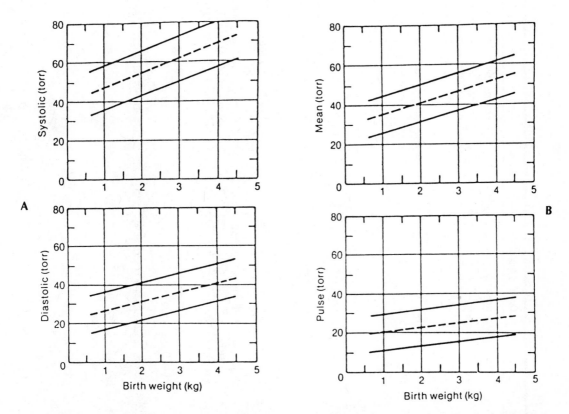

Fig. C-2. A, Linear regressions (broken lines) and 95% confidence limits (solid lines) of systolic (top) and diastolic (bottom) aortic blood pressures on birth weight in 61 healthy newborn infants during the first 12 hours after birth. For systolic pressure, y = 7.13x + 40.45; r = .79. For diastolic pressure, y = 4.81x + 22.18; r = .71. For both, n = 413 and P < .001. **B,** Linear regressions (broken lines) and 95% confidence limits (solid lines) of mean pressure (top) and pulse pressure (systolic-diastolic pressure amplitude) (bottom) on birth weight in 61 healthy newborn infants during the first 12 hours after birth. For mean pressure, y = 5.16x + 29.80; n = 443; r = .80. For pulse pressure, y = 2.31x + 18.27; n = 413; r = .45. For both, P < .001. (From Versmold, H.T., Kitterman, J.A., and others: Aortic blood pressure during the first 12 hours of life in infants with birth weight 610 to 4,220 grams, Pediatrics **67:**607-613, 1981. Copyright American Academy of Pediatrics, 1981.)

Table C-2. Commonly used drugs

Generic name	Trade name	Dose	Route	How supplied
Acetaminophen	Tempra, Tylenol, Liquiprin	10-15 mg/kg/dose q4h	PO, PR	Drops: 60 mg/0.6 ml Syrup: 120 mg/5 ml Chewable: 80 mg/tablet Suppository: 125, 300, and 600 mg
Adrenal corticosteroids	See Table C-3			
Aluminum hydroxide gel	Amphojel	15-30 ml q4h	PO (gavage)	Suspension: 320 mg/5 ml
Aluminum hydroxide gel with magnesium hydroxide	Maalox	15-30 ml q4h	PO (gavage)	Suspension: 2.5 mg/5 ml
Antibiotics	See Tables 41-4, 43-4, and 45-2			
Aspirin		10-15 mg/kg/dose q4h		Drops: 60 mg/0.6 ml Syrup: 120 mg/5 ml Suppository: 120, 300, and 600 mg
Calcium gluconate		50-100 mg/kg/dose	IV	Ampule: 10 ml, 10% Tablet: 1 g
Carbamazepine	Tegretol	10-20 mg/kg 24 hr in 3 divided doses	PO	Tablet: 200 mg
Chloral hydrate	Noctec	Sedative: 10-20 mg/kg (single dose) Hypnotic: 50 mg/kg	PO, PR	Capsule: 250 and 500 mg Syrup: 500 mg/5 ml Suppository: 350, 500, 650, 1300 mg Elixir: 500 mg/ml
Chlorpromazine hydrochloride	Thorazine	0.5-1.0 mg/kg/dose	IV	Ampule: 1 or 2 ml; 25 mg/ml Vial: 10 ml; 25 mg/ml
Cimetidine	Tagamet	25 mg/kg/24 hr in 4 divided doses 300 mg q6h (adult)	PO	Tablet: 300 mg
Codeine		0.5-1.0 mg/kg	IV IM, PO	Vial: 2 ml; 300 mg Vial: 1 ml; 30 mg/ml Tablet: 15, 30, and 60 mg
Curare	Tubocurarine	0.5 mg/kg/dose	IV	Vial: 10 ml; 3 mg/ml
Diazoxide	Hyperstat	5 mg/kg/dose	IV	Ampule: 15 mg/ml
Digoxin	See Table 13-1			
Dioctyl sodium sulfosuccinate	Colace	5 mg/kg/24 hr	PO (gavage)	Capsule: 50, 100, and 250 mg Liquid: 10 and 50 mg/ml Syrup: 20 mg/5 ml

Drug	Trade name	Dosage	Route	Supplied
Diphenhydramine hydrochloride	Benadryl	0.5-1.5 mg/kg/dose in 4 divided doses (maximum daily dose 5 mg/kg)	PO, IV	Capsule: 25 and 50 mg Ampule: 1 ml; 50 mg/ml Vial: 10 and 30 ml; 10 mg/ml Elixir: 12.5 mg/5 ml
Emergency drugs	See Table C-4			
Epinephrine, racemic	Vaponefrin	<20 kg: 0.25 ml in 3-5 ml 0.9% NaCl solution 20-40 kg: 0.5 ml in 3-5 ml 0.9% NaCl solution >40 kg: 0.75 ml in 3-5 ml 0.9% NaCl solution		
Furosemide	Lasix	1 mg/kg/dose	IV, IM, PO	Tablet: 20 and 40 mg Ampule: 2 and 10 ml; 10 mg/ml
Glycerol		1 g/kg over 30 min q2h		
Hydralazine hydrochloride	Apresoline	0.2-0.5 mg/kg/dose q4h	PO, IM, IV	Tablet: 10, 25, 50, and 100 mg Ampule: 1 ml; 20 mg/ml
Hydroxyzine	Atarax, Vistaril	0.5 mg/kg q6h	PO, IM	Tablets: 10, 25, 50, and 100 mg Capsules, 25 and 50 mg Syrup: 25 mg/5 ml Vial: 25 and 50 mg/ml
Inhaled medications	See Chapter 101			
Insulin	See Chapter 48			
Magnesia magma	Milk of magnesia	0.5 ml/kg/dose q1-2h	PO (gavage)	
Mannitol		0.5-1.0 g/kg over 30 min q4-6h	IV	Ampule: 50 ml, 25% (12.5 g/50 ml)
Meperidine hydrochloride	Demerol	1-2 mg/kg q4h	IM, PO	Ampule: 0.5, 1, 1.5, and 2 ml; 50, 75, and 100 mg/ml Syrup: 50 mg/5 ml Tablet: 50 and 100 mg
Methyldopa	Aldomet	10-50 mg/kg/day in 2 divided doses	IV, PO	Vial: 5 ml; 250 mg/5 ml Tablet: 125, 250, and 500 mg
Morphine sulfate		0.1-0.2 mg/kg/dose q4h	IM, IV	Ampule: 1 ml; 8, 10, and 15 mg/ml Vial: 20 ml; 15 mg/ml
Neomycin sulfate		100 mg/kg	PO (gavage)	Tablet: 500 mg
Nitroprusside	Nipride	See Table C-5		
Pancuronium	Pavulon	0.1 mg/kg/dose	IV	Ampule: 2 and 5 ml; 2 mg/dl Vial: 10 ml; 1 mg/ml
Paraldehyde		0.3 ml/kg/dose	PR	Ampule: 5 ml (1 g/ml)
Phenobarbital		Loading, 10 mg/kg Maintenance, 5 mg/kg/24 hr in 2 divided doses	IV IV, PO	Vial: 1 ml; 65 mg/ml Powder: dilute with 1 ml; 130 mg/ml Suspension: 20 mg/5 ml Tablet: 15, 30, 60, and 100 mg
Phentolamine	Regitine	See Table C-5		

Continued.

Table C-2. Commonly used drugs—cont'd

Generic name	Trade name	Dose	Route	How supplied
Phenytoin	Dilantin	Loading, 10 mg/kg Maintenance, 5 mg/kg/24 hr	IV, PO	Suspension: 30 and 125 mg/5 ml Capsule: 30 and 100 mg Ampule: 2 and 5 ml; 50 mg/ml Tablet: 50 mg
Poisonings	See Table C-6			
Promethazine hydrochloride	Phenergan	0.5 mg/kg	IM, IV	Ampule: 1 ml; 25 mg/ml
Propranolol hydrochloride	Inderal	0.5-2.0 mg/kg/24 hr in 3 divided doses (0.01 mg/kg/dose); if IV, slower than 1 mg/kg/min	PO, IV	Ampule: 1 ml; 1 mg/ml Tablet: 10, 40, and 80 mg
Sodium polystyrene sulfonate	Kayexalate	1 g/kg	PO (gavage), PR	Jar: 453.6 g; 25% suspension in sorbitol solution
Spironolactone	Aldactone	3.3 mg/kg/day in 2 divided doses	PO	Tablet: 25 mg (must be made into suspension)
Succinylcholine chloride	Anectine	1.0-2.0 mg/kg/dose	IV	Vial: 10 ml; 20 mg/ml
Sucralfate	Carafate	1 g 4 times daily (adult dose)	PO	Tablet: 1 g
Thiopental sodium	Pentothal	2-4 mg/kg/dose	IV	
Tolazoline hydrochloride	Priscoline	See Table C-5		
Valproic acid	Depakene	10-30 mg/kg	PO	Capsule: 250 mg Vial: 250 mg/5 ml
Vasopressin	Pitressin	15-60 mU/hr	IV	20 units/ml
Vitamin K	Aquamephyton	1-5 mg	IM, IV	Ampule: 1 and 2.5 ml; 10 mg/ml or 5 and 0.5 ml; 1 mg/ml

Table C-3. Adrenal corticosteroids*

Generic name	Trade name	Glucocorticoid activity	Mineralocorticoid activity	Route	Duration of action	How supplied
Cortisone acetate, USP	Cortone	100 mg	100 mg	IV PO IM	6 hr (half-life 60-90 min) 6 hr 3 days	Vial: 25 and 50 mg/ml Tablet: 5, 10, and 25 mg
Hydrocortisone sodium succinate	Solu-Cortef	80 mg	80 mg	IV	4-6 hr (half-life 60-90 min)	Vial: 100, 250, and 500 mg
Hydrocortisone, USP	Cortef	80 mg	80 mg	PO	24-36 hr	Tablet: 5, 10, and 20 mg
Prednisone, USP		20 mg	100 mg	PO	6-8 hr	Tablet: 1, 2.5, 5, 20, and 50 mg
Prednisolone	Delta-Cortef	20 mg	100 mg	PO	24-36 hr	Tablet: 5 mg Vial: 25 and 50 mg
Methylprednisolone sodium succinate	Solu-Medrol	16 mg	No effect	IV IM	4-6 hr 4-6 hr	Vial: 40, 125, 500, and 1000 mg
Methylprednisolone acetate	Depo-Medrol	16 mg	No effect	IM	1-7 days	Vial: 20, 40, and 80 mg/ml
Dexamethasone	Decadron Hexadrol Dexameth	2 mg	No effect	PO	8-12 hr	Tablet: 0.25, 0.5, 0.75, 1.5, and 4 mg Liquid: 0.5 mg/5 ml Vial: 4 and 10 mg/ml
Desoxycorticosterone	Doca Percorten Cortrate Decortin	No effect	2 mg	IM SC SL	24 hr 8-12 months	Vial: 5 mg/ml Pellet: 125 mg Tablets: 2 and 5 mg
Fludrocortisone acetate	Florinef	No effect	20 mg	PO	24 hr	Tablet: 0.1 mg

*The dosages of adrenal corticosteroids are extremely varied, and therefore the reader is referred to specific chapters for this information.

Table C-4. Emergency drugs

Generic name	Trade name	Dose	Route	How supplied
Aminophylline		4-6 mg/kg/dose over 20 min q6h	IV	Ampule: 10 ml; 25 mg/ml
Atropine sulfate		0.01 mg/kg/dose	IV, IM	Ampule: 1 ml; 1 mg/ml
Calcium chloride (10%)		0.25 ml/kg/dose (25 mg/kg/dose)	IV	Ampule: 10 ml; 10% calcium
Defibrillation		1-2 watt-sec/kg		
Dextrose (25%)		2 ml/kg (0.5 g/kg)	IV	Vial: 50 ml; 50% dextrose
Diazepam	Valium	For seizures, 0.3 mg/kg/dose	IV	Ampule: 2 ml; 5 mg/ml
Diazoxide	Hyperstat	5 mg/kg fast IV push	IV	Ampule: 20 ml; 15 mg/ml
Epinephrine hydrochloride (1:10,000 bolus)	Adrenalin	Bolus, 0.1 ml/kg/dose (10 μg/kg/dose)	IV, IC	Ampule: 1 ml 1:1000 (1 mg)
Human albumin (25%)		1 g/kg	IV	Vial: 50 ml; 25%, 1 g/4 ml
Lidocaine	Xylocaine	1 mg/kg/dose	IV	Vial: 20 ml; 1%, 10 mg/ml
Methylprednisolone sodium succinate	Solu-Medrol	For shock, 30 mg/kg/dose	IV	Vial: 2 ml; 67.5 mg/ml
Naloxone	Narcan	5-10 μg/kg/dose	IV	Ampule: 1 ml; 0.02 mg/ml and 0.4 mg/ml
Oxygen		2-10 L/min	Inhaled	Wall line at 60 psi or tanks (E cylinders)
Phenobarbital		10 mg/kg/loading dose	IV	Vial: 1 ml; 65 mg/ml
Sodium bicarbonate (0.9%)		1 mEq/kg; may repeat 1-2 times (or 0.3 × kg × base deficit)	IV, IC	Vial: 50 ml; 1 mEq/ml
Vasoactive and inotropic drugs	See Table C-5			

Table C-5. Vasoactive and inotropic drugs

Generic name	Trade name	Dose	Route	How supplied
Dobutamine	Dobutrex	2.5-10.0 μg/kg/min	IV	Vial: 250 mg powder
Dopamine	Intropin	0.5-20.0 μg/kg/min	IV	Ampule: 5 ml; 40 mg/ml
		Dopaminergic, 0.5-2.0 μg/ kg/min		
		Dopaminergic + β, 2.0-10.0 μg/kg/min		
		α and β, 10.0-20.0 μg/kg/min		
		α, >20.0 μg/kg/min		
Epinephrine hydro-chloride infusion	Adrenalin	0.05-1.0 μg/kg/min	IV	Ampule: 1 ml 1:1000 (1 mg)
Isoproterenol	Isuprel	0.05-1.0 μg/kg/min	IV	Ampule: 1 and 5 ml; 1 mg/5 ml
Nitroprusside	Nipride	0.5-8.0 μg/kg/min	IV	Vial: 5 ml; 10 mg/ml
Norepinephrine bitartrate	Levophed	0.01-1.0 μg/kg/min	IV	Ampule: 4 ml; 1 mg/ml
Phentolamine	Regitine	1-20 μg/kg/min	IV	Vial: 1 ml; 5 mg/ml
Tolazoline hydro-chloride	Priscoline	1 mg/kg/dose or 2 mg/kg/hr (33 μg/kg/min)	IV	Vial: 10 ml; 25 mg/ml

Table C-6. Guide to drug dosages in poisoning

Drug	Dose
Acetazolamide (Diamox)	10-30 mg/kg/day PO in 3 doses
N-Acetylcysteine (Mucomyst)	140 mg/kg PO followed by 70 mg/kg q4h to a total of 18 doses
Apomorphine	0.1 mg/kg or 3 mg/m² IM
Atropine sulfate	0.01 mg/kg IV, IM, SC for bradycardia
	0.02-0.05 mg/kg IV, IM, SC for atropinization
Carthartics	
Magnesium sulfate	0.25 g/kg/dose PO
Milk of magnesia	0.5 ml/kg/dose PO
Sodium sulfate	200 ml/kg/dose PO
Charcoal, activated, USP	1 g/kg in 250 ml water PO
	or
	5-10 parts for each part toxin
Chelating agents	
BAL (dimercaprol)	3 mg/kg IM q4h for 2 days, 2.5 mg/kg IM q6h for 1 day, and 2.5 mg/kg IM q12h for 12 days
	or
	5 mg/kg IM q4h for 1 day and 2 mg/kg IM q8h for 2 days
Ca EDTA	75 mg/kg/24 hr IV maximum dose
	or
	50 mg/kg/24 hr IV in 2-3 doses for 5-7 days

Continued.

Table C-6. Guide to drug dosages in poisoning—cont'd

Drug	Dose
Desferrioxamine (Desferal)	20 mg/kg IM q6h for 2-3 days (maximum dose 3.5 mg/m²/day) followed by 10 mg/kg IM q4-12h *or* 40 mg/kg IV over 4 hr (rate not to exceed 15 mg/kg/hr), repeat in 4-6 hr; 20 mg/kg drip over 8-12 hr
DTPA	0.5-1.0 g as 25% solution IV
D-Penicillamine (Cuprimine)	40 mg/kg/day PO free base *or* 50 mg/kg/day PO hydrochloride *or* 25 mg/kg q6h for 5 days with maximum dose not to exceed 1 g/kg/day
Ethyl alcohol (100 proof)	1 mg/kg IV as 5% in 0.9% NaCl solution
Ipecac, syrup of	15-30 ml PO, repeat once
Lavage fluids	
Ammonia water	5 ml in 500 ml water
Calcium lactate (gluconate)	15-30 g in 1 L water
Magnesium hydroxide	25 g in 1 L water
Milk	
Potassium permanganate	1:10,000 solution
Sodium bicarbonate, 5%	
Sodium chloride, 0.9%	
Starch solution	80 g in 1 L water
Tannic acid	30-50 g in 1 L water
Mannitol	1 g/kg/dose IV, repeat q4-6h
Naloxone (Narcan)	5-10 μg/kg/dose
Olive oil	30-60 ml PO
Physostigmine (Antilirium)	0.01-0.03 mg/kg/dose IV, IM (rate not to exceed 0.1 mg/kg/min)
Phytonadione (vitamin K)	1-5 mg IV for bleeding 25-150 mg IV as antidote
Pralidoxime (Protopam)	25-50 mg/kg IV over 15-30 min (rate not to exceed 7-10 mg/kg/min) q8h
Prednisone	2 mg/kg/day PO or equivalent IV
Sodium bicarbonate	2-4 mEq/kg/dose to alkalinize urine
Sodium nitrite	0.005-0.01 mg/kg IV over 3-4 min
Sodium thiosulfate	150-200 mg/kg IV over 10 min

Index

A

Reintubation, common problems necessitating, 586
Relatives, distraught, and pediatric intensive care unit staff, 450
Relaxants, 321
Renal anomalies, congenital, 113
Renal artery thrombosis, bilateral, 111-112
Renal dysplasia, severe, 113
Renal failure
  acute
    bilateral renal artery thrombosis as prerenal cause of, 111-112
    bilateral vein thrombosis as prerenal cause of, 112
    biochemical indications for peritoneal dialysis in, 613
    calcium imbalance in, 118
    diagnosis of, 113-114
    dialysis fluid for, 617
    fluid balance in, 114-115
    hyperkalemia in, 116-118
    hyperphosphatemia in, 118
    hypertension in, 115-116
    hypocalcemia in, 118
    intrarenal causes of, 112-113
    nonmedical management of, 119
    nutritional aspects of management of, 118-119
    peritoneal dialysis for, 612-613
    phosphorus imbalances in, 118
    postrenal causes of, 113
    prerenal causes of, 111-112
    prognosis in, 119
  after cardiothoracic surgery, 339-340
Renal system in hyperbilirubinemia, 380
Renal vein thrombosis, bilateral, 112
Renal-metabolic system, 11-13
  in acute adrenocortical insufficiency, 305-306
  in acute hepatic failure, 132-133
  in acute renal failure, 114
  in altered states of consciousness, 33
  in central diabetes insipidus, 313-314
  in congestive heart failure, 65
  in diabetic ketoacidosis, 301
  in diaphragmatic hernia, 366
  in gastroschisis, 356, 358
  in Guillain-Barré syndrome, 152, 154
  in hyaline membrane disease, 227-228
  in hypoxia, 170-171
  in imperforate anus, 359-360
  in intestinal atresia, 359-360
  in lightning injuries, 173-175
  in meconium inhalation syndrome, 237
  in myasthenia gravis, 163, 166
  in near-drowning, 182
  in necrotizing enterocolitis, 348
  in neonatal asphyxia, 241-243
  in neonatal polycythemia, 256, 257
  in omphalocele, 356, 358
  in organophosphate insecticide poisoning, 430
  in peritonitis, 287-289
  in persistent pulmonary hypertension of newborn, 267
  in Reye's syndrome, 146-148

Renal-metabolic system—cont'd
  in salicylism, 403
  in status epilepticus, 42
Repolarization, 474
Residual volume, 184, 649
Resinoids, 413, 414, 415
Resorcinol, 423
Respiration, monitoring, in cardiothoracic surgery, 328
Respiratory acidemia in acute severe asthma, 186
Respiratory centers, physiologic integration of, 208-212
Respiratory distress syndrome, 71-72, 181, 182
  as indication for tracheostomy, 587
Respiratory failure
  acute, 58-62
  as indication for intubation, 536
Respiratory fatigue, 71
Respiratory injury, postburn, 176-178
Respiratory instability, factors influencing, 210-211
Respiratory isolation, 270
Respiratory monitors, 474-478
Respiratory obstruction in epiglottitis, 205-206
Respiratory reflexes during suctioning, 569
Respiratory support in neonatal asphyxia, 241
Respiratory syncytial virus, 218
  as causative viral agent in croup, 197
Respiratory system
  in acute hepatic failure, 134
  in acute respiratory failure, 61
  in acute severe asthma, 187
  in altered states of consciousness, 33
  anaphylaxis in, 90
  in epiglottitis, 205
  in gastroesophageal reflux, 373
  in Guillain-Barré syndrome, 151-154
  in hyaline membrane disease, 226-230
  and increased intracranial pressure, 49
  during intubation, 195
  in lightning injuries, 172-174
  in meconium inhalation syndrome, 234-237
  in myasthenia gravis, 159-160, 165-166
  in near-drowning, 182
  in organophosphate poisoning, 429-430
  in persistent pulmonary hypertension of newborn, 265-266
  in petroleum distillate ingestion, 418-420
  in poisoning, 390
  in Reye's syndrome, 146-148
  in salicylism, 403
  in status epilepticus, 42
Respiratory therapists in pediatric intensive care unit, 4
Respiratory treatment equipment and procedures, 531-597
Respiratory waveform, cardiac output in, 477
Responses, reflex, in altered states of consciousness, 31
Resuscitation
  cardiopulmonary; see Cardiopulmonary resuscitation
  equipment for, emergency, 26
  technique of, 18-25
Retrolental fibroplasia in hyaline membrane disease, 226
Reverse isolation, 271